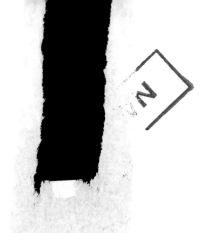

Pain

D1331418

50646618

50646618

Commissioning Editor: Rita Demetriou-Swanwick
Development Editor: Catherine Jackson
Project Manager: Srividhya Vidhyashankar
Designer/Design Direction: Miles Hitchen
Illustration Manager: Jennifer Rose
Illustrator: Ethan Danielson

Pain
A textbook for health professionals

Second Edition

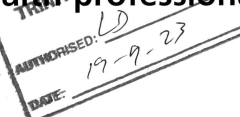

WITHDRAWN
THE LIBRARY OF
TRINITY COLLEGE DUBLIN
AUTHORISED: LD
19-9-23
DATE:

Edited by

Hubert van Griensven

Research Fellow in Musculoskeletal Physiotherapy, University of Brighton, Eastbourne,
East Sussex, UK, and
Consultant Physiotherapist, Southend University Hospital
NHS Foundation Trust, Essex, UK

Jenny Strong

Professor of Occupational Therapy, Division of Occupational Therapy,
School of Health and Rehabilitation Sciences, The University of Queensland, Brisbane, Australia

Anita M. Unruh

Associate Dean (Research & Academic), Academic Integrity Officer, Faculty of Health Professions,
Dalhousie University, Halifax, Canada

Foreword by
Ronald Melzack

Professor Emeritus, Department of Psychology, McGill University, Montreal, Quebec, Canada

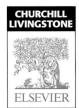

CHURCHILL
LIVINGSTONE

ELSEVIER

Edinburgh London New York Oxford Philadelphia St Louis Sydney Toronto 2014

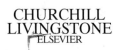

WITHDRAWN

Trinity Library Dublin JSML

© 2014 Elsevier Ltd. All rights reserved.

No part of this publication may be reproduced or transmitted in any form or by any means, electronic or mechanical, including photocopying, recording, or any information storage and retrieval system, without permission in writing from the publisher. Details on how to seek permission, further information about the Publisher's permissions policies and our arrangements with organizations such as the Copyright Clearance Center and the Copyright Licensing Agency, can be found at our website: *www.elsevier.com/permissions*.

This book and the individual contributions contained in it are protected under copyright by the Publisher (other than as may be noted herein).

First edition 2002
Second edition 2014
  Reprinted 2014 (twice), 2016

ISBN: 978 0 7020 3478 7

British Library Cataloguing in Publication Data
A catalogue record for this book is available from the British Library

Library of Congress Cataloging in Publication Data
A catalog record for this book is available from the Library of Congress

TRINITY LIBRARY
10 NOV 2016
WITHDRAWN
DUBLIN

Notices

Knowledge and best practice in this field are constantly changing. As new research and experience broaden our understanding, changes in research methods, professional practices, or medical treatment may become necessary.

Practitioners and researchers must always rely on their own experience and knowledge in evaluating and using any information, methods, compounds, or experiments described herein. In using such information or methods they should be mindful of their own safety and the safety of others, including parties for whom they have a professional responsibility.

With respect to any drug or pharmaceutical products identified, readers are advised to check the most current information provided (i) on procedures featured or (ii) by the manufacturer of each product to be administered, to verify the recommended dose or formula, the method and duration of administration, and contraindications. It is the responsibility of practitioners, relying on their own experience and knowledge of their patients, to make diagnoses, to determine dosages and the best treatment for each individual patient, and to take all appropriate safety precautions.

To the fullest extent of the law, neither the Publisher nor the authors, contributors, or editors, assume any liability for any injury and/or damage to persons or property as a matter of products liability, negligence or otherwise, or from any use or operation of any methods, products, instructions, or ideas contained in the material herein.

ELSEVIER
your source for books, journals and multimedia in the health sciences

www.elsevierhealth.com

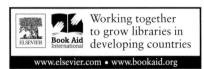

Working together
to grow libraries in
developing countries

www.elsevier.com • www.bookaid.org

The Publisher's policy is to use **paper manufactured from sustainable forests**

Printed in China

Last digit is the print number: 10 9 8 7 6 5 4

SJ
616.047
R43j3

Contents

Contents

Foreword

Pain research has made revolutionary advances in the past half-century. The traditional concept of pain as a specific sensation has evolved into a broader concept of pain as comprising sensory, affective and cognitive dimensions. Many people suffer severe chronic pain that is out of proportion to any detectable physical cause, which forces us to explore neural programs in the brain, where subjective experience occurs. Research on the language of pain has produced questionnaires that allow us to evaluate subjective pain experience.

The revolution in pain management has taken us from surgical section of a "pain pathway" to multiple interacting approaches. Countless drugs, ranging from aspirin to morphine, are used to produce relief of severe acute pains, postoperative pain, and even persistent pain from cancer and arthritis that destroy body tissue. Cancer pain, for example, can be greatly diminished, sometimes abolished entirely, by appropriate doses of morphine or other opioid drugs. Yet despite the best efforts in hospitals with outstanding facilities, 5-10% of patients with cancer continue to have moderate to high levels of pain.

Chronic pain is the most challenging type of pain. When it follows an earlier injury, it is out of proportion to the injury or other pathology, and persists long after healing is complete. The traditional assumption that a spinal pathway must be causing the pain has led to the use of spinal anaesthetic blocks to stop the pain. Sometimes severe chronic pains are diminished or even abolished. More often, however, the pain returns to its former intensity.

Forty-plus years of active research based on the traditional "bottom-up" theory of pain has yet to discover any major new classes of drugs. Aspirin, acetaminophen and morphine are still the first line of attack on all pains and many variants of these drugs with fewer undesirable side-effects have been produced. Most remarkable, however, is the discovery of two new classes of drugs that were originally developed for other purposes. Drugs that were prescribed to control depression were unexpectedly found to produce significant relief of several forms of chronic pain. Similarly, drugs developed to control epilepsy were found to relieve severe chronic pains associated with diseases of nerves. Recently developed variants of both classes of drugs are more effective and have fewer side-effects. These drugs, which evolved from the "top-down" approach based on patients' subjective descriptions of their pain, opened the gate to a new pharmacology of chronic pain focussed on the brain. Both classes of drugs are now major sources of relief for many severe, previously intractable chronic pains.

Despite the advances, chronic pains remain difficult to treat. For example, backaches and pelvic pains may be relieved in some patients by spinal blocks or some combination of drugs, but no widely effective treatment has yet been found. Similarly, excellent new drugs are effective for some kinds of chronic headache, but not for all. The most terrible chronic pains that are rarely relieved are "central pains" due to strokes or other neurological diseases.

The recognition that pain is a multidimensional experience determined by psychological as well as physical factors has broadened the scope of pain therapies. Patients with chronic pain as well as terminally ill cancer patients with intense pain need every bit of the armamentarium to battle the pain. John Bonica, a brilliant American anaesthesiologist, played a huge role in these developments. The gate control theory, published in 1965, provided a scientific foundation for Bonica's contention that chronic pain is not a "symptom" but a syndrome in its own right, and requires a pain clinic that includes therapists from a wide range of disciplines. At the same time, Cicely Saunders in England recognized the importance of psychological approaches as part of palliative care for dying patients in addition to effective levels of morphine. Bonica and Saunders argued that unrelenting pain is an evil to be abolished by every available means.

The rapid rise of non-drug therapies is a major result of the new concept of pain. Psychological therapies, which were once used as a last resort when drugs or neurosurgery failed to control pain, are now an integral part of pain management strategies. The recognition that pain is the result of multiple contributions gave rise to a variety of psychological approaches such as relaxation, hypnosis, and cognitive therapies. So too, transcutaneous electrical nerve stimulation (TENS) and physical therapy procedures evolved rapidly, bringing substantial pain relief to large numbers of people.

The pain revolution has taken us from a direct-line pain pathway to an open biological system that comprises multiple sensory inputs, memories of past experiences, personal and social expectations, genetic contributions, gender, aging, and stress patterns involving the endocrine, autonomic and immune systems. Pain is now universally recognized as a major challenge for medicine, psychology, physical therapy, occupational therapy and all other health sciences and professions. Every aspect of life, from birth to dying, has characteristic pain problems. Genetics, until recently, was rarely considered relevant to understanding pain, but sophisticated epidemiological and laboratory studies have established genetic predispositions related to pain as an essential component of the field. The study of pain, therefore, has broadened and now incorporates research in epidemiology and medical genetics as well as sociological and cultural studies.

The authors of this book are highly respected practitioners as well as university and hospital teachers and scientists. They have the knowledge and wisdom of years of practice. I commend them for the excellent organization and valuable information they provide in this volume.

Ronald Melzack
McGill University

Contributors

Gordon J.G. Asmundson
Fellow of Royal Society of Canada,
CACBT Certified in Cognitive Behaviour Therapy,
President's Chair in Adult Mental Health Research,
Professor of Psychology,
Editor-in-Chief (NA) Cognitive Behaviour Therapy,
Department of Psychology,
University of Regina,
Saskatchewan, Canada

Karl S. Bagraith
Occupational Therapist - Senior,
Occupational Therapy Department,
Royal Brisbane and Women's Hospital and,
School of Health and Rehabilitation Sciences,
The University of Queensland,
Brisbane, Australia

Sally Bennett
Senior Lecturer in Occupational Therapy,
School of Health and Rehabilitation Sciences,
University of Queensland,
Brisbane, Australia

Annette Bishop
NIHR Research Fellow,
Arthritis Research UK Primary Care Research Centre,
Keele University,
Keele, UK

Emma Briggs
King's Teaching Fellow/Lecturer,
Department of Postgraduate Research,
Florence Nightingale School of Nursing & Midwifery,
King's College London,
London, UK

R. Nicholas Carleton
Assistant Professor,
Department of Psychology,
University of Regina,
Saskatchewan, Canada

Ann Carter
Education Co-Lead,
Integrative Therapies Unit,
Christie NHS Trust,
Manchester, UK

Jill MacLaren Chorney
Assistant Professor,
Departments of Anesthesiology,
Pain Management and Perioperative Medicine
and Psychology,
Dalhousie University,
Complex Pain Team,
IWK Health Centre,
Halifax, Canada

Nicola U. Cook
British Accredited Hand Therapist,
Sydney Hand Therapy and Rehabilitation,
Australia

Kenneth D. Craig
Professor Emeritus of Psychiatry,
Department of Psychology,
University of British Columbia,
Vancouver, Canada

Diarmuid Denneny
Pain Management Physiotherapist,
University College London Hospitals,
NHS Foundation Trust,
London, UK

Krysia Dziedzic
NIHR Research Professor of Musculoskeletal Health in
Primary Care,
Arthritis Research UK Primary Care Research Centre,
Keele University,
Keele, UK

Samantha R. Fashler
Associate Faculty Member,
Department of Psychology,
York University,
Toronto, Canada

Contributors

Nadine E. Foster
NIHR Research Professor of Musculoskeletal Health
in Primary Care,
Arthritis Research UK Primary Care Research Centre,
Keele University,
Keele, UK

Mary P. Galea
Professor Fellow,
Department of Medicine (Royal Melbourne Hospital),
The University of Melbourne,
Parkville, Australia

Libby Gibson
School of Health and Rehabilitation Sciences,
University of Queensland,
Brisbane, Australia

Stephen J. Gibson
Deputy Director,
National Ageing Research Institute,
Royal Melbourne Hospital and Professor,
Department of Medicine,
University of Melbourne and Director of Research,
Caulfield Pain Management and Research Centre,
Caulfield, Australia

Lydia Gomez-Perez
Sessional Lecturer of Psychology,
Department of Psychology,
University of Regina,
Saskatchewan, Canada

Hubert van Griensven
Research Fellow in Musculoskeletal Physiotherapy,
University of Brighton,
Eastbourne,
East Sussex, UK, and
Consultant Physiotherapist,
Southend University Hospital NHS Foundation Trust,
Essex, UK

Sarah E. Henderson
School of Clinical Sciences,
College of Medicine and Veterinary Medicine,
University of Edinburgh,
Edinburgh, UK

Melanie A. Holden
Research Fellow in Applied Osteoarthritis,
NIHR Research Professor of Musculoskeletal Health
in Primary Care,
Arthritis Research UK Primary Care Research Centre,
Keele University,
Keele, UK

Anna Huguet
Research Associate,
IWK Health Centre,
Halifax, Canada

Mark I. Johnson
Professor of Pain and Analgesia,
Faculty of Health and Social Sciences,
Leeds Metropolitan University and Leeds Pallium Research Group,
Leeds, UK

Peter A. Mackereth
Clinical Lead Supportive Care & Tobacco Control,
Christie NHS Trust and Honorary Lecturer,
Manchester Metropolitan University,
Manchester, UK

Tsipora Mankovsky-Arnold
Department of Psychology,
McGill University,
Montreal, Canada

Chris McCarthy
Lead Orthopaedic Physiotherapy Practitioner,
Imperial College Healthcare,
St Mary's Hospital,
Paddington,
London, UK

Patrick J. McGrath
Vice-President of Research,
IWK Health Centre; Canada Research Chair,
Dalhousie University;
Professor of Psychology,
Paediatrics and Psychiatry,
Dalhousie University,
Halifax, Canada

Danuta Mendelson
Professor of Law (Research),
School of Law,
Deakin University,
Burwood, Australia

George Mendelson
Adjunct Clinical Associate Professor,
School of Psychology and Psychiatry,
Faculty of Medicine,
Nursing and Health Sciences,
Monash University, Victoria, and
Australia and Honorary Research Fellow,
Caulfield Pain Management and Research,
Caulfield Hospital,
Caulfield, Australia

Harold Merskey
Professor Emeritus of Psychiatry,
University of Western Ontario,
Ontario, Canada

Geoffrey Mitchell
Professor of General Practice and Palliative Care,
University of Queensland,
Brisbane, Australia

Arjun Muralidharan
The University of Queensland,
Centre for Integrated Preclinical Drug Development & School
of Pharmacy,
St Lucia Campus,
Brisbane, Australia

Mandy Nielsen
Research Officer,
School of Health and Rehabilitation Sciences,
University of Queensland,
Brisbane, Australia

Carole A. Paley
Airedale NHS Foundation Trust,
West Yorkshire, and Leeds Metropolitan University and Leeds
Pallium Research Group,
Leeds, UK

Esther M. Pogatzki-Zahn
Department of Anesthesiology,
Intensive Care and Pain Medicine,
University Hospital Muenster,
Albert-Schweitzer-Campus 1,
Münster, Germany

Ashley A. Richter
Research Associate,
Department of Psychology,
Louisiana State University,
Baton Rouge,
LA, USA

Stephan A. Schug
Professor and Chair of Anaesthesiology,
University of Western Australia,
Perth, Australia

Maree T. Smith
The University of Queensland,
Centre for Integrated Preclinical Drug Development & School
of Pharmacy,
St Lucia Campus,
Brisbane, Australia

Jenny Strong
Professor of Occupational Therapy,
Division of Occupational Therapy,
School of Health and Rehabilitation Sciences,
The University of Queensland,
Brisbane, Australia

Jacqui Stringer
Clinical Lead for Supportive Care,
Christie NHS Trust & Honorary Lecturer,
University of Manchester,
Manchester, UK

Michael J.L. Sullivan
Departments of Psychology,
Medicine and Neurology,
Canada Research Chair in Behavioural Health,
McGill University,
Montreal, Canada

Anita M. Unruh
Associate Dean (Research & Academic),
Academic Integrity Officer,
Faculty of Health Professions,
Dalhousie University,
Halifax, Canada

Deborah Shan Boughay Watson
Consultant Anaesthetist,
Department of Anaesthesia,
Fremantle Hospital,
Perth, Western Australia

Chapter | 1 |

Introduction to pain

Anita M. Unruh, Jenny Strong and Hubert van Griensven

OVERVIEW

Pain is a serious and often debilitating problem for people who live with it, their families and our society. Yet pain is a common occurrence in all of life. As an early warning system of possible harm, pain alerts the person experiencing it of danger and the need to withdraw from the situation. Pain is frequently associated with the bumps and bruises of childhood, health procedures and unintentional injuries, as well as illnesses and diseases that may occur over a normal lifespan. Despite its association with injury and disease, pain is a subjective symptom that cannot be objectively measured in the way that temperature can be measured with a thermometer. That subjectivity is part of its presenting challenge. Many other factors aside from pain, such as age, gender, underlying disability, and social or cultural contexts, shape how we communicate about pain to others. For all of these reasons, pain is an intensely personal experience with biological, psychological and social components, existing where a person says it exists and when a person says it exists (McCaffery & Beebe 1989).

This book was initially written in 2002 as a textbook for occupational therapists and physiotherapists who are involved in caring for and treating people who live with pain. In this revised book, we have prepared an interprofessional text on pain for students in any health profession. In this chapter, we will briefly examine what pain is, the experience of the person confronted with ongoing pain, the healthcare team that is involved in pain management, and the roles and responsibilities of health professionals within this team. To prepare, go to Reflective exercise 1.1, and complete the questions.

Reflective exercise 1.1

Gather some blank white paper and a set of coloured markers. Think about a pain experience that you have had in the past 3 weeks. The pain can be minor or more troublesome.

♦ What caused the pain?

♦ Was it familiar or something unexpected?

♦ Were you alone or with others?

♦ How did being alone or being with others affect how you felt and what you did about the pain?

♦ What factors affected whether you were concerned about the pain or saw it as of no great consequence?

♦ What did you do to make the pain better? Was it effective?

On the paper, draw a picture of your pain. If we could see it what would it look like?

© 2014 Elsevier Ltd.

WHAT IS PAIN?

The International Association for the Study of Pain (IASP) defined pain as, 'an unpleasant sensory and emotional experience associated with actual or potential tissue damage, or described in terms of such damage' (Merskey & Bogduk 1994, p. 210). This definition highlights the duality of pain as a physiological and psychological experience. It is a physiological event within the body that is dependent on subjective recognition, that is, without psychological awareness pain cannot exist. The definition also highlights several other important aspects of the pain experience. Pain is usually perceived as a warning signal of actual or potential tissue damage. Nevertheless, pain can occur in the absence of tissue damage, even though the experience may be described by the individual as if damage had occurred. The assumption that pain is linked with tissue damage is protective, reflexive and ingrained biologically, psychologically and socially in human nature. It is thus a very strongly held and deeply embedded assumption, which is difficult to break when pain persists in the absence of treatable tissue pathology.

Acute pain usually stops long before healing is completed, a process that may take a few days or a few weeks (Loeser & Melzack 1999). Chronic pain is often considered as pain that persists for more than 3–6 months. Pain may be present and persistent for many reasons, as detailed further in Chapters 5 and 6. The IASP definition of chronic pain is:

'A persistent pain that is not amenable, as a rule, to treatments based upon specific remedies, or to the routine methods of pain control such as non-narcotic analgesics.'

(Merskey & Bogduk 1994, p. xii)

Loeser & Melzack (1999, p. 1609) concluded:

'It is not the duration of pain that distinguishes acute from chronic pain but, more importantly, the inability of the body to restore its physiological functions to normal homeostatic levels.'

These distinctions between acute and chronic pain have important implications for pain assessment and intervention. Acute pain signals tissue damage, but chronic pain that is not associated with disease is markedly disassociated from tissue damage and may be out of proportion to any initiating pathology or tissue damage.

Pain is a highly subjective experience. The best measure of pain is a reliable and valid self-report measure of pain (see Chapter 7) for persons who can provide self-report, and validated behavioural measures of pain for individuals who are unable to self-report. While such measures provide important information about pain, many people who live with chronic pain, if not most, confront at some time disbelief and doubt from health professionals, family, friends or colleagues due to the subjectivity of pain and its invisibility to an observer.

THE PERSON WHO LIVES WITH PAIN

The experience of living with chronic pain and the suffering with which it may be associated is not readily grasped by those living outside the experience. As pain is inherently a warning signal of harm to the person receiving it, turning attention away from pain is difficult. Accepting its ongoing presence is elusive, difficult and often physically, emotionally and spiritually overwhelming. It can isolate individuals and push a person to the edge, as Heather and Greg share in their comments below:

'During the times when it was most severe I felt completely detached from my family and from life in general.'

(Heather Davulcu in Unruh 2008, p. 199)

'I think I have come to simply accept that the pain's here and it is unlikely to go away. I try to accept it as a part of my being right now, because I really have only two choices: to endure it or die. Thus far, I've chosen to exist, but sometimes just basically accept.'

(Lum 1997, p. 66)

People who live with chronic pain may struggle to reconcile themselves with the reality of their experience. Acceptance that pain may be ongoing can be a starting point to regaining control over its impact on life and balancing it with hope for pain relief (see Chapters 4, 8 and 9).

'No matter how bad it is, accepting is the starting place. Whether it's being okay with where you are, it's accepting, it's realizing, it's realizing the truth, it's realizing where you are.'

(Participant in Tull et al 2011, p. 439.)

'I don't think that accepting means giving up, and I think that we can always keep that little bit of hope. I mean there's still maybe better medication that might come out and it doesn't necessarily mean that it will, or it will happen in our lifetime, but it might happen.'

(Madison F M in LaChapelle et al 2008, p. 204)

Acceptance is an individual journey. Many factors contribute to it. Inevitably, it may include facing losses due to pain and if possible finding new avenues to restore meaning and purpose in life despite pain. Ladonna and Helen in the comments below found alternative ways to construct a self-identity, despite pain, that was still consistent with who they were before they were sidelined by pain. Both Helen and Heather above also found that painting opened up a world that took them away from pain.

'Life without ballet. What could I do? Who would I be? Would anyone love me if I couldn't dance? Would I be desirable, if I had no gift to offer, no special talent? It may seem silly now, but I had known nothing else for my entire lifetime ... My identity as a ballerina had provided me with a sense of belonging and understanding of my place in the world. Without that identity, I felt lost. It took me years to realize that in losing my identity I had not lost who I am. Perhaps I would have, had I not found a new way to manifest the essential qualities of my original gift. The gift was not simply the physical ability to execute the steps. Rather it was the ability to bring to life an expression of great emotion. That gift remains mine.'

(Ladonna in Kielhofner 2002, p. 134–135)

'When I was sidelined by pain I began to think my world was shrinking, but when I became involved with NACPAC, CPS and the Canadian Pain Coalition, I saw that I still had something to offer. I became a nurse to help others. That desire was still there and I could fulfill it in this way.'

(Helen Tupper in Unruh 2008, p. 199)

The patient's voice is explored more fully in Chapter 2.

A competent and compassionate pain management team can do a great deal to reduce the distress and suffering that may be associated with exposure to painful procedures and living with ongoing pain. The focus of the health professionals concerned with pain is to treat and manage any underlying treatable pathology, to reduce pain as much as possible, to enhance function and to enable living meaningfully and productively despite pain.

THE INTERPROFESSIONAL PAIN TEAM

There is abundant evidence that the best approach to the management of chronic pain is multidimensional, that is, when a person has multiple pain management strategies at their disposal. These strategies typically include medication, cognitive–behavioural processes, attention to physical activity and modification to lifestyle to maintain function and reduce pain and disability. Depending on the person's age and life context, pain management may also involve liaison with school teachers, with employers and the workplace, and meetings with family. This work is likely to be at its best with a multiprofessional pain team that collaborates together in an interprofessional context respecting each others' training as well as the overlapping boundaries that often occur in professional roles and responsibilities. Below is a brief and general overview of the health professionals that make up the core of a pain team: the physician, the nurse, the psychologist, the physiotherapist and the occupational therapist. All of these professions have roles and responsibilities that are set out by their professional associations in any given jurisdiction in a particular country. Some professional roles may evolve in particular and local ways within a team, particularly when a team works interprofessionally. For example, in some clinics, an occupational therapist may be the most skilled in using distraction to manage pain during acute procedures. In other clinics, this skill and responsibility may lie with another health professional. The reader is advised to consult professional standards and guidelines for practice in their own jurisdiction.

THE PHYSICIAN

Multiple physicians are commonly involved in the health care of a person living with pain. Typically the first health professional is the family physician. The family physician is likely to begin the initial process of assessment and screening to insure that other conditions can be ruled out, and may prescribe medication and other lifestyle modifications that may assist the person to decrease pain and limit disability, monitor for side effects, and advise on the use of complementary alternative therapies (Bope et al 2004). The patient may be referred to other medical specialties based on assessment outcomes and the person's response to interventions.

Anaesthesiologists are involved in acute pain management, particularly in surgery and other procedures that require airway management and analgesia. In chronic pain, the anaesthesiologist is often the medical director of the pain clinic, but this role has also been assumed by other medical specialists such as neurologists, psychiatrists, rheumatologists and/or psychiatrists. The medical director is responsible for overall medical care of the person, assessment of pain and determining the need for medical, surgical and/or pharmacological interventions. A physician who specializes in pain management may also use pain education, cognitive–behavioural interventions and counselling to support goals related to function.

Sources for more information:

- Bope et al (2004)
- Stewart & Kostash (1998)
- Swerdlow et al (1978).

THE NURSE

The responsibilities of a nurse involved in pain management are often diverse, depending on the context of the patient's care, and the nurse's level of training and specialization. In acute care, the nurse will have primary responsibility for pain assessment, the administration of medications, and patient advocacy to ensure the adequacy of pain management. A nurse practitioner may also prescribe medications, including controlled substances, but this role may be restricted in some parts of a country or in some countries. In some countries such as the USA, Sweden and others, the nurse may be specialized as a nurse anaesthetist to provide intraoperative management of surgical patients and pre- and post-operative pain management (Stomberg et al 2003). Beyond pharmacological management, nurses also have the skills to enable and support a patient to use psychological interventions to manage pain (Twycross 2002). Nurses promote sleep and assist the patient to use meditation, relaxation, distraction and humour (Pellino et al 2002). In chronic pain, the nurse's role may focus on pain education for the patient and family, the use of social and psychological strategies to manage pain, and coordination of the patient's care to maximize medication treatment and other strategies. The goal is to reduce the need for the patient to require emergency services. In some pain clinics, the nurse may have the primary liaison role with schools and employers. For nurses who have advanced practice roles (clinical nurse specialist) there will be additional responsibilities related to policy and programme development and implementation related to pain, as well as education and support of staff nurses and other health are professionals in their care of the patient. They provide consultation on the best methods of pain assessment, non-pharmacological strategies to reduce pain and maximizing medications as ordered.

Sources for more information:

- Carr & Layzell (2010)
- Hamric et al (2009) Advanced Practice Nursing: An Integrated Approach.
- Kazanowski & Laccetti (2008)
- MacLellan (2006)
- McCaffery & Pasero (1999)
- Pellino et al (2002)
- Stomberg et al (2003).

THE PSYCHOLOGIST

Psychology is the study of behaviour and its correlates. Psychologists study normal behaviour and aberrant behaviour. They examine the relationship of what people do (their behaviour) respective to their emotions, genetic make-up, brain activity, social context, families, law, culture and work. Psychologists use observation and self-reporting of behaviour, measurement of physiological responses, brain activity, social activity and changes in the environment in assessment.

Psychology is both a profession and a discipline. Psychologists are trained to a doctoral level. The most common qualification for clinical psychology, the profession, is a PhD, which combines a high level of research training and extensive professional training.

Some clinical psychologists take a PsyD, which is usually focused more on professional practice than research. In North America (the USA and Canada) the 5 or 6 years of graduate training for a clinical psychologist are followed by a year-long residency or internship. There are many psychology subspecialities. At one time, different schools (e.g. Freudian, Skinnerian) dominated but nowadays they have much less influence and the focus is on the evidence for different approaches. Clinical psychologists are the most likely subspecialty to be involved in pain care.

Their goal is to understand behaviour in order to change it. Psychological interventions are discussed in detail in Chapters 8 and 9.

Sources for more information:

- Eccleston (2001)
- Simon & Folen (2001)
- Main et al (2008).

THE PHYSIOTHERAPIST (PHYSICAL THERAPIST)

Physiotherapists apply a wide range of physical and behavioural treatments to reduce pain and prevent or overcome dysfunction. Physiotherapy assessment focuses initially on the evaluation of impairments related to the client's presenting condition, as well as undertaking a detailed appraisal of various aspects of the client's pain report, such as temporal patterns of pain and those activities that specifically aggravate or relieve pain. A major focus is assessing and quantifying motor and sensory impairments. The assessment extends to consider secondary biomechanical and or behavioural factors that contribute to pain, pain–activity interactions and overall function. A physiotherapy treatment programme is developed to provide pain relief, modify the effects of primary and secondary factors contributing to pain, reduce or reverse specific impairments, promote healing and repair, and minimize the influence of factors that may lead to recurrence of pain.

Physiotherapy interventions strategies may include education, exercise, manual therapy, movement facilitation techniques and application of electrophysical agents. Increasingly, physiotherapists working in pain settings adopt a cognitive–behavioural approach. Educational approaches focus on understanding pain, on improving posture, body mechanics and gait, and on minimizing contributing factors. Exercise may be used by physiotherapists to activate specific muscle groups, re-educate motor control skills, increase muscle endurance, strengthen specific muscle groups and counteract the effects of generalized deconditioning. Movement may be used to control and decrease pain, and increase mobility.

Sources for more information:

- Chevan & Clapis (2012)
- Doliber (1984)
- Main et al (2008)
- Stetts & Carpenter (2012)
- Sluka (2009).

THE OCCUPATIONAL THERAPIST

Occupational therapists are concerned with the psychosocial and environmental factors that contribute to pain and the impact of pain on everyday life. Occupational therapists assess the impact of pain on looking after oneself (self-care, enjoying life (leisure) and contributing to the social and economic fabric of their communities (productivity).

Occupational therapists assess the impact of pain on self-care, paid and unpaid work, interests and leisure pursuits, customary habits and routines, and family relationships. Assessment includes evaluation of psychosocial and environmental factors aggravating pain in the home and workplace. Occupational therapists work collaboratively with the person to develop an occupational therapy programme to increase self-esteem, restore self-efficacy and promote optimal occupational function despite pain. Intervention strategies may include assistive devices and equipment, purposeful and productive, activities and vocational rehabilitation or work hardening to improve endurance and work skills, and re-establish the roles and routines of everyday life. Education about pain and supportive individual, family or group counselling are utilized as needed.

Sources for more information:

- Canadian Association of Occupational Therapists (2012)
- Robinson et al (2011)
- Skjutar et al (2010)
- Strong (1996)
- Traines (1994).

OTHER HEALTHCARE PROVIDERS

Although the health professions noted above are the core of a pain management team, they are not the only healthcare providers who have such roles and responsibilities. Many other healthcare personnel have responsibility for procedures that can cause discomfort or pain (e.g. venipunctures, mammograms, dental care, etc.). Beyond the conventional health care provided in hospitals, many complementary or alternative health practitioners have roles and responsibilities for pain assessment and management. Chiropractors, acupuncturists, osteopaths and massage therapists are frequently seen by people who are living with chronic pain or have an acute episode of pain. Together, all of these professionals become responsible for ensuring the optimal pain management of a person living with pain.

Reflective exercise 1.2: Roles and responsibilities

Subjective experiences like pain can be difficult for other people to understand. For this exercise, think about a time when you consulted a health professional about a pain problem.

- Did the health professional believe you and take your pain complaint seriously?
- How did belief or doubt about your pain affect the type and quality of the care that you received?
- Were you satisfied with the response that you received?

Unfortunately, pain research has demonstrated that people are frequently given inadequate care for their pain. The subjectivity of pain can complicate pain assessment and intervention (see Reflective exercise 1.2). Health professionals make clinical judgements about the veracity of a person's pain story. These judgements are based on many factors, such as professional experience, research familiarity, involvement in continuing education about pain and personal beliefs about how people should respond to pain. Health professionals can be also be caught between perceived obligations to an employer and obligations to the person living with pain (Merskey & Teasell 2007). Employers may expect the health professional to be particularly attentive to detect people who may not have real pain or may be exaggerating pain complaints for economic gain or to obtain medication for reasons other than pain relief. In other situations pain behaviour or disability may seem higher than what might be anticipated based on underlying physical factors. Such discordances often lead to negative judgement about the individual. Health professionals worry about whether or not to believe a person's complaint of pain. On the other hand, people expect to be believed when they complain of pain and to receive appropriate assessment and care. McCaffery & Beebe (1989) argued that:

'Pain is subjective and being fooled is simply a reality in dealing with something that can never be proved or disapproved. This point must be acknowledged by all members of the health team. The risk of being fooled does not justify doubting the patient or withholding

pain relief. No matter which approach we use in responding to the patient's report of pain, we will eventually make a mistake. If we doubt some patients and withhold treatment, we may avoid being fooled by the minority who are addicts, abusers or malingerers, but we will eventually fail to help someone who does have pain. On the other hand, if we give everyone the benefit of the doubt and try to relieve pain in all who say they have it, we will be fooled by some who are addicts, abusers, or malingerers, but we will never fail to help someone who does have pain. Either way we will make a mistake. Therefore we must address our professional responsibility and consider which mistake we can afford.'

(McCaffery & Beebe 1989, p. 8)

Inevitably, health professionals must constantly challenge themselves about the quality of their relationships with people living with pain to be certain that the care they provide is competent and optimal in managing pain. Regardless of specific professional roles, the central responsibility of a health professional caring for a person in pain is a compassionate response.

ACKNOWLEDGEMENTS

The authors express their gratitude to Drs Allen Finley and Paula Forgeron for reviewing sections pertaining to the roles of members of the team.

REFERENCES

Bope, E.T., Douglass, A.B., Gibovsky, A., et al., 2004. Pain management by the family physician: the family practice pain education project. J. Am. Board Fam. Pract. 17, S1–S12.

Canadian Association of Occupational Therapists, 2012. CAOT Position Statement: Pain management and occupational therapy. Online. Available: http://www.caot.ca/position%20statements/Pain%20management%20and%20occupational%20therapy%20position%20statement%20.pdf.

Carr, E., Layzell, M., 2010. Advancing nursing practice in pain management. Blackwell Publishing, Oxford.

Chevan, J., Clapis, P., 2012. Physical therapy management of low back pain. Jones & Bartlett Learning, Burlington, MA.

Doliber, C.M., 1984. Role of the physical therapist at pain treatment centers: a survey. Phys. Ther. 64, 905–909.

Eccleston, C., 2001. Role of psychology in pain management. Br. J. Anaesth. 87, 144–152.

Hamric, A.B., Spross, J.A., Hanson, C.M., 2009. Advanced practice nursing: an integrated approach, fourth ed. Elsevier Saunders, Edinburgh.

Kazanowski, M.K., Laccetti, M., 2008. Quick look nursing: pain management, second ed. Jones & Bartlett Learning, Burlington, MA.

Kielhofner, G., 2002. Dimensions of doing. In: Kielhofner, K. (Ed.), Model of human occupation. third ed. Lippincott, Williams and Wilkins, Baltimore MA, pp. 124–144.

LaChapelle, D.L., Lavoie, S., Boudreau, A., 2008. The meaning and process of pain acceptance: perceptions of women living with arthritis and fibromyalgia. Pain Res. Manag. 13, 201–210.

Loeser, J., Melzack, R., 1999. Pain: an overview. Lancet. 353 (May 8), 1607–1609.

Lum, G., 1997. Prisoner of pain. In: Young-Mason, J. (Ed.), The patient's voice: experiences of illness. F A Davis, Philadelphia, pp. 63–71.

MacLellan, K., 2006. Management of pain: expanding nursing and health care practice series. Nelson Thornes, Cheltenham.

Main, C., Sullivan, M., Watson, P., 2008. Pain management. Practical applications of the biopsychosocial perspective in clinical and occupational settings, second ed. Churchill Livingstone, Edinburgh.

McCaffery, M., Beebe, A., 1989. Pain: a clinical manual for nursing practice. Mosby, St Louis.

McCaffery, M., Pasero, C., 1999. Pain: A clinical manual, second ed. Mosby, St Louis.

Merskey, H., Bogduk, N., 1994. Classification of chronic pain. Definitions of Chronic Pain Syndromes and Definition of Pain Terms, second ed. International Association for the Study of Pain, Seattle.

Merskey, H., Teasell, R.W., 2007. Problems with insurance-based research on chronic pain. Med. Clin. North Am. 91, 31–43.

Pellino, T.A., Willens, J., Polomano, R.C., et al., 2002. The American Society of Pain Management Nurses practice analysis: role delineation study. Pain Manag. Nurs. 3, 2–15.

Robinson, K., Kennedy, N., Harmon, D., 2011. Review of occupational therapy for people with chronic pain. Australian Journal of Occupational Therapy 58, 74–81.

Simon, E.P., Folen, R.A., 2001. The role of the psychologist on the multidisciplinary pain management team. Professional Psychology: Research and Practice 32, 125–134.

Skjutar, A., Schult, M.L., Christensson, K., et al., 2010. Indicators of need for occupational therapy in patients with chronic pain: occupational therapists' focus groups. Occup. Ther. Int. 17, 93–103.

Sluka, K., 2009. Mechanisms and management of pain for the physical therapist. IASP Press, Seattle.

Stetts, D.M., Carpenter, G., 2012. Physical therapy management of patients with spinal pain; an evidence based approach. Jones & Bartlett Learning, Burlington, MA.

Stewart, J.C., Kostash, M.A., 1998. Anaesthetists as pain management consultants. Curr. Opin. Anaesthesiol. 11, 429–433.

Stomberg, M.W., Sjöström, B., Haljamäe, H., 2003. The role of the nurse anaesthetist in the planning of postoperative pain management. AANA J. 71, 197–202.

Strong, J., 1996. Chronic pain: the occupational therapists perspective. Churchill Livingstone, Edinburgh.

Swerdlow, M., Mehta, M.D., Lipton, S., 1978. The role of the anaesthetist in chronic pain management. Anaesthesia 33, 250–257.

Traines, M.A., 1994. Occupational therapy intervention in the relief of foot pain. American Occupational Therapy Association, Rockville, MD.

Tull, Y., Unruh, A.M., Dick, B.D., 2011. Yoga for chronic pain management: a qualitative exploration. Scand. J. Caring Sci. 25, 435–443.

Twycross, A., 2002. Educating nurses about pain management: the way forward. J. Clin. Nurs. 11, 705–714.

Unruh, A.M., 2008. Pain in women. Pain Res. Manag. 13, 199–200.

Chapter | 2 |

The patient's voice

Mandy Nielsen

LEARNING OBJECTIVES

At the end of this chapter readers will have an understanding of:

1. The importance of listening to the patient's story.
2. The impact that chronic pain can have across varied life domains.
3. The link between the individual experience of pain and the social environment.
4. The association between healthcare provider–patient communication and health outcomes.

OVERVIEW

This chapter is concerned with the importance and value of listening to the patient's voice in our practice with people in pain. Living with pain involves so much more than managing the pain sensation. Pain has the potential to affect every domain of an individual's life, as well as that of their family and others close to them. Listening and responding to a patient's story can be more than a sympathetic gesture. It can have direct consequences for the relevance and quality of health research and health delivery, and may influence post-consultation outcomes. In this chapter we will explore the experience of living with chronic pain to establish why listening to the patient's voice is important. To facilitate this we will be hearing from four patients with different pain conditions throughout the chapter: Ron, Catherine, Beth and Mat.

THE EXPERIENCE OF LIVING WITH CHRONIC PAIN

Understanding illness begins with an understanding of illness as it is lived (Johansson et al 1999, p. 1800).

The excerpt from the interview with Ron (Box 2.1) clearly demonstrates that living with pain involves much more than managing the sensation of pain. In this short passage we can see that the experience of persistent pain has had a significant impact on a number of aspects of Ron's life, including his sense of self, career, family relationships, and social and recreational activities. Honkasalo aptly described chronic pain as 'an intruder or thief that takes away the most precious things in life. Pain discontinues stories, interrupts life projects, it messes up life plans' (Honkasalo 2001).

One of the difficulties associated with pain, however, is that each individual's experience is unique. Ron's experience of living with fibromyalgia will not mirror the experience of someone else. It is important therefore to acknowledge the heterogeneity of people living with pain, recognizing that it is not possible to apply a 'one size fits all' treatment or management framework, however desirable this may be. The full impact that living with pain has on a person's life can only begin to be understood by talking

© 2014 Elsevier Ltd.

Box 2.1 **One patient's voice: Ron**

'I still continue with regular bouts of chronic fatigue and very, very defined muscle, joint and, I would say, bone pain. My career has ground to a halt, I've been to lots of specialists, and now I reside at home. I'm pretty stuffed I suppose, stuffed in many ways. The consequences of it are, I've lost my career, I'm a lousy father in the sense of my ability to handle the kids for more than an hour at a time, there's no football, running on beaches, the ability to socialise, all those sorts of things I can't do because movement aggravates pain, any movement aggravates muscle and joint pain. The fatigue denies me any ability to keep my brain alive, so going out to dinner and talking to someone is generally just not on. By about three in the afternoon I start winding down, by five I'm pretty uncomfortable, by seven I'm asleep on the sofa or very quiet watching TV somewhere. Life has ground to a halt. So my circumstances are aggravated beyond my physical symptoms to now include emotional and psychological ones, because my relationship with life in the context of a family and career is distorted from I suppose expectations, or what you try to achieve or what you dream for. So now I'm an invalid, I don't leave the house much, I drive the kids to school occasionally, go to the shops and get some milk and bread and those sorts of things, go to doctors, but I've become socially isolated, and it's difficult. I'm in my 40s, but it's like I'm living a life in my 80s, and my mind and emotions aren't prepared for it or still comfortable with it, so a natural depression comes out of that, a difficulty relating to life, trying to find your place in it. My mindset has always been, be useful, or in other words, don't be a nuisance in life, so relying on a partner to do a lot of the domestic work, and not being able to step forward and take an equal, or even a lead role is very difficult. The kids are, as kids are, very accommodating. It's great that Dad gets up, helps them with a bit of breakfast and goes back to bed. Dad doesn't join them at the beach or on social occasions, and they seem to adjust. But from my point of view, there's a disconnection and missing out, and I suppose a degree of deficiency as a parent. I've been a hard worker for the last 25 odd years, and so not working is...I was built for working, I spent 25 years training and skilling myself up, and so what do you do with your mind? Life becomes very internalised and contemplative. It is very difficult, and you become disconnected from a degree of reality...you're socially removed. I do try to socially join in, but I find that I'm brain dead or very uncomfortable in my body pain wise or fatigue wise, that I'm not a very good conversationalist. So that sort of gives a viewpoint of where I am.'

(Excerpt from narrative interview with Ron, 3 years after the onset of a chronic condition diagnosed as chronic fatigue syndrome and/or fibromyalgia.)

---

with them about what they are experiencing, and what pain means to them. As practitioners, we need to give patients the time and the permission to 'tell their story' (Neilsen et al 2009).

Adopting the practice of listening to patients as the departure point for our work with people in pain may, however, create a sense of uncertainty. Is this a completely unmapped journey we are embarking on, or are there some signposts to provide a bit more direction for improved practice with this patient group? Fortunately, by considering the phenomenological research in this area it is possible to identify some similarities of experience, knowledge of which will help us when listening to patients' stories. Three key themes within this literature relevant to our discussion are the search for restoration, loss and stigma.

THE SEARCH FOR RESTORATION

'I said is it in my head or is there something wrong? Because it doesn't show anything on the CAT scan. And he said, 'Well it's definitely not in your head.' But nobody can tell me what it is!'

Mat

Not surprisingly, when people first experience pain they try to relieve or stop it. For most of us, there is an expectation of what Hilbert (1984) described as 'normal' pain, reflecting the sociocultural expectation that, with the exception of particular identifiable conditions, pain is temporary and treatable, and 'normal' life will soon be restored. This expectation is continually reinforced through, for example, the advertising of medications and other products purported to quickly eliminate pain.

If pain does not resolve as expected, most people will embark on an often long and convoluted search for a diagnosis and cure for their pain. In contemporary industrialized societies this search typically focuses on resources within the biomedical healthcare system, involving consultations often with multiple medical practitioners and allied health professionals. The search can sometimes stretch over a number of years, and it is not uncommon for people to list 10 or more health professionals they have consulted in the quest to eradicate pain from their lives. This journey can be not only time-consuming and expensive, but the process of retelling their story multiple times may be overwhelming and demoralizing, particularly when it does not result in a 'cure' for the pain. In addition, patients may receive as many different diagnoses as consultations they have attended. As one research participant said, 'It takes a lot to have to keep repeating your story over and over again. . .all these medical people come from their own little sides of the fence and put their take on things. And they still don't really even get the whole picture of what's going on'. It is important to acknowledge to patients, therefore, that you are aware that they may have been on a frustrating journey searching for pain relief. While it may not be possible to avoid a retelling of the story, demonstrating an awareness of the journey they have been on is an important part of developing a therapeutic relationship with the patient.

It is not uncommon for people who have consulted numerous healthcare professionals to become frustrated and angry when this process does not result in a diagnosis or effective treatment for their pain. As healthcare professionals we may experience what on the surface appears to be undeserved anger being directed at us. Often much of a patient's anger is the emotional consequence of previous treatment experiences, experiences related to legal or compensation processes associated with the injury or accident which precipitated the pain, or the impact that their pain is having on their family and social relationships. It is important to allow patients to talk about these experiences and the emotions associated with them. Avoid 'individualizing' the anger and attributing it to particular individual characteristics. By listening to the patient's story and considering the individual within their social context, we can avoid 'blaming the victim' and develop a more constructive relationship with the patient.

While one factor contributing to patients' frustration and anger may be the failure of healthcare professionals to eliminate their pain, research suggests that an additional trigger can be the way people are dealt with during the healthcare encounter (Holloway et al 2000; McGowan et al 2007; Nielsen 2009; Warwick et al 2004). This can be particularly so in cases where an identifiable cause of ongoing pain cannot be found, as the reality of the pain may be implicitly or explicitly questioned, resulting in feelings of delegitimation. The term 'delegitimation' describes the experience when an individual's perceptions and knowledge of their pain are 'systematically disconfirmed or discounted' (Garro 1994, p. 788). Delegitimation is a recurring theme in phenomenological research with chronic pain sufferers, and can have wide-ranging effects. These include people becoming reluctant to disclose their chronic pain condition due to concern that others will not understand and will label them as 'malingerers', or the possibility that this could have a negative impact on a work situation, or the perception that stigmatization that has affected their access to, or the quality of, medical treatment. People may disengage from a healthcare system that they feel is not only unable to ameliorate their pain, but is also doubting the reality of their pain at all.

An important starting point in practice with chronic pain patients is to confirm the legitimacy of their pain and to normalize their experiences. Therapists should clearly state their belief in the reality of the pain that patients are experiencing. It is also important to let people know that they are not alone in this experience – what they are feeling and thinking is commonly reported by other people with chronic pain conditions.

LOSS

'. . .there are all sorts of big deal things that I feel like I've lost, that while they're not exactly about my pain, they're all sort of linked. . .There's so many things to grieve about.'

Catherine

Chronic pain, particularly when combined with impairment, often results in a series of losses across numerous life domains, including employment and income, family and social relationships, lifestyle and interests, social status, and plans for the future (Large et al 2002, p. 431). In their research with people with chronic back pain, Walker and colleagues identified 'a catalogue of socioeconomic and other material and psychological losses' (Walker et al 2006, p. 204), including loss of abilities and roles, employment-related losses, financial losses, relationship losses, and loss of identity and hope.

Loss of employment

Loss of employment is frequently identified as a consequence of chronic pain (Access Economics 2007; Crooks 2007; Howden et al 2003; Patel et al 2007; Raak & Wabren 2006). People will often describe a long process of trying to return successfully to work after an accident or illness. Mat, for example, was seriously injured in a car accident in 1991. After 9 months of rehabilitation he returned to his job driving a sugar cane harvester:

'It was hard. Like I used to ache and I couldn't jump up and down off the machines anymore. Eventually it got that way I couldn't drive a harvester or bin out anymore, it was too rough, just the shakin'. . .'

When he could no longer deal with the physical demands of cane harvesting, Mat started driving taxis for a living. He described this as '. . .alright for a couple of years, but you work such long hours. And from the constant driving I got to the point I was up at the doctor's more times than I was actually working', and again he gave up the job due to his pain. Despite this, Mat managed to earn a living for a further 10 years, until he reached a point when he finally had to admit he could no longer work and applied for 'the thing', as he called the government disability pension. Mat was so ashamed at having to do this that he had difficulty saying what 'the thing' was, let alone discussing it further.

Catherine, a healthcare professional, was told she could not come back to work until she was '100% fit'. Although she tried to return to work on two occasions, she said lack of support and understanding by supervising staff and consequent legal proceedings led her to eventually resign.

These examples point to the enabling or constraining potential of the workplace to affect the lives of people with chronic pain. Research has highlighted a number of social environmental factors that can contribute to loss of employment, including attitudes of employers and lack of flexibility in employment arrangements (Nielsen 2009). The fluctuating levels of pain and incapacity that are often a feature of chronic pain can make work capacity difficult to predict and manage (Patel et al 2007). Ideally, therefore, employment policies and programmes should enable people with chronic pain to negotiate employment arrangements in ways that meet their changing needs and abilities (Crooks 2007). Initiatives such as increased flexibility and support within the workplace could perhaps transform this situation and contribute to a reduction in the social suffering experienced by people with chronic pain. This contention is supported by recent Australian research, which suggested that support such as job flexibility could significantly reduce lost productivity costs due to chronic pain (Access Economics 2007, p. 25).

The broader individual and social outcomes resulting from loss of employment are evident when the associated loss of income is considered. The financial impact of unemployment is frequently articulated by people with chronic pain (Nielsen 2009). The ongoing financial cost of having chronic pain, in terms of visits to health practitioners and accessing services or equipment which provides relief and aids functioning, can be an additional financial burden. For some people, loss of income due to unemployment means they cannot afford treatment or therapies which alleviate their pain. Catherine, for example, felt she was in a Catch-22 situation in that she was being advised by her GP and physiotherapist to stop working, but she needed an income to continue to afford services such as physiotherapy, which she believed decreased her pain and increased her functional capacity.

Research indicates that having a disability increases the risk of poverty and hardship (Saunders 2006), and identifies a link between chronic pain and lower socioeconomic status (Access Economics 2007). While loss of employment due to chronic pain may be seen as an individual crisis, lack of flexibility in employment arrangements and inadequate financial support for those receiving a government pension demonstrates the broader social aspect of the suffering that job loss can engender.

Loss of social and family roles

Living with chronic pain can also limit social activities, with a subsequent loss of valued roles in this domain. On one level, people with chronic pain may not feel physically able or comfortable to participate in social activities due to factors such as difficulty walking or sitting for any length of time, associated fatigue and medication side effects, or the all-consuming effort of managing their pain. This was illustrated in the earlier excerpt from the interview with Ron, when he described himself as 'brain dead' and 'not a very good conversationalist'. Similarly, Beth described life in general as becoming 'sort of non-existent' after the onset of her pain:

> 'For the last almost two years it's just been working full time and managing my pain, seeing medical people. So I haven't had a lot of social life. And even, like with the pain, it's hard to drive sometimes. And because of my back I haven't been able to go to the movies until recently because I haven't been able to sit for two hours. So the pleasurable things in life sort of became non-pleasurable because of the pain that was involved.'

Lack of involvement in social activities can contribute to people becoming socially isolated. While in part this can be due to the mechanics of being in pain, it can also be related to what Hilbert (1984) has described as the 'acultural' aspect of chronic pain. When the search for restoration does not result in a cure for their pain, people find themselves experiencing pain they cannot understand, and which others in society do not understand or talk about. Chronic pain is not a problem that can be put aside to be dealt with later; it is, as Hilbert described it, an ongoing, ever present somatic reminder that 'things are not as they should be:

> 'At home, at work, and in their social life generally, sufferers are saddled with an insoluble dilemma, of paramount concern to them, in the presence of others for whom no such priority exists. This preoccupation further documents in sufferers' minds their isolation and estrangement from the society around them.'

(Hilbert 1984, p. 370).

While a common way of dealing with a problem in our society is to talk it over with others, the acultural nature of chronic pain may serve to isolate sufferers even further due to a lack of understanding and the prospect of delegitimation, as discussed earlier in this chapter. Social isolation is compounded by an inability to communicate what is a major issue in sufferers' lives. Beth described pain as 'a lonely thing': 'If somebody says "How are you going?" or "How are you?", they don't really want to know. This is a perfect opportunity to whinge about all your aches and pains. But normally you don't burden other people with that sort of thing...You just keep it to yourself.'

People with chronic pain therefore can experience not only loss of physical participation in social activities, but also the loss of a previously taken-for-granted social membership. Hilbert identified this as a form of suffering 'which transcends physical pain' and can result in what he describes as 'falling out of culture':

'. . . sufferers, though living within a society and within a culture, are precariously and continuously approaching the amorphous frontier of non-membership'

(Hilbert 1984, p. 375).

In addition to the impact on social relationships, living with chronic pain can also have a significant impact on family relationships. People with children will often talk about their guilt about not being able to play with and do things with their children. Ron described himself as 'a lousy father', while Mat talked of being 'stuffed for a week' if he spent half an hour playing cricket in the backyard with his kids. While Beth said she had been very involved in her children's activities, she identified 'the one big downer' of her life with pain as being the impact it had had on her experience as a parent:

'The saddest part of having a bad back is when your children are little and they're sick, they don't call for Mum, because they know Mum can't come and pick them up. . .Dad was the one they called for when they were sick.'

People with chronic pain also talk about the impact pain has had on relationships with their partners. Ron described his partner as a wonderful person who had passionately stood by him. However, he felt his pain experience had done a lot of damage to this relationship:

'Needless to say, being personal, sexuality is a no-go area, as much on my part, as much on her part. It's just when you're dealing with such [pain related] issues all the time, it's not an easy comfortable dynamic.'

Beth described her partner as 'really really good' but her pain had changed their relationship, as he now does the majority of the household activities, which she found very frustrating. She also identified the importance of having a loving family: '. . .it was a dreadful thought but it was quite often, if I didn't have a loving family I wouldn't want to go on. Knowing it [the pain] is going to be there forever.' Not all people with chronic pain will experience such support from their partners. Living with someone with chronic pain in the family can have a detrimental impact on the partners and families of those with pain. Strunin & Boden (2004), for example, found that partners and children took over the family responsibilities previously undertaken by the person with pain, and that this led to stress within family relationships. These findings are reflected in other qualitative studies (Ostlund et al 2001; Richardson et al 2007; Seers & Friedli 1996; Strong et al 1994).

As well as identifying numerous functional limitations as a consequence of pain, people will often express regret and distress at these losses. It may be beneficial, therefore, to explore these individual experiences of loss with clients. Walker and colleagues have suggested that the experience of loss may have implications for existing cognitive-based therapies for pain, such as relaxation techniques, changing negative pain beliefs and 'catastrophizing', and problem-solving strategies, which are based on the premise that pessimistic beliefs are a result of 'cognitive distortion' and/or a pre-existing psychological 'vulnerability' (Walker et al 2006, p. 204). They propose an alternative perspective: that negative cognitive beliefs may represent *realistic* appraisals of tangible losses and negative social consequences, rather than some form of 'latent personal vulnerability' that pre-existed in the individual prior to the development of chronic pain. Helping people come to terms with tangible losses may therefore be an important precursor to pain management strategies aimed at cognitive change and functional improvement.

Loss of 'self'

Long-term interference with social roles, combined with changing perceptions of personal attributes, has been shown to have an impact on a person's identity or 'sense of self' (Harris et al 2003). From a sociological perspective, the self is developed and maintained through social relations; that is, one's identity is fundamentally social in nature (Charmaz 1983, p. 170). Charmaz (1983) identified 'loss of self' as a fundamental form of suffering experienced by people who are chronically ill. She contended that serious chronic illness 'results in spiraling consequences such as loss of productive function, financial crises, family strain, stigma, and a restricted existence' and that 'suffering such losses results in a diminished self':

'Chronically ill persons frequently experience a crumbling away of their former self-images without simultaneous development of equally valued new ones. The experiences and meanings upon which these ill persons had built former positive self-images are no longer available to them. . .Over time, accumulated loss of formerly sustaining self-images without new ones results in a diminished self-concept.'

(Charmaz 1983, p. 168)

The previous discussion regarding the impact of chronic pain on social and family roles illustrates that people with chronic pain can experience the 'spiraling consequences' that Charmaz described. Living with pain, and with the associated restrictions this can place on quality of life, can challenge pre-pain self identities; people experience the 'crumbling away' of their former self, without developing an acceptable alternative identity. This sense of loss of identity will often become apparent when people with chronic pain talk about their 'before-pain' self and their 'after-pain' self. The before-pain self is usually physically, intellectually and/or socially active. Mat and Ron described energetic before-pain selves, involved in sport or other physical activities. For example, Mat said he used to do whatever he liked before the accident: 'Did everything. Rode motorbikes. Now I couldn't. Last time I rode a bike, which was about 20 minutes, I was in bed for three days. So I don't ride bikes anymore…now I can barely walk from here to the shop.' Mat described his post-pain self as 'useless'. Similarly, Ron described himself as 'pretty stuffed in many ways…there's no football or running on beaches.'

Clients also commonly identify a loss of identity and purpose associated with no longer being able to work. Catherine described the loss of her nursing position as being more than the loss of a job; it was more a loss of who she was:

> '…when I'm trying to sleep at night I think about so many things that I've lost; it's not just I've lost a fully functioning arm, I've lost my career, I've lost the other thing that was probably the thing that gave me joy in life, music and playing the piano, and I did that as a semi-professional, which I can't do anymore. So you know, there are all sorts of big deal things that I feel like I've lost…'

Beth also talked about a loss of identity, although for her the cognitive impact of living with pain had more salience: 'You feel as if you're brain dead. I used to consider myself as reasonably intelligent, now I have to really think about everything I'm doing.' Ron described himself as going from being 'rather successful' to 'stuffed'; living like an invalid and trying to find his 'place in life.'

Chronic pain can therefore have an impact on people's identities in varying ways – their physical, intellectual, social and emotional selves. Charmaz (1983) has identified the 'loss of self' suffered by people with chronic illness generally as leading to a continued struggle to lead valued lives and maintain or develop positive and worthwhile definitions of self.

STIGMA

In the previous section, the 'crumbling away' of the former self through loss of social roles and personal attributes was discussed in terms of the impact this has on the individual with pain and their family. As therapists it is also important that we look beyond the individual in pain to consider the social environment in which they live, as this can have a powerful influence on how chronic pain is experienced (Box 2.2).

When telling the story of their pain, clients often spend relatively little time describing the location and bodily

---

Box 2.2 What is the 'social environment'?

'Human social environments encompass the immediate physical surroundings, social relationships, and cultural milieus within which defined groups of people function and interact. Components of the social environment include built infrastructure; industrial and occupational structure; labour markets; social and economic processes; wealth; social, human and health services; power relations; government; race relations; social inequality; cultural practices, the arts; religious institutions and practices; and beliefs about place and community…Embedded within contemporary social environments are historical social and power relations that have become institutionalised over time.'

(Barnett & Casper 2001, p. 465)

---

sensation of the pain per se. Rather, their focus will be on the process of trying to cope with the pain on a daily basis, and the impact of the pain on their life as a whole. As the previous discussion on loss illustrates, clients can experience a form of suffering which, while experienced by the individual, is partly a consequence of political, economic and institutional structures outside their control. Kleinman and colleagues refer to this as 'social suffering', where the focus widens from the individual experience to include 'what political, economic and institutional power does to people, and, reciprocally…how these forms of power themselves influence responses to social problems' (Kleinman et al 1996, p. XI).

While there may be many aspects of social suffering that are not in our power as therapists to address, social suffering is an important concept to be aware of when listening to clients' stories, as it will help us consider the experience of living with chronic pain as a whole, rather than focusing on an individual body part or functional activity. One aspect of social suffering which may be in the therapist's capacity to effect is the experience of stigma.

The relationship between stigma and chronic pain is increasingly being recognised (Holloway et al 2007; Nielsen 2012; Slade et al 2009). Stigmatization of people with chronic pain is a cumulative and social process that can have serious consequences for the person with pain and their family. It is therefore important that therapists have an understanding of how this process occurs so that they can avoid it in their own practice *and* challenge it in the practice of other health professionals when they see it occurring.

For many people with chronic pain, the lack of diagnosis and a clear treatment path leads them to acquire a label of 'different' or 'difficult'. This, combined with the open-ended nature of chronic pain, means they cannot perform the role of the socially acceptable sick person, that is, actively participate in the recommended treatment regime and then return to normal duties (Parsons 1958). Additionally, as Bodwell (2010) has pointed out, people with chronic pain cannot tell the preferred 'restitution story of illness', where they become sick, receive treatment and recover. Clients may find themselves negatively stereotyped because of their chronic pain. A 'heart sink patient' and 'malingerer' are two not uncommon stereotypes used to describe people with chronic pain who present for treatment. Research indicates that many people with chronic pain believe that health professionals, and society more generally, question the reality of their pain in the absence of an identifiable cause or an observable manifestation of disability. As Beth said: 'If it's not explained by a blood test or an x-ray or whatever, it doesn't exist.' Stereotyping of the client with chronic pain in this way may indeed result in more than stigmatization; Chibnall and Tait's body of work suggests that biomedical evidence has an 'inordinate amount of influence' on physician pain judgements, and may contribute to the under-treatment of pain (Chibnall et al 1997, 2000; Chibnall & Tait 1999; Tait & Chibnall 1997).

Stereotyping people with chronic pain as somehow different from 'us' constructs a rationale for devaluing and excluding people within society. This process, which Link & Phelan (2001) have termed 'separation', can mean that the reactions of others produce a sense of being devalued or disrespected, or in some way different in a negative way to others in society. Many people with chronic pain will describe this process of separation as they talk about their gradual recognition that their pain was somehow atypical, as it didn't conform to the previously discussed expectation of 'normal' pain. The omnipresent nature of chronic pain, which can't be left at home for a good night out, can create and continually reinforce a sense of isolation and estrangement from society.

This experience of separation can be greatly exacerbated if clients feel they are being negatively stereotyped by healthcare professionals. In telling the story of his pain, Ron deliberately structured his narrative to include a section which he introduced as 'how the medical profession has dealt with me'. He described being treated with cynicism and suspicion, particularly when requesting pain-relieving medication. Catherine said she believed she had been considered 'a liar and a cheat' in her dealings with some healthcare professionals and with her employer. Without a socially condoned diagnosis for their pain, it is easy for chronic pain sufferers to be positioned in a negative stereotype that separates them not only from society as a whole, but also from more 'deserving' people with legitimate health problems. This can be related to what Holloway and colleagues (2007) have termed 'moral stigma'; that is, chronic pain sufferers are labelled as 'morally weak' when there is a lack of congruity between their pain report and biomedical findings.

It is critically important that therapists do not fall into the 'practice trap' of labelling and stereotyping clients with chronic pain in this way. Not only may it compromise the strength of the relationship and the trust between the therapist and their client, there is also evidence that there is an association between healthcare provider–patient communication and patient health outcomes. The value of listening and responding to the client's story, therefore, goes beyond the immediate consultation period, and it is to this issue that we now turn.

THE VALUE OF THE PATIENT'S VOICE

'I really think doctors need to learn to listen to people who know their own body. You know when it's not quite right, you know when things aren't working properly, and you try to explain it to them and they just, it seems to go in one ear and out the other, or they just totally dismiss it.'

Beth

Research has demonstrated an association between healthcare provider–patient communication and patient health outcomes (Street et al 2009). In a review of literature concerned with doctor–patient communication and patient health outcomes, Stewart (1995) concluded that patient health outcomes can be improved with good doctor–patient communication. The studies reviewed suggested that good communication can have a positive influence on the emotional health of patients, as well as symptom resolution, functional and physiological status, and pain control. Other research has suggested that interpersonal communication processes between patients and healthcare providers can influence patient satisfaction with the care provided, adherence to treatment recommendations, retention of information and understanding of health conditions, and improvement in health (Duggan 2006; Ong et al 1995; Street 2001; Vranceanu et al 2009).

What is it about communication between healthcare practitioners and their patients which improves healthcare outcomes? More specifically, what makes for 'good communication'? The importance of practitioners and patients talking with each other is, at a basic level, fairly obvious, in the sense that people tell the practitioner what their symptoms are and the practitioner applies their knowledge and experience to identify a correct diagnosis and appropriate treatment or management regime. However, effective communication between practitioners and their patients is more complex than this seemingly simple information exchange process, particularly in situations where there is no clear diagnosis, as is the case in many instances of chronic pain.

15

Box 2.3 Features of the 'good back consultation' (Laerum et al 2006)

- To be taken seriously (be seen, heard and believed).
- To be given an understandable explanation of what is wrong.
- To have patient-centred communication (seeking patients' perspectives and/or preferences).
- To receive reassurance and, if possible, be given a favourable prognosis.
- To be told what can be done (by the patient him/herself and by the healthcare provider).

In a study by Laerum and colleagues (2006), patients with chronic low back pain were asked what they considered were the most important characteristics of a 'good back consultation'. The results, ranked according to the frequency, emphasis and stated importance by patients, are presented in Box 2.3. The findings of this study emphasize that one of the most important aspects of effectively communicating with people with chronic pain is listening and valuing what they say about their experience.

It is also important to integrate client beliefs and knowledge into a pain management partnership between the therapist and the client. This practice will contribute to improved congruency between the patient and the healthcare provider. Lack of congruency, particularly with regard to beliefs about the causes of pain, treatment preferences and desired outcomes, may have a negative effect on the therapeutic relationship and health outcomes (Brown 2003). Patient beliefs and expectations have been identified as being at the core of the therapeutic consultation process, particularly in terms of having the potential to influence adherence to recommended management regimes and as mediators of outcomes (Main et al 2010).

It is therefore critical to explicitly discuss with clients, at an early stage of the therapeutic relationship, why they think they have pain and what they want to achieve from their involvement with the therapist. Be aware that what the client wants out of a therapeutic programme may differ from what the therapist wants, but it is necessary to privilege the client's outcomes to ensure the development of interventions that are individually meaningful, appropriate and acceptable (Brown 2003).

It may be that the client will hold beliefs about the reason for their ongoing pain which are not supported by the current scientific knowledge in this area. Alternatively, clients may have no idea why they have persistent pain, and are frustrated and distressed by this. By identifying these issues early, it is possible for the therapist to address specific concerns expressed by the client, and to explore and clarify beliefs that are not supported by the available evidence. Main and colleagues (2010) suggest that all patients should be given a credible but simple explanation of differences between acute and chronic pain, the role of central pain mechanisms, and the development of disability. As a therapist, it is necessary to provide such an explanation using language that the client will understand. Research has indicated that while it is possible for patients to understand the neurophysiology of pain if it is explained appropriately, healthcare professionals often underestimate patients' ability to understand and may therefore not include appropriate explanations in their practice with chronic pain patients (Moseley 2003).

SHARED VOICES: THE VALUE OF CONSUMER GROUPS

'There is a great need for somewhere where you can be recognised and supported, and it's not psychology services, it's a step back from that...All the [internet] blogs I am on, probably the most outstanding thing people are saying is "I have lost all my family, I have lost all my social network, I have lost all my employment, I have lost all that and mostly I can't deal with x, y, and z aspects of my life because they still don't believe or recognise that this is not just me making it up".'

Ron

As discussed earlier in this chapter, living with chronic pain often results in feelings of social isolation and estrangement. The acultural nature of chronic pain can result in people feeling that they have what Hilbert (1984) described as 'an extreme personal idiosyncrasy' that cannot be shared with others in society. Kotarba's (1983) early work with professional athletes and 'blue-collar manual labourers' suggests that where pain is an inherent part of a particular profession or group, a shared language and understanding may develop, providing sufferers with a sense of belonging and strategies for managing and living with pain. In this final section of the chapter, the potential benefits of creating networks of 'shared voices' for people living with chronic pain will be discussed.

Pain consumers form and join groups for different reasons. One reason may be to meet with and obtain support from other people living with chronic pain. In an online survey of people living with chronic pain in Australia, 66% of the 587 participants indicated that they would be interested in joining a support group of some kind (Nielsen 2009). In a study of a consumer-led support group for people with chronic non-malignant pain,

---

Box 2.4 Reported benefits of support group participation (Subramaniam et al 1999)

- Additional information on pain management.
- Enhanced adaptation to the challenges of chronic pain.
- Increased functional activity.
- Enhanced social networks and peer support.
- Improved self-esteem and morale.
- A more positive appraisal of difficulties.

Box 2.5 Advocacy and chronic pain

Advocacy is about supporting another person's cause. There are a number of ways of doing this, including:
- individual advocacy
- systemic advocacy.

Individual advocacy involves actively promoting a person's welfare and rights, for example assisting someone with chronic pain negotiate reasonable accommodation in the work place. An outcome of individual advocacy may also be assisting an individual to advocate for themselves (self advocacy).

Systemic advocacy is primarily concerned with influencing and changing the system in ways that will benefit people with chronic pain as a group within society. Systems advocates will encourage changes to the law, government and service policies, and community attitudes. Lobbying politicians for increased funding for community-based pain management resources is an example of systemic advocacy.

(Adapted from http://qla.org.au/PDFforms/Forms/Advocacy%20Info%2020Dec07.pdf)

Subramaniam and colleagues (1999) found that participants identified a number of benefits from participating in a monthly face-to-face group (see Box 2.4). In addition, participants reported contact with 21% fewer healthcare services in the 3 months prior to a 5-month follow-up interview, and significantly less functional disability at the 5-month follow-up interview. These findings may indicate that participants were obtaining support from their peers, rather than seeking this support through their general practitioners (Subramaniam et al 1999, p. 380). Other potential benefits of participating in a consumer-led support group can include legitimization of the chronic pain condition and feeling understood by others (Friedberg et al 2005).

Not everyone with chronic pain will be want to or be able to attend a face-to-face support group. One of the potential problems with consumer-led pain support groups is the difficulty actively participating in such groups can present for people with ongoing pain and/or limited resources. In a study involving active and inactive members of chronic fatigue syndrome and fibromyalgia support groups, nearly 30% of the 135 members who had become inactive or dropped out of a group cited being too sick as the reason for their non-attendance. Other frequently reported reasons for non-attendance were inconvenient location (37.8%) or time (37.0%) (Friedberg et al 2005). Therapists should therefore not automatically assume that a person with chronic pain will be interested in attending a support group. It is useful to consider other social networking options, such as chat rooms, email discussion groups or blogs. Most importantly, talk with people to identify if they would like more support and, if so, what form such support should take.

Consumers may also form or join a group with the aim of improving the lives of people with chronic pain through healthcare policy and practice change. This type of consumer group is more focused on individual, group and/or systemic *advocacy*, rather than individual support (Box 2.5).

Of course it is possible for a consumer group to have both a support *and* advocacy focus. Whether or not people with chronic pain are involved in support and/or advocacy groups, they may appreciate some assistance from healthcare professionals. This could be in the form of helping with transport to and from group meetings, providing administrative support, or talking about specific topics at meetings. It is important, however, to talk with consumers to determine whether assistance is required and, if so, what form this could take. Do not assume that consumer groups will always want or need healthcare professional involvement or that, as therapists, we will know what sort of assistance will be helpful.

CONCLUSION

Listening and responding to the patient's story is integral to the successful management of chronic pain. Actively listening to their story validates the patient's experience and provides the basis for a trusting and effective healthcare partnership. It is only by listening to the patient's voice that the therapist will develop a true understanding of what living with pain means to individual clients, how it has affected their lives and the lives of their family members, and what they hope to achieve from their involvement with the therapist.

Respecting and incorporating the patient's voice into practice requires a shift in the balance of power between the healthcare provider and the patient. The client is the expert in their pain; the therapist's role is to provide resources and facilitate appropriate and relevant pain management practices. This can be challenging, but to neglect or devalue the patient voice will affect the potential for successful health outcomes. It is not so difficult. To give Mat the final word:

'Don't call people liars. Look and talk to them like they're people, not an x-ray walking through the door. And listen to what they have to say.'

Q | **Study questions/questions for revision**

1. What aspects of a person's life can be affected by chronic pain?
2. Why is it important to allow the patient to tell their story?
3. What is meant by the term 'delegitimatise' and why is it important?
4. List some losses that a person may experience as a consequence of chronic pain.
5. How can health outcomes be affected by patient–provider communication?

REFERENCES

Access Economics, 2007. The High Price of Pain: The Economic Impact of Persistent Pain In Australia. Access Economics, Sydney.

Barnett, E., Casper, M., 2001. A definition of 'social environment'. Am. J. Public Health 91 (3), 465.

Bodwell, M.B., 2010. How to listen in chronic pain narratives. In: Fernandez, J. (Ed.), Making Sense of Pain: Critical and Interdisciplinary Perspectives. Proceedings of the First Global Conference on Making Sense of Pain. Inter-disciplinary Press, Oxford. Available: http://www.inter-disciplinary.net/wp-content/uploads/2010/10/pain2010ever11007102.pdf.

Brown, C.A., 2003. Service users' and occupational therapists' beliefs about effective treatments for chronic pain: a meeting of the minds or the great divide? Disabil. Rehabil. 25 (19), 1115–1125.

Charmaz, K., 1983. Loss of self: a fundamental form of suffering in the chronically ill. Sociol. Health Illn. 5 (2), 168–195.

Chibnall, J.T., Tait, R.C., 1999. Social and medical influences on attributions and evaluations of chronic pain. Psychology and Health 14, 719–729.

Chibnall, J.T., Tait, R.C., Ross, L.R., 1997. The effects of medical evidence and pain intensity on medical student judgements of chronic pain patients. J. Behav. Med. 20, 257–271.

Chibnall, J.T., Dabney, A., Tait, R.C., 2000. Internist judgements of chronic low back pain. Pain Med. 1 (3), 231–237.

Crooks, V.A., 2007. Women's experiences of developing musculoskeletal diseases: employment challenges and policy recommendations. Disabil. Rehabil. 29 (14), 1107–1116.

Duggan, A., 2006. Understanding interpersonal communication processes across health contexts: Advances in the last decade and challenges for the next decade. J. Health Commun. 11, 93–108.

Friedberg, F., Leung, D.W., Quick, J., 2005. Do support groups help people with chronic fatigue syndrome and fibromyalgia? A comparison of active and inactive members. J. Rheumatol. 32 (12), 2416–2420.

Garro, L.C., 1994. Narrative representations of chronic illness experience: Cultural models of illness, mind, and body in stories concerning the Temporomandibular joint (TMJ). Soc. Sci. Med. 38 (6), 775–788.

Harris, S., Morley, S., Barton, S.B., 2003. Role loss and emotional adjustment in chronic pain. Pain. 105, 363–370.

Hilbert, R.A., 1984. The acultural dimensions of chronic pain: flawed reality construction and the problem of meaning. Soc. Probl. 31 (4), 365–378.

Holloway, I., Sofaer, B., Walker, J., 2000. The transition from well person to 'pain afflicted' patient: The career of people with chronic back pain. Illness, Crisis & Loss. 8 (4), 373–387.

Holloway, I., Sofaer-Bennett, B., Walker, J., 2007. The stigmatisation of people with chronic back pain.

Disabil. Rehabil. 29 (18), 1456–1464.

Honkasalo, M., 2001. Pain, Self and the body. American Journal of Semiotics. 17 (4), 9–31.

Howden, S., Jones, D., Martin, D., et al., 2003. Employment and chronic non-cancer pain: Insights into work retention and loss. Work. 20, 199–204.

Johansson, E.E., Hamberg, K., Westman, G., et al., 1999. The meanings of pain: an exploration of women's descriptions of symptoms. Soc. Sci. Med. 48, 1791–1802.

Kleinman, A., Das, V., Lock, M., 1996. Introduction. Daedalus. 125 (1), XI–XX.

Kotarba, J.A., 1983. Chronic Pain: Its Social Dimensions. Sage, Beverly Hills, CA.

Laerum, E., Indahl, A., Skouen, J.S., 2006. What is 'the good back consultation'? A combined qualitative and quantitative study of chronic low back pain patients' interaction with and perceptions of consultations with specialists. J. Rehabil. Med. 38, 255–262.

Large, R.G., New, F., Strong, J., et al., 2002. Chronic pain and psychiatric problems. In: Strong, J., Unruh, A.M., Wright, A., Baxter, G.D. (Eds.), Pain: A Textbook for Therapists. Churchill Livingstone, Sydney.

Link, B.G., Phelan, J.C., 2001. Conceptualizing stigma. Annual Review of Sociology. 27, 363–385.

Main, C.J., Buchbinder, R., Porcheret, M., et al., 2010. Addressing patient beliefs and expectations in the consultation. Best Pract. Res. Clin. Rheumatol. 24, 219–225.

McGowan, L., Luker, K.A., Creed, F., et al., 2007. 'How do you explain a pain that can't be seen?': The narratives of women with chronic pelvic pain and their disengagement with the diagnsotic cycle. Br. J. Health Psychol. 12, 261–274.

Moseley, L., 2003. Unraveling the barriers to reconceptualisation of the problem in chronic pain: The actual and perceived ability of patients and health professionals to understand neurophysiology. Journal of Pain. 4 (4), 184–189.

Nielsen, A., 2009. 'It's a whole lot more than just about my pain': Understanding and responding to the social dimension of living with chronic pain. University of Queensland, Brisbane.

Nielsen, A., 2012. Journeys with chronic pain: Acquiring stigma along the way. In: McKenzie, H., Quintner, J., Bendelow, G. (Eds.), At The Edge of Being The Aporia of Pain. Inter-Disciplinary Press, Oxford.

Nielsen, A., Copleston, P., Wales, C., 2009. Pain Is Not Invisible Project Interim Report: Chronic Pain. Unpublished.

Ong, L.M.L., Haes, C.J.M., Hoos, A.M., et al., 1995. Doctor–patient communication: A review of the literature. Soc. Sci. Med. 40 (7), 903–918.

Ostlund, G., Cedersund, E., Alexanderson, K., et al., 2001. 'It was really nice to have someone' – lay people with musculoskeletal disorders request supportive relationships in rehabilitation. Scand. J. Public Health. 29, 285–291.

Parsons, T., 1958. Definitions of health and illness in the light of American values and social structure. In: Gartly Jaco, E. (Ed.), Patients, Physicians and Illness. Free Press, Glencoe, IL.

Patel, S., Greasley, K., Watson, P.J., 2007. Barriers to rehabilitation and return to work for unemployed chronic pain patients: A qualitative study. Eur. J. Pain. 11 (8), 831–840.

Raak, R., Wabren, L.K., 2006. Health experiences and employment status in subjects with chronic pain: A long-term perspective. Pain Manag. Nurs. 7 (2), 64–70.

Richardson, J.C., Ong, B.N., Sim, J., 2007. Experiencing chronic widespread pain in a family context: giving and receiving practical and emotional support. Sociol. Health Illn. 29 (3), 347–365.

Saunders, P., 2006. The Costs of Disability and the Incidence of Poverty. The Social Policy Research Centre, Sydney.

Seers, K., Friedli, K., 1996. The patients' experiences of their chronic non-malignant pain. J. Adv. Nurs. 24, 1160–1168.

Slade, S.C., Molloy, E., Keating, J.L., 2009. Stigma experienced by people with nonspecific chronic low back pain: a qualitative study. Pain Med. 10 (1), 143–154.

Stewart, M.A., 1995. Effective physician-patient communication and health outcomes: A review. Can. Med. Assoc. J. 152 (9), 1423–1433.

Street, R.L., 2001. Active Patients as Powerful Communicators. In: Robinson, W.P., Giles, H. (Eds.), The New Handbook of Language and Social Psychology. John Wiley & Sons, Chichester, pp. 541–560.

Street, R.L., Makoul, G., Arora, N.K., et al., 2009. How does communication heal? Pathways linking clinician-patient communication to health outcomes. Patient Educ. Couns. 74, 295–301.

Strong, J., Ashton, R., Chant, D., et al., 1994. An investigation of the dimensions of chronic low back pain: the patients' perspectives. British Journal of Occupational Therapy. 57 (6), 204–208.

Strunin, L., Boden, L.I., 2004. Family consequences of chronic back pain. Soc. Sci. Med. 58, 1385–1393.

Subramaniam, V., Stewart, M.W., Smith, J.F., 1999. The development and impact of a chronic pain support group: A qualitative and quantitative study. J. Pain. Symptom. Manage. 17 (5), 376–383.

Tait, R.C., Chibnall, J.T., 1997. Physician judgments of chronic pain patients. Soc. Sci. Med. 45 (8), 1199–1205.

Vranceanu, A., Cooper, C., Ring, D., 2009. Integrating patient values into evidence-based practice: Effective communication for shared decision-making. Hand Clin. 25, 83–96.

Walker, J., Sofaer, B., Holloway, I., 2006. The experience of chronic back pain: Accounts of loss in those seeking help from pain clinic. Eur. J. Pain. 10, 199–207.

Warwick, R., Joseph, S., Cordle, C., et al., 2004. Social support for women with chronic pelvic pain: What is helpful from whom? Psychology and Health 19 (1), 117–134.

Chapter 3

Social determinants of pain

Kenneth D. Craig and Samantha R. Fashler

LEARNING OBJECTIVES

On completion of this chapter readers will have:

1. A social determinants framework of the experience of pain.
2. An evidence-based theoretical framework encompassing these social determinants and a social communication model of pain.
3. An understanding of the application of social determinants to innovative prevention, assessment and intervention strategies.

OVERVIEW

The social contexts of people's lives, past and present, are powerful determinants of pain. Social factors determine whether people will experience pain, what they think, feel and sense during the experience, and how they behave and communicate their distress to others. Thus, presence, perception, expression, maintenance, exacerbation and respite from pain all have sources in social factors. In this chapter, we provide a theoretical framework with its supporting evidence to argue that social determinants of pain have a strong causal bearing on pain experience. By examining social determinants we redress the overwhelming, yet narrow, emphasis on biological processes in contemporary efforts to understand and control pain.

Focusing on the causal role of social determinants provides important information about prevention of pain across the life span, the impact of opportunities to learn about pain and novel perspectives on treatment. Attending to how care for people in pain is structured and delivered in occupational, familial, medical and other environments has the potential to mitigate pervasive inadequate and unsuccessful treatment of pain. Understanding the social sources of pain provides a necessary basis for transforming and enhancing interventions, thereby extending the armamentarium beyond standard medical interventions of drugs, surgery and other biologically oriented approaches.

Seeking 'social causes' of pain is consistent with the long history of interest in aetiological mechanisms for pain. Identifying causes of pain leads to more effective interventions. Causes conventionally have been approached through diagnosis of disease and injury, an approach endorsed by many researchers, healthcare professionals and parties responsible for health care and public policy. This approach is conventional wisdom and expected by patients in pain or living with chronic pain. Typical questions are 'What injury or disease accounts for the pain?' or 'Is the source nociceptive or neuropathic?'. Such questions demonstrably neglect alternative major sources of pain and do not lead to numerous safe and efficacious interventions. The biopsychosocial

© 2014 Elsevier Ltd.

model of health offers a broader approach which posits that all biological, psychological and social factors must be considered in understanding human health or illness (Engel 1977). Despite the substantial evidence supporting this position as it applies to pain (Gatchel et al 2007; Turk & Okifuji 2002), attention to biological phenomena overwhelms the field. Psychologically based approaches are often ignored by people with strong biomedical orientations, and social determinants of pain have received minimal attention (Blyth et al 2007; Morris 2010; Skevington & Mason 2004).

There are conceptual and logistic problems with attributing causal importance to social factors. Powerful experimental designs that randomly assign research participants to variations in social factors (e.g. gender, ethnicity, socioeconomic status) typically cannot be undertaken for ethical and logistic reasons. Thus, accounts of some of the predictive relationships described below should be recognized as based on correlations that do not permit causal conclusions; the direction of the relationship is unclear and other unidentified variables could be more important causal factors. Any incident of pain must be recognized as having multiple determinants. Proximate and distal causes often can be described when attempting to prioritize causal factors to manage intervention. Injury and disease are frequently, but not always, proximal causes of pain. When present, they are an immediate target for intervention. Nevertheless, social factors often play a more important causal role than is typically recognized. Workplace safety programmes provide a good example – prevention of painful injuries dramatically reduces the personal and institutional costs of accidents. Distal interventions, including those that are preventive, may be the most important and cost-effective.

The position advocated here acknowledges the fundamental biological nature of pain. There have been major advances in understanding the cell biology consequences of tissue damage, genetic variability as a source of individual differences, biological transduction in nociceptive systems, peripheral and central nervous system impacts, and medical diagnosis and therapy for acute and intractable conditions. The dominant mechanistic theories of pain (specificity theory, pattern theory, summation theory, gate control theory, the neuromatrix perspective, neural plasticity and central sensitization, etc.) focus on these phenomena (Cope 2010). It is the search for complementary social causes of pain that occupies this chapter.

The focus on social processes appears particularly important in understanding human pain. Diverse patterns of adaptive behaviour supporting survival are evident across species, as biological systems evolve to sustain functioning in unique environments. In all animals, pain serves to warn about tissue damage and to motivate escape or avoidance behaviour. But pain can also come to acquire social functions and roles. Non-human mammals demonstrate an emergent capacity to utilize the social environment as a means of recognizing and avoiding danger and providing protective care (de Waal 2009). Human capacities for social engagement extend the likelihood that the social environment is particularly important in providing protection from pain. It is not clear whether the human brain evolved because of the challenges of life in complex social environments or an evolved brain permitted the complex adaptations of human attachment, cooperation and communal living, but these are integral features of all facets of human experience and living. One unique feature of the human brain is its ability to allow penetrating inferences concerning the emotions and intentions of other persons. Human adaptations reflect the necessity and complexity of interpersonal interaction, including its challenges and opportunities. The provision of care incorporating complex technological and healthcare system arrangements perhaps epitomizes social engineering in the interests of minimizing pain and suffering. It is not surprising that these unique human social capabilities should be integrated with pain experience and its expression, and one would expect the human pain system to have adapted accordingly.

Biomedical approaches to understanding and controlling pain have become progressively more microscopic as advances in genetics, cell biology and biophysics have extended the scope of the biological sciences. We argue that there are substantial grounds for shifting the focus from fine-grained analysis of biological functions to understanding the whole person in the sociocultural, political and economic environments that govern their behaviour.

THE SOCIAL COMMUNICATION MODEL OF PAIN

The social communication model of pain provides a detailed framework for understanding the complex interactions among the biological, psychological and social factors of pain (Craig 2009) (see Fig. 3.1). The following features of the model are examined here in sequence: sources of pain, the experience of pain, how pain is communicated to others and how others recognize, interpret and respond to information about the person's pain. The process is recognized as dynamic and recursive. Each stage has an impact on whether the individual or others come to control the pain and whether the pain persists. Intrapersonal (biological and psychological) and interpersonal (social) factors are important at each stage. Unlike most models of pain, attention is devoted to the role of the caregiver and the social and healthcare policies they represent, given their importance if care is to be provided to the person in pain. At all stages, attention to social processes provides opportunities to delivering preventive care or interventions. One could attend to those social circumstances that lead to the presence of pain, its exacerbation, over- or under-reaction to the event, the intentional or

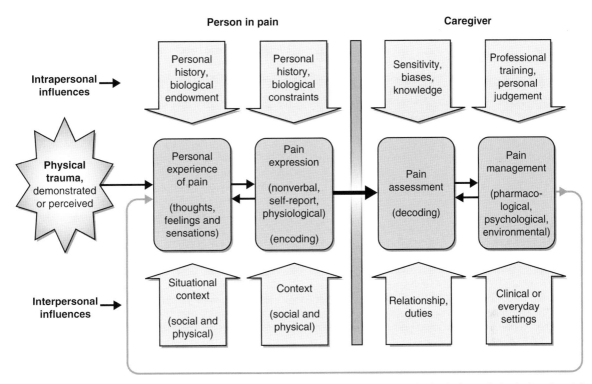

Fig. 3.1 The social communication model of pain. A conceptual model integrating biological, psychological and social perspectives at the level of interaction between the person in pain and persons present.
Adapted from Craig K D, Korol C T 2008 Developmental issues in understanding, assessing, and managing pediatric pain. In: Walco G, Goldschnieder K (eds) Pain in Children: a practical guide for primary care, pp 9–20, fig 2.1. Humana Press Inc, With kind permission of Springer Science + Business Media.

unintentional infliction of pain by others, or the failure to use interventions that would minimize pain and suffering, among many other possibilities.

SOURCES OF PAIN: OPPORTUNITIES FOR PREVENTION

Social circumstances often dictate whether people will be exposed to injury or disease. Therein lie opportunities for engaging in primary prevention, precluding the likelihood of pain before it happens. Epidemiological approaches to studying the distribution and determinants of pain have identified sociodemographic variations, social risk factors and population health trends in the prevalence and care of diverse painful conditions (von Korff & LeResche 2005). In establishing the complex web of causation, opportunities for prevention emerge. For example, oestrogen therapy for postmenopausal adult women is associated with increased risk of temporomandibular disorder (LeResche et al 1997). Awareness of this relationship contributes to cost–benefit analysis of hormone replacement

therapy, perhaps decreasing the incidence of this painful condition. In this manner, social factors, public awareness and policy may have an impact on use of a biomedical intervention strategy for chronic pain.

Characterization of social origins or risk factors has received minimal attention, despite interests of epidemiologists in risk and ecological factors (Dworkin et al 1992). Major categories of social risk factors can be conceptualized (see Box 3.1). The illustrations are not exhaustive; they are designed to highlight potential social causes of pain across the major social contexts of people's lives. The balance between interpersonal and intrapersonal control of these sources of pain is not always evident. Some events may be the consequence of personal decisions of the person in pain, such as risk taking in dangerous sports, but social pressures and constraints influence such decisions. Pain imposed by others in the interests of the person, but entered voluntarily, is perhaps best typified by medical procedures, including medical prophylaxis, diagnosis and treatment (including surgery). Medical pain usually is construed as an undesirable, but inevitable, event. Nevertheless, recent interpretations increasingly characterize pain as an adverse event and argue that more should be done

Box 3.1 **Social actions antecedent to pain**

Delivery of medical services (prophylactic, diagnostic, treatment)

Early childhood play and accidents

Risk taking (sports, recreational activities, motor vehicles)

Exposure to danger at work or in domestic settings

Social rituals (circumcision, adolescent rites)

Intentional aggression (criminal acts, police or military action, corporal punishment)

Self-inflicted pain (tattooing, piercing, branding, cutting, masochistic acts)

to preclude or mitigate pain (Chorney et al 2010). Pharmaceutical, psychological and environmental interventions can prevent or minimize immediate pain and the long-term consequences arising from medical procedures. For example, substantial neonatal exposure to pain is often characterized as the inevitable consequence of risk factors associated with preterm delivery, very low birth weight or congenital conditions. Nevertheless, there is reason to believe that exposure to pain is often unnecessarily excessive and disposes to adverse pain experience and behaviour later in life (Grunau & Tu 2007). Similarly, early life experience of dental pain predisposes children and adults to dental fears and avoidance of treatment (Versloot & Craig 2009). Thus, social factors again appear responsible for the risks associated with painful exposure and its consequences early in life.

Many other sources of pain outside health care are shaped by social factors. Pain may be a consequence of intentional, aggressive acts, such as in domestic violence, criminal behaviour and police enforcement or military action. Harm can also be the consequence of unintentional or voluntary exposure to risky settings in work, domestic and community environments if protective procedures, training or equipment are not provided or utilized. For example, workplace safety standards depend on policies and procedures and the subsequent compliance by employers and employees. Similarly, major risks associated with driving a motor vehicle have been diminished by programmes designed to enhance vehicular safety, such as use of child restraints, highway engineering, improved signage and markings, and reducing driving under the influence of alcohol. Both illustrate how social interventions can prevent painful injury.

Similar consideration should be given to prevention of pain that is socially sanctioned in the absence of malicious intent and conducted with or without the full consent of the individual, as seen with male and female circumcision. The interaction between social events and the experience of pain is further complicated by consensual painful actions in which people undergo severe discomfort for cosmetic purposes (e.g. piercings, tattoos, branding or scarification)

or for the sensation derived from the painful experience itself, as seen in masochism or self-inflicted injury. Similarly, neglecting to treat or assuage painful conditions with available resources is another form of socially derived pain.

Painful experiences also may be maintained or exacerbated by social events. Stress accompanies both daily life and periods of major social adjustment, and can contribute directly to psychophysiological disorders, lower immune functioning and promote tumour growth. This may compromise healing, thereby contributing to the manifestation, exacerbation and preservation of painful diseases and injuries (Antoni et al 2006). Stressful family, employer or other relationships tend to have a negative impact on coping and result in increased healthcare utilization. Under this strain, there is potential for vicious circles of family conflict, dysfunctional relationships, unemployment and social isolation that in turn perpetuate stress and pain. Alleviating circumstances creating stress for the individual can have an impact on the experience and expression of pain.

In general, healthcare systems that promote health provide a multifaceted and sustainable means of addressing pain. The major advances in preventive health care, including immunization programmes and public sanitation, dramatically diminish exposure to pain and suffering associated with infectious diseases. Similarly, injury prevention programmes are effective in reducing the incidence of painful injury (Pike et al 2010). Advertising campaigns, legal regulations and required certification and training all serve as preventive measures to diminish exposure to pain. Many examples of socially oriented programmes, such as ensuring a safe food supply and reducing tobacco use and alcohol abuse, have yielded long-term benefits, including reduction of health costs and the experience of pain. Thus, attention to healthcare policies and public education can be of considerable importance.

THE EXPERIENCE OF PAIN

An individual's life history and current social environment determine the thoughts and feelings experienced during a painful event. Substantial, and sometimes dramatic, variations in how people describe and react to apparently comparable disease and injuries are well documented (Fillingim 2010; Mogil 1999). This variability is usually represented as unidimensional; some people respond with considerable stoicism whereas others react with hysterical distress. Such representation fails to reflect the richness of the cognitive, emotional and sensory features of painful experience (Williams et al 2010). Complex thoughts reflecting prior experiences, the current context and solutions to the challenges invariably accompany all painful experiences, including 'What's happening to me?', 'How serious is this?', 'Will it last long?' and 'What can I do?'

People vary in the extent to which they attend to bodily sensations, perceive painful experiences as varying in severity, and use personal and social schema to interpret their experiences. In addition, emotional distress, such as anxiety or depression, greatly varies among patients. Of particular importance are maladaptive patterns of thinking, such as catastrophizing (Sullivan et al 2004), and hypervigilance (Van Damme et al 2010) or emotional reactions, such as anxiety or fear avoidance (Vlaeyen & Linton 2000), which exacerbate and maintain dysfunctional pain and pain-related disability, and influence the ability to benefit from treatment.

Although individual variations are popularly described in terms of intrapersonal factors (e.g. 'the person is "anxious" or "catastrophizing"'), these emotional reactions can have origins in biological inheritance and life experience. The biological features of pain are of unquestioned importance (Mogil 1999). They can be 'hardwired', as exemplified by the capacity of even the prematurely born neonate to signal pain (Craig et al 1993; Grunau & Craig 1987). Such signalling patterns probably have social origins because of the success of cry, facial expression and other non-verbal behaviour in capturing parental attention, thereby enhancing the likelihood of survival. In humans, the biological systems reflect remarkable flexibility and transform with maturity and life experience.

Humans have adapted to remarkably different physical environments across the globe, as well as to social environments that vary dramatically in cultural customs and practices, socioeconomic opportunity, discrimination and prejudice, and access to health care (Keefe et al 2005). Cultural variation includes differences in beliefs and practices concerning pain, reflecting unique histories in adapting to ecosystems and discovery of solutions to the challenges of physical danger (Craig & Pillai 2003). Culture-specific practices in the manner in which we appraise and react emotionally to pain dominate peoples' lives from birth to death (Bates 1987; McCracken et al 2001; Nayak et al 2000; Zborowski 1969). In Western societies 30 years ago, infants were deemed to be insensitive to pain, and doctors responded in a culturally specific way by not using anaesthetics during surgical procedures. The substantial shift in analgesic use in infants and young children carries strong emotional implications; today, using less anaesthetic would be deemed primitive and inhumane, even though it was deemed appropriate in the near past (American Academy of Pediatrics/Canadian Pediatric Society 2006). At the opposite end of the age range, elderly people, particularly those with cognitive impairment, were deemed relatively insensitive to pain (Hadjistavropoulos et al 2007). Recent development of pain measures independent of self-report capability now indicate the capacity to experience pain is not impaired even though the ability to self-report is diminished by dementias and other impairments (Hadjistavropoulos et al 2000; Kunz et al 2007).

Human adaptive capabilities support adjustment to those family, ethnic and cultural environments in which the individual is born and raised. Maternal factors contribute to individual differences in infant behaviour very early in life (Pillai Riddell et al 2007). Culture and family specific dispositions to the challenges of pain are transferred through social learning to children, thereby determining the dynamics and structure of the painful experiences of succeeding generations. The intergenerational transfer of acquired meanings of pain appears to be intuitive, but has a strong basis in social experience (Goubert et al 2011). Pain cannot be experienced without using these meanings; they become an integral feature of the experience.

Life experience provides ample opportunities to learn ways of experiencing and expressing pain through direct and vicarious experience. The inevitable physical trauma of early childhood includes frequent opportunities for minor pain as a result of falls, sprains, cuts, burns and pain inflicted by age peers and adults (Fearon et al 1996; von Baeyer et al 1998). Direct experience vigorously instructs in hazards for painful experience and the consequences of exposure, including strategies for avoiding and minimizing painful distress. The reactions of others to the child at risk or in pain also represent a major source of sociocultural influence as parents and significant others endeavour to shape the child's reactions in accordance with familial and cultural expectations (Chambers et al 2002; McMurtry et al 2010). Children's safety motivates parents to impose strong protective control. Parental appraisals and expectancies are enforced by constructing safe environments, providing physical guidance and intense supervision for infants and younger children, giving plentiful verbal instruction to older children, and progressively reducing scrutiny and supervision as children mature and acquire personal skills. The supervision is prompted by the considerable risks infants and young children confront when unsupervised and the traumatic consequences for the children (and the responsible adults) should injurious accidents occur. Parental preoccupation with danger and safety lead to instruction on personal safety through physical guidance, warnings, verbal instruction, reinforcement for behaviour conforming to parental expectations, and reprimands, criticism and other forms of punishment for failure to conform to strict demands.

Observational learning greatly expands occasions for this type of learning without direct exposure to pain (Craig 1986; Goubert et al 2011). Most human skills are acquired through social modelling experiences (Bandura 1977). The benefits of this form of instruction are easily observed in non-human mammals (Mineka & Zinbarg 2006). In humans, social modelling represents a foundation for intergenerational transmission of cultural knowledge. Observational learning provides opportunities to learn without personal threat about dangerous circumstances and the events leading to them. An observer notes what happens to others when they are not prudent or protected by others, the physical, psychological and social consequences of injury, and how the person in pain behaves (effectively and ineffectively). Also noted is how others react to the person's distress and injuries. What is demonstrated and what is perceived reflects beliefs, expectancies, illness role models and accepted practices for expressing pain and providing for those in pain based on familial, community and cultural circumstances. Children exposed to atypical pain in the family, including excessive, recurrent or persistent pain, become vulnerable to atypical patterns of pain display (Craig 1986; Hermann 2006).

Successful socialization leads to the development of the skills needed for self-management of pain. People may learn realistic ways of interpreting pain, acquire a sense of self-efficacy when confronting pain and develop emotional control appropriate to the situation. They come to understand social norms for various patterns of coping response and learn satisfactory coping skills. Experiences within the family, in contact with peers or even broader socialization through use of media (at present internet communication is important) can also convey misinformation, maladaptive beliefs, misinterpretation of pain symptoms, adverse ways of thinking and coping with pain, emotional distress, fear and hypervigilance. Sullivan et al (2004) have proposed a communal coping model of pain catastrophizing, demonstrating that the intrapersonal trait should be interpreted from an interpersonal perspective. The cognitive pattern (pain magnification, rumination and feelings of helplessness) serves social communication functions in that overt expressions solicit empathic responses and social support. Goubert et al (2011) have similarly proposed a primarily observational learning account of the origins of destructive fear of pain. In this manner, the subjective experience of pain is shaped by the individual's history of social experiences related to pain, with the current social context cueing subjective patterns of response.

HOW PAIN IS COMMUNICATED TO OTHERS

Pain is a far more social phenomenon than is usually acknowledged. It has been argued that pain is wholly a private experience, with one person's pain unknowable to others (Illich 1976). In reality, behavioural reactions are very difficult to inhibit entirely and public manifestations typically provide access to the experience by others. Relatively stereotyped patterns of protective and communicative behaviour are observable in people in pain (Revicki et al 2009). Some reactions indirectly communicate pain because they reflect efforts to protect against pain by disengaging from contact with the noxious event; this withdrawal may be unconscious, such as in the case of

nociceptive flexion reflexes, pulling one's hand away from an object that is red hot, or more deliberate, such as limping, which is a more complex integrated response typically used to control pain. Other actions directly communicate distress (and protect indirectly) by engaging the assistance of others through behaviours such as crying, facial grimaces and pleas for help (Sullivan 2008).

These behavioural reactions reflect underlying neuroregulatory systems that can be characterized as automatic or controlled. Automatic reactions tend to be reflexive, unintentional and unconscious, whereas controlled reactions are voluntary, conscious and goal-oriented (Hadjistavropoulos & Craig 2002). Automatic reactions can be either immediately protective (e.g. defensive reflexes permitting escape from a source of pain) or communicative (e.g. facial grimaces of pain or certain vocalizations). Controlled reactions similarly include both protective actions (e.g. using analgesic medication) and communicative behaviour (e.g. verbal report of pain). Controlled reactions are more likely to reflect socialization experiences. McCrystal et al (2011) found observers had little difficulty distinguishing immediate, reflexive and spontaneous reactions (primarily facial expression and paralinguistic features of speech) from purposeful and controlled expressions (verbal behaviour, instrumental behaviour requiring organized responses). The capacity to distinguish behaviour in this way discloses implicit observer dispositions to organize cues signalling pain in others into these well-defined categories.

Some features of painful expression are biologically inherited reflexes, whereas others are acquired in the course of socialization in familial and cultural contexts. Newborn infants readily communicate painful distress through facial action and cry. It can be argued that these reflexive responses have ancient social origins because of their adaptive value for the infant (Darwin 1871). Facial action becomes increasingly amenable to voluntary control as a child matures and acquires life experience, although the basic structure of the facial expression of pain is consistent throughout the life span (Craig et al 2011). Vocalizations are similar; newborns cry reflexively in response to painful events. The cry subsequently acquires linguistic overtones as the capacity for language emerges. Thus, reflexive cry transforms to become a speech act.

The use of language to convey painful distress to others is slowly acquired in the course of the first years of life (Franck et al 2010; Stanford et al 2005). Language is typically culture specific, modelled within the child's family and community, and slowly refined as an effective communication tool. Developmental processes are important in understanding the expression of pain, with maturation of motor, cognitive, emotional and social capabilities subjected to the influence of life experience, social and otherwise (Craig & Korol 2008). It is noteworthy that automatic expression comprises both inherited reflexes and over-learned skills that no longer require purposeful or conscious decision making (Craig et al 2010). The automatic manifestations appear to be most often observed during moderate to severe acute pain and exacerbations of chronic pain. Chronic pain patients not experiencing paroxysmal pain become dependent on controlled expression, including self-report and convincing depictions of painful distress, when interviewed about their current symptomatic status (Werner & Malerud 2003).

Both verbal and non-verbal behaviours have automatic and voluntary features. While verbal behaviour typically requires social skills and conscious deliberation, non-linguistic features of verbalizations (pitch, amplitude, overtones and other features) are less subject to purposeful control. Self-report of pain is often described as the gold standard for pain assessment, but it cannot be interpreted as a mirror of subjective experience. It invariably includes the person's efforts to influence others (Schiavenato & Craig 2010). As a result, people are quite variable in whether they report symptoms or not (Mechanic 1986; Pennebaker 1982). Non-verbal behaviour tends to be seen by others as less subject to personal control, but a competent adult can effectively feign persuasive non-verbal expression (Hadjistavropoulos et al 1996; Poole & Craig 1992) with skills acquired in the course of childhood (Larochette et al 2006). Thus, people use both verbal and non-verbal expression to achieve personal objectives. Incentives for faked or exaggerated pain may be financial (long-term disability payments, the outcome of litigation), access to potent drugs, avoidance of work or domestic duties, or manipulation of others through use of the sick role. Alternatively, people can suppress pain expression to avoid social disapprobation (appearing weak or complaining), denial of usual roles (e.g. parent, worker, athlete), conformity to social demands and fearing sick role imposition (and its stigma), diagnoses, drugs, needles or other invasive procedures.

Acquisition of linguistic and social skills in pain expression is imperative if the individual is to be successful in persuading others to provide the best pain relief possible. The importance of this skill is perhaps most conspicuous among people who do not have the social and/or communication competence observed in other adults (Hadjistavropoulos et al 2010). This large group includes those who are critically ill, infants and young children, and people with cognitive and motor impairments. They frequently lack the skills to effectively access health care, and are handicapped further by current emphasis on self-report as the gold standard of pain assessment (Schiavenato & Craig 2010). Consequently, substantial evidence indicates that seniors with dementia are significantly under-treated for their pain compared to other seniors (Tsai & Chang 2004; van Herk et al 2007; Zwakhalen et al 2006), even though they do not differ in the prevalence of chronic health conditions that lead to pain (Hadjistavropoulos et al 2007; Herr et al 2006; Smith 2005). Judgements of pain in children with autism similarly share this misinformed assumption. Standard reference manuals and scholarly descriptions describe them as relatively insensitive to pain. In contrast, systematic evidence indicates they react more vigorously to painful situations than typical children, although this is commonly overlooked due to the strong emphasis on self-report (Nader et al 2004). Achieving access to healthcare systems can be a greater challenge than is commonly acknowledged.

Pain expression is also contingent on the audience. This sensitivity perhaps reflects the evolutionary benefit of different responses in the presence of predators, enemies and friends. Vulnerability can be dangerous in the presence of predators and enemies, leading to at least the pretence of strength and resilience when in pain. The evidence suggests that stoical presentation is more common in the presence of others, particularly strangers, with people more expressive when alone (Badali 2008). In the clinic, it is clear that patients must present in a convincing manner if a physician is to provide access to care. These resources can be considerable, ranging from provision of medical care, including access to analgesics, psychotropics or surgery, as well as the diagnoses necessary to justify time off work or domestic duties, disability income, workers' compensation, insurance settlements, etc. The challenge is perhaps greatest for patients with chronic pain when physical pathology does not legitimize their needs (Werner & Malerud 2003).

Socialization in pain expression will vary with the characteristics of individuals and their social contexts. In the former category, gender differences in pain expression are not accounted for wholly by differences in the painful conditions experienced by men and women or genetic factors (Fillingim 2010; Mogil 1999). Differences in familial and ethnic expectations, interpersonal dynamics and traditions contribute to different socialization practices. Amongst the most salient ethnocultural variations are standards for when one should complain of pain. In general, people tend to inhibit complaining, although the degree varies across cultures. Thus, role models of stoical forbearance seem to prevail, with the rules as to when one should complain varying across persons and social contexts.

HOW OTHERS RECOGNIZE, INTERPRET AND RESPOND TO THE PERSON'S PAIN

A major social determinant of pain is access to provision of care. Providing care requires recognition of pain, skills in assessment and treatment, and the physical resources necessary to accomplish required tasks. Successful recognition that a person is suffering from pain often appears to be difficult to accomplish. In many cases, all the requisite cues are present: the person reacts vigorously verbally and non-verbally, attempts are made to escape the noxious event, the source can be identified and tissue damage is evident. Often one or more of these sources of information are absent and people may be suppressing, exaggerating or faking pain (Poole & Craig 1992). The absence of tissue pathology is perceived as especially suspicious and is a common barrier for receiving proper treatment in chronic and non-malignant pain patients.

The neuroregulatory systems responsible for automatic and controlled pain expression also play a role in observer reactions (Craig et al 2010). Witnessing others displaying pain provokes major peripheral and central nervous system activity, as demonstrated by studies of autonomic arousal (Craig & Prkachin 1978) and brain imaging (Jackson et al 2006; Ochsner et al 2008; Simon et al 2006). People are remarkably responsive to the emotional experiences of others (Norris et al 2004). The biological response to observing someone in pain has some of the same features as a personal experience of pain, but they are not identical, as indicated by autonomic (Craig 1968) and brain measures (Jackson et al 2006; Ochsner et al 2008; Simon et al 2006). The differentiation of personal and vicarious experiences is consistent with engagement of higher-level processes when observers seek to understand another person's distress. The observer is not beset by painful distress to the same extreme. There is an opportunity to learn about what constitutes potentially painful circumstances, how other people respond (thoughts, feelings and behaviour) to the pain and how other observers react to a person's distress, behaviour and circumstances. Observer reactions are likely to depend on the relationship between the person in pain and the observer. Kin, friends, strangers, enemies, combatants and professionals will be motivated differently. Kin and friend motivation would reflect inherent biological dispositions to provide care, enemies to exacerbate or exploit distress and healthcare practitioners may or may not be motivated to intervene, depending on professional duties and financial incentives.

A model of empathic reactions to others in pain (Goubert et al 2005) distinguishes 'bottom-up' input to the observer's reaction (the expressive reaction of the person in pain as well as salient situational events, including the source of pain and evidence of tissue damage) from 'top-down' processing of this information, whereby the observer appraises and comes to understand the person's predicament. The observer brings to the situation not only ancient, intuitive dispositions to react emotionally, but human capacities to arrive at a considered judgement as to what is happening. This may reflect rational and probabilistic understanding, perhaps a consequence of professional education and training, but understanding is also vulnerable to vagaries of personal experience, idiosyncratic belief and attitudinal systems, and subculture myths and personal biases. In consequence, the observer may overreact (Goubert et al 2009) or under-react, as is evident in widespread tendencies to underestimate pain in others (Chambers et al 1999; Kappesser et al 2006; Prkachin et al 2007). Both response patterns have immediate and long-term consequences for the person in pain.

Observer decisions lead to differences in the delivery of care. These will reflect personal life experience and practitioner training among other factors. Efforts to provide relief for people in pain are documented from prehistoric times and display considerable diversity. Ancient forms of treatment include trepanation, acupuncture, cupping, moxibustion, bloodletting, purging, application of topical and oral herbs, prayer and religious practices. Treatment fads persist in modern culture, with pharmacological approaches to pain control currently the most fashionable treatment method. The scope of potential interventions has broadened to include psychological and environmental interventions.

Social policy and health service delivery

The capabilities of people providing care and the likelihood of care for pain being made available are largely determined by broader social policies concerning health care and the social and cultural environments (Rashiq et al 2008). Systems factors representing standards of care and public policy are important determinants of care for people in pain. Healthcare politics and ideologies (e.g. socialized medicine vs business models), socioeconomic resources (national and regional economic disparities; Bonham 2001) and dominant beliefs concerning various forms of treatment (e.g. use of opioids, requirements for empirically supported interventions) are powerful determinants of access to care. These determinants are informed to the extent that research has been available to establish innovative and superior practices. Given the large numbers of people for whom pain research and pain management have failed to relieve pain (Resnik et al 2001), it is increasingly evident that current healthcare policies are ineffective for many patients. This problem can be described as widespread discrimination against these patients. Patients, their families and significant others often become angry and frustrated about the inadequacies of public policies, compensation and insurance programmes, and healthcare providers regarding unresolved chronic pain (Walker et al 2007).

CONCLUSION

Pain is suffered by the individual, but it always occurs in a complex social context driven by family, vocational, community, political and cultural factors. These factors determine whether or not pain is suffered, how it is suffered and expressed to others, and whether or not care will be provided. Dissatisfaction with care has led to pressures for change in the current system of delivery of health services. The social determinants of pain must receive attention in examining the nature and quality of services for people in pain to ensure optimal care for everyone. Social causes of pain are under the control of more people in the community than those responsible for medical interventions. There are many possibilities for improvement, including preventive interventions prior to pain-instigating situations, changing how people self-regulate painful experiences and enhancing their capacity to accurately communicate personal distress, as well as improving the judgemental and decision-making capacities of those available to deliver care and improving public and institutional policies, standards and practices for the delivery of care.

REFERENCES

American Academy of Pediatrics/ Canadian Pediatric Society, 2006. Prevention and management of pain in the neonate. Pediatrics. 118, 2231–2241.

Antoni, M.H., Lutgendorf, S.K., Cole, S.W., et al., 2006. The influence of bio-behavioural factors on tumour biology: pathways and mechanisms. Nat. Rev. Cancer. 6, 240–248.

Badali, M.A., 2008. Experimenter Audience Effects on Young Adults' Facial Expressions during Pain. Unpublished doctoral dissertation, University of British Columbia, Columbia, Vancouver, BC.

Bandura, A., 1977. Social Learning Theory. General Learning Press, New York.

Bates, A.M.S., 1987. Ethnicity and pain: a biocultural model. Soc. Sci. Med. 24, 47–50.

Blyth, F.M., Macfarlane, G.J., Nicholas, M.K., 2007. The contribution of psychosocial factors to the development of chronic pain: the key to better outcomes for patients? Pain. 129, 8–11.

Bonham, V.L., 2001. Race, ethnicity, and pain treatment: striving to understand the causes and solutions to the disparities in pain treatment. J. Law Med. Ethics. 29, 52–68.

Chambers, C.T., Reid, G.J., Craig, K.D., et al., 1999. Agreement between child and parent reports of pain. Clin. J. Pain. 14, 336–342.

Chambers, C.T., Craig, K.D., Bennett, S.M., 2002. The impact of maternal behavior on children's pain experiences: an experimental analysis. J. Pediatr. Psychol. 27, 293–301.

Chorney, J.M., McGrath, P., Finley, G.A., 2010. Pain as the neglected adverse event. Can. Med. Assoc. J. 182, 732.

Cope, D.K., 2010. Intellectual milestones in our understanding and treatment of pain. In: Fishman, S.M., Ballantyne, J.C., Rathnell, J.P. (Eds.), Bonica's Management of Pain. Wolters Kluwer/Lippincott Williams & Wilkins, Philadelphia, PA, pp. 1–12.

Craig, K.D., 1968. Physiological arousal as a function of imagined, vicarious and direct stress experiences. J. Abnorm. Psychol. 73, 513–520.

Craig, K.D., 1986. Social modeling influences: pain in context. In: Sternbach, R.A. (Ed.), The Psychology of Pain. second ed. Raven Press, New York, pp. 67–96.

Craig, K.D., 2009. The social communication model of pain. Canadian Psychology/Psychologie Canadienne. 50 (1), 22–32.

Craig, K.D., Korol, C.T., 2008. Developmental issues in understanding, assessing, and managing pediatric pain. In: Walco, G., Goldschnieder, K. (Eds.), Pediatric Pain Management in Primary Care: A Practical Guide. Humana Press Inc, Totowa NJ, pp. 9–20.

Craig, K.D., Pillai, R., 2003. Social influences, ethnicity, and culture. In: Finley, G.A., McGrath, P.J. (Eds.), The Context of Pediatric Pain: Biology, Family, Society, and Culture. IASP Press, Seattle WA, pp. 159–182.

Craig, K.D., Prkachin, K.M., 1978. Social modeling influences on sensory decision theory and psychophysiological indexes of pain. J. Pers. Soc. Psychol. 36 (8), 805–815.

Craig, K.D., Whitfield, M.F., Grunau, R.V.E., et al., 1993. Pain in the pre-term neonate: behavioural and physiological indices. Pain. 52, 287–299.

Craig, K.D., Versloot, J., Goubert, L., et al., 2010. Perceiving others in pain: automatic and controlled mechanisms. J. Pain. 11, 101–108.

Craig, K.D., Prkachin, K.M., Grunau, R.V.E., 2011. The facial expression of pain. In: Turk, D., Melzack, R. (Eds.), Handbook of Pain Assessment. third ed. Guilford, New York, pp. 117–133.

Darwin, C., 1871. The Descent of Man. Appleton and Company, New York.

de Waal, F., 2009. The Age of Empathy. Harmony Books, New York.

Dworkin, S.F., Von Korff, M., LeResche, L., 1992. Epidemiologic studies of chronic pain: a dynamic-ecologic perspective. Ann. Behav. Med. 14, 3–11.

Engel, G.L., 1977. The need for a new medical model: a challenge for biomedicine. Science. 196 (4286), 129–136.

Fearon, I., McGrath, P.J., Achat, H., 1996. 'Booboos': the study of everyday pain among young children. Pain. 68, 55–62.

Fillingim, R.B., 2010. Individual differences in pain: the roles of gender, ethnicity and genetics. In: Fishman, S.M., Ballantyne, J.C., Rathnell, J.P. (Eds.), Bonica's Management of Pain. Wolters Kluwer/ Lippincott Williams & Wilkins, Philadelphia PA, pp. 86–97.

Franck, L., Noble, G., Liossi, C., 2010. From tears to words: the development of language to express pain in young children with everyday minor illnesses and injuries. Child Care Health Dev. 36, 524–533.

Gatchel, R.J., Peng, Y.B., Peters, M.L., et al., 2007. The biopsychosocial approach to chronic pain: scientific advances and future directions. Psychol. Bull. 133 (4), 581–624.

Goubert, L., Craig, K.D., Vervoort, T., et al., 2005. Facing others in pain: the effects of empathy. Pain. 118, 286–288.

Goubert, L., Vervoort, T., Cano, A.M., et al., 2009. Catastrophizing about their children's pain is related to higher parent-child congruency in pain ratings: an experimental investigation. Eur. J. Pain. 13, 196–201.

Goubert, L., Vlaeyen, J.W.S., Crombez, G., et al., 2011. Learning about pain from others: an observational learning account. J. Pain. 12, 167–174.

Grunau, R.V.E., Craig, K.D., 1987. Pain expression in neonates: facial action and cry. Pain. 28, 395–410.

Grunau, R.E., Tu, M.T., 2007. Long-term consequences of pain in human neonates. In: Anand, K.J.S., Stevens, B.J., McGrath, P.J. (Eds.), Pain in Neonates. third ed. Elsevier Science, Amsterdam, pp. 45–55.

Hadjistavropoulos, T., Craig, K.D., 2002. A theoretical framework for understanding self-report and observational measures of pain: a communications model. Behav. Res. Ther. 40, 551–570.

Hadjistavropoulos, H.D., Craig, K.D., Hadjistavropoulos, T., et al., 1996. Subjective judgments of deception in pain expression: Accuracy and errors. Pain. 65, 251–258.

Hadjistavropoulos, T., LaChapelle, D.L., MacLeod, et al., 2000. Measuring movement exacerbated pain in cognitively impaired frail elders. Clin. J. Pain. 16, 54–63.

Hadjistavropoulos, T., Herr, K., Turk, D.C., et al., 2007. An interdisciplinary expert consensus statement on assessment of pain in older persons. Clin. J. Pain. 23 (Suppl. 1), 1–43.

Hadjistavropoulos, T., Breau, L., Craig, K.D., 2010. Pain assessment in adults and children with limited ability to communicate. In: Turk, D.C., Melzack, R. (Eds.), Handbook of pain assessment, third ed. Guilford Press, New York, pp. 260–282.

Hermann, C., 2006. Modeling, social learning in pain. In: Schmidt, R.F., Willis, W.D. (Eds.), The Encyclopedia of Pain. Springer Publishing, Berlin, pp. 1168–1170.

Herr, K., Bjoro, K., Decker, S., 2006. Tools for assessment of pain in nonverbal older adults with dementia: a state of the science review. J. Pain Symptom. Manage. 31, 170–192.

Illich, I., 1976. Medical Nemesis: The Expropriation of Health. Random House, New York.

Jackson, P.L., Rainville, P., Decety, J., 2006. To what extent do we share the pain of others? Insight from the neural bases of pain empathy. Pain. 125, 5–9.

Kappesser, J., Williams, A.C., Prkachin, K.M., 2006. Testing two accounts of pain underestimation. Pain. 124, 109–116.

Keefe, F.J., Dixon, K.E., Pryor, R.W., 2005. Psychological contributions to the understanding and treatment of pain. In: Merskey, H., Loeser, J.D., Dubner, R. (Eds.), The paths of pain 1975–2005. IASP Press, Seattle, pp. 403–420.

Kunz, M., Scharmann, S., Hemmeter, U., et al., 2007. The facial expression of pain in patients with dementia. Pain. 133, 221–228.

Larochette, A.C., Chambers, C.T., Craig, K.D., 2006. Genuine, suppressed and faked facial expressions of pain in children. Pain. 126, 64–71.

LeResche, L., Saunders, K., Von Korff, M., et al., 1997. Use of exogenous hormones and risk of temporomandibular disorder pain. Pain. 69, 153–160.

McCracken, L.M., Matthews, A.K., Tang, T.S., et al., 2001. A comparison of blacks and whites seeking treatment for chronic pain. Clin. J. Pain. 17, 249–255.

McCrystal, K.N., Craig, K.D., Versloot, J., et al., 2011. Perceiving others in pain: Validation of a dual processing model. Pain. 152, 1083–1089.

McMurtry, C.M., Chambers, C.T., McGrath, P.J., et al., 2010. When 'don't worry' communicates fear: children's perceptions of parental reassurance and distraction during a painful medical procedure. Pain. 150, 52–58.

Mechanic, D., 1986. The concept of illness behavior: culture, situation and personal predisposition. Psychol. Med. 16, 1–7.

Mineka, S., Zinbarg, R., 2006. A contemporary learning theory perspective on the etiology of anxiety disorders: it's not what you thought it was. Am. Psychol. 61, 10–26.

Mogil, J.S., 1999. The genetic mediation of individual differences in sensitivity to pain and its inhibition. Proc. Natl. Acad. Sci. U. S. A. 96, 7744–7751.

Morris, D.G., 2010. Sociocultural dimensions of pain management. In: Fishman, S.M., Ballantyne, J.C., Rathnell, J.P. (Eds.), Bonica's Management of Pain. Wolters Kluwer/ Lippincott Williams & Wilkins, Philadelphia PA, pp. 133–144.

Nader, R., Oberlander, T.F., Chambers, C.T., et al., 2004. The expression of pain in children with autism. Clin. J. Pain. 20, 88–97.

Nayak, S., Shiflett, S.C., Eshun, S., et al., 2000. Culture and gender effects in pain beliefs and the prediction of pain tolerance. Cross-Cultural Research. 34, 135–151.

Norris, C.J., Chen, E., Zhu, D.C., et al., 2004. The interaction of social and emotional processes in the brain. J. Cogn. Neurosci. 16, 1818–1829.

Ochsner, K.N., Zaki, J., Hanelin, J., et al., 2008. Your pain or mine? Common and distinct neural systems supporting the perception of pain in self and other. Social Cognitive and Affective Neuroscience. 3, 144–160.

Pennebaker, J.W., 1982. The psychology of physical symptoms. Springer-Verlag, New York.

Pike, I., Macpherson, A., Warda, L., et al., 2010. Measuring injury matters: Injury indicators for children and youth in Canada. University of British Columbia, Vancouver, BC.

Pillai Riddell, R., Stevens, B., Cohen, L., et al., 2007. Predicting maternal and behavioural measures of infant pain: the relative contribution of maternal factors. Pain. 133, 138–149.

Poole, G.D., Craig, K.D., 1992. Judgments of genuine, suppressed and faked facial expressions of pain. J. Pers. Soc. Psychol. 63, 797–805.

Prkachin, K.M., Solomon, P.A., Ross, A.J., 2007. The underestimation of pain among health-care providers. Canadian Journal of Nursing Research. 39, 88–106.

Rashiq, S., Schopflocher, D., Taenzer, P. et al., (Eds.), 2008. Chronic pain: A health policy perspective. Wiley-VCH, Weinheim.

Resnik, D.B., Rehm, M., Minard, R.B., 2001. The under-treatment of pain: scientific, clinical, cultural, and philosophical factors. Med. Health Care Philos. 4, 277–288.

Revicki, D.A., Chen, W.H., Harnam, N., et al., 2009. Development and psychometric analysis of the PROMIS pain behavior item bank. Pain. 146, 158–169.

Schiavenato, M., Craig, K.D., 2010. Pain assessment as a social transaction: beyond the 'Gold Standard'. Clin. J. Pain. 26, 667–676.

Simon, D., Craig, K.D., Miltner, W.H.R., et al., 2006. Brain responses to dynamic facial expressions of pain. Pain. 126, 309–318.

Skevington, S.M., Mason, V.L., 2004. Social influences on individual differences in responding to pain. In: Hadjistavropoulos, T., Craig, K.D. (Eds.), Pain: Psychological perspectives. Lawrence Erlbaum Associates, Mahwah, NJ.

Smith, M., 2005. Pain assessment in nonverbal older adults with advanced dementia. Perspect. Psychiatr. Care. 41, 99–113.

Stanford, E.A., Chambers, C.T., Craig, K.D., 2005. A normative analysis of the development of pain-related vocabulary in children. Pain. 114, 278–284.

Sullivan, M.J.L., 2008. Toward a biopsychomotor conceptualization of pain: implications for research and intervention. Clin. J. Pain. 24, 281–290.

Sullivan, M.J.L., Adams, H., Sullivan, M.E., 2004. Communicative dimensions of pain catastrophizing: social cueing effects on pain behaviour and coping. Pain. 107, 220–226.

Tsai, P., Chang, J.Y., 2004. Assessment of pain in elders with dementia. Medsurg Nurs. 13, 364–370.

Turk, D.C., Okifuji, A., 2002. Psychological factors in chronic pain: Evolution and revolution. J. Consult. Clin. Psychol. 70 (3), 678–690.

Van Damme, S., Legrain, V., Vogt, J., et al., 2010. Keeping pain in mind: a motivational account of attention to pain. Neuroscience and Biobehavioral Research. 34, 204–213.

van Herk, R., van Dijk, M., Baar, F.P.M., et al., 2007. Observation scales for pain assessment in older adults with cognitive impairments or communication difficulties. Nurs. Res. 56, 34–43.

Versloot, J., Craig, K.D., 2009. The communication of pain in paediatric dentistry. Eur. Arch. Paediatr. Dent. 10, 61–66.

Vlaeyen, J.W.S., Linton, S.J., 2000. Fear-avoidance and its consequences in chronic musculoskeletal pain: a state of the art. Pain. 85, 317–332.

von Baeyer, C.L., Baskerville, S., McGrath, P.J., 1998. Everyday pain in 3–5 year old children in day care. Pain Res. Manag. 3, 111–116.

von Korff, M., LeResche, L., 2005. Epidemiology of pain. In: Merskey, H., Loeser, J.D., Dubner, R. (Eds.), The paths of pain 1975–2005. IASP Press, Seattle, pp. 339–352.

Walker, L.S., Smith, C.A., Garber, J., et al., 2007. Appraisal and coping with daily stressors by pediatric pain patients and well children. J. Pediatr. Psychol. 32, 206–216.

Werner, A., Malerud, K., 2003. It is hard work behaving as a credible patient: encounters between women with chronic pain and their doctors. Soc. Sci. Med. 57, 1409–1419.

Williams, C.M., Maher, C.G., Hancock, M.J., et al., 2010. Low back pain and best practice care. Arch. Intern. Med. 170, 271–277.

Zborowski, M., 1969. People in pain. Jossey-Bass, San Francisco.

Zwakhalen, S.M., Hamers, J.P., Abu-Saad, H., et al., 2006. Pain in elderly people with severe dementia: a systematic review of behavioural pain assessment tools. BMC Geriatr. 6, 3.

Section | 1 |

Overview: what is pain?

Chapter | 4 |

The psychology of pain: models and targets for comprehensive assessment

Gordon J.G. Asmundson, Lydia Gomez-Perez, Ashley A. Richter and R. Nicholas Carleton

LEARNING OBJECTIVES

On completing this chapter readers will have an understanding of the following:

1. The distinction between pain and chronic pain.
2. Gate control theory.
3. Biopsychosocial models of pain.
4. Cognitive constructs associated with beliefs, mood, anxiety and fear.
5. Behavioural constructs related to avoidance, activity limitation, coping behaviour, pain and suicide.
6. Environmental influences of family, culture and ethnicity, socioeconomic factors and work.

OVERVIEW

In this chapter we review the current state of knowledge regarding the psychology of pain as it can be applied to assessment planning and case conceptualization. We provide definitions of pain and chronic pain, summarize important features of a historical model that provided the foundation for contemporary biopsychosocial approaches to understanding pain, selectively highlight important cognitive constructs and pain behaviours as well as environmental influences, and conclude with a summary of important considerations in assessment planning and case conceptualization. This approach is predicated on the position that assessment and case conceptualization should be a conceptually driven process (Asmundson & Hadjistavropoulos 2006; Taylor & Asmundson 2004); as such, empirically supported theoretical constructs and applications form the foundation upon which assessment, case conceptualization and subsequent treatment plans are built. Throughout we refer to current empirical findings and, as appropriate, incorporate examples to illustrate salient points.

PAIN AND CHRONIC PAIN DEFINED

The traditional biomedical model of pain dates back to Descartes (1596–1650), who suggested that pain is a sensory experience resulting from stimulation of specific noxious receptors, usually from physical damage due to injury or disease. Consistent with Cartesian dualism (i.e. the idea that mind and body are non-overlapping entities), the model is both reductionistic (i.e. all disease is directly linked to specific physical pathology) and exclusionary (i.e. social, psychological, behavioural mechanisms of illness are not of primary importance). Applications of the traditional biomedical model to diagnosis, assessment and treatment are generally straightforward. Physical pathology would be confirmed by data from objective tests of physical damage, and interventions would then be directed toward rectifying the damage and associated

© 2014 Elsevier Ltd.

limitations in physical functioning. The experience of pain would not be viewed as significant but, rather, as a secondary reaction to or symptom of physical damage that would diminish with healing.

Pain is now understood to involve more than a pure sensory experience arising from physical injury or other pathology. Over the past half century a number of pain models that incorporate biological as well as psychological (e.g. perception, cognition, affect), behavioural (e.g. avoidance) and social (e.g. cultural) factors have been proposed. These models, described in more detail below, have dramatically improved the understanding of pain and the ability to assess and effectively intervene in cases where it is intense, unremitting or both intense and unremitting.

Pain is currently defined as a complex perceptual phenomenon that involves a number of dimensions, including, but not limited to, intensity, quality, time course and personal meaning (Merskey & Bogduk 1994). It is adaptive in the short term, facilitating the ability to identify, respond to and resolve physical pathology or injury. Unfortunately, a significant number of people experience pain for periods that substantially exceed expected times for physical healing (e.g. Waddell 1987). When pain persists for 3 months or longer, it is considered chronic (e.g. International Association for the Study of Pain (IASP) 1986) and, while not necessarily maladaptive (Asmundson et al 1998; Turk & Rudy 1987), often leads to physical decline, limited functional ability and emotional distress. These pain experiences are also associated with an increased probability of experiencing comorbid psychopathology (McWilliams et al 2003; for review, see Asmundson & Katz 2009), inappropriate use of medical services, reduced work performance or absenteeism, and high cost insurance claims (Spengler et al 1986; Stewart et al 2003). Translated into a dollar value, common chronic pain conditions cost the USA and Canada, respectively, approximately US$60 billion and CAN$6 billion dollars annually.

MODELS PERTINENT TO UNDERSTANDING PAIN

There are several contemporary pain models that are important in the context of assessment and case conceptualization. These models are similar in that they all recognize the interplay between biological, psychological and sociocultural factors in the pain experience. Below we highlight one model of considerable historical significance as well as primary features of various contemporary biopsychosocial models. Detailed descriptions of the social influences on pain are provided by Craig in this volume (Chapter 3).

Gate control theory

Melzack and colleagues' seminal papers on the gate control theory of pain (Melzack & Casey 1968; Melzack & Wall 1965) are frequently cited as the first to integrate biological and psychological mechanisms of pain within the context of a single model. Melzack & Wall (1965) suggested that the passage of ascending nociceptive (pain) information from the body to the brain was controlled by a hypothetical gating mechanism within the dorsal horn of the spinal cord. The gating mechanism works as follows. Excitation along the large-diameter, myelinated fibres of the spinal cord closes the gate, whereas excitation along the small-diameter, unmyelinated fibres opens the gate. Transmissions about current cognition and mood descending from the brain to the gating mechanism also influence whether the gate is closed or opened. In short, the summation of information travelling along the different types of ascending fibres from the body with that travelling on descending fibres from the brain determines whether the gate is open or closed and, thereby, influences the perception of pain. Melzack & Casey (1968) further proposed that three different neural networks (i.e. sensory–discriminative, motivational–affective and cognitive–evaluative) influence the modulation of sensory input. The addition of these networks to the model allowed for 'perceptual information regarding the location, magnitude, and spatiotemporal properties of the noxious stimulus, motivational tendency toward escape or attack, and cognitive information based on analysis of multimodal information, past experience, and probability of outcome of different response strategies' (pp 427–428).

Time and empirical effort have led to advances in understanding the anatomy and structure of the gating mechanism proposed by Melzack and Wall (Price 2000; Wall 1996), as well as to elaborations of the neural network model (Melzack 1999; Melzack & Katz 2004; please refer to Chapter 6). Notwithstanding, the gate control theory challenged the primary assumptions of the traditional biomedical models. Rather than being exclusively conceptualized as sensation arising from physical damage, the experience of pain came to be viewed as a combination of both pathophysiology and psychological factors. As such, pain as well as pain-related cognitions and mood were no longer viewed as secondary reactions to physical damage. Instead, the pathophysiology of pain was conceptualized as having a reciprocal influence on cognitions and mood, and vice versa. It is this foundation from which contemporary biopsychosocial models emerged.

Biopsychosocial models

The biopsychosocial approach holds that the experience of pain is determined by the interaction between biological, psychological (e.g. cognition, behaviour, mood) and social (e.g. cultural) factors. A number of specific biopsychosocial models have been proposed over the past 35 years, including several behaviourally based models (Fordyce 1976; Fordyce et al 1982), as well as the more comprehensive cognitive–behavioural Glasgow (Waddell 1987; Waddell et al

1984) and biobehavioural (Turk 2002; Turk & Flor 1999; Turk et al 1983) models. Detailed descriptions of these models of pain are provided elsewhere (e.g. Asmundson et al 2004a; Asmundson & Wright 2004).

Despite differences with respect to specificity regarding behavioural and cognitive influences on pain, all of the biopsychosocial models share a common focus – the focus is not on *disease* per se but on *illness*, where illness is viewed as a type of behaviour (Parsons 1951). The concept of illness behaviour (Mechanic 1962) implies that individuals may differ in perception of and response to bodily sensations and changes (e.g. pain, nausea, heart palpitations), and that these differences can be understood in the context of psychological and social processes. For example, whereas one person may perceive pain as indicative of a potentially serious malady and solicit reassurances or assistance from others in even the most rudimentary of daily activities, another person may perceive similar pain as discomforting but harmless and work through the discomfort. Illness behaviour is considered a dynamic process, with the role of biological, psychological and social factors changing in relative importance as the condition evolves. While a condition may be initiated by biological factors, such as physical injury or pathology, the psychological and social factors may come to play a primary role in maintenance and exacerbation; indeed, the focus often shifts from pain to significant concern and anxiety about personal health and well-being (see, for example, Hadjistavropoulos et al 2001).

This focus is also shared in the more recent fear–avoidance models of chronic pain (Asmundson et al 1999, 2004a; Vlaeyen & Linton 2000), wherein pain-related fear and anxiety are suggested to play primary roles in the development and maintenance of disabling chronic pain. The fear–avoidance models are predicated on long-standing observations that fear and anxiety appear to be critical elements in the pain experience. Indeed, the association between fear and pain dates back to at least as early as Aristotle, who, over 2000 years ago, stated 'Let fear, then, be a kind of pain or disturbance resulting the imagination of impending danger, either destructive or painful', and is an important consideration in each of the biopsychosocial models described above. Since fear–avoidance models have stimulated some of the most recent developments with respect to assessment and case conceptualization for individuals who have pain lasting beyond the time typical for physical healing, we provide a more detailed description here.

Contemporary fear-avoidance models of chronic pain are based primarily on the writings of several scholars (Asmundson et al 1999; McCracken et al 1992; Vlaeyen et al 1995; Waddell et al 1993), each of whom provided slightly different conceptualizations of the role of fear, anxiety, and avoidance in perpetuating pain. Subtle differences aside, the primary postulates of each of these scholars are captured in the model proposed by Vlaeyen & Linton

(2000), and illustrated in Figure 4.1. This model can be summarized as follows. On perceiving pain, people make an appraisal of the meaning or purpose of the pain (pain experience). Most people appraise the pain to be unpleasant and discomforting but not indicative of serious threat to their well-being (no fear). These people then engage in appropriate behavioural restriction and graduated increases in activity (confrontation) until they have healed (recovery). However, some people appraise the pain as being indicative of a serious threat to their well-being (pain catastrophizing) and, influenced by predispositional and current psychological factors, spiral into a self-perpetuating cycle characterized by fear (i.e. fear of pain, fear of (re) injury), activity limitations, disability and pain. It is this latter group of people who experience pain that lasts beyond the time expected for normal healing.

This model has served as a useful platform upon which considerable amounts of empirical research and related practical applications have been based (for review of findings current to the beginning of this millennium, see Vlaeyen & Linton 2000; for review of more recent findings, see Leeuw et al 2007; for review of empirically supported treatment options, see Bailey et al 2010). In addition to advances in empirical findings and practical applications to this field of inquiry, there has been continuing refinement of the contemporary fear-avoidance model (e.g. Asmundson et al 2004a; Norton & Asmundson 2003).

Summary

The models described above provide comprehensive conceptualizations of pain and chronic pain, with varying degrees of emphasis on cognitive, behavioural and environmental constructs. It is these constructs that form the basis of conceptually driven assessment and treatment planning. Below we provide an overview of some of the most important cognitive, behavioural and environmental constructs and how these are assessed.

COGNITIVE CONSTRUCTS

Beliefs

Pain beliefs are a broad category of ideations, often catastrophic in nature, held by all people, not just those with chronic pain (van Damme et al 2002; Sullivan et al 2001). An individual forms pain beliefs, which are relatively stable across time, based on past experiences and cultural norms (Turner et al 2004; Werner et al 2005). There have been several tools designed to measure pain beliefs (e.g. Edwards et al 1992; Waddell et al 1993; Wallston et al 1978; Williams & Thorn 1989), any of which can be used to provide a reliable and valid assessment of the nature of a person's beliefs about pain.

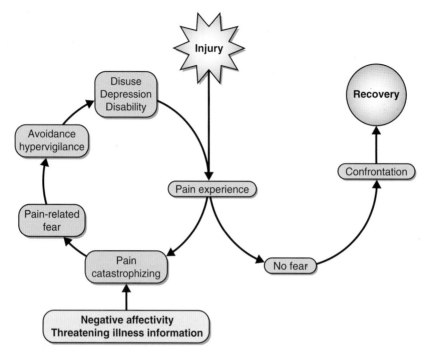

Fig. 4.1 Fear-avoidance model.

Reprinted from Vlaeyan, J.W.S., and Linton, S.J., Fear avoidance and its consequences in chronic musculoskeletal pain: a state of the art. PAIN® 2000, April 85(3); 317-332. This figure has been reproduced with permission of the International Association for the study of Pain® (IASP). The figure may not be reproduced for any other purpose without permision.

Pain beliefs are commonly divided into two subcategories, *organic* and *psychological* (Edwards et al 1992). Organic pain beliefs centre on the notion that pain indicates immediate or imminent physical harm (e.g. 'Pain is the result of damage to the tissues of my body'). In contrast, psychological pain beliefs centre on the notion that pain is mediated by internal and external factors (e.g. 'Thinking about pain makes it worse'). Pain beliefs have been associated uniquely and independently with disability and depression (Turner et al 2000).

There is more than two decades of evidence suggesting a relationship between organic pain beliefs and physical disability for patients with chronic pain (Jensen et al 1991; Sloan et al 2007), but the relationship with pain intensity has been minimal (Edwards et al 1992). In short, persons who have disabling chronic pain tend to strongly endorse organic pain beliefs and are less likely than people without chronic pain to endorse psychological pain beliefs (Edwards et al 1992; Walsh & Radcliffe 2002). Because pain beliefs are learned (Turner et al 2004; van Damme et al 2002; Werner et al 2005), they are also modifiable. Increasing a person's belief that pain involves a significant psychological component tends to be associated with decreases in disability and, often, reports of reduced pain intensity (Bailey et al 2010; de Jong et al 2005; Jensen et al 2001; Walsh & Radcliffe 2002).

Mood

Depression symptoms have been associated with increased pain behaviour (e.g. guarding, bracing, rubbing, grimacing, sighing), reduced individual, social and occupation activity, as well as increased use of medical services (Arnow et al 2009; Asmundson et al 2008; Keefe et al 1986; Ratcliffe et al 2008; Smith et al 1998; Worz 2003). In chronic pain samples, prevalence rates of clinically significant depression vary based on the criteria used for assessment (Geisser et al 1997; Pincus & Williams 1999), but often exceed 28% (Morley et al 2002; Polatin et al 1993; Poole et al 2009; Worz 2003); in contrast, lifetime and 12-month community prevalence rates for depression are approximately 17% and 7%, respectively (Kessler et al 2005a,b). Persons with one pain site are nearly twice as likely to be depressed than persons with no pain, whereas persons with more than one pain site are nearly four times as likely to be depressed (Gureje et al 2008). In addition, the longer a person is in pain, or the more intense the pain, the more likely the person is to experience depressive symptoms (Krause et al 1994; Odegard et al 2007). Depressive symptoms do not necessarily impede treatment outcomes, however, and treating depression itself may provide reductions in disabling pain symptoms (Glombiewski et al 2010; Teh et al 2009).

Assessment of depression symptoms in persons with chronic pain should be ongoing, as there is evidence that pain is associated with fluctuations in mood over time (Krause et al 1994; Odegard et al 2007). In addition to structured clinical interviews (e.g. First et al 1996), there is a variety of standardized self-report tools that can measure ongoing depression symptoms (e.g. Beck et al 1988; Radloff 1977). Given the probability of low mood resulting from ongoing pain, the high rates of comorbidity with depression, and the associated personal and economic costs, ongoing depression symptom assessment should occur for all patients with disabling chronic pain.

Anxiety and fear

As with depression, persons with one pain site are nearly twice as likely to have clinically significant levels of anxiety compared to persons with no pain, whereas persons with more than one pain site are more than three times as likely to be anxious (Gureje et al 2008). Findings from community-dwelling adults in 17 countries ($n = 85,088$) indicate that those with back or neck pain are two to three times more likely to have current (i.e. past 12 months) panic disorder, agoraphobia or social anxiety disorder, and almost three times more likely to have generalized anxiety disorder (GAD) or post-traumatic stress disorder (PTSD) (Demyttenaere et al 2007). Data on lifetime prevalence show similar patterns. For example, community-dwelling women with fibromyalgia are four to five times more likely to have had a lifetime diagnosis of obsessive–compulsive disorder, PTSD or GAD than those without (Raphael et al 2006). In people seeking treatment for pain, some but not all studies indicate elevated prevalence of any current (25–29%) and lifetime (28%) anxiety disorder relative to the general population (18%) (Kessler et al 2005a,b), with specific elevations in the prevalence of current seasonal affective disorder, GAD, panic disorder and PTSD (for review, see Asmundson & Katz 2009).

Fear and anxiety related to pain are also pertinent issues. The constructs of pain-related anxiety and pain-related fear are often used interchangeably, but there is theory and evidence that suggests the two are distinct (Carleton & Asmundson 2009). Specifically, pain-related anxiety represents a response to anticipated *future* encounters with pain-related threats that drives avoidance behaviours; in contrast, pain-related fear represents a response to a *current* encounter with a pain-related threat that drives escape behaviours. There are differing opinions about whether pain-related fear is focused on painful sensations (Lethem et al 1983; Vlaeyen & Linton 2000), activities associated with those sensations (e.g. Waddell et al 1993) or

painful reinjury (Kori et al 1990), or whether it is best subsumed by a fear of somatic sensations and changes (Asmundson et al 1999; Greenberg & Burns 2003). Despite the potential utility of clearly distinguishing between pain-related anxiety and pain-related fear, additional empirical study is required; as such, in the current text, pain-related anxiety will be used to refer to both constructs.

The structure of pain-related anxiety appears to be multidimensional (i.e. comprising cognitive, behavioural and physiological components; McCracken et al 1993) and continuous (i.e. occurring along a continuum ranging from low to high; Asmundson et al 2007). Accordingly, there is also evidence that pain-related anxiety is ubiquitous in the population (Carleton & Asmundson 2007; Carleton et al 2009). There have been several tools designed to measure pain-related anxiety (e.g. McCracken & Dhingra 2002; McNeil & Rainwater 1998; Melzack 1983) and ongoing assessment provides clinicians with information about a key cognitive component in the maintenance of disabling chronic pain.

Spirituality

Exploration of the relationship between religion, spirituality and chronic pain remains relatively novel. In a recent review, religious and spiritual beliefs were found to represent important components of the chronic pain experience (Rippentrop 2005; Unruh 2007). Many people with chronic pain report that religious and spiritual beliefs function as coping mechanisms that facilitate their continued activity (Büssing et al 2009), but the available evidence suggests that religious and spiritual beliefs do not directly impact pain intensity or pain interference (Rippentrop et al 2005). Research to date suggests most people with chronic pain reporting a religious affiliation neither feel abandoned nor punished as a function of their religious and spiritual beliefs, and that most report prayer to be an important coping strategy (Glover-Graf et al 2007). While additional investigation into the impact of religious and spiritual beliefs on the pain experience is warranted, there is sufficient evidence to suggest that religious and spiritual beliefs be considered as a component of comprehensive assessment. Several general and well-established measures of religious and spiritual beliefs are available (e.g. Cloninger et al 1994; Piedmont 1999) and more specific measures have been developed recently (e.g. Glover-Graf et al 2007).

BEHAVIOURAL CONSTRUCTS

Avoidance behaviour

The cognitive constructs described above often serve to influence the way in which a person with chronic pain behaves. Perhaps the most significant pain-related behaviour is that of avoidance (Asmundson et al 2004b). Indeed, avoidance behaviours are intrinsically appropriate components of pain (Larsen et al 1997; McCracken et al 1992; Osman et al 1994). Relatively higher levels of pain-related anxiety facilitate avoidance that, from the perspective of the person with chronic pain, provides a protective function (Vlaeyen et al 2004); in short, anticipated pain and additional harm are skirted. The challenge associated with avoidance is that it does serve a protective function as part of the recovery process, but only in the short term. When anxiety drives avoidance beyond the time required for healing, its once protective functions become maladaptive (Asmundson et al 2004b). Maladaptive avoidance behaviours can be driven by pain-related beliefs (Waddell et al 1993), anxiety (McCracken & Dhingra 2002) or fear of re-injury (Kori et al 1990). Avoidance behaviours have been associated with self-reported disability (Crombez et al 1999; McCracken & Gross 1995; Osman et al 2001), non-specific physical complaints (McCracken et al 1998) and reduced physical capacity (Burns et al 2000). Consequently, assessment of avoidance behaviour warrants careful attention.

Activity limitation for secondary gain

There is a lack of clarity associated with the terms 'malingering' and 'secondary gain' (Craig et al 1999; Main 2003), particularly as clinicians attempt to reconcile both terms with exaggerations of legitimate symptoms as attempts to receive help (Rogers & Neumann 2003). Secondary gain has been defined as 'acceptable or legitimate interpersonal advantages that result when one has the symptom of a physical disease' (Fishbain 1994; Fishbain et al 1995). In contrast, malingering is defined as the false or fraudulent exaggeration or simulation of physical or mental disease. Secondary gains are necessary for malingering to occur, but secondary gains can occur independent of malingering (Fishbain et al 2004).

Pain behaviours, particularly activity limitations, can produce positive consequences, such as receiving attention, decrease of responsibilities or economic compensation, all of which constitute secondary gains that can aggravate or maintain pain (Walker et al 2002; Worzer et al 2009). In addition, litigation (DeBerard et al 2001; Epker & Block 2001; LaCaille et al 2005; Taylor et al 2000) and insurance or worker's compensation (Deyo et al 2005; Epker & Block 2001; Mannion & Elfering 2006; Taylor et al 2000) are associated with poor surgical outcome (Bruns & Disorbio 2009). Despite the available research, meta-analytic reviews accounting for severity of pain or disability have been mixed. Some reviews find more abnormalities and disability in patients who have financial incentives than in those without (Binder & Rohling 1996), while other meta-analytic reviews have found minimal effects of compensation (Rohling et al 1995). Recent longitudinal research suggests that the absence of compensation may be associated with better post-surgical outcomes (Atlas et al 2010) and less healthcare utilization (Blyth et al 2003); similarly, patients appear to recover faster post injury when compensation for pain and suffering is not available (Cassidy et al 2000). In any case, the historical evidence suggests that chronic pain is associated with many more losses than gains (Fishbain 1994).

Pain coping behaviours

Individual beliefs, attitudes and appraisals pertaining to pain impact pain perception and coping behaviours (Unruh 1996; Unruh et al 1999). When pain is perceived as challenging or threatening, pain behaviours often include information seeking, healthcare utilization, seeking social support, problem solving and increased or decreased use of distraction strategies (for review, see Taylor & Asmundson 2004). Discussion of the various pain coping behaviours is beyond the scope of this chapter, but it is important it note that the effectiveness of these various strategies is often dependent on situational and individual difference factors. To illustrate, research into the effectiveness of cognitive control strategies, such as distraction or suppression of pain-related thoughts, has been equivocal (for review, see Asmundson et al 2010). Some studies have supported the use of distraction, particularly for children's procedural or acute pain, but most indicate that directing attention away from pain increases pain sensitivity and pain-related disability. Directing attention towards the sensory quality of pain (i.e. somatic focus) may actually reduce pain sensitivity, but the effect may depend on the sex of the person in pain (Keogh et al 2000). The disparate findings also may relate to psychological individual difference variables, such that distraction is less effective in persons who catastrophize about pain (Goubert et al 2004; Hadjistavropoulos et al 2000; Heyneman et al 1990; Roelofs et al 2004). These individuals may instead benefit from increasing somatic focus (Hadjistavropoulos et al 2000; Keogh & Mansoor 2001; Roelofs et al 2004).

Pain and suicide

Risk of suicide increases when chronic pain becomes overwhelming. Relative to persons without chronic pain, those with chronic pain are three times more likely to experience suicidal ideations and twice as likely to attempt suicide (Tang & Crane 2006). Up to half of all people with chronic pain have considered suicide (Hitchcock et al 1994), but ideation appears more frequent than forming a plan for or attempting suicide (Smith et al 2004). Chronic pain appears to play an important role in successful suicides (Fishbain et al 1991), particularly for older adults, who are highly susceptible to both psychiatric illness and physical health conditions (Manthorpe & Illife in press). That said, the most common method of suicide among people with chronic pain is prescription overdose (Smith et al 2004), which may be associated with increased access to prescription medications. A more comprehensive discussion of the current state of knowledge regarding suicide in people with various chronic pain conditions is provided by El-Gabalawy et al (2011).

ENVIRONMENTAL INFLUENCES

Pain is experienced and acted on within the context of the environment in which a person operates on a daily basis. Consequently, pain and pain-related cognitions and behaviours are influenced by numerous aspects of the environment. Here we provide an overview of the influence of family, culture and ethnicity, socioeconomics, and work factors on pain.

Family

Family appears to influence pain experiences through both genetic and social learning mechanisms. An association between some genes (i.e. the CMT and GTP ciclohydroxilase genes) and pain perception and chronic pain has been found (Diatchenko et al 2005; Tegeder et al 2006), but genetic influences are, at minimum, shaped by social learning. Parents experiencing pain appear to be effective models of illness behaviours in their children (Osborne et al 1989). This is illustrated by Goodman & McGrath (2003), who exposed three groups of children to their mother's behaviour during a cold pressor task. The mothers were assigned to three different conditions, including an exaggerated pain condition (i.e. instructions to exaggerate pain response), a minimized pain condition (i.e. instructed to minimize pain response) and a control condition without specific instructions. Children of the mothers instructed to exaggerate their pain response had lower pain thresholds and more exaggerated facial responses to cold pressor than did children of mothers in the control group.

Spouses and significant others (e.g. family members, friends) can likewise influence the pain and pain behaviour of the person experiencing pain (for review, see Leonard et al 2006). To illustrate, a spouse may unwittingly contribute to the persistence of pain by rewarding (e.g. providing attention or sympathy) pain expression and passively sanctioning avoidance of unwanted responsibilities or undesirable activities, by expressing negative emotion toward pain behaviours and by responding negatively to well behaviours (Raichle et al 2011). However, the effects of pain on the family need not be negative. Pain might act for some as a stabilizing force and play a substantive role in maintaining family homeostasis (Turk et al 1992). In the context of assessment and case conceptualization, it is important that the therapist be mindful of both negative and positive influences of family on the pain experience and pain reports.

Culture and ethnicity

Culture can be understood as the knowledge through which groups of people interpret their lives and direct their behaviours (Turner 2005). Some aspects of the culture of an individual can influence how pain is experienced. For example, those from the Mexican American culture are generally obligated to bear pain stoically (Villareul 1995). This expectation may influence both their experience of pain and the way they communicate pain to others. Culture can have important influences on the way in which pain assessment and treatment are conceptualized and practiced. Mind–body dualism, focus on disease versus illness and biases toward cure versus care can substantively hinder successful treatment of pain; as such, some theorists (Crowley-Matoka et al 2009) have called for general movement towards biopsychosocial models of pain.

Ethnicity–cultural groupings traditionally defined by a common language, religion, nationality or heritage (Shavers et al 2010) are also related to the way in which pain is experienced and communicated. Indeed, the prevalence of chronic pain has been demonstrated to be significantly higher for some ethnic groups in North America, as are adverse outcomes related to pain (for review, see Anderson et al 2009). For example, Day & Thorn (2010) found that African Americans report significantly higher pain intensity and pain interference compared to Caucasian Americans. Others studies suggest that the relationship between ethnicity and pain is better explained by socioeconomic differences, as the association between ethnicity and pain outcomes are attenuated when socioeconomic factors are controlled (Fuentes et al 2007; Stanaway et al 2011).

Craig (Chapter 3) provides a comprehensive discussion of the influences of culture and ethnicity on pain. In the context of assessment and case conceptualization, it is important that the therapist be mindful of potential cultural and ethnic influences on pain experience and pain reports. It is likewise important that he or she be mindful of the way in which pain-related information from patients is received and interpreted; indeed, minorities are rated by their providers as having less severe pain, less likely to receive opioid medications and less likely to receive comprehensive assessment and treatment when compared non-Hispanic Caucasian people (Shavers et al 2010).

Socioeconomics

Socioeconomic status (SES) represents a dynamic, multidimensional construct that is a robust determinant of health. SES has a clear association with pain. Low neighbourhood SES (i.e. a high percentage of households below the poverty line, a high percentage of people 25 years old with less than a high-school education and a high percentage of people in the labour force who are unemployed) has been shown to be associated with increased pain, both sensory and affective, as well as disability and mood disorders in adults with chronic low back pain (Fuentes et al 2007). Similarly, recent findings indicate that those attending an emergency room were more likely to self-report chronic illness and chronic pain if they were homeless, had family income less than $25 000 and perceived a lack of access to primary care (Hanley et al 2010). Cano et al (2006) suggest that pain coping strategies may be dependent on cognitive skills that are potentially enhanced by higher education and primary literacy levels; thus, those with lower SES may be less likely to cope effectively with pain and, as a consequence, be more prone to persistence of their pain experience.

Work

Characteristics of work and the work environment have emerged as predictors of back pain and disability, even after controlling for a host of other psychosocial, demographic and health-related variables (for reviews, see Crook et al 2002; Hoogendoorn et al 2000; Linton 2001; Shaw et al 2001, 2009). In a recent 2-year longitudinal study performed with neck pain patients, pain was predicted not only by mechanical factors (e.g. working with arms raised) but also social factors (e.g. job demands, decision control, role conflict, empowering leadership) (Christensen & Knardahl 2010). High work demands (e.g. long work hours, repetitive work, fatigue), biomechanical factors (e.g. repetitive and sustained work posture), and low work support and job satisfaction have been identified as significant contributing factors to musculoskeletal injury and pain (Crowther & Quayle 2010; for review, also see Macfarlane et al 2009). The Decade of the Flag Working Group has recently identified seven workplace variables that have been shown to contribute to back pain and pain-related disability: heavy physical demands, ability to modify work, job stress, social support, job satisfaction, expectations for resuming work and fear of re-injury (Shaw et al 2009). Consequently, comprehensive assessment of pain may necessitate consideration of physical, psychological and social factors of work and the work place.

KEY CONSIDERATIONS IN ASSESSMENT AND CASE CONCEPTUALIZATION

Assessment and case conceptualization

Careful and comprehensive assessment of pain is a necessary component of any treatment plan and any empirical pursuit wherein pain is of interest, and is covered in detail in Chapter 7. It is beyond the scope of this chapter to review the potential complexities associated with a comprehensive

assessment of pain. Instead, we provide some general guidelines to facilitate a comprehensive and multidimensional assessment approach (see also Dworkin et al 2005; Tait 1999), all predicated on the notion that assessment is a conceptually driven process. First, we recommend that assessment include consideration of pain severity or intensity, pain location and distribution, as well as pain stability (e.g. intermittent vs persistent) and durations. Second, we recommend that some measure of physical functioning be included in assessment. The experience of chronic pain is not homogenous and, as such, some people with chronic pain function well whereas others do not. The extent of functional limitation, which may or may not be associated with pain severity or intensity (Turk 2002), is important for directing treatment. Third, we recommend consideration of the various empirically supported and theoretically relevant cognitive, behavioural and environment influences described above. Person-specific circumstances can aid in tailoring selection of constructs for assessment, for example one's living circumstances, religious beliefs and current work status may dictate whether measures related to these areas are used. Consideration of convenience and time commitments for the patient and assessor are also important in selecting constructs that will be assessed. Is there expertise to assess comorbid psychopathology? Is there time to do so? If so, there are several structured clinical interviews that a trained clinician can use for this purpose. If not, there are a variety of self-report and clinician-administered measures that can be used to screen for significant symptoms of psychopathology which, in turn, can be more thoroughly evaluated as necessary. Finally, we recommend selection of a core set of measures that can be used to gauge progress over time. This core set of measures should tap the pain experience, physical functioning and psychosocial factors associated with pain.

Treatment overview

Across the available treatment alternatives, the overwhelming evidence for more than two decades suggests that multidisciplinary treatments (i.e. those involving biological and psychosocial interventions) result in better treatment outcomes than unimodal treatments (i.e. biological interventions or physical therapy) for patients with chronic pain (for review, see Flor et al 1992). Reviews of multidisciplinary treatment programmes suggest that they are not only therapeutically effective, but also cost-effective (for review, see Gatchel & Okifuji 2006). Irrespective of specific underlying causes, there is growing evidence that pain-related anxiety and fear can both be reduced using exposure-based therapies that encourage confronting anxiety- and fear-related stimuli (Asmundson et al 2004b; Bailey et al 2010; McCracken 1997; McCracken et al 1992). For discussion about psychological interventions see Chapters 8 and 9 in this text.

CONCLUSION

Contemporary biopsychosocial approaches to understanding pain provide a sound foundation on which comprehensive assessment, case conceptualization and treatment planning can be based. While each case may involve consideration of different biological, psychological and social factors in the context of the pain experience, it is careful consideration of these factors that will ultimately lead to the best outcomes for those disabled by pain.

REFERENCES

Anderson, K.O., Green, C.R., Payne, R., 2009. Racial and ethnic disparities in pain: Causes and consequences of unequal care. J. Pain. 10, 1187–1204.

Arnow, B.A., Blasey, C.M., Lee, J., et al., 2009. Relationships among depression, chronic pain, chronic disabling pain, and medical costs. Psychiatr. Serv. 60, 344–350.

Asmundson, G.J.G., Hadjistavropoulos, H.D., 2006. Addressing shared vulnerability for PTSD and chronic pain: A cognitive-behavioral perspective. Cognitive and Behavioral Practice 13, 8–16.

Asmundson, G.J.G., Katz, J., 2009. Understanding the co-occurrence of anxiety disorders and chronic musculoskeletal pain: The state-of-the-art. Depress. Anxiety 26, 888–901.

Asmundson, G.J.G., Wright, K.D., 2004. Biopsychosocial approaches to pain. In: Hadjistavropoulos, T., Craig, K.D. (Eds.), Pain: Psychological Perspectives. Erlbaum, New Jersey, pp. 35–57.

Asmundson, G.J.G., Norton, G.R., Allerdings, M.D., et al., 1998. Posttraumatic stress disorder and work-related injury. J. Anxiety Disord. 12, 57–69.

Asmundson, G.J.G., Norton, P.J., Norton, G.R., 1999. Beyond pain: The role of fear and avoidance in chronicity. Clin. Psychol. Rev. 19, 97–119.

Asmundson, G.J.G., Norton, P.J., Vlaeyen, J.W.S., 2004a. Fear-avoidance models of chronic pain: An overview. In: Asmundson, G.J.G., Vlaeyen, J.W.S., Crombez, G. (Eds.), Understanding and Treating Fear of Pain. Oxford University Press, Oxford, pp. 3–24.

Asmundson, G.J.G., Vlaeyen, J.W.S., Crombez, G., 2004b. Understanding and treating fear of pain. Oxford University Press, Oxford.

Asmundson, G.J.G., Collimore, K.C., Bernstein, A., et al., 2007. Is the latent structure of fear of pain continuous or discontinuous among pain patients? Taxometric analysis of the pain anxiety symptoms scale. J. Pain 8, 387–395.

Asmundson, G.J.G., Abrams, M.P., Collimore, K.C., 2008. Pain and anxiety disorders. In: Zvolensky, M.J., Smits, J.A.J. (Eds.), Health behaviors and physical illness in anxiety and its disorders: Contemporary theory and research. Springer, New York, pp. 207–235.

Asmundson, G.J.G., Peluso, D., Carleton, R.N., et al., 2010. Chronic Musculoskeletal Pain and Related Health Conditions. In: Zvolensky, M.J., Bernstein, A., Vujanovic, A.A. (Eds.), Distress Tolerance: Theory, Research, and Clinical Applications. Guilford Publications, New York, pp. 221–244.

Atlas, S.J., Tosteson, T.D., Blood, E.A., et al., 2010. The impact of workers' compensation on outcomes of surgical and nonoperative therapy for patients with a lumbar disc herniation SPORT. Spine 35, 89–97.

Bailey, K.M., Carleton, R.N., Vlaeyen, J.W.S., et al., 2010. Treatments addressing pain-related fear and anxiety in patients with chronic musculoskeletal pain: A preliminary review. Cogn. Behav. Ther. 39, 46–63.

Beck, A.T., Epstein, N., Brown, G., et al., 1988. An inventory for measuring clinical anxiety: Psychometric properties. J. Consult. Clin. Psychol. 56, 893–897.

Binder, L.M., Rohling, M.L., 1996. Money matters: A meta-analytic review of the effects of financial incentives on recovery after closed-head injury. Am. J. Psychiatry 153, 7–10.

Blyth, F.M., March, L.M., Nicholas, M.K., et al., 2003. Chronic pain, work performance and litigation. Pain 103, 41–47.

Bruns, D., Disorbio, J.M., 2009. Assessment of biopsychosocial risk factors for medical treatment: a collaborative approach. J. Clin. Psychol. Med. Settings 16, 127–147.

Burns, J.W., Mullen, J.T., Higdon, L.J., et al., 2000. Validity of the Pain Anxiety Symptoms Scale (PASS): Prediction of physical capacity variables. Pain 84, 247–252.

Büssing, A., Michalsen, A., Balzat, H., et al., 2009. Are spirituality and religiosity resources for patients with chronic pain conditions? Pain Med. 10, 327–339.

Cano, A., Mayo, A., Ventimiglia, M., 2006. Coping, pain severity, interference, and disability: the potential mediating and moderating roles of race and education. J. Pain 7, 459–468.

Carleton, R.N., Asmundson, G.J.G., 2007. Review of cognitive-behavioral therapies for trauma, 2nd edn. Canadian Psychology/Psychologie Canadienne 48, 201–203.

Carleton, R.N., Asmundson, G.J.G., 2009. The multidimensionality of fear of pain: Construct independence for the Fear of Pain Questionnaire-Short Form and the Pain Anxiety Symptoms Scale-20. J. Pain 10, 29–37.

Carleton, R.N., Abrams, M.P., Asmundson, G.J.G., et al., 2009. Pain-related anxiety and anxiety sensitivity across anxiety and depressive disorders. J. Anxiety Disord. 23, 791–798.

Cassidy, J.D., Carroll, L.J., Côté, P., et al., 2000. Effect of eliminating compensation for pain and suffering on the outcome of insurance claims for whiplash injury. N. Engl. J. Med. 342, 1179–1186.

Christensen, J.O., Knardahl, S., 2010. Work and neck pain: A prospective study of psychological, social, and mechanical risk factors. Pain 151, 162–173.

Cloninger, R.C., Przybeck, T.R., Svrakic, D.M., et al., 1994. The Temperament and Character Inventory (TCI): A guide to its development and use. Center for Psychobiology of Personality, Washington University, St Louis, MO.

Craig, K.D., Hill, M.L., McMurty, B.W., 1999. Detecting deception and malingering. In: Block, A.R., Kramer, E.F., Fernandez, E. (Eds.), Handbook of pain syndromes: biopsychosocial perspectives. Lawrence Erlbaum, Mahwah, New Jersey, pp. 41–58.

Crombez, G., Vlaeyen, J.W.S., Heuts, P.H.T.G., et al., 1999. Pain-related fear is more disabling than pain itself: Evidence on the role of pain-related fear in chronic back pain disability. Pain 80, 329–339.

Crook, J., Milner, R., Schultz, I.Z., et al., 2002. Determinants of occupational disability following a back injury: A critical review of the literature. J. Occup. Rehabil. 12, 277–295.

Crowley-Matoka, M., Saha, S., Dobscha, S.K., et al., 2009. Problems of quality and equity in pain management: exploring the role of biomedical culture. Pain Med. 10, 1312–1324.

Crowther, I.E., Quayle, L., 2010. Women's health at work program. Musculoskeletal pain experience by women of Chinese background working on market gardens in the Sydney basin. Work 36, 129–140.

Day, M.A., Thorn, B.E., 2010. The relationship of demographic and psychosocial variables to pain-related outcomes in a rural chronic pain population. Pain. http://dx.doi.org/10.1016/j.pain.2010.08.015.

DeBerard, M.S., Masters, K.S., Colledge, A.L., et al., 2001. Outcomes of posterolateral lumbar fusion in Utah patients receiving workers' compensation: A retrospective cohort study. Spine 26, 738–746.

de Jong, J.R., Vlaeyen, J.W., Onghena, P., et al., 2005. Fear of movement/(re) injury in chronic low back pain: education or exposure in vivo as mediator to fear reduction? Clin. J. Pain 21, 9–17.

Demyttenaere, K., Bruffaerts, R., Lee, S., et al., 2007. Mental disorders among persons with chronic back or neck pain: results from the World Mental Health Surveys. Pain 129, 332–342.

Deyo, R.A., Mirza, S.K., Heagerty, P.J., et al., 2005. A prospective cohort study of surgical treatment for back pain with degenerated discs; study protocol. BMC Musculoskelet. Disord. 6, 24.

Diatchenko, L., Slade, G.D., Nackley, A.G., et al., 2005. Genetic basis for individual variations in pain perception and the development of a chronic pain condition. Hum. Mol. Genet. 14, 135–143.

Dworkin, R.H., Turk, D.C., Farrar, J.T., et al., 2005. Core outcome measures for chronic pain clinical trials: IMMPACT recommendations. Pain 113, 9–19.

Edwards, L.C., Pearce, S.A., Turner-Stokes, L., et al., 1992. The Pain Beliefs Questionnaire: an investigation of beliefs in the causes and consequences of pain. Pain 51, 267–272.

El-Gabalawy, R., Asmundson, G.J.G., Sareen, J., 2011. Suicide and chronic pain. In: Pompili, M., Berman, L. (Eds.), Suicide Risk and Physical Illness. American Association of Suicidology, Washington, DC, pp. 75–86.

Epker, J., Block, A.R., 2001. Presurgical psychological screening in back pain patients: A review. Clin. J. Pain 17, 200–205.

First, M., Spitzer, R., Gibbon, M., et al., 1996. Structured Clinical Interview for DSM-IV Axis I Disorders – Patient edition. New York State Psychiatric Institute, Biometrics Research Department, New York.

Fishbain, D.A., 1994. Secondary gain concept: Definition problems and its abuse in medical practice. APS Journal 3, 264–273.

Fishbain, D.A., Goldberg, M., Rosomoff, R.S., et al., 1991. Case Reports: Completed Suicide in Chronic Pain. Clin. J. Pain 7, 29–36.

Fishbain, D.A., Rosomoff, H.L., Cutler, R., et al., 1995. Do chronic pain patients' perceptions about their preinjury jobs determine their intent to return to the same type of job post-pain facility treatment? Clin. J. Pain. 11, 267–278.

Fishbain, D.A., Cutler, R.B., Lewis, J., et al., 2004. Do the Second-Generation 'Atypical Neuroleptics' have analgesic properties? A structured evidenced-based review. Pain Med. 5, 359–365.

Flor, H., Fydrich, T., Turk, D.C., 1992. Efficacy of multidisciplinary pain treatment centers: a meta-analytic review. Pain 49, 221–230.

Fordyce, W.E., 1976. Behavioral methods for chronic pain and illness. Mosby, St Louis, MO.

Fordyce, W.E., Shelton, J.L., Dundore, D.E., 1982. The modification of avoidance learning pain behaviors. J. Behav. Med. 5, 405–414.

Fuentes, M., Hart-Johnson, T., Green, C.R., 2007. The Association among Neighborhood Socioeconomic Status, Race and Chronic Pain in Black and White Older Adults. J. Natl. Med. Assoc. 99, 1160–1169.

Gatchel, R.J., Okifuji, A., 2006. Evidence-based scientific data documenting the treatment and cost-effectiveness of comprehensive pain programs for chronic nonmalignant pain. J. Pain 7 (11), 779–793.

Geisser, M.E., Roth, R.S., Robinson, M.E., 1997. Assessing depression among persons with chronic pain using the Center for Epidemiological Studies – Depression Scale and the Beck Depression Inventory: a comparative analysis. Clin. J. Pain 13, 163–170.

Glombiewski, J.A., Hartwich-Tersek, J., Rief, W., 2010. Depression in chronic back pain patients: Prediction of pain intensity and pain disability in cognitive-behavioral treatment. Psychosomatics 51, 130–136.

Glover-Graf, N.M., Marini, I., Baker, J., et al., 2007. Religious and spiritual beliefs and practices of persons with chronic pain. Rehabilitation Counseling Bulletin 51, 21–33.

Goodman, J.E., McGrath, P.J., 2003. Mothers' modeling influences children's pain during a cold presor task. Pain 104, 559–565.

Goubert, L., Crombez, G., Van Damme, S., 2004. The role of neuroticism, pain catastrophizing and pain-related fear in vigilance to pain: a structural equations approach. Pain 107, 234–241.

Greenberg, J., Burns, J.W., 2003. Pain anxiety among chronic pain patients: specific phobia or manifestation of anxiety sensitivity? Behav. Res. Ther. 41, 223–240.

Gureje, O., Von Korff, M., Kola, L., et al., 2008. The relation between multiple pains and mental disorders: Results from the World Mental Health Surveys. Pain 135, 82–91.

Hadjistavropoulos, H.D., Hadjistavropoulos, T., Quine, A., 2000. Health anxiety moderates the effects of distraction versus attention to pain. Behav. Res. Ther. 38, 425–438.

Hadjistavropoulos, H.D., Owens, K.M.B., Hadjistavropoulos, T., et al., 2001. Hypochondriasis and health anxiety among pain patients. In: Asmundson, G.J.G., Taylor, S., Cox, B.J. (Eds.), Health Anxiety: Clinical and research perspectives on hypochondriasis and related conditions. John Wiley & Sons, Toronto, pp. 298–323.

Hanley, O., Miner, J., Rockswold, E., et al., 2010. The relationship between chronic illness, chronic pain, and socioeconomic factors in the ED. Am. J. Emerg. Med. http://dx.doi.org/10.1016/j.ajem.2009.10.002.

Heyneman, N.E., Fremouw, W.J., Gano, D., et al., 1990. Individual differences and the effectiveness of different coping strategies for pain. Cogn. Behav. Ther. 14, 63–77.

Hitchcock, L.S., Ferrell, B.R., McCaffery, M., 1994. The experience of chronic nonmalignant pain. J. Pain Symptom. Manage. 9, 312–318.

Hoogendoorn, W.E., van Poppel, M.N., Bongers, P.M., et al., 2000. Systematic review of psychosocial factors at work and private life as risk factors for back pain. Spine. 25, 2114–2125.

International Association for the Study of Pain, 1986. Classification of chronic pain: Descriptions of chronic pain syndromes and definitions of pain terms. Pain. (Suppl. 3), 1–222.

Jensen, M.P., Turner, J.A., Romano, J.M., et al., 1991. Coping with chronic pain: A critical review of the literature. Pain. 47, 249–283.

Jensen, M.P., Turner, J.A., Romano, J.M., 2001. Changes in beliefs, catastrophizing, and coping are associated with improvement in multidisciplinary pain treatment. J. Consult. Clin. Psychol. 69, 655–662.

Keefe, F.J., Wilkins, R.H., Cook Jr., W.A., et al., 1986. Depression, pain, and pain behavior. J. Consult. Clin. Psychol. 54, 665–669.

Keogh, E., Mansoor, L., 2001. Investigating the effects of anxiety sensitivity and coping on the perception of cold pressor pain in healthy women. Eur. J. Pain 5, 11–22.

Keogh, E., Hatton, H., Ellery, D., 2000. Avoidance versus focused attention and the perception of pain: differential effects for men and women. Pain 85, 225–230.

Kessler, R.C., Berglund, P., Demler, O., et al., 2005a. Lifetime prevalence and age-of-onset distributions of DSM-IV disorders in the National Comorbidity Survey Replication. Arch. Gen. Psychiatry 62, 593–602.

Kessler, R.C., Chiu, W.T., Demler, O., et al., 2005b. Prevalence, severity, and comorbidity of 12-month DSM-IV disorders in the National Comorbidity Survey Replication. Arch. Gen. Psychiatry 62, 617–627.

Kori, S.H., Miller, R.P., Todd, D.D., 1990. Kinesiophobia: A new view of chronic pain behavior. Pain Management 3, 35–43.

Krause, S.J., Weiner, R.L., Tait, R.C., 1994. Depression and pain behavior in patients with chronic pain. Clin. J. Pain 10, 122–127.

LaCaille, R.A., DeBerard, M.S., Masters, K.S., et al., 2005. Presurgical biopsychosocial factors predict multidimensional patient outcomes of interbody cage lumbar fusion. Spine J. 5 (1), 71–78.

Larsen, D.K., Taylor, S., Asmundson, G.J.G., 1997. Exploratory factor analysis of the Pain Anxiety Symptoms Scale in patients with chronic pain complaints. Pain 69, 27–34.

Leeuw, M., Peters, M.L., Wiers, R.W., et al., 2007. Measuring fear of movement/(re)injury in chronic low back pain using implicit measures. Cogn. Behav. Ther. 36, 52–64.

Leonard, M.T., Cano, A., Johansen, A.B., 2006. Chronic pain in a couples context: a review and integration of theoretical models and empirical evidence. J. Pain 7, 377–390.

Lethem, J., Slade, P.D., Troup, J.D., et al., 1983. Outline of a fear-avoidance model of exaggerated pain perception: I. Behav. Res. Ther. 21, 401–408.

Linton, S.J., 2001. Occupational psychological factors increase the risk for back pain: a systematic review. J. Occup. Rehabil. 11, 53–66.

Main, C.J., 2003. The nature of chronic pain: a clinical and legal challenge. In: Hallingan, P.W., Bass, C., Oakley, D.A. (Eds.), Malingering and Illness Deception. Oxford University Press, New York, pp. 171–183.

Macfarlane, G.J., Pallewatte, N., Paudyal, P., et al., 2009. Evaluation of work-related psychosocial factors and regional musculoskeletal pain: results from a EULAR Task Force. Annual of Rheumatic Diseases 68, 885–891.

Mannion, A.F., Elfering, A., 2006. Predictors of surgical outcome and their assessment. Eur. Spine J. 15, S93–S108.

Manthorpe, J., Illife, S., in press Suicide in later life: public health and practitioner perspectives. Int. J. Geriatr. Psychiatry 25, 1230–1238.

McCracken, L.M., 1997. 'Attention' to pain in persons with chronic pain: a behavioral approach. Behaviour Therapy 28, 271–284.

McCracken, L.M., Dhingra, L., 2002. A short version of the pain anxiety symptoms scale (PASS-20): Preliminary development and validity. Pain Res. Manag. 7, 45–50.

McCracken, L.M., Gross, R.T., 1995. The pain anxiety symptoms scale (PASS) and the assessment of emotional responses to pain. In: VandeCreek, L., Knapp, S., Jackson, T.L. (Eds.), Innovations in clinical practice: a sourcebook. Professional Resources Press, Sarasota, FL, pp. 309–321.

McCracken, L.M., Zayfert, C., Gross, R.T., 1992. The pain anxiety symptoms scale: Development and validation of a scale to measure fear of pain. Pain 50, 67–73.

McCracken, L.M., Zayfert, C., Gross, R.T., 1993. The pain anxiety symptoms scale (PASS): a multimodal measure of pain-specific anxiety symptoms. Behavior Therapist 16, 183–184.

McCracken, L.M., Faber, S.D., Janeck, A.S., 1998. Pain-related anxiety predicts nonspecific physical complaints in persons with chronic pain. Behav. Res. Ther. 36, 621–630.

McNeil, D.W., Rainwater, A.J., 1998. Development of the fear of pain questionnaire-III. J. Behav. Med. 21, 389–410.

McWilliams, L.A., Cox, B.J., Enns, M.W., 2003. Mood and anxiety disorders associated with chronic pain: an examination in a nationally representative sample. Pain 106, 127–133.

Mechanic, D., 1962. The concept of illness behavior. J. Chronic Dis. 15, 189–194.

Melzack, R., 1983. The McGill Pain Questionnaire. In: Melzack, R. (Ed.), Pain Measurement and Assessment. Raven Press, New York, pp. 41–47.

Melzack, R., 1999. From the gate to the neuromatrix. Pain (Suppl. 6), S121–S126.

Merskey, H., Bogduk, N., 1994. Classification of chronic pain: descriptions of chronic pain syndromes and definitions of pain terms, second ed. IASP Press, Seattle.

Melzack, R., Casey, K.L., 1968. Sensory, motivational and central control determinants of pain. In: Kenshalo, D.R. (Ed.), The Skin Senses. CC Thomas, Springfield, IL, pp. 423–439.

Melzack, R., Katz, J., 2004. The gate control theory: Reaching for the Brain. In: Craig, K.D., Hadjistavropoulos, T. (Eds.), Pain: Psychological Perspectives. Lawrence Erlbaum, Mahwah, NJ, pp. 303–322.

Melzack, R., Wall, P.D., 1965. Pain mechanisms: a new theory. Science 150, 971–979.

Morley, S., Williams, A.C., Black, S., 2002. A confirmatory factor analysis of the Beck Depression Inventory in chronic pain. Pain 99, 289–298.

Norton, P.J., Asmundson, G.J.G., 2003. Amending the fear-avoidance model of chronic pain: What is the role of physiological arousal? Behav. Ther. 34, 17–30.

Odegard, S., Finset, A., Mowinckel, P., et al., 2007. Pain and psychology health status over a 10 year period in patients with recent onset rheumatoid arthritis. Ann. Rheum. Dis. 66, 1195–1201.

Osborne, R.B., Hatcher, J.W., Richtsmeier, A.J., 1989. The role of social modeling in unexplained pediatric pain. J. Pediatr. Psychol. 14, 43–61.

Osman, A., Barrios, F.X., Osman, J.R., et al., 1994. The Pain Anxiety Symptoms Scale: psychometric properties in a community sample. J. Behav. Med. 17 (5), 511–522.

Osman, A., Breitenstein, J.L., Barrios, F.X., et al., 2001. The fear of pain questionnaire-III: further reliability and validity with nonclinical samples. J. Behav. Med. 25, 155–173.

Parsons, T., 1951. The Social System. Free Press, New York.

Piedmont, R.L., 1999. Does spirituality represent the sixth factor of personality? Spiritual transcendence and the five-factor model. J. Pers. 67, 985–1013.

Pincus, T., Williams, A., 1999. Models and measurements of depression in chronic pain. J. Psychosom. Res. 47, 211–219.

Polatin, P.B., Kinney, R.K., Gatchel, R.J., et al., 1993. Psychiatric illness and chronic low-back pain. The mind and the spine – which goes first? Spine 18, 66–71.

Poole, H., White, S., Blake, C., et al., 2009. Depression in Chronic Pain Patients: Prevalence and Measurement. Pain Pract. 9, 173–180.

Price, D.D., 2000. Psychological and neural mechanisms of the affective dimension of pain. Science. 288, 1769–1772.

Radloff, L.S., 1977. The CES-D Scale: A self-report depression scale for research in the general population. Applied Psychological Measurement. 1, 385–401.

Raichle, K.A., Romano, J.M., Jensen, M.P., 2011. Partner responses to patient pain and well behaviors and their relationship to patient pain behavior, functioning, and depression. Pain 152, 82–88.

Raphael, K.G., Janal, M.N., Nayak, S., et al., 2006. Psychiatric comorbidities in a community sample of women with fibromyalgia. Pain 124, 117–125.

Ratcliffe, G.E., Enns, M.W., Belik, S.L., et al., 2008. Chronic pain conditions and suicidal ideation and suicide attempts: An epidemiologic perspective. Clin. J. Pain 24, 204–210.

Rippentrop, E.A., 2005. A review of the role of religion and spirituality in chronic pain populations. Rehabilitation Psychology 50, 278–284.

Rippentrop, E.A., Altmaier, E.M., Chen, J., et al., 2005. The relationship between religion/spirituality and physical health, mental health, and pain in a chronic pain population. Pain 116, 311–321.

Roelofs, J., Peters, M.L., van der Zijden, M., et al., 2004. Does fear of pain moderate the effects of sensory focusing and distraction on cold pressor pain in pain-free individuals? J. Pain 5, 250–256.

Rogers, R., Neumann, C.S., 2003. Conceptual issues and explanatory models of malingering. In: Halligan, P.W., Bass, C., Oakley, D.A. (Eds.), Malingering and illness deception: Clinical and theoretical perspectives. Oxford University Press, Oxford, pp. 71–82.

Rohling, M.L., Binder, L.M., Langhirinrichsen-Rohling, J., 1995. Money matters: a meta-analytic review of the association between financial compensation and the experience and treatment of chronic pain. Health Psychol. 14, 537–547.

Shavers, V.L., Bakos, A., Sheppard, V.B., 2010. Race, Ethnicity, and Pain among the US Adult Population. J. Health Care Poor Underserved 21, 177–220.

Shaw, W.S., Pransky, G., Fitzgerald, T.E., 2001. Early prognosis for low back disability: intervention strategies for health care providers. Disabil. Rehabil. 23, 815–828.

Shaw, W.S., van der Windt, D.A., Main, C.J., et al., the Decade of the Flags Working Group, 2009. Early Patient Screening and Intervention to Address Individual-Level

Occupational Factors ('Blue Flags') in Back Disability. J. Occup. Rehabil. 19, 64–80.

Sloan, T.J., Gupta, R., Zhang, W., et al., 2007. Beliefs about the causes and consequences of pain in patients with chronic inflammatory or noninflammatory low back pain and in pain-free individuals. Spine 33, 966–972.

Smith, W.B., Gracely, R.H., Safer, M.A., 1998. The meaning of pain: Cancer patients' rating and recall of pain intensity and affect. Pain 78, 123–129.

Smith, M.T., Edwards, R.R., Robinson, R.C., et al., 2004. Suicidal ideation, plans, and attempts in chronic pain patients: factors associated with increased risk. Pain 111, 201–208.

Spengler, D.M., Bigos, S.J., Martin, N.A., 1986. Back injuries in industry: A retrospective study. 1. Overview and cost analysis. Spine 11, 241–245.

Stanaway, F.F., Blyth, F.M., Cumming, R.G., et al., 2011. Back pain in older male Italian-born immigrants in. The importance of socioeconomic factors. Eur. J. Pain, Australia http://dx.doi.org/10.1016/j.ejpain.2010.05.009.

Stewart, W.F., Ricci, J.A., Chee, E., et al., 2003. Lost productive time and cost due to common pain conditions in the US workforce. J. Am. Med. Assoc. 290, 2443–2454.

Sullivan, M.J.L., Thorn, B., Haythornthwaite, J.A., et al., 2001. Theoretical perspectives on the relation between catastrophizing and pain. Clin. J. Pain 17, 52–64.

Tait, R., 1999. Evaluation of treatment effectiveness in patients with intractable pain: Measures and methods. In: Gatchel, R.J., Turk, D.C. (Eds.), Psychosocial factors in pain: Critical perspectives. Guilford Press, New York, pp. 457–480.

Tang, N.K.Y., Crane, C., 2006. Suicidality in chronic pain: a review of the prevalence, risk factors and psychological links. Psychol. Med. 36, 575–586.

Taylor, S., Asmundson, G.J.G., 2004. Treating health anxiety: A cognitive-behavioral approach. Guilford Press, New York.

Taylor, V.M., Deyo, R.A., Ciol, M., et al., 2000. Patient-oriented outcomes from low back surgery: A community-based study. Spine 25, 2445–2452.

Tegeder, I., Costigan, M., Griffin, R.S., et al., 2006. GTP cyclohydrolase and tetrahydrobiopterin regulate pain sensitivity and persistence. Nat. Med. 12, 1269–1277.

Teh, C.F., Zaslavsky, A.M., Reynolds, C.F., et al., 2009. Effect of depression treatment on chronic pain outcomes. Psychosom. Med. 72, 61–67.

Turk, D.C., 2002. A diathesis-stress model of chronic pain and disability following traumatic injury. Pain Res. Manag. 7, 9–19.

Turk, D.C., Flor, H., 1999. The biobehavioral perspective of pain. In: Gatchel, R.J., Turk, D.C. (Eds.), Psychosocial factors in pain. Clinical perspectives. Guilford Press, New York, pp. 18–34.

Turk, D.C., Rudy, T.E., 1987. IASP taxonomy of chronic pain syndromes: Preliminary assessment of reliability. Pain 30, 177–189.

Turk, D.C., Meichenbaum, D., Genest, M., 1983. Pain and behavioral medicine: A cognitive-behavioral perspective. Guilford Press, New York.

Turk, D.C., Kerns, R.D., Rosenberg, R., 1992. Effects of marital interaction on chronic pain and disability: Examining the down side of social support. Rehabilitation Psychology 37, 259–274.

Turner, L., 2005. From the local to the global: bioethics and the concept of culture. J. Med. Philos. 30, 305–320.

Turner, J.A., Jensen, M.P., Romano, J.M., 2000. Do beliefs, coping, and catastrophizing independently predict functioning in patients with chronic pain? Pain 85, 115–125.

Turner, J.A., Mancl, L., Aaron, L.A., 2004. Pain-related catastrophizing: a daily process study. Pain 110, 103–111.

Unruh, A.M., 1996. Gender variations in clinical pain experience. Pain 65, 123–167.

Unruh, A.M., 2007. Spirituality, religion and pain. Can. J. Nurs. Res. 39, 66–86.

Unruh, A.M., Ritchie, J.A., Merskey, H., 1999. Does gender affect appraisal of pain and pain coping strategies? Clin. J. Pain 15, 31–40.

Van Damme, S., Crombez, G., Bijttebier, P., et al., 2002. A confirmatory factor analysis of the pain catastrophizing scale: invariant factor structure across clinical and non-clinical populations. Pain 96, 319–324.

Villareul, A.M., 1995. Mexican-American cultural meanings, expressions, self-care and dependent-care actions associated with experiences of pain. Res. Nurs. Health 18, 427–436.

Vlaeyen, J.W.S., Linton, S.J., 2000. Fear-avoidance and its consequences in chronic musculoskeletal pain: A state of the art. Pain 85, 317–332.

Vlaeyen, J.W.S., Kole-Snijders, A.M., Boeren, R.G., et al., 1995. Fear of movement/(re)injury in chronic low back pain and its relation to behavioral performance. Pain 62, 363–372.

Vlaeyen, J.W.S., de Jong, J., Leeuw, M., et al., 2004. Fear reduction in chronic pain: graded exposure in vivo with behavioral experiments. In: Asmundson, G.J., Vlaeyen, J.W.S., Crombez, G. (Eds.), Understanding and treating fear of pain. Oxford University Press, Oxford.

Waddell, G., 1987. A new clinical model for the treatment of low back pain. Spine 12, 623–644.

Waddell, G., Main, C.J., Morris, E.W., et al., 1984. Chronic low-back pain, psychologic distress, and illness behavior. Spine 9 (2), 209–213.

Waddell, G., Newton, M., Henderson, I., et al., 1993. A Fear-Avoidance Beliefs Questionnaire (FABQ) and the role of fear-avoidance beliefs in chronic low back pain and disability. Pain 52, 157–168.

Walker, L.S., Claar, R.L., Garber, J., 2002. Social consequences of children's pain: When do they encourage symptom maintenance? J. Pediatr. Psychol. 27, 689–698.

Wall, P.D., 1996. Comments after 30 years of the gate control theory of pain. Pain Forum 5, 12–22.

Wallston, K.A., Wallston, B.S., DeVellis, R., 1978. Development of the multidimensional health locus of control (MHLC) scale. Health Educ. Monogr. 6, 525.

Walsh, D.A., Radcliffe, J.C., 2002. Pain beliefs and perceived physical disability of patients with chronic low back pain. Pain 97, 23–31.

Werner, E.L., Ihlebaek, C., Skouen, J.S., et al., 2005. Beliefs about low back pain in the Norwegian general population: are they related to pain experiences and health professionals? Spine. 30, 1770–1776.

Williams, D.A., Thorn, B.E., 1989. An empirical assessment of pain beliefs. Pain 36, 351–358.

Worz, R., 2003. Pain in depression – depression in pain. Pain Clinical Updates (IASP) XI (1), 1–4.

Worzer, W.E., Kishino, N.D., Gatchel, R.J., 2009. Primary, secondary, and tertiary losses in chronic pain patients. Psychology, Injury, and Law 2, 215–224.

Chapter | 5 |

Neuroanatomy of the nociceptive system

Mary P. Galea

LEARNING OBJECTIVES

At the end of this chapter readers will:

1. Appreciate the different types of peripheral nociceptors and their associated axons.
2. Understand the organization of the dorsal horn and the termination patterns of afferent inputs.
3. Understand the pathways involved in transmitting nociceptive information within the nervous system.
4. Understand the areas of the nervous system involved in the perception, integration and response to nociception.

OVERVIEW

This chapter is concerned specifically with the nervous system structures involved in nociception. The historical framework for studying pain has implied that there is a sensory channel for pain in the manner of sensory channels for other sensations (Willis & Coggeshall 1991). It will be clear from the following review that this is not the case, and that pain is a complex, multidimensional phenomenon, with pain signals being transmitted to many different regions of the nervous system. Melzack and Casey (1968) suggested that pain needs to be considered in three interacting dimensions: sensory–discriminative, cognitive–evaluative and motivational–affective. The sensory dimension refers to the capacity to analyse the intensity, location, quality and behaviour of pain. The cognitive–evaluative dimension is concerned with the phenomena of anticipation, attention, suggestion and the influence of previous experience and knowledge. Finally, the motivational–affective dimension is the emotional response (fear, anxiety) that controls responses to the pain. A study of the anatomical connections of the nociceptive system provides a framework for understanding how all these dimensions of pain are registered and interact within the nervous system.

The physiological basis of nociception, particularly the mechanisms of signalling and modulating nociceptive stimuli, will be covered more specifically in the next chapter.

STRUCTURE AND FUNCTION OF PERIPHERAL NOCICEPTORS

A receptor is specialized nervous tissue sensitive to a particular change in the environment. A change in the

© 2014 Elsevier Ltd.

environment provides the stimulus. Normally, a receptor responds preferentially only to one type of stimulus, called the *adequate stimulus*, not in the sense of magnitude, but rather in its specificity to that receptor. Receptors convert the physical energy of the adequate stimulus into electro-chemical energy that activates the associated neuron.

Nociceptors are a class of peripheral receptors that respond to tissue-damaging or potentially tissue-damaging stimuli (from Latin *nocere*, to injure). The skin is densely innervated by nociceptors, which are present in other body tissues, including bone, muscle, joint capsules, viscera and blood vessels, as well as the meninges and peripheral nerve sheaths. Nociceptors have not been found in articular cartilage, synovial membranes, lung parenchyma, visceral pleura, pericardium, brain or spinal cord tissue. The sim-plest type of sensory receptor is called the free nerve end-ing, which terminates in a naked unmyelinated ending in cutaneous or other tissue. Historically, free nerve end-ings have been believed to subserve only pain, but this is not the case. Moreover, more recent studies of the ultra-structure of these receptors have indicated that their struc-ture is more complex than this descriptive term implies. Its terminals remain ensheathed by Schwann cell processes until they penetrate the epidermal basal lamina (Kruger et al 1981).

The inference that specialized nociceptors existed was made on the basis of experiments on peripheral nerves in humans using graded electrical stimulation and differential nerve blocks (Adrian 1931; Bessou & Perl 1969; Burgess & Perl 1967). These experiments also indicated that pain was signalled by two sets of afferent fibres:

- *small-diameter thinly myelinated fibres (Aδ)* with a conduction velocity of 5–30 m/s – activation of these fibres is associated with well-localized sensations of sharp, pricking pain.
- *small-diameter, unmyelinated C fibres* that conduct slowly (0.5–2 m/s) – these fibres carry diffuse pain sensations that can be dull, poorly localized and persistent (Torebjörk & Ochoa 1980). A class of C fibres, called C-tactile afferents, are present only in hairy skin, and mediate pleasant touch (Löken et al 2009).

This terminology is used in relation to cutaneous and visceral axons (Erlanger & Gasser 1937). A different termi-nology applies in the case of muscle and joint nerves (Table 5.1).

Nociceptors

Nociceptors are complex structures that have heteroge-neous properties, responding to multiple stimulus modal-ities (polymodal). Investigation of responses of specific nociceptors is fraught with difficulty, as a lack of response may indicate a failure to apply a sufficient intensity of stim-ulation. Moreover, application of the stimulus may induce long-term changes in the response properties of the noci-ceptor (Meyer et al 2006).

Aδ nociceptors, although polymodal, can be divided into two main classes on the basis of response to mechanical stimuli, leading to a distinction between mechanically sensitive afferents (MSA) and mechanically insensitive afferents (MIA).

Table 5.1 Classifications of mammalian nerve fibres					
Fibre type (Erlanger/ Gasser)	**Function**	**Group (Lloyd)**	**Function**	**Average fibre diameter (μm)**	**Average conduction velocity (m/s)**
Aα	Primary muscle spindle afferents, motor fibres to motor neurons	I	Primary muscle spindle afferents	15	95
Aβ	Cutaneous touch and pressure afferents	II	Afferents from tendon organs, afferents from cutaneous mechanoreceptors	8	50
Aγ	Motor fibres to muscle spindles			6	20
Aδ	Cutaneous temperature and pain afferents	III	Afferents from deep pressure receptors in muscle	3	15
B	Sympathetic preganglionic fibres			3	7
C	Cutaneous pain afferents (unmyelinated); sympathetic post-ganglionic fibres	IV	Unmyelinated nerve fibres	0.5	1

Type I Aδ nociceptors were initially called high-threshold mechanoreceptors (HTM; Burgess & Perl 1967) because they respond with a slowly adapting discharge to strong punctate pressure and were thought to be unresponsive to heat. However, they have been shown to have very high heat thresholds, usually 53°C or higher (Treede et al 1991). With maintained heat stimuli, HTM receptors will respond and become sensitized with tissue injury (Basbaum et al 2009). Meyer et al (1994) have suggested that the Aδ Type I receptors be termed A-fibre mechano-heat sensitive receptors (AMHs), as they are responsive to both mechanical and heat stimuli. Heat sensitivity in AMHs is mediated by the vanilloid receptor-like protein 1 (TRPV2) receptors (Caterina et al 1999). These units are densely distributed in hairy and glabrous skin (Campbell et al 1979). Their receptive fields are distinctive, consisting of a series of sensitive points that may be spread evenly over an area of several square centimetres in proximal areas. In distal areas, such as the glabrous skin of the hands and feet, or on the face, receptive fields are smaller and may comprise only a single point. These units have myelinated axons (Aδ) with a conducting speed of 5–25 m/s, with a few conducting more quickly in the A–β range (55 m/s). They mediate the 'first' response to pinprick and other intense mechanical stimuli (Basbaum et al 2009).

Type II Aδ nociceptors have a lower heat threshold than Type 1 units, but have very high mechanical thresholds, so they are termed *heat-responsive MIAs*. Mean conduction velocity is 15 m/s. These mediate the 'first' acute pain response to noxious heat. They have been reported in the knee joint (Schaible & Schmidt 1985), viscera (Häbler et al 1990) and cornea (Tanelian 1991). Some of the cutaneous MIAs may be chemospecific receptors, while others may respond to intense cold or heat stimuli (Meyer et al 1991). MIAs are not found in glabrous skin. These receptors may become sensitized to mechanical stimuli after injury.

The *unmyelinated C fibres* are heterogeneous. Most C fibres are polymodal, responding to both mechanical and heat stimuli, hence the term C-fibre mechano-heat sensitive receptor (CMH). Bessou and Perl (1969) have shown that these are the predominant type of C-fibre nociceptor in mammalian skin, comprising about 90% of all afferent C fibres.

The heat responsive terminals of CMHs lie at varying depths beneath the skin (between 20 and 570 μm) and so their heat threshold is dependent on the temperature at the heat responsive terminal and not on the rate of temperature increase (Tillman et al 1995). Mechanical nociceptors with C-axons have a slowly adapting response to mechanical stimuli. They lack the distinctive multipoint receptive fields of the A-fibre units; instead their fields usually consist of a small zone of uniform sensitivity (Iggo 1960; Lynn 1984).

C-tactile fibres are low-threshold mechanoreceptors found in hairy skin. They have small receptive fields (Wessberg et al 2003) and respond vigorously to slow and light stroking (Bessou et al 1971; Vallbo et al 1999).

These fibres mediate pleasant touch sensation, i.e. the affective dimension of sensation.

The chemosensitivity of C-polymodal nociceptors has not been studied as much as their sensitivity to heat and pressure. They can be excited by potassium, histamine, serotonin, bradykinin, capsaicin, mustard oil, acetylcholine and dilute acids, by various means (topical application, intradermal injection, arterial injection) and all in doses that would be painful in humans (see Willis & Coggeshall 1991 for review). Chemicals act on nociceptors by altering the conductance of ion channels in the cell membrane and causing depolarization (Rang et al 1991). This may result in sensitization of the nociceptors, such that they have an increased responsiveness to stimulation. Further information on peripheral sensitization will be presented in Chapter 6.

Cold nociceptors, transmitting along C fibres, have been reported in monkeys (LaMotte & Thalhammer 1982) and in humans (Campero et al 1996). These respond strongly to prolonged cooling of the skin by ice and weakly to strong pressure, but are not responsive to heat. The threshold for cold pain is about 14°C. Because of the delay in response between the onset of the stimulus and report of pain, it has been suggested that cold pain is subserved by deeper receptors than heat pain. The sense of cooling is subserved by primary afferents called cold fibres, which are predominantly Aδ in type. However, cold fibres do not faithfully encode stimuli that induce cold pain (Meyer et al 2005). Cutaneous Aδ nociceptors have ongoing activity at room temperature. They also respond to temperatures below 0°C and encode stimulus intensity (Simone & Kajander 1997). Cold pain is thought to be mediated by nociceptors located in cutaneous veins (Klement & Arndt 1992).

Another way of classifying nociceptors is through identification of neuroanatomical and molecular characteristics (Snider & McMahon 1998). A peptidergic population releases neuropeptides such as substance P and calcitonin gene-related peptide (CGRP), as well as the TrkA neurotrophin receptor. A non-peptidergic population expresses the Ret tyrosine kinase receptor and is sensitive to glial-derived neurotrophic factor (GDNF). These two populations of nociceptors have different central projection patterns. The peptidergic population terminates in lamina I and the outer part of lamina II of the dorsal horn, while the non-peptidergic group terminates in the inner part of lamina II. The functional difference between the two populations is not yet clear (Snider & McMahon 1998).

Skeletal muscle nociceptors

The terminology of Lloyd (1943) is usually used in relation to muscle and joint nerves (Table 5.1). Group III afferent fibres are small-diameter myelinated fibres; group IV fibres are unmyelinated and constitute the majority of muscle nociceptors. Numerous unencapsulated endings can be located in the connective tissue and in the wall of arterioles in skeletal

51

muscle, and can be subdivided into mechanical and polymodal types (Stacey 1969). Effective stimuli are high-intensity mechanical forces, as well as endogenous pain-producing substances such as bradykinin, serotonin and potassium ions. Hypoxia and impaired metabolism following trauma or unaccustomed exercise and increased levels of adrenaline may also activate nociceptors (Kieschke et al 1988; Mense 1993). Group III afferent fibres are responsive to mechanical stimulation of muscle, including stretch (Mense & Stahnke 1983), and many would be activated by exercise and therefore probably function as ergoreceptors. However, a significant proportion of these are nociceptive. Some group III afferents are responsive to the injection of chemicals such as hypertonic sodium chloride (Abrahams et al 1984). Approximately 40% of group IV afferents are classified as low-threshold mechanosensitive (LTM) units and respond to gentle muscle stretch or contraction (Hoheisel et al 2005). These non-nociceptive units control the adjustment of circulation and respiration to the demands of physical exercise (McCloskey & Mitchell 1972). The remaining proportion of group IV afferents are activated with tissue-threatening mechanical stimulation, e.g. when muscle contractions occur during ischaemia (Mense & Meyer 1985), and are called HTM units (Mense 2009). Many are readily activated by pain producing chemicals (Mense & Meyer 1988) or thermal stimuli (Hertel et al 1976).

One of the most relevant chemical causes of muscle pain is a drop in tissue pH (an increase in proton concentration), possibly related to tonic contractions leading to ischaemia or accumulation of lactic acid (Mense 2009). The mechanism is related to the large number of acid-sensing ion channels (ASICs) in the membrane of muscle nociceptors (Hoheisel et al 2004; Sluka et al 2003). Another cause is a release of adenosine triphosphate (ATP) resulting from damage to muscle cells or an increase in permeability of the muscle cell membrane (Burnstock 2007). Other chemical factors are bradykinin, formed in damaged tissue, and serotonin, prostaglandins and nerve growth factor, which have a sensitizing action of group IV afferents (see Mense 2009 for review).

Joint nociceptors

Nociceptors in joints are located in the joint capsule and ligaments, bone, periosteum, articular fat pads and around blood vessels, but not in the joint cartilage. They have been studied predominantly in the knee joint. The terminals of group III and group IV sensory nerve endings comprise multiple axonal beads ensheathed by Schwann cell processes except for some areas of exposed axon membrane containing structural specializations characteristic of receptive sites. The beads thus represent multiple receptive sites (Heppelmann et al 1990). Some of these receptors may be nociceptive.

Joint nociceptors can be classified as:

- high-threshold units that discharge only in response to noxious pressure or extreme joint movement (Bessou & Laporte 1961)

- units that respond to strong pressure but not to movement
- units that do not respond to any mechanical stimulus in the normal joint (MIAs or silent nociceptors) (Schaible & Schmidt 1988).

In the normal joint, only the first type are activated, but all joint afferents become sensitized if the joint becomes inflamed (see Chapter 6).

Visceral nociceptors

In somatic tissue such as skin and muscle there is a clear distinction between mechanorecptive and nociceptive afferents. However, this is not the case in visceral tissue, for which pain may not be reported even in response to tissue-damaging stimuli. Nociceptors are located in visceral organs, including the heart, gastrointestinal tract and reproductive organs, and in the walls of blood vessels. Pain-producing stimuli in the viscera include inflammation, distension of hollow muscular-walled organs such as the gastrointestinal tract, the urinary tract and the gall bladder, ischaemia in organs such as the heart, and traction in the mesentery. Inflammation of visceral organs can induce central sensitization (see Chapter 6) of dorsal horn neurons and may lead to referred hyperalgesia.

Visceral nociceptors are also sensitive to irritating chemicals. Afferent nociceptive fibres in viscera are found in association with both sympathetic and parasympathetic efferents (Meyer et al 1994).

NON-NEURONAL CELLS

It has been increasingly recognized that non-neuronal cells such as immune cells (macrophages and lymphocytes) and glial cells in the peripheral nervous system (Schwann cells and satellite cells) and central nervous system (astrocytes and microglia) play a critical role in chronic pain processing (see Milligan & Watkins 2009 for review). Nerve injury induces substantial changes in both microglia and astrocytes in the spinal cord (Ji et al 2006).

ANATOMY OF REFERRED PAIN

Pain from stimulation of viscera is frequently localized to the surface of the body, a phenomenon termed *referred pain*. This may be explained by the convergence of nociceptive input for deep and cutaneous tissues onto common somatosensory spinal neurons that also receive afferents from topographically separate body regions (the so-called projection–convergence theory; Ruch 1946). There are no separate ascending spinal pathways dedicated to the signalling of sensations from the viscera. These sensations are represented within the known somatosensory pathways. The level of the spinal cord to which visceral afferent fibres from the internal organs project depends on their embryonic innervation. Many viscera migrate well away from their embryonic origin during development, and therefore referred pain from the viscera may be perceived at locations remote from the actual site of the stimulus. For example, the heart is derived from endoderm in the neck and upper thorax, with the result that nociceptive afferents from the heart enter the spinal cord through the dorsal roots C3–T5 rather than lower down. Similarly, afferents from the gall bladder enter the spinal cord at T9 rather than at L1, its location later in life. The pain signals carried by these fibres may be referred to the areas of skin via Aδ fibres to the same segment of the spinal cord. Hence, a heart attack causing ischaemia of cardiac muscle can often present as pain in the left shoulder passing into the left arm (the cutaneous segments supplied by C3–T5). In the same way, an inflamed gall bladder can frequently cause pain at the tip of the right scapula, supplied by T9.

Pain may also be referred from tissues other than viscera, and frequently occurs in musculoskeletal conditions. This type of referred pain has been explained with reference to patterns of dermatomal, myotomal and sclerotomal territories. However, there is enormous individual variation in these territories, as well as variability in presenting symptoms (Grieve 1994).

DORSAL ROOT GANGLION CELLS

The somas of nociceptive afferents are located in the dorsal root ganglia (DRG) and the equivalent ganglia of cranial nerves V, VII, IX and X. DRG cells are pseudo-unipolar neurons conveying information from the periphery into the spinal cord. These cells can be grouped into two classes based on variations in soma size, diameter of axons, morphology of peripheral terminals and site of central terminations. The division into two size classes has a functional correlate in that, generally, large cells giving rise to large-diameter axons relay low-threshold mechanical and proprioceptive stimuli, and small cells relay nociceptive and thermal stimuli (Lawson 1992). Small DRG cells stain intensely and contain many organelles and peptides, including substance P (SP), somatostatin, calcitonin gene-related peptide (CGRP), vasoactive intestinal peptide (VIP) and galanin (Willis & Coggeshall 1991).

PRIMARY AFFERENTS

As primary afferent fibres in peripheral nerves travel towards the spinal cord, they group together to form spinal nerves, each spinal nerve supplying a discrete area of skin (dermatome), and overlapping to a greater or lesser degree the dermatomes of neighbouring spinal nerves. Each spinal nerve splits to form a ventral and dorsal root. The dorsal roots are purely sensory, but a considerable number of small-diameter unmyelinated afferent fibres are located in the ventral root (ventral root afferents; Coggeshall et al 1974; Light & Metz 1978). The majority of these fibres appear to end blindly, with the rest either looping within the ventral roots or branching into the dorsal root (Willis & Coggeshall 1991). The function of the ventral root afferents is, as yet, unclear.

Sorting of primary afferent fibres occurs in the dorsal roots in primates (Snyder 1977). Large-diameter afferents subserving mechanoreception enter the spinal cord in the medial division of the dorsal root, while small-diameter fibres form a lateral bundle. The fibres enter the cord at the dorsal root entry zone. The bundle of small-diameter fibres contains those involved in nociception, together with fibres involved in temperature and visceral sensation. They divide into short ascending and descending branches that run longitudinally in the dorsolateral fasciculus of Lissauer. Within several segments they leave the tract to synapse on neurons in the dorsal horn.

THE DORSAL HORN

The dorsal horn of the spinal cord is the first site for integration and processing of incoming sensory information. The dorsal horn has historically been divided into three broad regions: the marginal zone, the substantia gelatinosa and the nucleus proprius. Rexed (1952, 1954) divided the grey matter of the dorsal horn into six laminae based on cytoarchitectural criteria, the most dorsal being lamina I (Fig. 5.1). Further anatomical and physiological studies have since confirmed functional differences in dorsal horn neurons in different laminae, as well as different patterns of projections. In addition, cells, axons and terminals in the different laminae of the dorsal horn have a distinctive chemical profile, which has been shown to change following a lesion (see Willis & Coggeshall 1991 for review).

Primary afferent fibres terminate in different laminae depending on their function (Fig. 5.2).

Lamina I (the marginal zone) contains a high density of projection neurons that process nociceptive information. There are *nociceptive-specific* neurons that are excited solely by nociceptors and *wide dynamic range* neurons (also in lamina V–VI) that respond to both nociceptive and mechanoreceptive input.

Lamina II is also called the substantia gelatinosa. The most prominent structures in lamina II are complex structures called *glomeruli* through which a primary afferent terminal can make synaptic contact with several peripheral dendrites, axonal terminals and cell bodies (Kerr 1975).

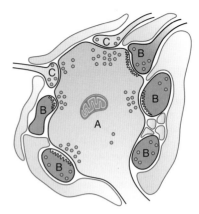

Fig. 5.3 Diagram of a glomerulus based on the work of Kerr (1975). A central terminal; B, dendrites; C, dendritic spines from lamina II neurons. Shaded areas represent glial processes.

Fig. 5.1 The laminae of the spinal cord based on the description of Rexed (1952, 1954). Laminae I–VI comprise the dorsal horn.

Glomeruli are key structures of the dorsal horn because they offer a morphological basis for both presynaptic and postsynaptic modulation of the primary afferent input. They comprise a central primary afferent terminal that makes contact with a group of between four and eight surrounding dendrites and other peripheral axon terminals, and are set apart from the surrounding tissue by glial processes (Fig. 5.3). Using morphological criteria, the peripheral terminals appear to have the characteristics of inhibitory synapses and may contain the inhibitory neurotransmitters γ-aminobutyric acid (GABA) or enkephalin. The central terminals have the characteristics of excitatory terminals and may contain CGRP, glutamate, SP, cholecystokinin or serotonin. The glomerulus therefore comprises a complicated arrangement of inhibitory synaptic terminals surrounding an excitatory primary afferent ending.

The neuropil of *lamina III* resembles that of lamina II, but has slightly larger cells and myelinated axons. *Laminae IV and V* are characterized by neurons of various sizes. Lamina IV has prominent large cells, while lamina V is

Fig. 5.2 The terminations of afferent fibres in the dorsal horn vary by depth. Large fibres (Aα and Aβ) enter in the medial division and small fibres (Aδ and C) enter in the lateral division of the dorsal root.

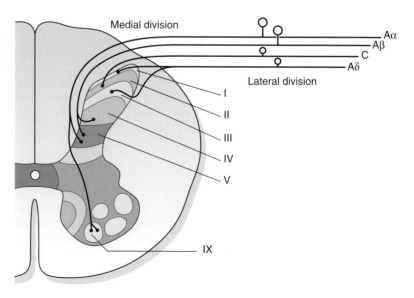

distinguished by longitudinally oriented myelinated axons. Laminae III, IV and the upper part of lamina V comprise most of the nucleus proprius.

Lamina VI is present only in cervical and lumbosacral enlargements and is a transition zone between the primary afferent-dominated dorsal horn and the ventral horn, with descending input predominating.

A population of neurons responding to noxious mechanical and thermal stimuli has been reported in *lamina X* in the vicinity of the central canal of the spinal cord. In addition to these high-threshold type cells, lamina X also contains neurons that are low threshold and have a wide dynamic range. Many of the cells have convergent input from visceral afferent fibres, and some of these respond only to visceral stimuli (Honda 1985; Honda & Perl 1985).

Terminations of afferent fibres in the dorsal horn

The incoming afferent fibres of all types establish a web of connections with dorsal horn neurons, exerting a changing pattern of excitatory and inhibitory inputs that determines the firing of dorsal horn projection neurons and of interneurons that mediate spinal reflex responses (Table 5.2). Normally there is a certain degree of segregation in the termination pattern for different afferent fibre classifications in the dorsal horn, but this may not be the case in pathological situations. Woolf et al (1992) showed that peripheral nerve injury triggers sprouting of myelinated afferents into lamina II, resulting in the possibility of functional contacts of low-threshold mechanoreceptive afferents with cells that normally have only C-fibre input.

Large-diameter myelinated fibres

Collaterals of the large Aβ fibres initially travel ventrally through the dorsal horn but reverse when they reach the deeper laminae, and break up to give rise to large flame-shaped arbors as they course dorsally. These terminations are dense in laminae III, IV and V. It has been shown that the distal parts of the arbors of

hair-follicle afferents enter the innermost part of lamina II (Brown 1981).

Small-diameter myelinated fibres

Collaterals of Aδ fibres terminate both superficially and deep within the dorsal horn. High-threshold afferents terminate profusely with arborizations in lamina I. Low-threshold hair afferents pass through lamina I to terminate in lamina V (Mense & Prabhakar 1986).

Unmyelinated fibres

Unmyelinated afferents terminate in the superficial dorsal horn. Lamina II is the site of termination of primary afferent fibres from the skin, with visceral afferents terminating in laminae I and II with some extension to lamina III (Gobel et al 1981; LaMotte 1977).

Peptidergic C fibres terminate in lamina I and the dorsal part of lamina II. Non-peptidergic fibres terminate in mid-lamina II. The ventral part of lamina II has excitatory interneurons expressing the gamma isoform of protein kinase C, which has been implicated in persistent pain post-injury (Malmberg et al 1997).

Visceral projections

Myelinated axons innervating abdominal and pelvic viscera can be classified into high- or low-threshold mechanoreceptive groups. They project to lamina I or deeper laminae V–VI (de Groat et al 1981; Morgan et al 1981).

Visceral afferent fibres terminate predominantly in lamina I, but have also been reported in laminae II, IV–V and X (Sugiura et al 1989).

Somatotopic organization of dorsal horn

The dorsal horn in the cervical and lumbar enlargements appears to be somatotopically organized with distal regions being represented medially and proximal areas laterally. There is a rostrocaudal representation of the digits, with the first digit being represented most rostrally and the fifth digit most caudally (Brown et al 1989; Florence et al 1988; Wilson et al 1986).

Response properties of dorsal horn neurons

Three major classes of dorsal horn neurons have been recognized (McMahon 1984):

1. low-threshold mechanosensitive (LTM), in which the cells are only excited by low-threshold innocuous stimuli such as hair movement, touching or brushing the skin

Table 5.2 Terminations of afferent fibres in the dorsal horn	
Afferents	**Terminal zones in dorsal horn**
Large diameter myelinated fibres	III, IV and V
Small diameter myelinated fibres (Aδ)	I and V
Unmyelinated fibres (C)	II, III
Visceral projections	II, IV–V and X

2. nociceptive-specific (NS), where only high-threshold noxious or near-noxious levels of peripheral stimulation excite the cells
3. wide dynamic range (WDR) or convergent cells, where the firing rate of the cells is increased by innocuous events, but further increased when stimulus intensity is raised to noxious levels.

This classification does not imply that each class of neurons is homogeneous. The properties of neurons in the dorsal horn depend to some extent on their location. A proportion of lamina I neurons is NS (Christensen & Perl 1970), but WDR cells form the largest population of neurons in this lamina. The dendrites of lamina I cells remain within the lamina and these cells give rise to an ascending projection to the thalamus (Trevino & Carstens 1975). Lamina II cells are predominantly of the WDR type, while lamina III cells are predominantly LTM.

Wall (1967) demonstrated that lamina IV cells were predominantly of the LTM type and often received input from large-diameter afferents only. Their receptive fields, located in distal regions of the body, tend to be smaller and have distinct edges. In lamina V, all three classes of cells are represented but the WDR type more frequently. Many of these cells have long ascending axons that reach supraspinal levels, some of them directly reaching the thalamus. WDR cells are excited by C fibres as well as by A fibres, and this input reaches them either via lamina II cells or by synapses on their distant dendrites. Many lamina V cells have dendrites which reach lamina II.

SPINAL CORD TRANSMISSION PATHWAYS

Ascending tracts

Somatosensory signals are conveyed along two major ascending systems in the spinal cord: the anterolateral system and the dorsal column-medial lemniscal system. The latter carries information about tactile sensation and limb proprioception. The anterolateral system relays information predominantly about pain and temperature, but also some tactile information. It comprises three pathways: the spinothalamic tract, the spinoreticular tract and the spinomesencephalic tract (Fig. 5.4).

The spinothalamic tract (STT) originates from neurons along the length of the spinal cord, with a particularly large concentration of STT cells in the uppermost cervical segments, including a large ipsilateral group of neurons in the ventral horn. Below this level, the majority of STT neurons are contralateral to their target. In the primate, STT neurons are located in three main regions: laminae I, IV–V and VII–VIII and comprise both nociceptive-specific

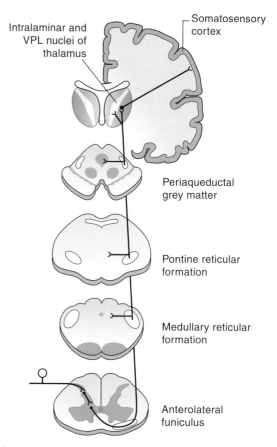

Fig. 5.4 Organization of the anterolateral system. Primary axons terminate in the dorsal horn. Second-order axons cross the midline and ascend in the anterolateral funiculus in the spinal cord and the spinal lemniscus in the brainstem to terminate in the thalamus. Collaterals of these axons terminate in the reticular formation (spinoreticular axons) and in the periaqueductal grey matter (spinomesencephalic axons) (shaded). Thalamocortical axons then project to the somatosensory cortex.

and wide dynamic range neurons. Some STT neurons are also in laminae II, III and X (Apkarian & Hodge 1989a). The axons cross the midline in the dorsal and ventral white commissures at a level near the cell body and ascend to the thalamus in the lateral funiculus on the contralateral side. While most of the axons occupy the ventral lateral quadrant of the spinal white matter, some axons, particularly those originating from lamina I cells, ascend in the dorsal lateral quadrant (Apkarian & Hodge 1989b). The STT in the lateral funiculus has a somatotopic organization. Axons from the most caudal regions of the spinal cord occupy the most dorsolateral position, with axons from progressively more rostral levels joining the tract in more ventromedial positions (Applebaum et al 1975). In the brain stem the STT passes dorsolateral to the inferior olivary nucleus in the medulla, then ascends dorsolateral to the medial lemniscus through higher levels of the brain stem to the thalamus. The spinothalamic tract transmits nociceptive and thermal information, as well as touch sensations.

The spinoreticular tract (SRT) in the primate originates from neurons in laminae VII and VIII, as well as the lateral part of lamina V. Some neurons are in lamina X. The majority of neurons giving rise to the SRT are in the uppermost cervical segments, although cells from all levels of the spinal cord are involved (Kevetter et al 1982). There are two components: a projection to the lateral reticular nucleus (a pre-cerebellar nucleus) and a projection to the pontine and medullary reticular formation, which gives rise to descending pathways to the spinal cord. Most of the projections from the cervical and lumbar enlargements cross the midline near the level of the cell bodies, but some axons originating from cervical segments remain uncrossed. They ascend in the ventral lateral column of the spinal cord with the STT and form a prominent bundle lateral to it in the brain stem. The SRT has no obvious somatotopic organization and terminates in the following nuclei of the reticular formation: nucleus medullae oblongatae centralis, lateral reticular nucleus, nucleus reticularis gigantocellularis, nucleus reticularis pontis caudalis and oralis, nucleus paragigantocellularis dorsalis and lateralis, and nucleus subcoeruleus (Mehler et al 1960).

The *spinomesencephalic tract* (SMT) is a collection of pathways from the spinal cord to several different midbrain nuclei. It originates primarily from neurons in laminae I, V, VII and X (Zhang et al 1990). The majority of axons cross the midline and ascend with the STT and SRT in the ventral lateral column. The SMT projects to the nucleus cuneiformis, the parabrachial nucleus, the intercollicular nucleus, the deep layers of the superior colliculus, the nucleus of Darkschewitsch, the anterior and posterior pretectal nuclei, the red nucleus, the Edinger–Westphal nucleus, the interstitial nucleus of Cajal and the periaqueductal grey (Yezierski 1988). The SMT is roughly somatotopically organized, with the projection from the cervical enlargement terminating more rostrally than that from the lumbosacral region. The periaqueductal grey contains neurons that are part of a descending pathway that regulates pain transmission.

Other tracts in the dorsolateral funiculus and the dorsal columns also convey nociceptive information (Fig. 5.5). The *spinocervical tract* (SCT) originates from laminae III and IV at all levels of the cord where neurons respond predominantly to tactile stimuli, but some are activated by noxious stimuli. The axons project ipsilaterally in the dorsolateral funiculus to the lateral cervical nucleus, located just ventrolateral to the dorsal horn in segments C1–C3. The lateral cervical nucleus is quite small in the primate (Mizuno et al 1967), and may be present in some humans, although it is possible that the nucleus may not be distinctly

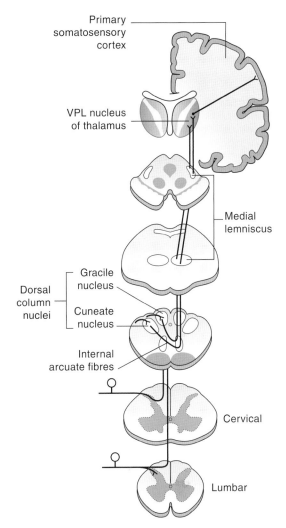

Fig. 5.5 Organization of the dorsal column-medial lemniscal system. Large-diameter axons enter the spinal cord and ascend in the dorsal columns to the medulla, where they synapse in the dorsal column nuclei (nucleus gracilis and nucleus cuneatus). Second-order axons cross the midline and ascend in the medial lemniscus to terminate in the VPL nucleus of the thalamus. Thalamocortical axons then project to the somatosensory cortex.

separate from the dorsal horn in some cases (Ha & Morin 1964; Kircher & Ha 1968; Truex et al 1965). Most of the neurons in the lateral cervical nucleus cross the midline in the ventral white commissure and ascend in the medial lemniscus to midbrain nuclei and to the thalamus.

The *dorsal column-medial lemniscal system* consists of branches of primary afferent fibres conveying tactile and proprioceptive information, as well as the axons of neurons in laminae IV–VI. There are also unmyelinated primary afferent fibres that synapse in the dorsal column nuclei, presumably arising from nociceptors (Patterson et al 1990). In addition, there is a visceral pain pathway ascending in the dorsal column (Al-Chaer et al 1998; Hirschberg et al 1996; Willis et al 1999). The medially located fasciculus gracilis contains a representation of the lower part of the trunk and lower extremity, whereas the fasciculus cuneatus lateral to it contains a representation of the upper part of the trunk and the upper extremity. This tract projects to the dorsal column nuclei in the medulla, from which axons ascend in the medial lemniscus to the thalamus. The sensory representation in the dorsal column nuclei is somatotopic with caudal parts of the body represented medially in the nucleus gracilis and the rostral regions laterally in the nucleus cuneatus. The trunk representation is in a region between the two nuclei. The distal extremities are represented dorsally and the proximal body ventrally (Johnson et al 1968).

TRIGEMINAL SYSTEM

Somatic sensation of the head and oral cavity is carried by four cranial nerves: the *trigeminal nerve* (innervates most of the head and oral cavity), the *facial, glossopharyngeal* and the *vagus* (innervate the skin of the external ear, pharynx, nasal cavity and middle ear). The meninges are innervated by the trigeminal and vagus nerves. The trigeminal nerve is the largest cranial nerve, with four nuclei: the motor nucleus, the main sensory nucleus, the spinal nucleus and the mesencephalic nucleus. As is the case with sensory inputs to the rest of the body, tactile sensation is mediated by large-diameter myelinated fibres, and pain and temperature sensations are mediated by small-diameter myelinated and unmyelinated fibres.

The sensory nuclei of the trigeminal nerve consist of three different parts. From caudal to rostral these are the *nucleus of the spinal tract*, the *main or principal sensory nucleus* and the *mesencephalic sensory nucleus* (Fig. 5.6). The fibres of the sensory root enter the pons and course dorsomedially towards the sensory nucleus. About half the fibres divide into ascending or descending branches as they enter the pons; the remainder ascend or descend without division. Many of the latter are very long and descend as the spinal tract of the trigeminal nerve to the caudal end of the medulla where it fuses with the dorsolateral tract of Lissauer in the spinal cord. As the tract descends, collaterals are given off to a long nucleus lying immediately medial to it, the *nucleus of the spinal tract*, which is continuous with the substantia gelatinosa of the dorsal horn. The *spinal nucleus* extends caudally through the whole length of the medulla and into the spinal cord as far as the second cervical segment. In the medulla, the tract and its nucleus are situated beneath the surface, with the upper part producing an elevation called the tuberculum cinereum.

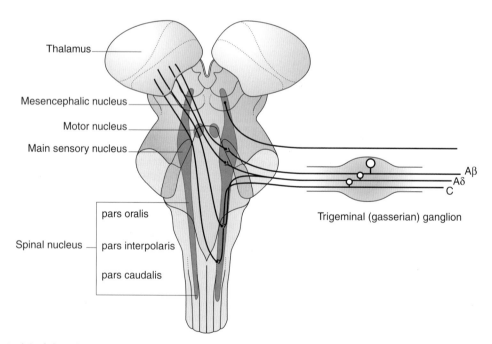

Fig. 5.6 Nuclei of the trigeminal nerve and their afferent connections. The cell bodies of most of the primary sensory neurons are in the trigeminal (Gasserian) ganglion, with the remainder in the mesencephalic nucleus. Small-diameter fibres subserving pain and temperature enter the spinal nucleus and synapse in the pars caudalis. Second-order axons cross the midline to form the trigeminothalamic tract.

Large-diameter axons of the trigeminal nerve terminate in the *main sensory nucleus*. The majority of neurons in the main sensory nucleus give rise to axons that decussate in the pons and ascend dorsomedial to fibres from the dorsal column nuclei in the medial lemniscus. These ascending fibres (the *trigeminal lemniscus*) synapse in the medial division of the ventral posterior nucleus of the thalamus (VPM). From here, the axons of the thalamic neurons project to the primary somatosensory cortex. This is the principal pathway for tactile perception in the face and is analogous to the dorsal column/medial lemniscal system. The main sensory nucleus of the trigeminal nerve is functionally similar to the dorsal column nuclei.

Pain and temperature are conveyed by smaller diameter fibres terminating in the spinal part of the nucleus. The spinal trigeminal nucleus can be divided into three morphologically different parts: the *nucleus caudalis*, the *nucleus interpolaris* and the *nucleus oralis*. The nucleus caudalis mediates facial sensation. Like the dorsal horn, it plays an important role in pain and temperature senses, including dental pain, and a lesser role in tactile sensation. The nucleus interpolaris plays a role in mediating sensation from the teeth and the nucleus oralis is thought to be involved with discriminative touch sensation. Structurally and functionally, the nucleus caudalis resembles the dorsal horn on the basis of a number of features: (a) morphology and lamination, (b) laminar distribution of afferent terminals and (c) laminar distribution of projection neurons. The caudal nucleus is sometimes called the medullary dorsal horn (Fig. 5.7) because its laminar organization is similar to the spinal dorsal horn (Dubner & Bennett 1983; Martin 1996).

Lamina I is equivalent to the marginal zone of the dorsal horn, and the portion of the spinal tract overlying lamina I of the spinal nucleus is the rostral extension of Lissauer's tract. Lamina II is equivalent to the substantia gelatinosa, and laminae III and IV, termed the magnocellular nucleus in the trigeminal system, are equivalent to the nucleus proprius. Each of these structures is associated with neurons responding to various types of stimuli. Those in the deep regions respond to both nociceptive and innocuous stimuli (wide dynamic range neurons), while neurons responding specifically to nociceptive or thermal stimuli are located in the substantia gelatinosa. There is an 'onion skin' pattern of representation of parts of the face in the spinal trigeminal nucleus, where regions around the mouth and nose are represented rostrally in the nucleus, while those in more lateral regions of the face are represented more caudally (Brodal 1981).

The ascending pathway from the spinal nucleus (especially the caudal and interpolar regions) mediates facial and dental pain. The organization of this pathway is similar to that of the anterolateral system. This pathway is called the *trigeminothalamic tract* and is predominantly crossed, ascending with the axons of the spinothalamic tract to the thalamus.

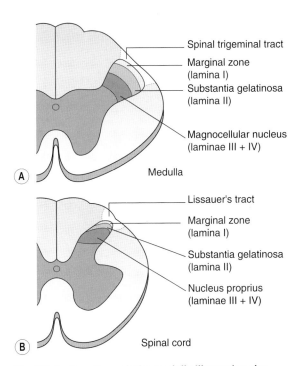

Fig. 5.7 **Section through the medulla illustrating the trigeminal dorsal horn in A. Corresponding areas of the spinal dorsal horn are shown in B.**

SYMPATHETIC NERVOUS SYSTEM

The responses of an organism during pain and stress, which consist of autonomic, neuroendocrine and motor responses, are integral components of an adaptive biological system. They are important for the organism to function in a dynamic, challenging and possibly dangerous environment. The typical autonomic responses consist of an activation of various sympathetic pathways to skeletal muscle, skin, heart and viscera, thus leading to an increase of blood flow through skeletal muscle, increased cardiac output, piloerection, sweating and a reduction of blood flow through skin and viscera (Jänig 1995). Under physiological conditions peripheral sympathetic pathways are distinct with respect to their target organs, and somatosensory pathways are functionally distinct with respect to the peripheral receptors and the corresponding sensations (Jänig 1992). However, following tissue damage this situation may radically change, such that the sympathetic and sensory channels are no longer separated (see below).

The *hypothalamus* has a major role in producing responses to emotional changes and needs, and is responsible for maintaining homeostasis. Through efferent pathways to autonomic ganglia in the brainstem and spinal cord, the hypothalamus controls sympathetic and para-sympathetic functions. The hypothalamus receives inputs from the reticular formation in the brainstem and the amygdala, a collection of nuclei in the temporal lobe that are considered to be part of the limbic system.

The sympathetic pathways from the hypothalamus descend through the brainstem and spinal cord to synapse in the intermediolateral columns of the spinal cord between T1 and L2. In this area are the cell bodies of the *preganglionic neurons*. The preganglionic axons are myelinated and short (white rami), leaving the CNS via the ventral root and synapsing in the paravertebral *sympathetic chain* (ganglia). The sympathetic chain extends from the base of the skull to the coccyx (Fig. 5.8). The *postganglionic axons* are unmyelinated (grey rami) and rejoin the spinal nerves (Fig. 5.9), accompanying the peripheral nerves to innervate the body

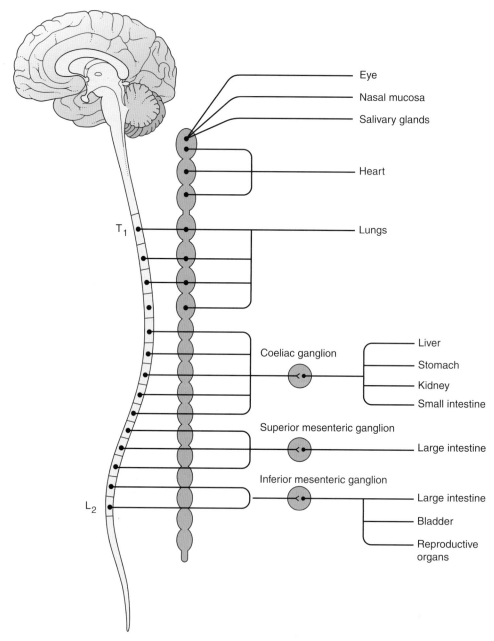

Fig. 5.8 Plan of the sympathetic nervous system. Preganglionic neurons are red, postganglionic neurons are blue. The innervation of blood vessels, sweat glands and piloerector muscles is not shown.

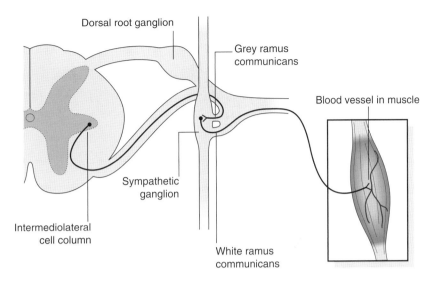

Fig. 5.9 Relationship of sympathetic axons with peripheral nerves.

wall and blood vessels. Sympathetic axons innervating the face and brain arise from the inferior, middle and superior cervical ganglia and follow the carotid and vertebral arteries to their targets.

Clinical observations of changes in skin blood flow and abnormal sudomotor activity affecting regions beyond the distribution of the injured part have implicated sympathetic hyperactivity as a factor in neuropathic pain, which is commonly associated with peripheral nerve injury (see Chapter 10). Sympathetic fibre sprouting and hyperactivity might act partly through abnormal connections between sympathetic and sensory neurons. Using an experimental peripheral nerve lesion model, McLachlan et al (1993) showed that noradrenergic axons in surrounding blood vessels sprout into dorsal root ganglia (on both injured and non-injured sides) and form basket-like structures around large-diameter sensory neurons. Following peripheral nerve injury, both intact sensory neurons (Sato & Perl 1991) and injured or regenerating axons (Wall & Gutnick 1974) develop an ectopic sensitivity to circulating adrenaline and noradrenaline released from post-ganglionic sympathetic nerve terminals, a process mediated by α-adrenoreceptors (Chen et al 1996) (see Chapter 10).

AREAS OF THE BRAIN INVOLVED IN THE PERCEPTION, INTEGRATION AND RESPONSE TO NOCICEPTION

Thalamus

The thalamus represents the final link in the transmission of impulses to the cerebral cortex, processing almost all sensory and motor information prior to its transfer to cortical areas. The thalamus consists of six groups of nuclei: lateral (ventral and dorsal), medial, anterior, intralaminar, midline and reticular (Fig. 5.10):

- The nuclei of the ventral tier of the lateral group are specific relay nuclei, each receiving specific sensory or motor input and projecting to specific regions of the cerebral cortex. Of this group of nuclei, the *ventral posterolateral (VPL)* and *ventral posteromedial (VPM)* nuclei are concerned with sensation from the body and the face, respectively, while the *ventral anterior (VA)* and *ventral lateral (VL)* nuclei are concerned with motor function.
- The nuclei of the dorsal tier of the lateral group and the nuclei of the medial group (*mediodorsal*) are association nuclei, projecting to association cortex (prefrontal association cortex, limbic association cortex, parietal-temporal-occipital association cortex).
- The *anterior nuclei* are specific relay nuclei, with connections to the hypothalamus and the cingulate gyrus.
- The *intralaminar, reticular* and *midline nuclei* are non-specific nuclei, with widespread connections. The intralaminar nuclei receive inputs from the reticular formation in the brainstem.

Termination of spinothalamic afferents in the thalamus

Two subdivisions of the thalamic nuclei receive nociceptive input from spinal projection neurons.

The lateral nuclear group

Spinothalamic afferents from the contralateral side of the spinal cord terminate throughout VPL (Berkley 1980; Boivie 1979; Burton & Craig 1983; Mantyh 1983;

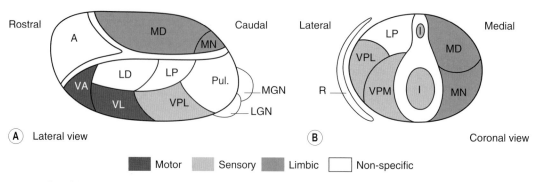

Fig. 5.10 Nuclei of the thalamus in lateral (A) and coronal (B) views. Nuclei associated with limbic functions: A, anterior nucleus; MD, mediodorsal nucleus; LD: lateral dorsal nucleus. Nuclei associated with motor functions: VA, ventral anterior nucleus; VL, ventral lateral nucleus. Nuclei associated with sensory functions: VPL, ventral posterolateral nucleus; VPM, ventral posteromedial nucleus; LGN lateral geniculate nucleus; MGN, medial geniculate nucleus. Nuclei associated with sensory integration: LP, lateral posterior; Pul, pulvinar. Non-specific nuclei: MN, midline nuclei; IL, intralaminar nuclei.

Ralston & Ralston 1992). The terminals of spinothalamic axons overlap with those of the medial lemniscus in VPL of monkeys (Mehler et al 1960) and extend into the ventral posterior inferior nucleus (VPI; Gingold et al 1991), rostrally into VL (Applebaum et al 1979; Berkley 1980; Boivie 1979; Burton & Craig 1983; Craig & Burton 1981) and caudally into the posterior nuclei (Ralston & Ralston 1992). There is a somatotopic organization of spinothalamic terminals in VPL, which appear to be arranged in clusters across the nucleus (Boivie 1979; Mantyh 1983; Mehler et al 1960). The receptive fields of thalamic neurons responsive to nociceptive stimuli are small and their discharge frequency can be related to the intensity and duration of the stimulus (Kenshalo et al 1980). These neurons mediate the sensory–discriminative aspects of pain. Neurons in VPI respond to innocuous mechanical stimuli (Kaas et al 1984) as well as to nociceptive stimuli (Casey & Morrow 1987). The spinothalamic inputs to the lateral thalamic nuclei, which have direct projections to the primary somatosensory cortex (Gingold et al 1991), are known as the *neo*-spinothalamic tract. This structure appears to be most prominently developed in primates.

The medial nuclear group

The medial group of thalamic nuclei, particularly the central lateral nucleus (CL), the intralaminar complex and the mediodorsal nucleus, receives collaterals of the spinothalamic and trigeminothalamic tracts, as well as inputs from the medullary and pontine reticular formation (Apkarian & Hodge 1989c; Burton & Craig 1983; Craig & Burton 1981; Mantyh 1983), the cerebellum (Asanuma et al 1983) and the globus pallidus (Nauta & Mehler 1966). Neurons in CL are responsive to the intensity and duration of nociceptive stimuli, and have large, often bilateral, receptive

fields (Dong et al 1978). Some spinothalamic tract axons project to both the intralaminar nuclei and VPL, and cells giving rise to these projections have small excitatory receptive fields, with surrounding larger inhibitory areas. Their discharge characteristics indicate that they could mediate discriminative aspects of noxious cutaneous stimulation, such as intensity, duration and localization. The receptive fields of cells giving rise to projections to the intralaminar nuclei alone have large bilateral receptive fields (Giesler et al 1981). The diffuse projections of the intralaminar nuclei to many different areas of the cortex have been considered to be part of a non-specific arousal system, but it is also possible that their role is concerned with affective states induced by a painful stimulus. These nuclei are characterized by significant numbers of opiate receptors (see Jones 1985 for review). Because these medial projections to the thalamus appeared first in vertebrate evolution, they have been termed the *paleo*-spinothalamic tract.

Brainstem

Periaqueductal grey matter

The periaqueductal grey matter (PAG) surrounds the cerebral aqueduct of the midbrain. Anatomically, the PAG can be divided into medial, dorsal, dorsolateral and ventrolateral regions, each region forming longitudinal columns that have a high degree of functional specificity (Bandler & Keay 1996; Bandler & Shipley 1994; Bandler et al 1991; Henderson et al 1998). Through these longitudinal columns the PAG has reciprocal connections with all levels of the nervous system and plays an important role in integrating a large number of functions that are critical to survival through its influence on the nociceptive, autonomic and motor systems (Bandler & Keay 1996; Bandler & Shipley 1994; Behbehani 1995; Bernard & Bandler 1998; Keay & Bandler

1993; Morgan et al 1998). Functions controlled by PAG include pain facilitation, analgesia, fear and anxiety, vocalization, sexual behaviour and cardiovascular control (Behbehani 1995; Bernard & Bandler 1998).

Pain modulation can be demonstrated from stimulation of various regions of the PAG. However, stimulation of the dorsolateral and ventrolateral subregions of the PAG produces different autonomic and motor responses (Lovick 1991; Morgan 1991) based on differing patterns of projections. In addition to the inputs from the spinal cord via the spinomesencephalic tract, the PAG also receives afferents from the parafascicular nucleus of the thalamus, the hypothalamus, the amygdala (Gray & Magnuson 1992), frontal and insular cortex (Hardy & Leichnetz 1981), the reticular formation, locus coeruleus (adrenergic projections) and other catecholaminergic nuclei in the brainstem (Herbert & Saper 1992). The ascending projections from the dorsolateral PAG are to the central lateral and paraventricular thalamic nuclei and the anterior hypothalamic area (Cameron et al 1995a). The descending projections are to the locus coeruleus the pericoerulear region and the nucleus paragigantocellularis (Cameron et al 1995b). The ventrolateral PAG, on the other hand, projects rostrally to the parafascicular and centromedian thalamic nuclei, the lateral hypothalamic area (Cameron et al 1995a) and the orbital frontal cortex (Coffield et al 1992). The descending projections are to the pontine reticular formation and the nucleus raphe magnus (Basbaum & Fields 1984; Cameron et al 1995b). Stimulation of the PAG or the nucleus raphe magnus inhibits spinothalamic tract cells (Fields & Basbaum 1994) (Fig. 5.11). This difference in anatomical connectivity between the dorsolateral and ventrolateral regions of the PAG may provide a basis for their distinct and opposite modulatory influences on pain, autonomic and motor function.

Reticular formation

The reticular formation comprises a number of morphologically and biochemically different groups of neurons distributed throughout the medulla, pons and midbrain. There is a projection from the reticular formation to the intralaminar nuclei of the thalamus (Peschanski & Besson 1984), which are known to be involved in the processing of nociceptive information (Kenshalo et al 1980), as well as a projection to the spinal cord. It is important to note that there are reciprocal connections between the reticular formation and the limbic system. As previously discussed, the nuclei of the reticular formation receive nociceptive inputs through the spinoreticular tract (Mehler et al 1960). The reticular formation is involved in several different functions: activation of the brain for behavioural arousal, modulation of segmental stretch reflexes via the reticulospinal tracts, control of breathing and cardiac functions, and modulation of pain.

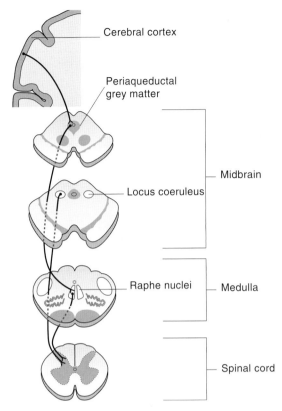

Fig. 5.11 The descending brainstem pathways from periaqueductal grey matter, raphe nucleus and locus coeruleus involved in pain inhibition.

Dorsolateral pontine tegmentum

Noradrenergic neurons of the pontine tegmentum, mainly from the locus coeruleus, contribute to pain modulation by inhibiting spinothalamic activity in the dorsal horn through binding of noradrenaline on the primary afferent neuron, which directly suppresses the release of substance P (Lipp 1991).

Rostral ventral medulla

Two nuclei that are widely implicated in descending control of nociception are the nucleus raphe magnus and the dorsal raphe nucleus. The nucleus raphe magnus receives inputs from the PAG and the dorsal raphe nucleus, and is believed to mediate some of the effects of PAG stimulation (Fig. 5.12). The raphe nuclei and adjacent nuclear groups contain serotonin (5HT) and project via the dorsolateral funiculus of the spinal cord to the superficial laminae of the dorsal horn, where the release of serotonin inhibits wide-dynamic range neurons (Lipp 1991). The dorsal raphe nucleus also has ascending projections to the thalamus and hypothalamus, the basal ganglia and the amygdala, and has been shown to modulate the activity

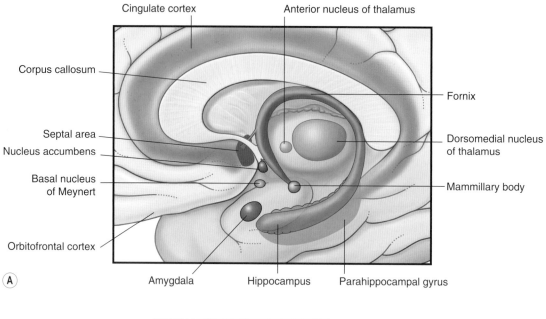

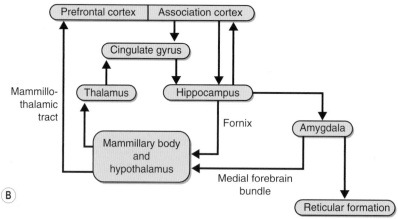

Fig. 5.12 **(A) Limbic areas of the brain. (B) Diagram of neural circuits within the limbic system.**

induced by noxious stimulation of neurons in the thalamus (Wang & Nakai 1994).

The nucleus paragigantocellularis in the ventromedial medulla also receives input from the PAG and gives rise to a large projection to the locus coeruleus, as well as to the nucleus raphe magnus and the spinal cord (Stamford 1995).

Limbic structures

Broca (1878) first described the *limbic lobe* as consisting of the cingulate gyrus, the parahippocampal gyrus as well as the subcallosal gyrus and the hippocampal formation. Papez (1937) suggested that the limbic lobe formed a neural circuit providing the anatomical substrate for emotion. It was MacLean (1955) who recommended the term *limbic*

system, which refers to a much more extensive complex of structures including the limbic lobe, the temporal pole, the anterior portion of the insula, the posterior orbital surface of the frontal lobe and a number of subcortical structures, such as the thalamus, hypothalamus, septal nuclei and the amygdala (Fig. 5.12).

Evidence from lesion studies seems to indicate that the limbic structures may provide a neural basis for the aversive behaviours that comprise the motivational dimension of pain. Studies of transections of the brain at different levels in the 1920s demonstrated the importance of the hypothalamus for the expression of emotional behaviour, both with respect to the somatic component (control of facial and limb muscles) and the visceral component (control of glands and muscles by the autonomic nervous system). Displays of intense emotional behaviour are accompanied by sympathetic responses, such as increased levels of adrenaline and noradrenaline, increased heart rate and piloerection, shunting of blood to the muscles and brain, and pupil dilation, in order to bring the animal to a high level of alertness and ready for any physical action. The hypothalamus causes the release of hormonal endorphins (β-endorphins) from the pituitary gland; these bind to opiate receptors in the brain and spinal cord and are a potent source of pain inhibition.

Ablation of the amygdala and overlying cortex in the cat cause changes in affective behaviour, including reduced responsiveness to noxious stimuli (Schreiner & Kling 1953). In humans, surgical section of the cingulum bundle, a tract connecting the frontal cortex with the hippocampus, was carried out to provide relief in cases of intractable pain, such as that from an inoperable carcinoma. Although still able to perceive the pain postoperatively, the patients seemed unconcerned about it. The aversive quality of the pain and the need to seek pain relief both appeared to be diminished.

Basal ganglia

Three large subcortical nuclei comprise the basal ganglia: *caudate*, *putamen* (together called the *corpus striatum*) and the *globus pallidus* (*external and internal components*). There are interconnections with the *subthalamic nucleus* and the *substantia nigra* (comprising the pars reticulata and the pars compacta), which are also considered to be part of the basal ganglia (Fig. 5.13). The basal ganglia have a markedly heterogeneous structure, structurally, neurochemically and

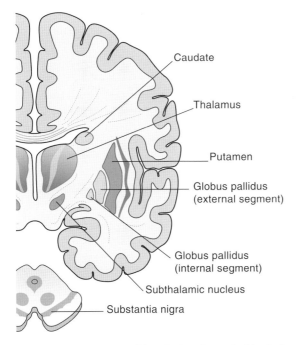

Fig. 5.13 **Structures comprising the basal ganglia (shaded).**

Labels on figure:
- Caudate
- Thalamus
- Putamen
- Globus pallidus (external segment)
- Globus pallidus (internal segment)
- Subthalamic nucleus
- Substantia nigra

functionally. Their role in movement control is evident from two common motor disorders affecting the basal ganglia, Parkinson's disease and Huntingdon's disease, both of which are caused by deficiencies in specific neurotransmitters.

The striatum receives afferent input from the entire cerebral cortex via the topographically organized corticostriate projection, as well as from other nuclei that comprise the basal ganglia, and projects to the ventral lateral, ventral posterior, mediodorsal and centromedian nuclei of the thalamus. Through this circuit there are projections back to different regions of the cerebral cortex. There are at least four open-loop circuits between the cerebral cortex and basal ganglia: a motor loop, concerned with regulation of movement, a cognitive loop, concerned with aspects of memory, a limbic loop concerned with emotional aspects of movement and an oculomotor loop concerned with the control of saccadic eye movements (Côté & Crutcher 1991). In the motor loop the putamen receives inputs from motor, somatosensory and parietal cortex, from the intralaminar nuclei of the thalamus, predominantly the centromedian nucleus and dopaminergic projections from the pars compacta of the substantia nigra. The putamen projects to the globus pallidus and substantia nigra and through these to the ventral anterior and ventral lateral nuclei of the thalamus, which in turn project to the prefrontal and premotor cortex. The cognitive loop passes between the association areas of cortex, through the caudate, globus pallidus and ventral anterior nucleus of the thalamus, which then projects to prefrontal cortex. The limbic loop passes between the cingulate gyrus, lateral orbitofrontal cortex and amygdala through the nucleus accumbens (ventral striatum) and the ventral globus pallidus, returning via the mediodorsal nucleus of the thalamus to the premotor cortex and supplementary motor cortex. This loop is likely to be involved in giving motor expression to emotions, e.g. smiling, gesturing, adoption of aggressive posture, etc.

The striatum is not a homogeneous collection of cells but is organized in compartments: islands of cell called striosomes, and the surrounding regions called matrix (Goldman & Nauta 1977). The majority of cortical projections to the striatum concerned with sensation and movement terminate in the matrix compartment. This compartment projects to the globus pallidus and the pars reticulata of the substantia nigra and inhibits the output from this region to the cortex via the ventral anterior and mediodorsal nuclei of the thalamus. The result is a disinhibition of the target cells in the cortex. The striosomes receive inputs from limbic regions, and project to the pars compacta of the substantia nigra where they inhibit dopaminergic cells which have a feedback loop onto matrix cells (Gerfen 1992). In primates there is a third compartment (matrisomes), which receive complex combinations of inputs from ipsilateral and contralateral motor and somatosensory areas (Flaherty & Graybiel 1993). Cells projecting to the globus pallidus, through which the basal ganglia project to the thalamus, are characterized by various neurotransmitters and neuropeptides. Those projecting to the external segment express GABA, enkephalin and the D2 receptors for dopamine, while those projecting to the internal segment express GABA, substance P, dynorphin and the D1 receptors for dopamine (Graybiel 1991). These parallel systems, each with a unique combination of connections and neurotransmitters, provide the structural basis for modulating the responsiveness of the basal ganglia to cortical inputs (Gerfen 1992).

Electrophysiological, metabolic and blood flow studies have demonstrated that neurons in the basal ganglia are responsive to noxious and non-noxious somatosensory information. Nociceptive neurons have been located in the substantia nigra, caudate, putamen and globus pallidus. There are neurons with large receptive fields that encode stimulus intensity, and another population of neurons responds selectively to noxious stimuli, but does not code stimulus intensity (Chudler et al 1993). Basal ganglia disease may be accompanied by changes in pain perception, and between 10 and 29% of patients with Parkinson's disease complain of pain symptoms not associated with motor dysfunction (Sandyk et al 1988). These observations, as well as the anatomical and neurochemical connections of the basal ganglia, have led to the suggestion that they have a role in the sensory–discriminative, affective and cognitive aspects of pain, as well as in the modulation of nociceptive information (Chudler & Dong 1995).

Cerebral cortex

The thalamocortical projections from the ventral posterolateral nucleus of the thalamus have as their target the primary somatosensory area of the cerebral cortex. This area (primary somatosensory, SI) of anthropoid primates is differentiable into three cytoarchitectonic subfields, areas 3, 1 and 2 of Brodmann. Each structurally distinctive cortical field subserves a specific function, that is, there are functionally different neuron populations in each of these areas, with area 3a receiving proprioceptive inputs from muscle spindles, areas 3b/1 receiving inputs from cutaneous receptors and area 2 receiving input from deep pressure receptors (Kaas et al 1979). The contralateral body surface is represented sequentially in each of these cortical areas. The regions of the body surface with the greatest tactile acuity, the face and the hand, are maximally represented in the cortical projection to the postcentral gyrus. These representational maps are dynamic and they change as a result of experience (Buonomano & Merzenich 1998).

Fewer than 25% of ascending thalamocortical axons are capable of relaying nociceptive and thermal information to SI, and these project predominantly from the VPL, VPI and CL nuclei (Gingold et al 1991). Nociceptive information is most likely to be transmitted to areas 3b and 1, relayed from neurons located along the dorsal and ventral regions of the medial part of VPL. The VPI has connections with SI and SII (Cusick & Gould 1990), but it is not known whether nociceptive inputs to VPI are relayed only to SI

or to both SI and SII. CL has diffuse cortical projections. Although stimulation of CL gives rise to motor responses (Schlag-Rey & Schlag 1984), spinothalamic projections to CL do not contact thalamocortical neurons projecting to primary motor cortex (Greenan & Strick 1986).

Cortical representation of pain

Many different imaging techniques have been used to investigate acute pain processing in healthy subjects. In addition to the SI cortex (Bushnell et al 1999), multiple cortical areas are activated by painful stimuli, including the SII, the anterior cingulate cortex (Talbot et al 1991), the insula, the prefrontal cortex (Treede et al 1999) and the supplementary motor area (Coghill et al 1994). Subcortical activity has been observed in the thalamus and cerebellum. There is a distributed cortical system, involving parietal, cingulate and frontal regions, involved in the dynamic coding of pain intensity over time (Porro et al 1998). These cortical regions also give rise to corticospinal projection (Galea & Darian-Smith 1994) and are also activated during active movement (Colebatch et al 1991; Deiber et al 1991; Matelli et al 1993; Seitz & Roland 1992). Pain-related activation is more widely dispersed across both thalamic and cortical regions than that produced by innocuous vibratory stimuli, which is focused on SI. This distributed cerebral activation reflects the complex nature of pain, involving discriminative, affective, autonomic and motor components (Coghill et al 1994). Parietal areas, including SI, are mainly involved in the sensory–discriminative aspects whereas frontal–limbic connections subserve the affective dimension of pain experience. For example, a study using positron emission tomography showed that hypnotic suggestion used to manipulate the unpleasantness of pain changed the regional cerebral blood flow (rCBF) response in the anterior cingulate region but not in SI (Rainville et al 1997).

Little is known about the central mechanisms responsible for integrating incoming nociceptive information that results in a motor response (Chudler & Dong 1995). An ongoing barrage of nociceptive input, as in the chronic pain situation, may potentially affect motor output and control. The opposite might also occur whereby active movement (exercise) could potentially modulate nociception, presumably through corticospinal pathways (see Chapter 13).

Corticospinal projections

Corticospinal projections are the only direct link between the sensorimotor cortex and the spinal cord. The origin of corticospinal projections in the primate cortex is more extensive than is commonly recognized. They comprise parallel, somatotopically organized projections to each level of the spinal cord with unique, though overlapping, patterns of termination. In addition to a dense projection from the motor cortex, corticospinal fibres arise from the premotor cortex, the postcentral cortex, especially the posterior parietal areas, the second somatosensory area and the caudal part of the insula. On the medial surface, there are extensive projections to the spinal cord from the supplementary motor area and the cortex within the cingulate sulcus (Dum & Strick 1991; Galea & Darian-Smith 1994) (Fig. 5.14).

Each of these cortical regions is distinguished not only by a characteristic cytoarchitecture, but also by a unique set of subcortical connections via the thalamus. The subcortical input to the precentral regions, including SMA and primary motor cortex, is mainly from the cerebellum and basal ganglia, whereas the input to the parietal corticospinal neuron populations is largely somatosensory (Darian-Smith et al 1990). The anterior cingulate cortex and insular cortex have connections with the limbic system (Baleydier & Maugiere 1980; Mesulam & Mufson 1982; Pandya et al 1981; Vogt & Pandya 1987), and may have particular relevance to avoidance behaviour (Shima et al 1991). Furthermore, the regions giving rise to corticospinal projections have complex, often reciprocal, cortico–cortical connections (Barbas & Pandya 1987; Cavada & Goldman-Rakic 1989; Preuss & Goldman-Rakic 1991). Both parietal and premotor cortical areas have converging inputs to the motor cortex (Leichnetz 1986; Matelli et al 1986; Muakkassa & Strick 1979; Petrides & Pandya 1984).

The direct cortical projections to the dorsal horn arise from postcentral cortical areas. However, there are corticospinal projections from other brain areas to other spinal cord laminae-containing spinothalamic neurons. Areas 3b/1 and 2/5 have projections to laminae III–VI, with the greatest concentration medially (Cheema et al 1984; Coulter & Jones 1977; Ralston & Ralston 1985). Cheema et al (1984) identified labelling in the superficial laminae of the dorsal horn (laminae I and II) after injections of WGA-HRP into the somatosensory cortex.

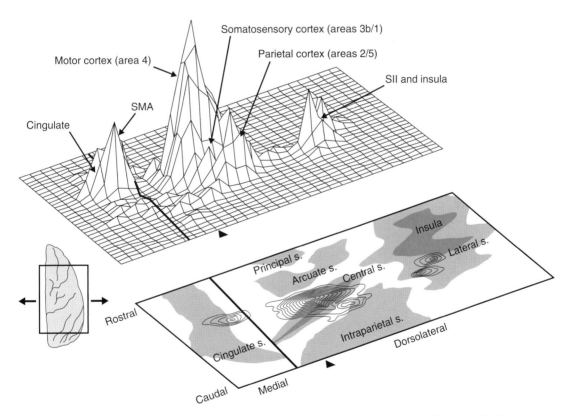

Fig. 5.14 Three-dimensional map and the corresponding contour map of the contralateral corticospinal soma distribution retrogradely labelled by a fluorescent dye injection at the cervical spinal cord. The contour map has been plotted onto the planar projection of the unfolded cortex. Sulci are indicated in light grey and are labelled in the middle map; area 3a and the insular cortex are shown in a darker shade of grey. The heavy black line indicated by the arrowhead represents the sagittal midline, with the medial surface to the left. The maps show the variation in density of corticospinal projections terminating at mid-cervical levels. The most dense projection is from the primary motor cortex in the dorsal bank of the central sulcus, with smaller projections arising from the medial surface (SMA and rostral cingulate cortex), posterior parietal and insular cortex (including SII). Note the reduction of the corticospinal projection from areas 3a and 3b, compared with that from adjacent areas 4 and 2/5.

The precentral cortical areas have a very wide pattern of termination. Area 4, classical motor cortex, projects predominantly to the intermediate zone (laminae VII and VIII), but the terminals extend into the lateral and medial regions of the ventral horn (lamina IX), as well as extensively, though more sparsely, into the deeper laminae of the dorsal horn (laminae V and VI). The supplementary motor cortex has a similar pattern of termination mainly in the intermediate zone and amongst the motor neuron pools (Galea & Darian-Smith 1997; Maier et al 1997). The dorsal caudal cingulate area projects to the dorsolateral portion of the intermediate zone of the spinal cord (where spinothalamic neurons are located) while projections from the ventral caudal cingulate area terminate in the dorsomedial region (in the region of neurons projecting to the dorsal columns). However, there are sparse terminations in the dorsolateral region of the ventral horn and in the dorsal horn (laminae III and IV). These projections appear to be more dense in the rostral segments of the cervical spinal cord (Dum & Strick 1996) (Fig. 5.15).

Role of corticospinal projections

The corticospinal projections form a parallel, distributed system arising from areas with complex interconnections and converging on different parts of the spinal circuitry. Their role in the modulation of activity in the dorsal horn, particularly in relation to pain, has not been investigated extensively.

Stimulation of SI and SII areas can result in primary afferent depolarization (PAD) in fibres of the dorsal root (group Ib and II muscle afferents and cutaneous afferents, but not group Ia afferents (Andersen et al 1964; Carpenter et al 1963). It appears that sensorimotor cortex stimulation depresses the response of superficial dorsal horn neurons to a subsequent stimulus from the Lissauer tract. This tract is therefore thought to mediate the PAD evoked from multiple neural pathways (Lidierth & Wall 1998). Stimulation of sensorimotor cortex can also elicit both excitatory and inhibitory responses in dorsal horn neurons, particularly in laminae IV and V (Fetz 1968; Lundberg et al 1962; Wall 1967). These cells receive a wide convergence of cutaneous input, as well as afferent information from muscle and joints. In a study in the monkey by Coulter et al (1974), stimulation of the pre- or post-central gyrus produced either a depression of the activity of neurons in the dorsal horn or an excitation followed by depression. Corticospinal projections from motor cortex may be excitatory to spinothalamic neurons, while those from postcentral cortex may inhibit them (Lidierth & Wall 1998; Ralston & Ralston 1985; Yezierski et al 1983). Corticospinal projections to the superficial laminae (arising predominantly from areas 3b/1) may directly modulate nociceptive-specific neurons (Cheema et al 1984).

Posterior parietal cortex has connections with the SI cortex and other polymodal association areas, including the limbic system (Cavada & Goldman-Rakic 1989) and is part of a general attentional system. Activation of this region

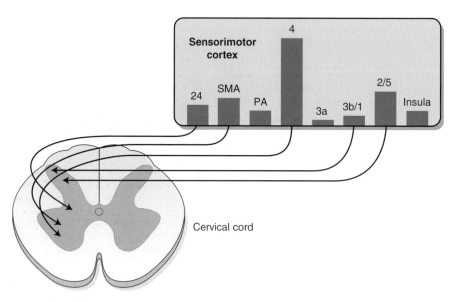

Fig. 5.15 **Representation of the known areas of termination of corticospinal projections from different cortical areas.**

may reflect hypervigilance or superattentiveness to the sensory information accompanying chronic pain. The role of corticospinal projections from this region on dorsal horn neurons is unknown.

The cingulate cortex is involved in the processing of painful stimuli (Hsieh et al 1995; Jones et al 1991; Treede et al 1999). The cingulate sulcus is a unique region of the limbic system, in that it appears to be involved in affect and regulating context-relevant motor behaviours (Devinsky et al 1995). It has been suggested that this region is critical for maintaining a working interaction between the limbic areas and motor areas of the cerebral cortex. Stimulation in the cingulate area (area 24) may also be involved in autonomic responses, such as changes in respiration and cardiovascular function (Hoff et al 1963; Lofving 1961). Its role might be in linking emotional, motivational and memory-related information generated in limbic areas directly to motor areas (Morecraft & van Hoesen 1998). The anterior cingulate cortex contains pain-anticipation related neurons (Koyama et al 1998) and therefore has a role in the anticipation of pain that precedes avoidance behaviour.

Neurons in SII and the granular insula (Ig) are responsive to a wide range of somatosensory stimuli (Burton & Robinson 1981). The corticospinal projections from these areas terminate in the dorsal horn, but their specific role is unknown. The majority of neurons in SII respond to rapid, transient stimuli such as light touch. 'Complex zones' have been described, which become active during the performance of complex tasks (Burton & Robinson 1981). The posterior insula (Ig) receives converging information about all five sensory modalities. Its efferent connections include the limbic system through the cingulate gyrus and amygdala (Mesulam & Mufson 1982), as well as the spinal cord (Galea & Darian-Smith 1994) therefore this area might have the function of providing the link between motivational and emotional states with relevant sensory information. Insular cortex is consistently activated by painful stimuli (Coghill et al 1999; Craig et al 2000). Noxious heat has been found to activate a region of the anterior insula (Id), which has connections with SI, SII and the cingulate region (area 24) (Mufson & Mesulam 1982) as well as with the amygdala and perirhinal cortex (Friedman et al 1986). Although stimulation of the anterior insula produces predominantly visceral sensations, it also evokes unusual somatic sensations, movements and sometimes a sense of fear (Penfield & Rasmussen 1955).

The corticospinal neuron populations can produce indirect effects on the dorsal horn through collaterals to the *dorsal column nuclei*, where the effect is to diminish the post-synaptic responses of the dorsal column nuclei to somatic sensory nerve stimulation (Magni et al 1959). In addition, there are collaterals to the PAG and the nucleus raphe magnus (Kuypers 1981), which have descending inhibitory connections with the spinal cord. Thus the cerebral cortex, through the corticospinal tract, may exert a modulatory effect on both motor and sensory functions, including pain.

CONCLUSION

This chapter has provided a review of the nervous system structures involved in nociception and their connections. Nociceptors are involved in signalling painful stimuli. There are several kinds of cutaneous nociceptors that can be activated by one or more kinds of noxious stimuli: mechanical, thermal or chemical. Other nociceptors are found in muscle, joints and viscera. Nociceptive and thermal signals are transmitted along unmyelinated (C) and small-diameter myelinated (Aδ) axons that synapse in the dorsal horn. Second-order neurons arise from different regions of the dorsal horn, cross the midline in the ventral commissure and ascend to the brainstem and thalamus in the anterolateral column. They synapse in a number of brainstem nuclei (including the reticular formation and the periaqueductal grey) and in several thalamic nuclei (VPL, VPI, CL and the intralaminar nuclei). From the thalamus, nociceptive and thermal stimuli are relayed mainly to the SI area of the cerebral cortex. Multiple cortical areas are activated by painful stimuli, including the SII cortex, the anterior cingulate cortex, the insula, the prefrontal cortex and the supplementary motor area. Pain signals may be modified through descending projections from the brainstem and cerebral cortex. The organization of these structures suggests that there is a distributed cortical system concerned with the perception of pain. This distributed cerebral activation reflects the complex nature of pain, involving discriminative, affective, autonomic and motor components. An understanding of this complexity can provide insights for the management of pain in the clinical setting.

> **Q** Study questions/questions for revision
>
> 1. What classes of axons convey nociceptive and temperature information?
> 2. In which ways could nociceptive information be modulated at the level of the dorsal horn?
> 3. What spinal cord pathways convey nociceptive information to the brain? What are their targets?
> 4. Which regions of the brain subserve the sensory–discriminative and motivational–affective aspects of pain? How do their connections differ?
> 5. Name the descending projections to the dorsal horn. What is their role?

REFERENCES

Abrahams, V.C., Lynn, B., Richmond, F.J.R., 1984. Organization and sensory properties of small myelinated fibres in the dorsal cervical rami of the cat. J. Physiol. 347, 177–187.

Adrian, E.D., 1931. The messages in sensory nerve fibres and their interpretation. Proceedings of the Royal Society Series B 109, 1–18.

Al-Chaer, E.D., Feng, Y., Willis, W.D., 1998. A role for the dorsal column in nociceptive visceral input into the thalamus of primates. J. Neurophysiol. 79, 3143–3150.

Andersen, P., Eccles, J.C., Sears, T.A., 1964. Cortically evoked depolarization of primary afferent fibers in the spinal cord. J. Neurophysiol. 27, 63–77.

Apkarian, A.V., Hodge, C., 1989a. Primate spinothalamic pathways: I. A quantitative study of the cells of origin of the spinothalamic pathway. J. Comp. Neurol. 288, 447–473.

Apkarian, A.V., Hodge, C., 1989b. Primate spinothalamic pathways: II. The cells of origin of the dorsolateral and ventral spinothalamic pathways. J. Comp. Neurol. 288, 474–492.

Apkarian, A.V., Hodge, C., 1989c. Primate spinothalamic pathways: III. Thalamic terminations of the dorsolateral and ventral spinothalamic pathways. J. Comp. Neurol. 288, 493–511.

Applebaum, A.E., Beall, J.E., Foreman, R.D., et al., 1975. Organization and receptive fields of primate spinothalamic tract neurons. J. Neurophysiol. 38, 572–586.

Applebaum, A.E., Leonard, R.B., Kenshalo, D.R., et al., 1979. Nuclei in which functionally identified spinothalamic tract neurons terminate. J. Comp. Neurol. 188, 575–586.

Asanuma, C., Thach, W.T., Jones, E.G., 1983. Anatomical evidence for segregated focal groupings of efferent cells and their terminal ramifications in the cerebellothalamic pathway of the monkey. Brain Research Reviews 5, 267–297.

Baleydier, C., Maugiere, F., 1980. The duality of the cingulate gyrus in

monkey: neuroanatomical study and functional hypothesis. Brain 103, 525–554.

Bandler, R., Keay, K.A., 1996. Columnar organization in the midbrain periaqueductal gray and the integration of emotional expression. Prog. Brain Res. 107, 285–300.

Bandler, R., Shipley, M.T., 1994. Columnar organization in the midbrain periaqueductal gray: modules for emotional expression? [published erratum appears in Trends Neurosci. 1994 Nov 17 (11), 445] Trends Neurosci. 17, 379–389.

Bandler, R., Carrive, P., Zhang, S.P., 1991. Integration of somatic and autonomic reactions within the midbrain periaqueductal gray: viscerotopic, somatotopic and functional organization. Prog. Brain Res. 87, 269–305.

Barbas, H., Pandya, D.N., 1987. Architecture and frontal cortical connections of the premotor cortex (area 6) in the rhesus monkey. J. Comp. Neurol. 256, 211–228.

Basbaum, A.I., Fields, H.L., 1984. Endogenous pain control systems: brainstem spinal pathways and endorphin circuitry. Annu. Rev. Neurosci. 7, 309–338.

Basbaum, A.I., Bautista, D.M., Scherrer, G., et al., 2009. Cellular and molecular mechanisms of pain. Cell 139 (2), 267–284.

Behbehani, M.M., 1995. Functional characteristics of the midbrain periaqueductal gray. Prog. Neurobiol. 46, 575–605.

Berkley, K., 1980. Spatial relationships between the terminations of somatic sensory and motor pathways in the rostral brainstem of cats and monkeys. I. Ascending somatic sensory inputs to lateral diencephalon. J. Comp. Neurol. 193, 283–317.

Bernard, J.F., Bandler, R., 1998. Parallel circuits for emotional coping behaviour: new pieces in the puzzle. J. Comp. Neurol. 401, 429–436.

Bessou, P., Laporte, Y., 1961. Étude des recepteurs musculaires innervés par les fibres afferentes du groupe III (fibres myelinisées fines), chez le chat. Arch. Ital. Biol. 99, 293–321.

Bessou, P., Perl, E.R., 1969. Response of cutaneous sensory units with unmyelinated fibres to noxious stimuli. J. Neurophysiol. 32, 1025–1043.

Bessou, P., Burgess, P.R., Perl, E.R., et al., 1971. Dynamic properties of mechanoreceptors with unmyelinated (C) fibers. J. Neurophysiol. 34, 116–131.

Boivie, J., 1979. An anatomical reinvestigation of the termination of the spinothalamic tract in the monkey. J. Comp. Neurol. 186, 343–370.

Broca, P., 1878. Anatomie comparée de circonvolutions cérébrales. Le grand lobe limbique et la scissure limbique dans le série des mammifères. Revue Anthropologique 1, 385–498.

Brodal, A., 1981. Neurological Anatomy in Relation to Clinical Medicine. Oxford University Press, New York.

Brown, A.G., 1981. Organization in the Spinal Cord. Springer, Berlin.

Brown, P.B., Brushart, T.M., Ritz, L.A., 1989. Somatotopy of digital nerve projections to the dorsal horn in the monkey. Somatosens. Mot. Res. 6, 309–317.

Buonomano, D.V., Merzenich, M.M., 1998. Cortical plasticity: from maps to synapses. Annu. Rev. Neurosci. 21, 149–186.

Burgess, P.R., Perl, E.R., 1967. Myelinated afferent fibres responding specifically to noxious stimulation of the skin. Journal of Physiology (London) 190, 541–562.

Burnstock, G., 2007. Physiology and pathophysiology of purogenic neurotransmission. Physiol. Rev. 87, 659–797.

Burton, H., Craig, A.D., 1983. Spinothalamic projections in cat, raccoon and monkey: a study based on anterograde transport of horseradish peroxidase. In: Macchi, G., Rustioni, A., Spreafico, R. (Eds.), Somatosensory Integration in the Thalamus. Elsevier, Amsterdam, pp. 17–41.

Burton, H., Robinson, C.J., 1981. Organization of the SII parietal cortex. Multiple somatic sensory representations within and near the second somatic sensory area of the cynomolgus monkeys. In:

Woolsey, C.N. (Ed.), Cortical Sensory Organization. Vol. 1. Multiple Sensory Areas. Humana Press, New Jersey, pp. 67–119.

Bushnell, M.C., Duncan, G.H., Hofbauer, R.K., et al., 1999. Pain perception: is there a role for primary somatosensory cortex? Proc. Natl. Acad. Sci. U. S. A. 96, 7705–7709.

Cameron, A.A., Khan, I.A., Westlund, K.N., et al., 1995a. The efferent projections of the periaqueductal gray in the rat: a Phaseolus vulgaris-leucoagglutinin study. I. Ascending projections. J. Comp. Neurol. 351, 568–584.

Cameron, A.A., Khan, I.A., Westlund, K.N., et al., 1995b. The efferent projections of the periaqueductal gray in the rat: a Phaseolus vulgaris-leucoagglutinin study. II. Descending projections. J. Comp. Neurol. 351, 585–601.

Campbell, J.N., Meyer, R.A., LaMotte, R.H., 1979. Sensitization of myelinated nociceptive afferents that innervate monkey hand. J. Neurophysiol. 42, 1669–1679.

Campero, M., Serra, J., Ochoa, J.L., 1996. C-polymodal nociceptors activated by noxious low temperature in human skin. J. Physiol. 497, 565–572.

Carpenter, D., Lundberg, A., Norrsell, U., 1963. Primary afferent depolarization evoked from the sensorimotor cortex. Acta Physiol. Scand. 59, 126–142.

Casey, K.L., Morrow, T.J., 1987. Nociceptive neurons in the ventral posterior thalamus of the awake squirrel monkey: observations in identification, modulation and drug effects. In: Besson, J.M., Guilbaud, D., Peschanksi, M. (Eds.), Thalamus and Pain. Elsevier, Amsterdam, pp. 211–226.

Caterina, M.J., Rosen, T.A., Tominaga, M., et al., 1999. A capsaicin-receptor homologue with a high threshold for noxious heat. Nature 398, 436–441.

Cavada, C., Goldman-Rakic, P.S., 1989. Posterior parietal cortex in rhesus monkey: II. Evidence for segregated corticocortical networks linking sensory and limbic areas with the frontal lobe. J. Comp. Neurol. 287, 422–445.

Cheema, S.S., Rustioni, A., Whitsel, B.L., 1984. Light and electron microscopic evidence for a direct corticospinal projection to superficial laminae of the dorsal horn in cats and monkeys. J. Comp. Neurol. 225, 276–290.

Chen, Y., Michaelis, M., Jänig, W., et al., 1996. Adrenoreceptor subtype mediating sympathetic-sensory coupling in injured sensory neurons. J. Neurophysiol. 76, 3721–3730.

Christensen, B.R., Perl, E.R., 1970. Spinal neurons specifically excited by noxious or thermal stimuli. J. Neurophysiol. 33, 293–307.

Chudler, E.H., Dong, W.K., 1995. The role of the basal ganglia in nociception and pain. Pain 60, 3–38.

Chudler, E.H., Sugiyama, K., Dong, W.K., 1993. Nociceptive responses of neurons in the neostriatum and globus pallidus of the rat. J. Neurophysiol. 69, 1890–1903.

Coffield, J.A., Bowen, K.K., Miletic, V., 1992. Retrograde tracing of projections between the nucleus submedius, the ventrolateral orbital cortex, and the midbrain in the rat. J. Comp. Neurol. 321, 488–499.

Coggeshall, R.E., Coulter, J.D., Willis, W.D., 1974. Unmyelinated axons in the ventral roots of the cat lumbosacral enlargement. J. Comp. Neurol. 153, 39–58.

Coghill, R.C., Talbot, J.D., Evans, A.C., et al., 1994. Distributed processing of pain and vibration by the human brain. J. Neurosci. 14, 4095–4108.

Coghill, R.C., Sang, C.N., Maisog, J.M., et al., 1999. Pain intensity processing within the human brain: a bilateral distributed mechanism. J. Neurophysiol. 82, 1934–1943.

Colebatch, J.G., Deiber, M.P., Passingham, R.E., et al., 1991. Regional cerebral blood flow during voluntary arm and hand movements in human subjects. J. Neurophysiol. 65, 1392–1401.

Côté, L., Crutcher, M.D., 1991. The basal ganglia. In: Kandel, E.R., Schwartz, J.H., Jessell, T.M. (Eds.), Principles of Neural Science, third ed. Elsevier, New York, pp. 647–659.

Coulter, J.D., Jones, E.G., 1977. Differential distribution of corticospinal projections from individual cytoarchitectonic fields in the monkey. Brain Res. 129, 335–340.

Coulter, J.D., Maunz, R.A., Willis, W.D., 1974. Effects of stimulation of sensorimotor cortex on primate spinothalamic neurons. Brain Res. 65, 351–356.

Craig, A.D., Burton, H., 1981. Spinal and medullary lamina I projection to nucleus submedius in medial thalamus: a possible pain center. J. Neurophysiol. 45, 443–466.

Craig, A.D., Chen, K., Bandy, D., et al., 2000. Thermosensory activation of insular cortex. Nat. Neurosci. 3, 184–190.

Cusick, C.G., Gould, H.J., 1990. Connections between area 3b of the somatosensory cortex and subdivisions of the ventroposterior nuclear complex and the anterior pulvinar in squirrel monkeys. J. Comp. Neurol. 292, 83–102.

Darian-Smith, C., Darian-Smith, I., Cheema, S.S., 1990. Thalamic projections to sensorimotor cortex in the macaque monkey: use of multiple retrograde tracers. J. Comp. Neurol. 299, 17–46.

de Groat, W.C., Nadelhaft, I., Milne, R., et al., 1981. Organisation of the sacral parasympathetic reflex pathways to the urinary bladder and large intestine. J. Auton. Nerv. Syst 3 (2–4), 135–160.

Deiber, M.P., Passingham, R.E., Colebatch, J.G., et al., 1991. Cortical areas and the selection of movement: a study with positron emission tomography. Exp. Brain Res. 84, 393–402.

Devinsky, O., Morrell, M.J., Vogt, B.A., 1995. Contributions of anterior cingulate cortex to behaviour. Brain. 118, 279–306.

Dong, W.K., Ryu, H., Wagman, I.H., 1978. Nociceptive responses in medial thalamus and their relationship to spinothalamic pathways. J. Neurophysiol. 41, 1592–1613.

Dubner, R., Bennett, G.J., 1983. Spinal and trigeminal mechanisms of nociception. Annu. Rev. Neurosci. 6, 381–418.

Dum, R.P., Strick, P.L., 1991. The origin of corticospinal projections from the premotor areas in the frontal lobe. J. Neurosci. 11, 667–689.

Dum, R.P., Strick, P.L., 1996. Spinal cord terminations of the medial wall motor areas in macaque monkeys. J. Neurosci. 16, 6513–6525.

Erlanger, J., Gasser, H.S., 1937. Electrical Signs of Nervous Activity. University of Pennsylvania Press, Philadelphia.

Fetz, E.E., 1968. Pyramidal tract effects on interneurons in the cat lumbar dorsal horn. J. Neurophysiol. 31, 69–80.

Fields, H.L., Basbaum, A.I., 1994. Central nervous system mechanisms of pain modulation. In: Wall, P.D., Melzack, R. (Eds.), Textbook of Pain. Churchill Livingstone, Edinburgh, pp. 243–257.

Flaherty, A.W., Graybiel, A.M., 1993. Two input systems for body representations in the primate striatal matrix: experimental evidence in the squirrel monkey. J. Neurosci. 13, 1120–1137.

Florence, S.L., Wall, J.T., Kaas, J.H., 1988. The somatotopic pattern of afferent projections from the digits to the spinal cord and cuneate nucleus in macaque monkeys. Brain Res. 452, 388–392.

Friedman, D.P., Murray, E.A., O'Neill, J.B., et al., 1986. Cortical connections of the somatosensory fields of the lateral sulcus of macaques: evidence of a corticolimbic pathway for touch. J. Comp. Neurol. 252, 323–347.

Galea, M.P., Darian-Smith, I., 1994. Multiple corticospinal neuron populations in the macaque monkey are specified by their unique cortical origins, spinal terminations and connections. Cereb. Cortex. 4, 166–194.

Galea, M.P., Darian-Smith, I., 1997. Corticospinal projection patterns following unilateral cervical spinal cord section in the newborn and juvenile macaque monkey. J. Comp. Neurol. 381, 282–306.

Gerfen, C.R., 1992. The neostriatal mosaic: multiple levels of compartmental organization. Trends Neurosci. 15, 133–139.

Giesler, G.J., Spiel, H.R., Willis, W.D., 1981. Organization of spinothalamic tract axons within the rat spinal cord. J. Comp. Neurol. 195, 243–252.

Gingold, S.I., Greenspan, J.D., Apkarian, A.V., 1991. Anatomic evidence of nociceptive inputs to primary somatosensory cortex: Relationship between spinothalamic terminals and thalamocortical cells in squirrel monkeys. J. Comp. Neurol. 308, 467–490.

Gobel, S., Falls, W.M., Humphrey, E., 1981. Morphology and synaptic connections of ultrafine primary axons in lamina I of the spinal dorsal horn: candidates for the terminal axonal arbors of primary neurones in unmyelinated (C) axons. J. Neurosci. 1, 1163–1179.

Goldman, P.S., Nauta, W.J.H., 1977. An intricately patterned prefronto-caudate projection in the rhesus monkey. J. Comp. Neurol. 171, 369–385.

Gray, T.S., Magnuson, D.J., 1992. Peptide immunoreactive neurons in the amygdala and the bed nucleus of the stria terminalis project to the midbrain central gray in the rat. Peptides 13, 451–460.

Graybiel, A.M., 1991. Basal ganglia: input, neural activity, and relation to the cortex. Curr. Biol. 1, 644–651.

Greenan, T.J., Strick, P.L., 1986. Do thalamic regions which project to rostral primate motor cortex receive spinothalamic input? Brain Res. 362, 384–388.

Grieve, G.P., 1994. Referred pain and other clinical features. In: Boyling, J.D., Palastanga, N. (Eds.), Grieve's Modern Manual Therapy, second ed. The Vertebral Column. Churchill Livingstone, Edinburgh.

Ha, H., Morin, F., 1964. Comparative anatomical observations of the cervical nucleus, N. cervicalis lateralis, of some primates. Anat. Record 148, 374–375.

Häbler, H.J., Jänig, W., Koltzenburg, M., 1990. Activation of unmyelinated fibres by mechanical stimuli and inflammation of the urinary bladder in the cat. Journal of Physiology (London) 425, 545–562.

Hardy, S.G.P., Leichnetz, G.R., 1981. Cortical projections to the periaqueductal gray in the monkey: a retrograde and orthograde horseradish peroxidase study. Neurosci. Lett. 22, 97–101.

Henderson, L.A., Keay, K.A., Bandler, R., 1998. The ventrolateral periaqueductal gray projects to caudal brainstem depressor regions: a functional-anatomical and physiological study. Neuroscience 82, 201–221.

Heppelmann, B., Messlinger, K., Neiss, W.F., et al., 1990. Ultrastructural three-dimensional reconstruction of group III and group IV sensory nerve endings ('free nerve endings') in the knee joint of the cat: evidence for multiple receptive sites. J. Comp. Neurol. 292, 103–116.

Herbert, H., Saper, C.R., 1992. Organization of medullary adrenergic and noradrenergic projections to the periaqueductal gray matter in the rat. J. Comp. Neurol. 314, 34–52.

Hertel, H.C., Howaldt, B., Mense, S., 1976. Responses of group IV and group III muscle afferents to thermal stimuli. Brain Res. 113, 201–205.

Hirschberg, R.M., Al-Chaer, E.D., Lawand, N.B., et al., 1996. Is there a pathway in the posterior funiculus that signals visceral pain? Pain 67, 291–305.

Hoff, E.C., Kell, J.F., Carroll, M.N., 1963. Effects of cortical stimulation and lesions on cardiovascular function. Physiology Review 43, 68–114.

Hoheisel, U., Reinöhl, J., Unger, T., et al., 2004. Acidic pH and capsaicin activate mechanosensitive group IV muscle receptors in the rat. Pain 110, 149–157.

Hoheisel, U., Unger, T., Mense, S., 2005. Excitatory and modulatory effects of inflammatory cytokines and neurotrophins on mechanosensitive group IV muscle afferents in the rat. Pain 114, 168–176.

Honda, C.N., 1985. Visceral and somatic afferent convergence onto neurons near the central canal in the sacral spinal cord of the cat. J. Neurophysiol. 53, 1059–1078.

Honda, C.N., Perl, E.R., 1985. Functional and morphological features of neurons in the midline region of the caudal spinal cord in the cat. Brain Res. 340, 285–295.

Hsieh, J.C., Belfrage, M., Stone-Elander, S., et al., 1995. Central representation of chronic ongoing neuropathic pain studied by positron emission tomography. Pain 63, 225–236.

Iggo, A., 1960. Cutaneous mechanoreceptors with C fibres.

Journal of Physiology (London) 152, 337–353.

Jänig, W., 1992. Pain and the sympathetic nervous system: pathophysiological mechanisms. In: Bannister, R., Mathias, C. (Eds.), Autonomic Failure. Oxford University Press, Oxford, pp. 231–251.

Jänig, W., 1995. The sympathetic nervous system in pain. Eur. J. Anaesthesiol. 12 (Suppl.10), 53–60.

Ji, R.R., Kawasaki, Y., Zhuang, Z.Y., et al., 2006. Posible role of spinal astrocytes in maintaining chronic pain sensitization: review of current evidence with focus on bFGF/JNK pathway. Neuron Glia Biology 2 (4), 259–269.

Johnson, J.I., Welker, W.I., Pubols, B.H., 1968. Somatotopic organization of raccoon dorsal column nuclei. J. Comp. Neurol. 132, 1–44.

Jones, E.G., 1985. The Thalamus. Plenum Press, New York.

Jones, A.K.P., Brown, W.D., Friston, K.J., et al., 1991. Cortical and subcortical localization of response to pain in man using positron emission tomography. Proceedings of the Royal Society, Series B 244, 39–44.

Kaas, J.H., Nelson, R.J., Sur, M., et al., 1979. Multiple representations of the body within the primary somatosensory cortex of primates. Science 204, 521–523.

Kaas, J.H., Nelson, R.J., Sur, M., et al., 1984. The somatotopic organization of the ventroposterior thalamus of the squirrel monkey, Saimiri sciureus. J. Comp. Neurol. 226, 111–140.

Keay, K.A., Bandler, R., 1993. Deep and superficial noxious stimulation increases Fos-like immunoreactivity in different regions of the midbrain periaqueductal gray of the rat. Neurosci. Lett. 154, 23–26.

Kenshalo, D.R., Giesler, G.J., Leonard, R.B., et al., 1980. Responses of neurons in primate ventral posterior lateral nucleus to noxious stimuli. J. Neurophysiol. 43, 1594–1614.

Kerr, F.W.L., 1975. Neuroanatomical substrates of nociception in the spinal cord. Pain 1, 325–356.

Kevetter, G.A., Haber, L.H., Yezierski, R.P., et al., 1982. Cells of origin of the spinoreticular tract in the monkey. J. Comp. Neurol. 207, 61–74.

Kieschke, J., Mense, S., Prabhakar, N.R., 1988. Influence of adrenaline and hypoxia on rat muscle receptors in vitro. In: Hamann, W., Iggo, A. (Eds.), Progress in Brain Research. Elsevier, Amsterdam, pp. 91–97.

Kircher, C., Ha, H., 1968. The nucleus cervicalis lateralis in primates including the human. Anat. Record 160, 376.

Klement, W., Arndt, J.O., 1992. The role of nociceptors of cutaneous veins in the mediation of cold pain in man. J. Physiol. 449, 73–83.

Koyama, T., Tanaka, Y.Z., Mikami, A., 1998. Nociceptive neurons in macaque anterior cingulate activate during anticipation of pain. Neuroreport 9, 2663–2667.

Kruger, L., Perl, E.R., Sedivec, M.J., 1981. Fine structure of myelinated mechanical nociceptor endings in cat hairy skin. J. Comp. Neurol. 198, 137–154.

Kuypers, H.G.J.M., 1981. Anatomy of the descending pathways. In: Brooks, V.B., Brookhart, J.M., Mountcastle, V.B. (Eds.), Handbook of Physiology Section 1: The Nervous System, Volume II, Motor Control, Part 1. American Physiological Society, Bethesda, pp. 597–666.

LaMotte, C., 1977. Distribution of the tract of Lissauer and dorsal horn root fibres in the primate spinal cord. J. Comp. Neurol. 172, 529–562.

LaMotte, R.H., Thalhammer, J.G., 1982. Response properties of high-threshold cutaneous cold receptors in the primate. Brain Res. 244, 279–287.

Lawson, S.N., 1992. Morphological and biochemical cell types of sensory neurons. In: Scott, S.A. (Ed.), Sensory Neurons: Diversity, Development and Plasticity. Oxford University Press, Oxford, pp. 27–59.

Leichnetz, G.R., 1986. Afferent and efferent connections of the dorsolateral precentral gyrus (area 4, hand/arm region) in the macaque monkey, with comparisons to area 8. J. Comp. Neurol. 254, 260–292.

Lidierth, M., Wall, P.D., 1998. Dorsal horn cells connected to the Lissauer tract and their relation to the dorsal root potential in the rat. J. Neurophysiol. 80, 667–679.

Light, A.R., Metz, C.B., 1978. The morphology of the spinal cord efferent and afferent neurons contributing to the ventral roots of the cat. J. Comp. Neurol. 179, 501–516.

Lipp, J., 1991. Possible mechanisms of morphine analgesia. Clin. Neuropharmacol. 14, 131–147.

Lloyd, D.P.C., 1943. Neuron patterns controlling transmission of ipsilateral hindlimb reflexes in cat. J. Neurophysiol. 6, 293–315.

Lofving, B., 1961. Cardiovascular adjustments induced from the rostral cingulate gyrus. Acta Physiol. Scand. 53, 1–82.

Löken, L.S., Wessberg, J., Morrison, I., et al., 2009. Coding of pleasant touch by unmyelinated afferents in humans. Nat. Neurosci. 12 (5), 547–548.

Lovick, T.A., 1991. Interactions between descending pathways from the dorsal and ventrolateral periaqueductal gray matter in the rat. In: Depaulis, A., Bandler, R. (Eds.), The Midbrain Periaqueductal Gray Matter. Plenum Press, New York, pp. 101–120.

Lundberg, A., Norrsell, U., Voorhoeve, P., 1962. Pyramidal effects on lumbosacral interneurons activated by somatic afferents. Acta Physiol. Scand. 56, 220–229.

Lynn, B., 1984. The detection of injury and tissue damage. In: Wall, P.D., Melzack, R. (Eds.), Textbook of Pain. Churchill Livingstone, Edinburgh, pp. 19–33.

MacLean, P.D., 1955. The limbic system ('visceral brain') and emotional behaviour. Arch. Neurol. Psychiatry 73, 130–134.

Magni, F., Melzack, R., Moruzzi, G., et al., 1959. Direct pyramidal influences on the dorsal column nuclei. Arch. Ital. Biol. 97, 357–377.

Maier, M.A., Davis, J.N., Armand, J., et al., 1997. Comparison of cortico-motoneuronal (CM) connections from macaque motor cortex and supplementary motor area. Society for Neuroscience Abstracts 23, 1274.

Malmberg, A.B., Chen, C., Tonegawa, S., et al., 1997. Preserved acute pain and reduced neuropathic pain in mice lacking PKC gamma. Science 278, 279–283.

Mantyh, P.W., 1983. The spinothalamic tract in the primate: a reexamination using wheatgerm agglutinin conjugated to horseradish peroxidase. Neuroscience 9, 847–862.

Martin, J.H., 1996. Neuroanatomy. Text and Atlas, second ed. Appleton & Lange, Stamford, CT.

Matelli, M., Camarda, R., Glickstein, M., et al., 1986. Afferent and efferent projections of the inferior area 6 in the macaque monkey. J. Comp. Neurol. 251, 281–298.

Matelli, M., Rizzolatti, G., Bettinardi, V., et al., 1993. Activation of precentral and mesial motor areas during the execution of elementary proximal and distal arm movements : a PET study. Neuroreport 4, 1295–1298.

McCloskey, D.I., Mitchell, J.H., 1972. Reflex cardiovascular and respiratory responses originating in exercising muscle. J. Physiol. 234, 173–186.

McLachlan, E.M., Jänig, W., Devor, M., et al., 1993. Peripheral nerve injury triggers noradrenergic sprouting within dorsal root ganglia. Nature 363, 543–546.

McMahon, S.B., 1984. Spinal mechanisms in somatic pain. In: Holden, A.V., Winlow, W. (Eds.), The Neurobiology of Pain. Manchester University Press, Manchester.

Mehler, W.R., Feferman, M.E., Nauta, W.J.H., 1960. Ascending axon degeneration following anterolateral cordotomy. An experimental study in the monkey. Brain 83, 718–751.

Melzack, R., Casey, K.L., 1968. Sensory, motivational, and central control determinants of pain. A new conceptual model. In: Kenshalo, R. (Ed.), The Skin Senses. Thomas, Springfield, IL, pp. 423–443.

Mense, S., 1993. Nociception from skeletal muscle in relation to clinical muscle pain. Pain 54, 241–289.

Mense, S., 2009. Algesic agents exciting muscle nociceptors. Exp. Brain Res. 196, 89–100.

Mense, S., Meyer, H., 1985. Different types of slowly conducting afferent units in cat skeletal muscle and tendon. J. Physiol. 363, 403–417.

Mense, S., Meyer, H., 1988. Bradykinin-induced modulation of the response behaviour of different types of feline group III and IV muscle receptors. J. Physiol. 398, 49–63.

Mense, S., Prabhakar, N.R., 1986. Spinal terminations of nociceptive afferent fibres from deep tissues in the cat. Neurosci. Lett. 66, 169–174.

Mense, S., Stahnke, M., 1983. Responses in muscle afferent fibres of slow conduction velocity to contractions and ischaemia in the cat. J. Physiol. 342, 383–397.

Mesulam, M.M., Mufson, E.J., 1982. Insula in the Old World monkey: efferent cortical output and comments on function. J. Comp. Neurol. 212, 38–52.

Meyer, R.A., Davis, K.D., Cohen, R.H., et al., 1991. Mechanically insensitive afferents (MIAs) in cutaneous nerves of monkey. Brain Res. 561, 252–261.

Meyer, R.A., Campbell, J.N., Raja, S.N., 1994. Peripheral neural mechanisms of nociception. In: Wall, P.D., Melzack, R. (Eds.), Textbook of Pain. Churchill Livingstone, Edinburgh, pp. 13–44.

Meyer, R.A., Ringkamp, M., Campbell, J.N., et al., 2006. Peripheral mechanisms of cutaneous nociception. In: McMahon, S.B., Koltzenburg, M. (Eds.), Wall and Melzack's Textbook of Pain, fifth ed. Elsevier, Philadelphia, pp. 3–34.

Milligan, E.S., Watkins, L.R., 2009. Pathological and protective roles of glia in chronic pain. Nature Reviews Neuroscience 10 (1), 23–36.

Mizuno, N., Nakano, K., Imaizumi, M., et al., 1967. The lateral cervical nucleus of the Japanese monkey (Macaca fuscata). J. Comp. Neurol. 129, 375–384.

Morecraft, R.J., van Hoesen, G.W., 1998. Convergence of limbic input to the cingulate motor cortex in the rhesus monkey. Brain Res. Bull. 45, 209–232.

Morgan, M.M., 1991. Differences in antinociception evoked from dorsal and ventral regions of the caudal periaqueductal gray matter. In: Depaulis, A., Bandler, R. (Eds.), The Midbrain Periaqueductal Gray Matter. Plenum Press, New York, pp. 139–150.

Morgan, C., Nadelhaft, I., de Groat, W.C., 1981. The distribution of visceral primary afferents from the pelvic nerve to Lissauer's tract and spinal gray matter and its relationship to the sacral parasympathetic nucleus. J. Comp. Neurol. 201 (3), 415–440.

Morgan, M.M., Whitney, P.K., Gold, M.S., 1998. Immobility and flight associated with antinociception produced by activation of the ventral and lateral/dorsal regions of the rat periaqueductal gray. Brain Res. 804, 159–166.

Muakkassa, K.F., Strick, P.L., 1979. Frontal lobe inputs to primate motor cortex: evidence for four somatotopically organized 'premotor' areas. Brain Res. 177, 176–182.

Mufson, E.J., Mesulam, M.M., 1982. Insula of the old world monkey. II Afferent cortical input and comments on the claustrum. J. Comp. Neurol. 212, 23–37.

Nauta, W.J.H., Mehler, W.R., 1966. Projections of the lentiform nucleus in the monkey. Brain Res. 1, 3–42.

Pandya, D.N., Van Hoesen, G.W., Mesulam, M.M., 1981. Efferent connections of the cingulate gyrus in the rhesus monkey. Exp. Brain Res. 42, 319–330.

Papez, J.W., 1937. A proposed mechanism of emotion. Arch. Neurol. Psychiatry. 38, 725–743.

Patterson, J.T., Coggeshall, R.E., Lee, W.T., et al., 1990. Long ascending unmyelinated primary afferent axons in the rat dorsal column: immunohistochemical localizations. Neurosci. Lett. 108, 6–10.

Penfield, W., Rasmussen, T., 1955. The Cerebral Cortex of Man. Macmillan, New York.

Peschanski, M., Besson, J.M., 1984. A spino-reticulo-thalamic pathway in the rat: an anatomical study with reference to pain transmission. Neuroscience 12, 165–178.

Petrides, M., Pandya, D.N., 1984. Projections to the frontal cortex from the posterior parietal region in the rhesus monkey. J. Comp. Neurol. 228, 105–116.

Porro, C.A., Cettolo, V., Francescato, M.P., et al., 1998. Temporal and intensity coding of pain in human cortex. J. Neurophysiol. 80, 3312–3320.

Preuss, T.M., Goldman-Rakic, P.S., 1991. Ipsilateral cortical connections of granular frontal cortex in the strepsirrhine primate Galago, with comparative comments on anthropoid primates. J. Comp. Neurol. 310, 507–549.

Rainville, P., Duncan, G.H., Price, D.D., et al., 1997. Pain affect encoded in human anterior cingulate but not somatosensory cortex. Science 277, 968–971.

Ralston, D.D., Ralston, H.J., 1985. The terminations of corticospinal tract axons in the macaque monkey. J. Comp. Neurol. 242, 325–337.

Ralston, H.J., Ralston, D.D., 1992. The primate dorsal spinothalamic tract: evidence for a specific termination in the posterior nuclei (Po/SG) of the thalamus. Pain 48, 107–118.

Rang, H.P., Bevan, S., Dray, A., 1991. Chemical activation of nociceptive peripheral neurons. Br. Med. Bull. 47, 534–548.

Rexed, B., 1952. The cytoarchitectonic organization of the spinal cord in the cat. J. Comp. Neurol. 96, 415–495.

Rexed, B., 1954. A cytoarchitectonic atlas of the spinal cord in the cat. J. Comp. Neurol. 100, 297–379.

Ruch, T.C., 1946. Visceral sensation and referred pain. In: Fulton, J.F. (Ed.), Howell's Textbook of Physiology, fifteenth ed. Saunders, Philadelphia, pp. 385–401.

Sandyk, R., Bamford, C.R., Iacono, R., 1988. Pain and sensory symptoms in Parkinson's disease. Int. J. Neurosci. 39, 15–25.

Sato, J., Perl, E.R., 1991. Adrenergic excitation of cutaneous pain receptors induced by peripheral nerve injury. Science. 251, 1608–1610.

Schaible, H.G., Schmidt, R.F., 1985. Effects of an experimental arthritis on the sensory properties of fine articular afferent units. J. Neurophysiol. 54, 1109–1122.

Schaible, H.G., Schmidt, R.F., 1988. Time course of mechanosensitivity changes in articular afferents during a developing experimental arthritis. J. Neurophysiol. 60, 2180–2195.

Schlag-Rey, M., Schlag, J., 1984. Visuomotor functions of central thalamus in monkey. I. Unit activity related to spontaneous eye movements. J. Neurophysiol. 51, 1149–1174.

Schreiner, L., Kling, A., 1953. Behavioural changes following rhinencephalic injury in cat. J. Neurophysiol. 15, 643–659.

Seitz, R.J., Roland, P.E., 1992. Learning of sequential and finger movements in man: a combined kinematic and positron emission tomography (PET) study. Eur. J. Neurosci. 4, 154–165.

Shima, K., Aya, K., Mushiake, H., et al., 1991. Two movement-related foci in the primate cingulate cortex observed in signal-triggered and self-paced forelimb movements. J. Neurophysiol. 65, 188–202.

Simone, D.A., Kajander, K.C., 1997. Responses of A-fiber nociceptors to noxious cold. J. Neurophysiol. 77, 2049–2060.

Sluka, K.A., Price, M.P., Breese, N.M., et al., 2003. Chronic hyperalgesia induced by repeated acid injections in muscle is abolished by the loss of the ASIC3, but not ASIC1. Pain 106, 229–239.

Snider, W.D., McMahon, S.B., 1998. Tackling pain at the source: new ideas about nociceptors. Neuron. 20, 629–632.

Snyder, R., 1977. The organization of the dorsal root entry zone in cats and monkeys. J. Comp. Neurol 174, 47–70.

Stacey, M.J., 1969. Free nerve endings in skeletal muscle of the cat. J. Anat. 105, 231–254.

Stamford, J.A., 1995. Descending control of pain. Br. J. Anaesth. 75, 217–227.

Sugiura, Y., Terui, N., Hosoya, Y., 1989. Difference in distribution of central terminals between visceral and somatic unmyelinated (C) primary afferent fibers. J. Neurophysiol. 62, 834–840.

Talbot, J.D., Marrett, S., Evans, A.C., et al., 1991. Multiple representations of pain in human cerebral cortex. Science 251, 1355–1358.

Tanelian, D.I., 1991. Cholinergic activation of a population of corneal afferent nerves. Exp. Brain Res. 86, 414–420.

Tillman, D.B., Treede, R.D., Meyer, R.A., et al., 1995. Response of C fibre nociceptors in the anaesthetized monkey to heat stimuli: estimates of receptor depth and threshold. J. Physiol. 485, 753–765.

Torebjörk, H.E., Ochoa, J.L., 1980. Specific sensations evoked by activity in single identified sensory units in man. Acta Physiol. Scand. 110, 445–447.

Treede, R.D., Meyer, R.A., Campbell, J.N., 1991. Classification of primate A-fiber nociceptors according to their heat response properties. Pflügers Archives 418 (Suppl. 1), R42.

Treede, R.D., Kenshalo, D.R., Gracely, R.H., et al., 1999. The cortical representation of pain. Pain 79, 105–111.

Trevino, D.L., Carstens, E., 1975. Confirmation of the location of spinothalamic neurons in the cat and monkey by the retrograde transport of horseradish peroxidase. Brain Res. 98, 177–182.

Truex, R.C., Taylor, M.J., Smythe, M.Q., et al., 1965. The lateral cervical nucleus of cat, dog and man. J. Comp. Neurol. 139, 93–104.

Vallbo, A.B., Olausson, H., Wessberg, J., 1999. Unmyelinated afferents constitute a second system coding tactile stimuli of the human hairy skin. J. Neurophysiol. 81, 2753–2763.

Vogt, B.A., Pandya, D.N., 1987. Cingulate cortex of the rhesus monkey : II Cortical afferents. J. Comp. Neurol. 262, 271–289.

Wall, P.D., 1967. The laminar organization of dorsal horn and effects of descending impulses. J. Physiol. 188, 403–423.

Wall, P.D., Gutnick, M., 1974. Ongoing activity in peripheral nerves: the physiology and pharmacology of impulses originating from a neuroma. Exp. Neurol. 43, 580–593.

Wang, Q.P., Nakai, Y., 1994. The dorsal raphe: an important nucleus in pain modulation. Brain Res. Bull. 34, 575–585.

Wessberg, J., Olausson, H., Fernstrom, K.W., et al., 2003. Receptive field properties of unmyelinated tactile afferents in the human skin. J. Neurophysiol. 89, 1567–1575.

Willis, W.D., Coggeshall, R.E., 1991. Sensory Mechanisms of the Spinal Cord, second ed. Plenum, New York.

Willis, W.D., Al-Chaer, E.D., Quast, M.J., et al., 1999. A visceral pathway in the dorsal column of the spinal cord. Proc. Natl. Acad. Sci. U. S. A. 96, 7675–7679.

Wilson, P., Meyers, D.E., Snow, P.J., 1986. The detailed somatotopic organization of the dorsal horn in the lumbosacral enlargement of the cat spinal cord. J. Neurophysiol. 55, 604–617.

Woolf, C.J., Shortland, P., Coggeshall, R.E., 1992. Peripheral nerve injury triggers central sprouting of myelinated afferents. Nature 355, 75–78.

Yezierski, R.P., 1988. Spinomesencephalic tract: projections from the lumbosacral spinal cord of the rat, cat, and monkey. J. Comp. Neurol. 267, 131–146.

Yezierski, R.P., Gerhart, K.D., Schrock, R.J., et al., 1983. A further examination of effects of cortical stimulation on primate spinothalamic tract cells. J. Neurophysiol. 49, 424–441.

Zhang, D., Carlton, S.M., Sorkin, L.S., et al., 1990. Collaterals of primate spinothalamic tract neurons to the periaqueductal gray. J. Comp. Neurol. 296, 277–290.

Chapter | 6 |

Neurophysiology of pain

Hubert van Griensven

LEARNING OBJECTIVES

By the end of this chapter readers should have an understanding of:

1. The neurophysiology underlying somatic and visceral pain.
2. Mechanisms of sensitization in the peripheral and central nervous system.
3. Ways in which the brain controls nociceptive processing.
4. Brain structures involved in the perception of pain.

OVERVIEW

Nociception, the perception of noxious stimuli arising in the body, is part of our biological protective mechanisms. It makes us avoid activities that may make the situation worse, and promotes behaviours that aid recovery, such as communication with others and adaptive postures.

During the period of recovery the peripheral and central sensory nervous system may become more sensitive as part of this adaptive process, but this sensitivity returns to normal as nociceptive input declines.

Chronic pain, however, is more than nociception. It is associated with longer-lasting functional changes in the nervous system that are maladaptive. As a result of these changes noxious stimuli become capable of causing higher levels of pain of longer duration (hyperalgesia), while normal (non-noxious) stimuli can start to cause or contribute to pain. Areas not involved in the original injury may become sensitized. In the longer term these adaptations can become structural within the central nervous system, so pain takes on more permanent features. The function and structure of the sensory nervous system are therefore powerful determinants of how physical stimuli are perceived, and how well perceptions correlate with what is happening in the body.

Interpretation of the pathophysiological aspects of a patient's symptoms requires that the clinician understands the sensory nervous system's function and plasticity. He also needs to be aware that pain, whatever its origin, tends to be interpreted by the patient as somatic and nociceptive. In other words, pain is usually subjectively felt in skin and musculoskeletal structures, even though it may be of, for instance, visceral or neurogenic origin. Additionally, the perception of pain and concomitant suffering is subject to changes in sensory processing. A grounding in pain physiology enables the clinician to consider whether a patient's pain is indeed likely to be somatic in nature, or whether other factors may be causing, maintaining or altering it. Leading pain psychologist Chris Main states that 'Disregard of the role of central pain-processing mechanisms leads to failure to integrate the contribution of

© 2014 Elsevier Ltd.

cognitive factors, pain memories and the emotional impact of pain into the explanation given to the patient of their pain experience' (Main 2009).

Finally, it is worth noting that most of the information in this chapter is based on laboratory findings. It is often plausible that these findings apply to the clinical situation because they closely resemble what we observe in and hear from patients. Clinicians must always be aware that human beings are extremely complex, however, and that laboratory research gives us models but no absolute certainty. Findings from experiments on a small part (e.g. dorsal horn cells in a rat) may or may not be reflected in the complex experience of live human beings. There is increasing call for translational pain research in order to bridge the gap between scientific research and clinical practice (Mao 2009).

NOCICEPTION OF SOMATIC AND VISCERAL ORIGIN

Different tissue types are associated with different sensory mechanisms. Of these, cutaneous sensation has been studied most and is the type of sensation that humans are most aware of. It will therefore be used as a general introduction into sensory physiology and nociception. After that, differences with deeper somatic tissues and viscera will be explored.

Cutaneous nociception

Generally, changes in the tissues such as pressure, heat or damage activate receptors at the peripheral terminal of sensory neurons. This activation produces one or more action potentials in the neurons, which are conducted to the central nervous system and eventually the brain. The brain receives precise information about tissue events because of the way stimuli are encoded and transmitted (Gardner et al 2000)[*]. First, most receptors are highly specialized for a specific type of stimulus. Second, the more intense the stimulus, the higher the frequency of the action potentials is. Finally, the way pathways in the central nervous system are organized reflects the origin of the stimuli (somatotopical organization).

Stimuli that are associated with actual or impending tissue damage are classed as noxious (see also Box 6.1). They activate sensory receptors called nociceptors, which have a high stimulation threshold and therefore only respond to stimuli outside the normal and healthy range. Nociceptors may be specialized for either extreme thermal or mechanical stimuli, or they may be polymodal (sensitive to extreme

---

[*]Although the above is true under normal circumstances, it will become clear in this chapter that persistent pain conditions are associated with plasticity in the nervous system.

> **Box 6.1 Nociception and pain**
>
> It is important to note that nociception does not necessarily equate with pain (Box 6.3); pain is an experience, as the IASP definition makes clear (see Glossary). Another definition makes this point even more strongly: 'Pain is whatever the patient says it is' (McCaffrey & Beebe 1989). There are no pain receptors, pain fibres or pain pathways as such, although unfortunately some textbooks continue to suggest there are. This text will use the term 'nociceptive pain' for pain resulting from tissue damage and inflammation. Unless associated with long-term inflammatory conditions, this may also be termed acute pain.

> **Box 6.2**
>
> Before technology enabled the identification of separate types of neuron, the British neurologist Henry Head called the different sensory systems epicritic (Aδ) and protopathic (C) (Head & Holmes 1920). He did, however, point out that this distinction only applied to the peripheral nervous system and not the spinal cord and above.
>
> The difference in sensation between the two systems can easily be demonstrated (Price 1999a, p. 73–74). When a limb 'falls asleep' due to nerve compression, for instance with crossed legs or by applying a pressure, the Aβ fibres which are most reliant on circulation stop functioning first. As soon as this happens (i.e. when sensitivity to touch disappears), a sharp pinch will mainly activate Aδ fibres and feel a little strange but immediate and sharp. This corresponds with the first pain. Once the Aδ neurons become blocked and the skin has become very numb, the same pinch will activate only C fibres. When the skin is pinched in this situation, even though it is numb, sensation arises mainly from C-fibre stimulation. It is delayed, feels dull and outlasts the pinch. This is similar to the second pain.

thermal and mechanical stimuli as well as chemicals. Once nociceptors are activated, they generate action potentials in unmyelinated C fibres and thin myelinated Aδ fibres.

Thermal and mechanical nociceptors form the terminals of Aδ neuronal fibres, while C fibres end in polymodal nociceptors (Basbaum & Jessell 2000). These fibres have different response characteristics and are associated with different aspects of pain (Box 6.2). Neurons of the Aδ type respond quickly and also have a short adaptation time, so they tend to be active only for the duration of the stimulation. They therefore produce a brief spike of activity. The pain associated with Aδ stimulation is sharp and brief. The receptive field is small so sensations are well localized. The conduction time of Aδ fibres is much faster than for C fibres, so their activity is perceived first (so-called first pain).

Box 6.3 Pain as an illusion of nociception

The fact that pain can arise under physiological conditions can be demonstrated by experiments with the thermal grill. One version of this device consists of 15 metal bars, each 1 cm wide, with a few millimetres in between bars (Basbaum & Jessell 2000). The temperature of uneven and even numbered bars can be controlled independently.

In the experiment, the subject puts their hand on the grill. When one set of bars is warmed just before the alternating

set is cooled down, the sensation of intense burning pain is created (Craig 2004). This happens despite the fact that neither the coolness nor the warmth are in the painful range. Non-noxious warming and cooling are mediated by C and Aδ fibres, respectively (Gardner et al 2000), but the illusory effect created by the thermal grill is the result of their combined processing in the central nervous system (Craig 2004).

On the other hand, brief stimulation of C fibres leads to a slow development of action potentials after Aδ activity has ceased. Low conduction speeds lead to a second pain, while the large receptive field means that this pain is diffuse, i.e. difficult to localize with precision. Acute localized trauma may therefore be felt as a sharp localized initial pain, followed by a wave of deep dull aching pain (van Cranenburgh 2000, pp 85–88).

Apart from enabling sensation, nociceptive neurons play an active role in the regulation of inflammation. Their peripheral terminals store neuropeptides that have been produced in the cell body. These peptides, called substance P (SP) and calcitonin gene-related peptide (CGRP), may be released when nociceptive fibres are activated (Basbaum & Jessell 2000). This produces vasodilation and therefore an area of redness and oedema (flare). This 'fuelling' of local inflammatory processes does not take place if the peripheral nerve is blocked proximally (LaMotte et al 1991) and is known as neurogenic inflammation. The neuropeptides are also responsible for peripheral sensitization of nociceptors in the area by stimulating local release of histamine from mast cells. This creates allodynia and hyperalgesia to mechanical stimuli and heat in the area of flare (Raja et al 1984). The mechanical sensations affected are stroking and sharpness, but not blunt pressure (Meyer et al 2006).

Deep somatic nociception

Joint structures and muscles are innervated by Aβ, Aδ and C fibres (for an extensive review see Schaible 2009). Aβ fibres have specialized mechanoreceptors responding to changes in position, movement and activity (Gardner et al 2000). On the other hand, the nociceptive Aδ and C fibres have free nerve endings, which will normally respond only to extreme mechanical stimuli such as end of range overpressures (Schaible 2006). They will also signal tissue damage and inflammation because of their sensitivity to inflammatory mediators such as bradykinin and prostaglandins. Some C fibres form an exception in that they have a low mechanical stimulation threshold. They terminate in socalled ergoceptors, which play a role in homeostatic

regulation in exercise (Mense 2008). Joint cartilage is not innervated.

Inflammation produces peripheral sensitization of nociceptors in the joint, producing mechanical allodynia (pain as a result of normally innocuous joint movements or stretch). Muscle nociceptors will respond to inflammation in a similar way, but also to muscle activity under ischaemic conditions. The latter applies to constriction induced in laboratory conditions, but probably also in exercise involving sustained or repetitive contractions. Mechanisms of central sensitization and descending control are probably similar to those described below, although the reader should be aware that research specifically addressing these processes is limited (Schaible 2006). There is evidence that repeated noxious unilateral muscle stimulation leads to central sensitization, which can last for several weeks after stimulation has ceased.

Visceral nociception

The viscera are very different from somatic structures in their innervation and pain perception, and there are differences between organs (refer to Mayer & Gebhart 1994 and Ness & Gebhart 1990 for reviews). Viscera have two sets of afferents: one set follows sympathetic nerves and parasympathetic sacral nerves back to the spinal cord, while the other follows the parasympathetic vagus nerve to the brain stem (Bielefeld & Gebhart 2006). It is important to note that the sympathetic and parasympathetic systems themselves are purely efferent, although they may be influenced by visceral afferents in the paravertebral ganglia or spinal cord.

Viscera are mostly innervated by Aδ and C fibres, which unlike cutaneous afferents respond to mechanical stimuli as well as the usual chemical and thermal sensations (Gebhart et al 2004). The types of stimuli which provoke pain are quite different from those causing somatic pain. For example, distention of the bowel and other hollow organs can be painful, while cutting the bowel does not cause any pain whatsoever (Cervero & Laird 1999).

Visceral activity is generally not perceived and nociceptive stimulation leads to diffuse pain that is difficult to localize

(Mayer & Raybould 1990). The pain refers to more superficial structures (see below) and can therefore be mistaken as being somatic in nature. This is an important point for clinicians to bear in mind when questioning and examining a patient; internal pathologies may masquerade as musculoskeletal ones. In functional pain disorders such as non-cardiac chest pain and irritable bowel syndrome, the responses to normal visceral stimuli become enhanced, leading to hyperalgesia and referred pain (see, for example, Mertz et al 1995 and Sarkar et al 2000). These changes are the result of changes in sensory processing in the peripheral and central nervous system, rather than in the organs themselves.

Referred pain

Referred pain is pain felt at a distance from and in tissues distinct from the origin of nociceptive stimulation. It is a phenomenon associated with a non-pathological intact nervous system and must therefore be distinguished from neurogenic pains such as nerve root pain. The exact mechanisms are as yet uncertain, but it is thought that changes in sensory processing in the dorsal horn are responsible (Mense 2008). Referred pain is not purely subjective and may be associated with measurable hyperalgesia in several studies (Coutinho et al 2000; Sarkar et al 2000).

Pain referral can be said to be from deep to superficial structures (Arendt-Nielsen et al 2000): visceral pain tends to be felt in musculoskeletal and cutaneous tissues, while muscle pain is referred to the skin. Cutaneous pain, on the other hand, does not refer to other tissues.

Two theories offer the most plausible explanation for referred pain (see Fig. 6.1; Arendt-Nielsen et al 2000; McMahon 1997). The convergence–projection theory suggests that afferents from deep tissues share second-order neurons with more superficial tissues. The brain therefore

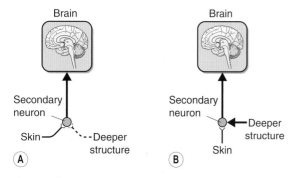

Fig. 6.1 The two main theoretical models of referred pain. (A) The convergence-projection model suggests that areas of skin and deeper tissues such as joints or viscera have an equal influence on the secondary neuron in the dorsal horn. (B) The convergence–facilitation model suggests that nociceptive stimulation from deeper structures creates pain by facilitating cutaneous input into secondary neurons in the dorsal horn.

has no way of establishing the exact origin of the pain. It interprets the pain as coming from the more superficial structures, presumably because this is where most sensation normally comes from. The convergence–facilitation theory poses that nociceptive input from deeper tissues may sensitize secondary neurons. Sensory input from superficial structures arriving at the same secondary neurons will be facilitated, so that innocuous sensations from those structures may now be perceived as painful.

There are two additional theories, each with their limitations. The thalamic convergence model suggests that sensory input from skin and viscera combines in the thalamus rather than the spinal cord. This model can account for several characteristics of referred pain, except its reduction following the application of a tourniquet or local anaesthetic (Laursen et al 1999). Projection of visceral afferents to the brain stem may therefore be partly responsible for referred pain. Finally, the axon reflex model is based on the assumption that some afferents are split to innervate both cutaneous and visceral structures. This type of axon is rare and therefore unlikely to be involved in the majority of cases of referred pain (McMahon 1997).

PERIPHERAL SENSITIZATION

It seems so intuitive that damaged or inflamed tissues will cause pain that few clinicians stop to wonder by what mechanism these processes stimulate sensory neurons. However, only if this is understood can a rational analysis be made of the possible origins of a patient's pain. Apart from damage to peripheral nerves, the subject of Chapter 10, damaged cells release chemicals such as histamine, bradykinin, serotonin and prostaglandin, some of which are inflammatory mediators released as part of the inflammatory response. These chemicals can either stimulate nociceptors directly (i.e. make them depolarize) or sensitize them (i.e. bring the membrane potential closer to depolarisation threshold) so that other stimuli are more likely to activate them. The latter is known as peripheral sensitization. An example is a fresh bruise, which may not be felt spontaneously but which is acutely sensitive to local pressure (mechanical allodynia). It will also be more sensitive to painful stimuli (primary hyperalgesia, as opposed to secondary hyperalgesia, which is the result of changes in the dorsal horn).

An overview of the mechanisms involved in peripheral sensitization follows (for a comprehensive review see McMahon et al 2006). The peripheral terminal of a nociceptive neuron has three types of receptors. Ligand-gated ion channels respond to hydrogen ions (present in acidic conditions), ATP, heat or capsaicin (an extract of chilli peppers) by opening, creating an ion flux which depolarizes the cell thus creating action potentials. Prostaglandins, bradykinin, epinephrine (adrenaline) and ATP bind to

G-protein receptors, which do not make the neuron fire but create internal chemical reactions. This leads to the sensitization of the ion channels as well as the sodium channels along the axon, thereby lowering the stimulation threshold and increasing the responsiveness of the neuron. Ligand-gated ion channels open in response to hydrogen ions (an extract of chilli peppers), creating an ion flux, which depolarizes.

The third type of receptor is tyrosine kinases, which respond to neurotrophic factors and cytokines. Small amounts of neurotrophic factors such as nerve growth factor (NGF) are released by tissues under normal conditions. They are important for the maintenance of the neurons and their make-up (see Chapter 10). Research suggests that NGF levels are increased during inflammation, sensitizing the nociceptive neurons and creating allodynia and hyperalgesia. The release of cytokines such as tumour necrosis factor-alpha (TNF-α) and interleukins (IL) also contributes to inflammatory pain. Their importance is confirmed by the efficacy of drugs that inhibit the action of TNF-α in the treatment of autoimmune diseases such as rheumatoid arthritis, ankylosing spondylitis and Crohn's disease. As they do not cross the blood–brain barrier, their action must be peripheral (Marchand et al 2005).

CENTRAL SENSITIZATION

Interestingly, in the injury model described above the area demonstrating mechanical hyperalgesia is considerably larger than the area of flare (Box 6.4). This is not the result of a spreading of sensitization within the tissues because it develops even if a tight band restricts fluid movement (LaMotte et al 1991). Instead it has been shown to be mediated by so-called central sensitization, a mechanism involving secondary sensory neurons in the dorsal horn. Central sensitization may develop as a result of persistent inflammation or peripheral nerve damage (Fig. 6.2). It is more

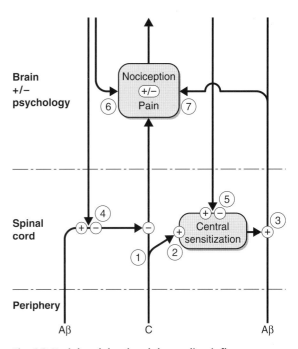

Fig. 6.2 Peripheral, local and descending influences on nociceptive processing in the dorsal horn. Nociceptive activity in C fibres can be attenuated at dorsal horn level by Aβ fibre stimulation (1). C-fibre stimulation feeds into central sensitization (2), which in turn can involve Aβ fibres in nociception (3). The extent to which Aβ stimulation influences nociception depends in part on descending influence from the brain, which may be either facilitating or inhibiting (4). Descending influences also impact on the development of central sensitization (5). Whether nociception becomes pain may rely on psychological and central pain controlling influences (6), as well as concurrent Aβ stimulation (7).

Box 6.4 **Mechanoreception and pain**

Central sensitization clearly enhances the response within the nociceptive system. In order to understand how it can lead to secondary hyperalgesia, it is important to briefly review sensory pathways in the dorsal horn. Primary nociceptive neurons synapse with secondary neurons that are either nociceptive specific (NS) or wide dynamic range (WDR). As the name implies, NS neurons transmit nociceptive information, while WDR neurons receive input from both nociceptive and Aβ fibres. When the WDR cell starts to change as a result of persistent nociceptive stimulation, this may affect the way Aβ mechanoreceptor information is processed.

Conversely Aβ fibre input affects the way nociceptive information is processed. Selective stimulation of

mechanoreceptors can have an inhibitory influence on the WDR cell, thereby reducing the excitation created by nociceptive stimulation. A simple example is rubbing or shaking a part of the body that is hurting. This mechanism is called segmental pain inhibition and may be partially responsible for some of the pain-relieving effect of stimulation therapies such as TENS and acupuncture (see Chapter 14).

Segmental inhibition was given recognition in Melzack and Wall's pain gate theory (Wall 1978). In addition, the architects of this model suggested that the pain gate might be influenced by higher centres (Melzack & Casey 1968). This is the subject of the section on descending inhibition and facilitation.

likely to develop as a result of nociceptive input from deep structures, e.g. joints and muscles, than from skin (Wall & Woolf 1984). As a consequence of central sensitization, input from mechanoreceptors and Aβ fibres into the dorsal horn will feed into or drive the nociceptive processing pathway (Woolf & Salter 2000). In other words, normal light stimuli will now feel unpleasant. Moreover, activity in the sensory nervous system will outlast the stimulus, so even a brief aggravation may be felt as pain for a long time (Box 6.5).

Key to understanding central sensitization is the fact that secondary neurons in the dorsal horn, even those classed as nociceptive specific or dedicated to nociception, receive low-level input from Aβ fibres and nociceptive fibres from regions surrounding their receptive field (Box 6.4; Latremoliere & Woolf 2009). Normally the input from these fibres is too low to activate the secondary neuron, i.e. their stimulus is not passed on beyond the dorsal horn and therefore not perceived. Once the secondary neuron becomes sensitized, however, these additional inputs start to contribute to nociception.

Classic diagrams of the sensory nervous system showing a single synapse pathway from periphery to spinal cord may be reasonably accurate in acute conditions. Clinicians ought to bear in mind that the dorsal horn contains a far more complex network of neurons, however, and that plasticity reduces sensory specificity. Patients may not be believed by clinicians ignorant of this, and some even doubt their own sanity because their symptoms are out of the ordinary. It is important to give them a realistic explanation (see Butler & Moseley 2003 and Nijs et al 2011 regarding educating patients in pain

physiology) and explore ways of addressing central sensitization.

Normally temporary nociceptive stimulation from, say, walking into the sharp corner of a metal desk will cause a primary neuron to release the excitatory neurotransmitter glutamate in its synapse in the dorsal horn (see Kandel & Siegelbaum 2000 for an overview). Glutamate binds to AMPA receptor channels on the post-synaptic membrane (second-order neuron) and opens them, thereby creating an influx of sodium and altering the membrane potential. Once stimulation threshold is reached an action potential is generated. A single impulse is normally not sufficient to generate an action potential; this requires either a train of impulses (temporal summation) or impulses from several primary neurons (spatial summation). This process stops as soon as nociceptive stimulation ends, i.e. no sensitization is involved.

If nociceptive input persists at sufficiently high intensity for at least tens of seconds, several processes occur which can increase and prolong the response of the second-order neuron (Latremoliere & Woolf 2009). The secondary membrane contains another type of glutamate receptor channel called NMDA. Normally the NMDA channel opens like the AMPA channel, but it does not let ions in because it is blocked by a magnesium ion, held in place by the voltage across the membrane. However, if prolonged or intensive stimulation reduces the membrane potential sufficiently, the magnesium ion is released. This is known as wind-up (Woolf & Salter 2000); the same amount of glutamate leads to an enhanced response, lowering of the threshold through AMPA receptors and an NMDA receptor-mediated influx of calcium.

Box 6.5 **Clinical conditions associated with altered sensory processing**

It is easy to think of central changes in sensory processing merely as abstract issues, but evidence increasingly suggests their importance in clinical conditions. Fibromyalgia, which foxed clinicians for years because of apparent inconsistencies in presentation, is now known to be associated with changes in sensory processing (Desmeules et al 2003; Staud et al 2004). Similarly, enhanced sensory processing has been demonstrated in patients with irritable bowel syndrome (Gebhart et al 2004). Interestingly, in this condition it is not just the bowel but also the skin that demonstrates an enhanced response to sensory stimulation (Verne et al 2001, 2003).

Central sensitization is associated not just with painful conditions which defy biomedical diagnosis. For example, in osteoarthritis of the knee there is poor correlation between radiological evidence of structural abnormality and pain (Creamer & Hochberg 1997). It is now clear that this condition may be associated with central sensitization in some patients (Arendt-Nielsen et al 2010). Other common conditions associated with possible central sensory changes

are headaches and temporo-mandibular disorder (Woolf 2010).

The fact that central sensitization plays a role in common painful conditions has implications for the clinical examination: both the local pathology and the processing status of the central nervous system need to be assessed when a patient presents with persistent pain (Dieppe & Lohmander 2005). The fact that processing changes have a strong genetic component (Woolf 2010) means that history taking should include questions about other painful conditions, both for the patient and within their family. A personal or familial history of seemingly unrelated painful conditions can give an initial indication of whether central sensitization may play a role. This can be explored further in the subjective and objective examination by gauging the irritability of the condition and the presence of heightened sensitivity in areas distant from the symptomatic area. Finally, fibromyalgia is likely to be associated with neurological signs and symptoms, so it is important not to jump to conclusions about the pain and carry out a full neurological examination (Watson et al 2009).

The increased concentration of calcium leads to a host of chemical processes inside the secondary neuron, reinforcing the maintenance of central sensitization. These are aided by activation of other receptors by excitatory neurotransmitters other than glutamate, for example substance P (SP) and calcitonin gene-related peptide (CGRP) (Latremoliere & Woolf 2009; Woolf & Salter 2000). In addition, more calcium may be released from within the cell itself. Together these changes enhance the response of the secondary neuron during stimulation and for some time after, up to several hours. Once established, central sensitization has been shown to be maintained for days by relatively low levels of C-fibre input (Koltzenburg et al 1992). This process is thought to play a role in maintaining pain in patients with inflammatory conditions such as rheumatoid arthritis.

With persistent nociceptive input, intracellular processes begin to alter the structure of the cell, making sensitization a more permanent feature of its response. First, AMPA proteins are transported from inside the cell and deposited in the membrane, increasing the number of glutamate receptors. At the same time some of the intracellular chemicals produced as a result of stimulation follow axonal transport back to the cell body. Here they change the transcription of DNA, leading to a change in the production of proteins. These proteins are transported back to the periphery of the cell, where they may be deposited as receptors. Now the response characteristics of the cell are changed on a more lasting basis.

Emerging research suggests that central sensitization is also mediated by microglia (Woolf & Salter 2006). These cells were previously thought to have a relatively passive role, but in fact they can release chemicals which affect neurons and mediate sensitization.

It may seem that persistent noxious stimulation or neuropathy will inevitably lead to the changes described above. Fortunately this is not the case because the influence of excitatory neurotransmitters is counteracted by inhibitory interneurons. They can release inhibitory neurotransmitters such as glycine. Whether a second-order neuron will generate an action potential or not depends on the sum of inhibitory and excitatory influences received. As described above, summation of excitation is required to make a nerve cell fire. Inhibition provides a subtraction to this process.

The dorsal horn is rich in populations of inhibitory interneurons, whose functions can be summed up as follows (Sandkühler 2009): they mute nociceptive neurons when there is no noxious stimulation and attenuate their response when there is. This ensures an appropriate level of response. When this mechanism fails, it leads to spontaneous pain and hyperalgesia. A further function is separating inputs from non-noxious Aβ fibres from nociceptive input, failure of which creates allodynia. Finally, they localize neuronal activation by controlling activation of neurons from other body regions. The inhibitory interneurons are in part under local control, but they are also powerfully influenced by descending inhibition, as discussed in the following section.

In the past some researchers have suggested that, if inhibitory mechanisms fail, the activity in the dorsal horn can eventually become permanent and independent of peripheral input. This so-called centralization of pain is now called into question (Basbaum 2008). Note also that this use of the term centralization is different from that used by physiotherapists when they refer to a reduction in peripheral spread of spinal pain as a condition improves.

DESCENDING INHIBITION AND FACILITATION

One of the most powerful discoveries in pain science is that the brain does not merely receive sensory information from the body and its surroundings, but it can select and modify its own input. Somehow this seems obvious when we think about closing our eyes or focusing on a conversation in a noisy room, but not when it comes to the perception of pain. Yet powerful mechanisms exist for the nervous system to either suppress or enhance the way nociceptive information is processed (Box 6.6; Fig. 6.2).

LeBars et al discovered that painful stimulation was able to inhibit nociceptive transmission by lumbar neurons receiving both Aβ and C fibres (i.e. WDR cells; Le Bars et al 1979a,b). They found that this effect only took place

---

Box 6.6 Nociceptive modulation and chronic pain

Laboratory evidence suggests that in inflammation and peripheral neuropathy, the brain's initial influence is facilitatory (Ossipov et al 2002; Porreca et al 2002). In fact, the development of secondary hyperalgesia as described above is mediated by this descending influence. Once inflammation resolves, descending inhibition starts to dampen down central sensitization (Dubner & Ren 2004). This responsive modulation of the way nociception is processed may have survival value:

following injury the brain initially stimulates protective behaviour. Once tissue damage resolves, awareness of the painful area is no longer necessary and may even be counterproductive so pain suppression mechanisms are activated. It is thought that this switch to inhibition does not happen in patients susceptible to chronic pain, and that plasticity in the RVM contributes to long-term pain enhancement (Porreca et al 2002).

with brain and spinal cord intact, and concluded that the effect had to be mediated by supraspinal processes. Because the inhibition could be brought on by painful stimulation even in areas not innervated by the lumbar segments, they called it the diffuse noxious inhibitory system (DNIC). It is now known that this is in part mediated by neurons in the caudal medulla (called the subnucleus reticularis dorsalis, SRD) whose activity increases according to the intensity of nociceptive stimulation received (Villanueva & Fields 2004, p. 224). They regulate activity in the thalamus (an important relay centre for nociceptive information), the deep dorsal horn (lamina V–VII) and several other regions (Villanueva & Fields 2004, p. 225). There is some evidence to suggest that the DNIC does not work well in patients with damage to caudal medulla (De Broucker et al 1990).

The DNIC-SRD network regulates nociceptive signals as they enter the spinal cord and also as they are processed in the brain stem. It is likely that they form the physiological basis of the clinical observation that one pain can inhibit another, so-called counter-irritation. For example, it is possible to apply TENS or acupuncture in this way (see Chapter 14). It is, however, important to note that the SRD's influence on the dorsal horn can be either inhibitory or facilitatory (Villanueva & Fields 2004, p. 225) and that the deciding factors are likely to be complex. Simply applying a painful stimulus may or may not have the desired effect.

Another network that has been shown to be important for the modulation of nociceptive processing involves the peri-aquaductal grey (PAG) and the rostral ventromedial medulla (RVM). Nociceptive stimulation can activate the PAG, which in turn stimulates neurons in the RVM. These neurons descend to the dorsal horn, where they inhibit firing of neurons in laminae I, II and V (Fields et al 2006). They do so through the release of serotonin (5-HT; Basbaum 2008). A similar pathway exists from the locus coeruleus (LC), which exerts its inhibitory influence on the dorsal horn by releasing noradrenaline (NA, norepinephrine) in the dorsal horn (Fields et al 2006). Clinical experiments have demonstrated that the PAG-RVM inhibition system acts specifically on the dorsal horn(s) where the nociceptive information is received (Benedetti et al 1999). It is able to suppress painful input very selectively.

The PAG-RVM network has also been shown to be activated in threatening situations (Fields et al 2006), producing what is known as stress-induced analgesia (Carlsson 2002). It is worth bearing in mind, however, that like the DNIC, the RVM can have not only an inhibitory but also a facilitatory influence on the dorsal horn. It has been implemented in the development of hypersensitivity (allodynia and hyperalgesia) in inflammation and neuropathy (Gardell et al 2003). This is because the RVM does not only contain descending neurons which inhibit nociceptive transmission (so-called off cells), but also cells that facilitate it (Fields et al 2006). The role of a third type, the neutral cell, is less clearly understood.

PROCESSING AND CONTROL BY HIGHER CENTRES

With the advent of modern recording and imaging techniques, it has become possible to find out which brain regions are involved when pain is experienced (Box 6.6). More importantly, the influence of cognitive and emotional factors such as distraction, anticipation and anxiety can be shown with relative accuracy. The findings can be correlated with the participant's subjective experience. The technology involved promises to bridge the gap between animal-based physiology research on one hand and human psychological and psycho-physical research on the other (Box 6.7; Jensen 2010). At present it is not yet clear to what extent brain imaging brings genuine insight or whether it represents a modern form of phrenology because observation of activity does not establish cause and effect (Moseley 2006). Moreover, it is not yet clear whether differences shown between individuals are the result of genetic differences or other factors (Tracey 2008).

Briefly, current imaging techniques utilize the fact that neuronal activity has a metabolic effect and is therefore associated with changes in blood flow and consumption of oxygen and glucose (Casey 2000). Blood oxygenation levels can be imaged using functional magnetic resonance imaging (fMRI). Positron emission tomography (PET) requires radioactive labelling of oxygen or neurotransmitters, which can then be traced. Other recording methods are electroencephalography (EEG) and magnetoencephalography (MEG). Each approach is indirect, and each has its own advantages and disadvantages. In terms of determining the involvement of brain regions, fMRI and PET offer higher spatial resolution, but encephalography represents temporal aspects more accurately (Lorenz & Tracey 2009).

Pain perception has many associations such as emotions, memories, thoughts, autonomic reactions and behaviours. Not surprisingly then, the brain's response is complex and involves many areas. The total of all regions involved has been called the pain matrix or cerebral signature (Tracey 2008). It is beyond the scope of this chapter to give a detailed description of the cerebral signature, but the main components are as follows. Lateral structures such as the primary and secondary somatosensory cortex (S1 and S2) and posterior insula seem to be involved with the sensory and discriminative aspects of pain, i.e. what is felt, where it is in the body and how intense it is. Activity in medial structures like the anterior cingulated cortex (ACC), prefrontal cortex (PFC) and anterior insula is associated with the affective and motivational components (Lorenz & Tracey 2009). The ACC can be said to be engaged with the pain's aspects of suffering, fear and taking action, while the insula can be viewed as a centre for overall well-being and homeostasis (Jensen 2010). Interestingly but perhaps not surprisingly,

Box 6.7 **Clinical application of brain neuroplasticity**

It is clear from brain-imaging studies and studies investigating descending pain control that inhibition of pain involves active physiological processes. For example, focusing attention on something other than pain does not mean that we simply look away from the pain, but that we activate circuitry that suppresses nociceptive processing. Anxiety does not accentuate pain merely because the patient imagines it to be worse than it is; it enhances sensory processing and amplifies the response.

Any intervention that reduces anxiety, enhances a sense of control, and enables relaxation and distraction can be viewed as a brain intervention with not only psychological but also physiological effects. Many years ago, Donald Hebb established the basic principle of neuroplasticity: nerves that fire together, wire together (LeDoux 2002 provides an excellent review). Neurons that are activated simultaneously on a regular basis will eventually form physical links and respond as a unit. In the case of pain, persistent nociceptive activity is likely to make pain felt more easily. Its associated thoughts, emotions and motor patterns can become permanent features; an activity that caused pain in the past activates neural circuits associated with that pain.

Because of neuroplasticity the opposite is also true. Repeated practice of positive emotions and pain management strategies gives a pain sufferer the chance to train the activation of the neural networks which control pain (see Dispenza 2007 for an in-depth exploration). Physical and psychological therapies, when approached in the right context, have the power to demonstrate to the patient that pain, negative emotions and activities are not inextricably linked. The elements of the pain experience can be disassociated from each other, for instance by allowing a patient to learn that a certain type of activity can be done without pain, and that a felt pain does not need to be linked with a learned emotional response. This dissociation is one of the objectives of mindfulness-based interventions (Grabovac et al 2011). An accessible discussion of this topic is provided in Buddha's Brain (Hanson & Mendius 2009).

these structures are also activated when a loved one experiences pain, while S1 remains unaffected (Singer et al 2004). As brain-imaging techniques developed, scientists expected to find differences in the activation of brain structures between acute and chronic pain. To date, this has not been demonstrated convincingly (Jones 2005).

With regards to pain control, research has demonstrated that the ACC has direct neural links with the PAG, both of which have high concentrations of opioid receptors (Petrovic & Ingvar 2002). The neurons controlling the PAG from the ACC and other regions like the lateral orbitofrontal cortex act by releasing the body's own types of opioids, known as endorphins (endogenous opioid peptides, of which there are three types: enkephalin, dynorphin and β-endorphin) and thereby activating PAG neurons. It is likely that the control of pain by the deliberate direction of attention, demonstrated in several studies, involves the activation of the descending inhibitory system by for instance the ACC (Bushnell et al 2004). Moreover, ACC and PAG have been shown to be activated by analgesia via either administered opioids (i.e. morphine) or placebo, while pain alone does not change their activity (Petrovic et al 2002). They are also involved in the modulation of pain perception by emotions (Villemure & Bushnell 2002).

The aforementioned study is further confirmation that placebo analgesia is not a purely subjective phenomenon, but that it has clear neurophysiological correlates (Price 1999b). In other words, the belief that pain will be relieved activates pain-suppressing pathways: the nervous system makes the belief real. This has been confirmed by repeating tests demonstrating the analgesic effects of placebo interventions and opioid drugs following the administration of naloxone (ter Riet et al 1998). Naloxone is a drug that in itself cannot be tasted or otherwise detected by the participant, but which blocks the body's opioid receptors, making them unresponsive to either endogenous or administered opioids. With naloxone in the system, placebo interventions and opioids no longer have any effect. The opioid system does not account for all aspects, however; some forms of conditioning producing placebo analgesia are not completely naloxone reversible and other mechanisms also play a role (Amanzio & Benedetti 1999).

More recent studies have demonstrated that placebo analgesia does not constitute a blanket suppression of nociceptive processing, but that it selectively targets the area of the body receiving the placebo intervention (Benedetti et al 1999). This suggests that there are pathways from the PAG to each level of the spinal cord, enabling it to control specific incoming signals.

CONCLUSION

Historically, clinicians have been prone to use an end organ model that is based on the assumption that pain felt in certain tissues must be the result of a pathology in those tissues (Mayer & Bushnell 2009). Clinical reality frequently challenges this model. Patients present with any number of symptoms, the internal relationship of which is often not clear. The clinician who decides what the primary pathology must be may be left with a dissatisfying range of unexplained co-morbidities. The difficulties become clear when confronted with a patient who demands a clear (end organ) explanation for their symptoms: how well do we fare when we have to explain back pain as non-specific?

This chapter has highlighted several ways in which functional changes in the nervous system can alter persistent pain. The relationship between stimulus and response changes, unaffected tissues become sensitive and previously innocuous stimuli become capable of generating pain. Armed with an understanding of the mechanisms underlying these changes the clinician can question and examine the patient from a different perspective (see van Griensven 2005, pp 181–199 for a discussion). Rather than trying to establish what the main pathology is, the first question is whether there indeed is a pathology, and to what extent changes in sensory processing and neural output may be contributing to the symptoms. In some cases taking away nociceptive input by treating the end organ, which is the traditional biomedical approach, may be sufficient. In many other cases it is the function of the nervous system and by extension the mental and emotional factors which need to be addressed.

An understanding of pain neurophysiology can help clinicians to interpret patient's symptoms, especially when signs and symptoms are confusing. It can enable them to give realistic explanations to patients, putting their minds at rest. Finally, it can be used to develop novel treatment strategies that may lead to pain relief for more people.

Q Questions for self-assessment

1. What is the difference between nociception and pain?
2. What pain characteristics would suggest that a nociceptive pain is mediated by Aδ fibres or by C fibres?
3. What are the mechanisms responsible for primary and secondary hyperalgesia?
4. If a patient has allodynia, what can give you an indication of whether it is due to primary or secondary hyperalgesia?
5. What is referred pain? How is it different from neuropathic pain?
6. Describe a physiological mechanism which explains how distraction can suppress nociceptive input.

REFERENCES

Amanzio, M., Benedetti, F., 1999. Neuropharmacological dissection of placebo analgesia: expectation-activated opioid systems versus conditioning-activated specific subsystems. J. Neurosci. 19 (1), 484–494.

Arendt-Nielsen, L., Laursen, R., Drewes, A., 2000. Referred pain as an indicator for neural plasticity. In: Sandkühler, J., Bromm, B., Gebhart, G. (Eds.), Nervous System Plasticity and Chronic Pain. Elsevier, Amsterdam, pp. 344–356.

Arendt-Nielsen, L., Nie, H., Laursen, M., et al., 2010. Sensitisation in patients with painful knee osteoarthritis. Pain 149, 573–581.

Basbaum, A., 2008. Pain: basic mechanims. In: Castro-Lopes, J., Raja, S., Schmelz, M. (Eds.), Pain 2008.An updated review. IASP Press, Seattle, pp. 3–12.

Basbaum, A., Jessell, T., 2000. The perception of pain. In: Kandel, E., Schwartz, J., Jessell, T. (Eds.), Principles of neural science, fourth ed. McGraw-Hill, New York, pp. 472–491.

Benedetti, F., Arduino, C., Amanzio, M., 1999. Somatotopic activation of opioid systems by target-directed expectations of analgesia. J. Neurosci. 19 (9), 3639–3648.

Bielefeld, K., Gebhart, G., 2006. Visceral pain: basic mechanisms. In: McMahon, S., Koltzenburg, M. (Eds.), Wall and Melzack's Textbook of Pain, fifth ed. Churchill Livingstone, Edinburgh, pp. 721–736.

Bushnell, M., Villemure, C., Duncan, G., 2004. Psychophysical and neurophysiological studies of pain modulation by attention. In: Price, D., Bushnell, M. (Eds.), Psychological methods of pain control: basic science and clinical perspectives. IASP Press, Seattle, pp. 99–116.

Butler, D., Moseley, G., 2003. Explain pain. NOIgroup, Adelaide.

Carlsson, C., 2002. Acupuncture mechanisms for clinically relevant long-term effects – reconsideration and a hypothesis. Acupunct. Med. 20 (2,3), 82–99.

Casey, K., 2000. The imaging of pain: background and rationale. In: Casey, K., Bushnell, M. (Eds.), Pain imaging. IASP Press, Seattle, pp. 1–29.

Cervero, F., Laird, J., 1999. Visceral pain. Lancet. 353, 2145–2148.

Coutinho, S., Su, X., Sengupta, J., et al., 2000. Role of sensitized pelvic nerve afferents from the inflamed rat colon in the maintenance of visceral hyperalgesia. In: Sandkühler, J., Bromm, B., Gebhart, G. (Eds.), Nervous System Plasticity and Chronic Pain. Elsevier, Amsterdam, pp. 375–387.

Craig, A., 2004. Insights from the thermal grill on the nature of pain and hyperalgesia in humans. In: Brune, K., Handwerker, H. (Eds.), Hyperalgesia: molecular mechanisms and clinical implications. IASP Press, Seattle, pp. 311–328.

Creamer, P., Hochberg, M., 1997. Why does osteoarthritis of the knee hurt – sometimes? Br. J. Rheumatol. 36 (7), 726–728.

De Broucker, T., Cesaro, P., Willer, J., et al., 1990. Diffuse noxious inhibitory controls in man. Involvement of the spinoreticular tract. Brain 113 (1223), 1234.

Desmeules, J., Cedraschi, C., Rapiti, E., et al., 2003. Neurophysiologic evidence for a central sensitisation in patients with fibromyalgia. Arthritis Rheum. 48 (5), 1420–1429.

Dieppe, P., Lohmander, L., 2005. Pathogenesis and management of pain in osteoarthritis. Lancet 365 (9463), 965–973.

Dispenza, J., 2007. Evolve your brain. The science of changing your mind. Health Communications, Deerfield Beach.

Dubner, R., Ren, K., 2004. Brainstem modulation of pain. In: Villanueva, L., Dickenson, A., Ollat, H. (Eds.), The pain system in normal and pathological states: a primer for clinicians. IASP Press, Seattle, pp. 107–120.

Fields, H., Basbaum, A., Heinricher, M., 2006. Central nervous system mechanisms of pain modulation. In: McMahon, S., Koltzenburg, M. (Eds.), Wall and Melzack's Textbook of Pain, fifth ed. Churchill Livingstone, Oxford, pp. 125–142.

Gardell, L., Vanderah, T., Gardell, S., et al., 2003. Enhanced evoked excitatory transmitter release in experimental neuropathy requires descending facilitation. J. Neurosci. 23 (23), 8370–8379.

Gardner, E., Martin, J., Jessell, T., 2000. The bodily senses. In: Kandel, E., Schwartz, J., Jessell, T. (Eds.), Principles of neural science, fourth ed. McGraw-Hill, New York, pp. 430–450.

Gebhart, G., Kuner, R., Jones, R., et al., 2004. Visceral hypersensitivity. In: Brune, K., Handwerker, H. (Eds.), Hyperalgesia: molecular mechanisms and clinical implications. IASP Press, Seattle, pp. 87–104.

Grabovac, A., Lau, M., Willett, B., 2011. Mechanisms of mindfulness: a Buddhist psychological model. Mindfulness 2 (3), 154–166.

Hanson, R., Mendius, R., 2009. Buddha's brain. The practical neuroscience of happiness, love & wisdom. New Harbinger, Oakland, CA.

Head, H., Holmes, G., 1920. Studies in neurology. Frowde; Stodder & Houghton, London.

Jensen, M., 2010. A neuropsychological model of pain: research and clinical implications. J. Pain 11 (1), 2–12.

Jones, A., 2005. The role of the cerebral cortex in pain perception. In: Justins, D. (Ed.), Pain 2005 – an updated review. IASP Press, Seattle, pp. 59–70.

Kandel, E., Siegelbaum, S., 2000. Synaptic integration. In: Kandel, E., Schwartz, J., Jessell, T. (Eds.), Principles of neural science, fourth ed.

McGraw-Hill, New York, pp. 207–228.

Koltzenburg, M., Lundberg, L., Torebjörk, E., 1992. Dynamic and static components of mechanical hyperalgesia in human hairy skin. Pain 51 (2), 207–219.

LaMotte, R., Shain, C., Simone, D., et al., 1991. Neurogenic hyperalgesia: psychophysical studies of underlying mechanisms. J. Neurophysiol. 66 (1), 190–211.

Latremoliere, A., Woolf, C., 2009. Central sensitisation: a generator of pain hypersensitivity by central neural plasticity. J. Pain 10 (9), 895–926.

Laursen, R., Graven-Nielsen, T., Jensen, T., et al., 1999. The effect of compression and regional anaesthetic block on referred pain intensity in humans. Pain 80 (12), 257–263.

Le Bars, D., Dickenson, A., Besson, J.M., 1979a. Diffuse noxious inhibitory controls (DNIC). 1. Effects on dorsal horn convergent neurones in the rat. Pain 6, 283–304.

Le Bars, D., Dickenson, A., Besson, J.M., 1979b. Diffuse noxious inhibitory controls (DNIC). 2. Lack of effect on non-convergent neurones, supraspinal involvement and theoretical implications. Pain 6, 305–327.

LeDoux, J., 2002. Synaptic self. Penguin, London.

Lorenz, J., Tracey, I., 2009. Brain correlates of psychological amplification of pain. In: Mayer, E., Bushnell, M. (Eds.), Functional pain syndromes: presentation and pathophysiology. IASP Press, Seattle, pp. 385–404.

Main, C.J., 2009. Talking about pain: What ever happened to Lumbago? Pain News Spring.

Mao, J., 2009. Translational pain research: achievements and challenges. J. Pain 10 (10), 1001–1011.

Marchand, F., Perretti, M., McMahon, S., 2005. Role of the immune system in chronic pain. Nat. Rev. Neurosci. 6, 521–532.

Mayer, E., Bushnell, M., 2009. Functional pain disorders: time for a paradigm shift? In: Mayer, E., Bushnell, M. (Eds.), Functional pain syndromes. Presentation and pathophysiology. IASP Press, Seattle, pp. 531–565.

Mayer, E., Gebhart, G., 1994. Basic and clinical aspects of visceral hyperalgesia. Gastroenterology 107, 271–293.

Mayer, E., Raybould, H., 1990. Role of visceral afferent mechanisms in functional bowel disorders. Gastroenterology 99, 1688–1704.

McCaffrey, M., Beebe, A., 1989. Pain: Clinical manual for nursing practice. Mosby, St Louis.

McMahon, S., 1997. Are there fundamental differences in the peripheral mechanisms of visceral and somatic pain? Behav. Brain Sci. 20, 381–391.

McMahon, S., Bennett, D., Bevan, S., 2006. Inflammatory mediators and modulators of pain. In: McMahon, S., Koltzenburg, M. (Eds.), Wall and Melzack's Textbook of Pain, fifth ed. Churchill Livingstone, Edinburgh, pp. 49–72.

Melzack, R., Casey, K., 1968. Sensory, motivational, and central control determinants of pain. In: Kenshalo, D. (Ed.), The skin senses. Charles C Thomas, Springfield, IL, pp. 423–443.

Mense, S., 2008. Peripheral and central mechanisms of musculoskeletal pain. In: Castro-Lopes, J., Raja, S., Schmelz, M. (Eds.), Pain 2008. An updated review. IASP Press, Seattle, pp. 55–62.

Mertz, H., Naliboff, B., Munakata, J., et al., 1995. Altered rectal perception is a biological marker of patients with irritable bowel syndrome. Gastroenterology 109, 40–52.

Meyer, R., Ringkamp, M., Campbell, J., et al., 2006. Peripheral mechanisms of cutaneous nociception. In: McMahon, S., Koltzenburg, M. (Eds.), Wall and Melzack's Textbook of Pain, fifth ed. Churchill Livingstone, Edinburgh, pp. 3–34.

Moseley, G., 2006. Making sense of S1 mania: Are things really that simple? In: Gifford, L. (Ed.), Topical issues in pain 5. CNS Press, Falmouth.

Ness, T., Gebhart, G., 1990. Visceral pain: a review of experimental studies. Pain 41, 167–234.

Nijs, J., van Wilgen, C., Van Oosterwijck, J., et al., 2011. How to explain central sensitisation to patients with 'unexplained' chronic musculoskeletal pain: practice guidelines. Manual Therapy. 16, 413–418.

Ossipov, M., Lai, J., Malan, T., et al., 2002. Tonic descending facilitation as a mechanism of neuropathic pain. In: Hansson, P., Fields, H.L., Hill, R.G. et al., (Eds.), Neuropathic Pain: Pathophysiology and Treatment. IASP Press, Seattle, pp. 107–124.

Petrovic, P., Ingvar, M., 2002. Imaging cognitive modulation of pain processing. Pain 95 (1,2), 1–5.

Petrovic, P., Kalso, E., Petersson, K., et al., 2002. Placebo and opioid analgesia-imaging a shared neuronal network. Science 295, 1737–1740.

Porreca, F., Ossipov, M., Gebhart, G., 2002. Chronic pain and medullary descending facilitation. Trends Neurosci. 25 (6), 319–325.

Price, D., 1999b. Placebo analgesia. In: Price, D. (Ed.), Psychological mechanisms of pain and analgesia. IASP Press, Seattle, pp. 155–181.

Price, D., 1999a. Psychological mechanisms of pain and analgesia. IASP Press, Seattle.

Raja, S., Campbell, J., Meyer, R., 1984. Evidence for different mechanisms of primary and secondary hyperalgesia following heat injury to the glabrous skin. Brain 107, 1179–1188.

Sandkühler, J., 2009. The role of inhibition in the generation and amplification of pain. In: Castro-Lopes, J. (Ed.), Current topics in pain. IASP Press, Seattle, pp. 53–72.

Sarkar, S., Aziz, Q., Woolf, C., et al., 2000. Contribution of central sensitisation to the development of non-cardiac chest pain. Lancet 356, 1154–1159.

Schaible, H., 2006. Basic mechanisms of deep somatic pain. In: McMahon, S., Koltzenburg, M. (Eds.), Wall and Melzack's Textbook of Pain, fifth ed. Churchill Livingstone, Oxford, pp. 621–633.

Schaible, H., 2009. Neuronal mechanisms of joint pain. In: Castro-Lopes, J. (Ed.), Current topics in pain. IASP Press, Seattle, pp. 115–138.

Singer, T., Seymour, B., O'Doherty, J., et al., 2004. Empathy for pain involves the affective but not sensory components of pain. Science 303 (5561), 1157–1162.

Staud, R., Price, D., Robinson, M., et al., 2004. Maintenance of windup of second pain requires less frequent stimulation in fibromyalgia patients compared to normal controls. Pain 110 (3), 689–696.

ter Riet, G., de Craen, A., de Boer, A., et al., 1998. Is placebo analgesia mediated by endogenous opioids? Pain 76 (3), 273–276.

Tracey, I., 2008. Imaging pain. Br. J. Anaesth. 101 (1), 32–39.

van Cranenburgh, B., 2000. Pijn – vanuit een neurowetenschappelijk perspectief. Elsevier Gezondheidszorg, Maarssen.

van Griensven, H., 2005. Putting it all together. In: van Griensven, H. (Ed.), Pain in practice. Theory and treatment strategies for manual therapists. Butterworth Heinemann, Edinburgh, pp. 181–199.

Verne, G., Robinson, M., Price, D., 2001. Hypersensitivity to visceral and cutaneous pain in the irritable bowel syndrome. Pain 93 (1), 7–14.

Verne, G., Himes, N., Robinson, M., et al., 2003. Central representation of visceral and cutaneous hypersensitivity in the irritable bowel syndrome. Pain 103, 99–110.

Villanueva, L., Fields, H., 2004. Endogenous central mechanisms of pain modulation. In: Villanueva, L., Dickenson, A., Ollat, H. (Eds.), The pain system in normal and pathological states: a primer for clinicians. IASP Press, Seattle, pp. 223–243.

Villemure, C., Bushnell, M., 2002. Cognitive modulation of pain: how do attention and emotion influence pain processing? Pain 95 (3), 195–199.

Wall, P., 1978. The gate control theory of pain mechanisms. A re-examination and re-statement. Brain 101, 1–18.

Wall, P., Woolf, C., 1984. Muscle but not cutaneous C-afferent input produces prolonged increases in the excitability of the flexion reflex of the rat. J. Physiol. 356 (1), 443–458.

Watson, N., Buchwald, D., Goldberg, J., et al., 2009. Neurologic signs and symptoms in fibromyalgia. Arthritis Rheum. 60 (9), 2839–2844.

Woolf, C., Salter, M., 2000. Neuronal plasticity: increasing the gain in pain. Science 288, 1765–1768.

Woolf, C., 2010. Central sensitisation: implications for the diagnosis and treatment of pain. Pain 152 (3), S2–S15.

Woolf, C., Salter, M., 2006. Plasticity and pain: the role of the dorsal horn. In: McMahon, S., Koltzenburg, M. (Eds.), Wall and Melzack's Textbook of Pain, fifth ed. Churchill Livingstone, Edinburgh, pp. 91–106.

Section | 2 |

Assessment and management of pain

Chapter 7

Assessing pain

Jenny Strong and Hubert van Griensven

LEARNING OBJECTIVES

At the end of this chapter readers will be able to:

1. Understand the differences between pain assessment and pain measurement.
2. Describe the types of pain evaluation commonly used.
3. Describe some of the most commonly used pain measurement tools.
4. Be aware of some consensus guidelines around pain assessment.
5. Understand the impact which culture, ethnicity, religion and gender can have on pain assessment.

OVERVIEW

In earlier chapters the multifaceted and all-encompassing experience of pain was discussed. It is not enough to ask 'How intense is your pain on a 0–10 scale?' A therapist must carefully assess the multidimensional aspects of the pain phenomenon to develop a comprehensive programme with the patient. In this chapter we will provide the novice

pain therapist with knowledge about pain assessment and measurement.

An overview of models and methods of assessing and measuring pain will be given. Broad, interdisciplinary models of pain assessment will be described, as well as profession or discipline-specific models. In particular, the occupational therapy model of occupational performance will be used as a guide to assessment by the occupational therapist, and the acute pain and orthopaedic models will be used to guide assessment by the physiotherapist.

Specific tools for measuring aspects of pain will be described. For each measure, utility, reliability and validity will be addressed. In conjunction with undertaking pain measurement for treatment, outcome measurement for determining therapy efficacy will also be reviewed. Lastly, we will consider other factors that may influence outcomes in the assessment and measurement of pain. Key terms are defined in Box 7.1

SOME IMPORTANT ISSUES IN THE MEASUREMENT OF PAIN

Assessment of an individual's pain is an important task for health professionals, yet pain is a subjective phenomenon that defies objective measurement (Unruh et al 2001). The perception, interpretation and assessment of a patient's pain are restricted, in theoretical, philosophical, diagnostic and practical terms, by the subjective nature of the pain experience. There have been many attempts to make a coherent objective assessment of pain (Beecher 1959; Noble et al 2005; Unruh et al 2002), including the application of numeric rating scales in clinical practice (Noble et al 1995). Most methods for assessing a person's pain have relied on a simple scale of pain magnitude or intensity (Gracely & Kwilosz 1988). A valuable channel

© 2014 Elsevier Ltd.

of information arises from the language used by the patient; that is, *by how they describe it* (Fernandez & Boyle 2001; Strong et al 2009).

The number of measurement tools available to assess and measure a person's pain has continued to increase over the past decade. Indeed, there is a plethora of literature about the measurement of pain experience. How does one decide what measures are suitable for a particular setting? There are three important considerations. The measure must have clinical utility. It must also be reliable, and it must be a valid measure of that aspect of pain for which it is intended. We will briefly discuss these three considerations before we discuss types of measures, and then measures for each of the four components of pain (description, temporal nature of the pain, response, impact). Additionally, we will look at the recommendations from some consensus guidelines about the necessary and sufficient dimensions and assessments of pain. Key terms are described in Table 7.1.

One other important aspect to be covered in this chapter is the impact of culture, ethnicity, religion and gender on pain assessment. As Fabrega and Tyma said, 'It follows logically that culture and language are inextricably bound together with the communication of pain' (Fabrega & Tyma 1976, pp 323–324). the assumption that one measurement tool, developed for a particular culture, has direct applicability to other cultures and languages will be examined.

Clinical utility

Clinical practice is often pragmatic or local in style, and may seem not to exactly match the theory on which a measure is based. Often, the primary consideration is that pain measurement must be clinically helpful to the setting in which it will be used. Voepel-Lewis et al (2010) argue that pain assessment tools are only useful when adaptable within busy settings, such as in intensive care situations. Most therapists find that there is a limit to the available time for assessment and measurement. Clinically useful measurement is therefore parsimonious; short, efficient measurements collecting the maximum useable information are preferred. For this reason, in order to be comprehensive and parsimonious, it is advisable to aim for only one measurement tool from each of the four dimensions (description of the pain, temporal nature of the pain, responses to the pain, impact of pain) unless more measurement is essential.

The usefulness of the measures we incorporate into our practice depends on the quality of their reliability and their validity. Measures about which the reliability and validity are unknown may provide quantitative information, they may be in common usage and may even be accepted by insurance companies, but they do not provide us with an accurate and confident assessment of the patient's pain experience. We do not really know that they measure what they claim to measure.

The use of many different outcome measures has meant that the results of different research trials have often been difficult to compare with each other and with results in clinical practice. In recent years efforts have been made to reach consensus on key pain measures to be used in research in order to improve consistency across clinical trials. The recommendations are referred to as the Initiative on Methods, Measurement, and Pain Assessment in Clinical Trials (IMMPACT; Dworkin et al 2005; Turk et al 2008). While they represent an important step in reducing the number of measures used, it is important to bear in mind that they are focused on research rather than clinical practice. Similar consensus was reached by a different group regarding a wider range of patient-reported health-related outcome measures. The Patient Reported Outcome Measurement Information System framework (PROMIS, see www.nihpromis.org) includes measures such as social health and social function, as well as pain, emotions and fatigue. Although its main focus is on research, the tools are likely to be useful to clinicians as well. Finally, the EuroQoL group have attempted to put together a simple health outcome measure which consists of six key questions including pain, the EQ-5D (see www.euroqol.org).

Reliability of pain measures

Reliable measures of pain provide consistent results from one time of use to the next. To illustrate, a reliable thermometer will give the same temperature from one hour to the next in a static thermal state. If there is much fluctuation in the temperature readings in the static thermal state, then the thermometer is not reliable. Of course, if circumstances change, such as the patient develops a fever, we would expect a reliable thermometer to measure this change. This property of a measurement tool is termed its responsiveness to change (Guyatt et al 1987). A reliable measure of pain also will provide similar information from one time to the next unless the pain changes (i.e. intra-rater reliability). The measure will also give the same results, or very close to the same, if two different therapists administer the measure (i.e. inter-rater reliability).

Data on the reliability of an instrument may be context specific. For example, the reliability may have been obtained in a population that may have specific characteristics (i.e. demographic, specific pain conditions or normal), which limits its use to that population. This is an issue that the therapist who is using the reliability data of an instrument should take into consideration.

How does the reliability of a pain measure relate to clinical usage for therapists? In selecting the most appropriate assessment or battery of assessments to use for any particular patient, the aim is to balance the need for psychometrically reliable data against the need for a measurement tool that can be administered efficiently. It may be that the most reliable measurement tool is very long and the patient has a short attention span, or requires so many other evaluations that a long one is impractical. In many clinical situations, the time available for completing an assessment is short. The measures that are used need to use time efficiently. For example, Krebs et al (2009) found that an ultrashort, three-item adaptation of the Brief Pain Inventory (BPI) (Payen et al 2001) was comparably valid for assessing pain among primary care and ambulatory clinic patients in relation to the original BPI.

The utility of a measurement is also limited by its complexity. In some situations, the most effective way to assess the quality of pain would be the McGill Pain Questionnaire (MPQ) (Melzack 1975), but if the patient speaks little English or any of the languages into which the MPQ has been translated, then a visual analogue scale (VAS) may be more useful. Other special populations, such as critically ill adults and children who are unable to report on their pain, have been shown to benefit from the use of the simple Face, Legs, Activity, Cry, Consolability (FLACC) behavioural tool (Voepel-Lewis et al 2010). This same study demonstrated correlation between FLACC results and those arising from 0–10 numeric rating scale usage, a measure which Jensen et al (1999) found to have sufficient reliability and validity for use with patients with chronic pain, especially in research involving large sample sizes.

Validity of pain measures

A pain measure is valid if the measure truly measures what it is supposed to measure and not something else. Knowing exactly what some pain measures are measuring may be more contentious than one would expect. The pain drawing (Parker et al 1995), for instance, may not simply describe areas where patients feel pain of various types. Sometimes anatomically and physiologically impossible distributions of pain are selected. Does the pain drawing describe the location of pain or does it measure something else, like psychological distress? In fact, it has been proposed that scoring systems for the pain drawing may be used to assess psychological distress, but efforts to do this have met with equivocal success (Parker et al 1995). Unusual drawings may convey psychological distress but they may also mean an unusual pain distribution (Waddell 2004).

When a measure is being developed, a prime concern is the content validity of the measure. However, if the measure is not reliable then it cannot be valid. A measure that provides inconsistent outcomes is giving information about something other than what it is intending to measure.

Types of pain measures

The distinction between categories of pain measures and their strengths and limitations will be assisted by completion of Reflective exercise 7.1.

Reflective exercise 7.1

Imagine you have a severe migraine. Your roommate has never had migraines. She observes that you are listening to some quiet music while you are trying a relaxation strategy on your bed. Suppose we want to measure how bad your migraine might be. We could ask you.
- What factors might influence the rating you give?

An alternative would be to ask your roommate to complete an observational pain measure.
- How accurate do you think her measurement of your pain would be?

A third way might be to record your pulse or rate of breathing.
- Do you think these measures would tell us anything about the severity of your migraine?

Self-report

As suggested in the Reflective exercise, there are three types of pain measures: self-report measures, observational measures and physiological measures (see Box 7.2). The first type is 'self-report'. The person with the pain provides the information to complete the measure about the pain. Self-report measures are used in many ways. They often involve rating pain on some kind of metric scale. A therapist might ask the patient to rate the worst pain, the least pain and the average pain in the past week. Diaries are another way to gain a prospective, subjective view of a patient's pain if the pain is persistent or chronic. It is a helpful way to measure the impact of the pain on the patient's life. Diaries can be relatively structured with the necessary information to record prepared in a format that is completed at regular intervals. Ratings of pain intensity, levels of rest and activity, and current mood and emotional or affective states can also be recorded.

Self-report is considered the gold standard of pain measurement because it is consistent with the definition of pain. Pain is a subjective experience, but the dilemma of self-report measures is exactly that subjective nature. They are based on the patient's perception of her or his pain and that perception may be influenced by other factors. To illustrate, the rating that you give about the severity of your migraine in Reflective exercise 7.1 is useful only to the extent that the therapist believes that you have given an honest response.

There has been controversy about the validity of self-report data; some work has shown the level of pain reported by patients with chronic pain was unrelated to their self-report of physical disability (Patrick & D'Eon 1996). The dilemma here is that we intuitively expect that the extent of disability should be proportionately related to the severity of the pain. When they are not related in this way, we are inclined to argue that the patient's self-report of pain intensity is exaggerated and invalid. This may be

Box 7.1 **Key terms defined**

In 1980, the World Health Organization (WHO) published the International Classification of Impairments, Disabilities and Handicaps (ICIDH) to help classify the consequences of injuries and diseases, and their implications for people. This taxonomy provides a useful framework for considering the functional difficulties faced by the patient with chronic pain. Harper and his colleagues (1992) utilized the ICIDH to develop a functional taxonomy of impairments, disabilities and handicaps associated with low back pain. In 1999 an updated draft document (ICIDH-2) was published (World Health Organization 1999). The concept of impairment was retained but concepts of disability and handicap were revised as noted in the definitions given below.

Impairment: Impairment is an objective, structural limitation that can be measured with a reasonable degree of accuracy and uniformity (Vasuderan 1989; Waddell & Main 1984; World Health Organization 1980, 1999). It may relate to psychological, anatomical or physiological structures.

Disability or activity limitations: The WHO (1980) defined disability as a restriction or lack of ability to perform an activity in the manner considered normal. The new WHO classification focuses on activity rather than disability. It defines activity as 'the performance of a task or action by an individual' and activity limitations as 'difficulties an individual may have in the performance of activities' (World Health Organization 1999, p. 14). Determining disability or activity limitation is complex. Jette's definition cited by Verbrugge (1990) as 'a gap between a person's capability and the environment's demand' is useful for therapists. The definition notes the importance

of the need for a fit between the person and the environment and the need to assess both components to fully understand activity limitations. Disability may be physical, mental or social.

Handicap or participation restrictions: Handicap is the extent to which the impairment and disability impinge on a person's normal vocational, social and family roles (World Health Organization 1980). ICIDH-2 defines participation as 'an individual's involvement in life situations' (World Health Organization 1999, p. 14), and participation restrictions as 'problems an individual may have in the manner or extent of involvement in life situations' (World Health Organization 1999, p. 14).

Reliability: Reliability is the extent to which a measurement is consistent, that is, it measures in the same way each time it is used even if some conditions have varied (the person administering it, the situation).

Validity: Validity is the extent to which a measurement actually measures what it claims to measure.

Function: Function is the output of active life skills based on precursor physical abilities (e.g. range of motion, strength, grip, gait) and psychosocial abilities (e.g. temperament, self-concept, organizational ability).

Self-efficacy: Self-efficacy is the belief in one's ability to successfully perform particular behaviours that are needed to produce particular outcomes (Bandura 1977; Council et al 1988; Jensen et al 1991; Strong 1995).

Pain behaviours: Pain behaviours are overt manifestations of pain and suffering, such as grimacing, limping, avoiding activity and moaning.

Box 7.2 **Types of pain measures**

1. Self-report measures (e.g. scales, drawings, questionnaires, diaries)
2. Observational measures (e.g. measure of behaviour, function, range or motion)
3. Physiological measures (e.g. heart rate, pulse)

so, but actual physical performance and perceived level of physical performance may be two entirely different constructs, each of which is valid clinical information about a patient with chronic pain. It has been identified that self-report validity is limited by the lack of a normative dataset, such as would standardize clinical interpretation of pain reportage from different patients (Nicholas et al 2008). Lastly, self-report measures rely on the person's ability to communicate about pain. Self-report is not possible for infants, young children or people with special needs that impair communication.

Observational measures

Observational measures are another method of pain measurement. Observational measures usually rely on a therapist, or someone well known to the patient, completing an observational measure of some aspect of pain experience, usually related to behaviour or activity performance. Observational measures can be useful to corroborate the self-reports given by the patient. They are also very useful to identify other areas of concern, particularly measurement of function and ergonomic factors that may exacerbate or cause work-related pain.

The subjective components may help in determining which type of treatment programme is most appropriate for which type of patient with pain (Strong et al 1994a). Nevertheless, observational measures may be relatively expensive as a technique since they require observation time. They may also be less sensitive to the subjective and affective components of the pain experience.

In research, observational measures have been shown to be most accurate for acute pain since pain behaviour tends to habituate as pain becomes more chronic

(McGrath & Unruh 1999). There is also no behaviour that is an indicator of pain and nothing else. Clutching the abdomen may be due to pain but it might also be a spasm of nausea. To know what the behaviour signifies one may need to ask the person and that is back to self-report. The advantage of collaborative reporting between patient and observer was noted in a study by Ahlers et al (2008), wherein ICU nurses were found to underestimate critically ill patients' level of pain in comparison to the patients' self-assessment using a numeric rating scale.

In this way, observational measures fail to provide solely objective pain measurement. Rather, they reflect the therapist's objective *and* subjective measurement of the patient's pain. The roommate's observational measurement of your migraine in Reflective exercise 7.1 may be affected by her or his inexperience with migraines and the observation that you are lying down and appear to be relaxing.

Physiological measures

The third category of pain measurement is physiological. Pain can cause biological changes in heart rate, respiration, sweating, muscle tension and other changes associated with a stress response (Turk & Okifuji 1999). These biological changes can be used as an indirect measure of acute pain, but biological response to acute pain may stabilize over time as the body attempts to recover its homeostasis. For example, your breathing or heart rate may have shown some small change at the outset of your migraine if the onset was relatively sudden and severe, but over time these changes are likely to return to before migraine rates even though your migraine persists. Physiological measures are useful in situations where observational measures are more difficult. For example, the Critical-Care Pain Observation Tool (C-CPOT) has been developed and tested for use with critically ill adults who cannot communicate verbally (Gélinas et al 2009).

In summary, self-report measures are considered the gold standard of pain measurement. After all, only you know how bad that migraine really is. Your roommate's measurement is also useful but her measurement is indirect. It is still very important to note here that all three categories of measures have some degree of error. They provide a part of the picture of the patient's pain experience but they do not have 100% accuracy. In the following sections we discuss the various measures that can be used to obtain a description of the pain, responses to the pain and the impact of pain on the person's life.

ASSESSMENT OF PAIN

Assessment of pain before intervention is important to ensure that the therapist and the pain team have a complete picture of the patient's needs and areas of difficulty.

Although the words assessment and measurement are related and they are often used interchangeably, their meaning is somewhat different. Assessment is the broader examination of the relationship between different components of the pain experience for a given patient, whereas measurement is the quantification of each component. Sometimes therapists measure components without an assessment framework, with the result that the information gathered may have minimal usefulness in determining whether an intervention programme was useful for the patient. Deciding what to measure depends on the therapist's assessment model and the assessment model depends on the therapist's practice frame of reference.

Assessment can be used to help with diagnosis, to assist in defining goals for clinical intervention and management, to help in evaluating the effectiveness of a treatment programme, to provide a picture of a patient's functional ability despite pain and to provide data for insurance, compensation and pension claims. If assessment of pain is to occur repeatedly for one patient, it is likely to follow the order just listed, that is, it will be for diagnostic (or exploratory) reasons first, and then to help in making treatment goals more precise and relevant.

In chronic pain, the World Health Organization (WHO) classifications of impairment, disability (activity and activity limitation) and handicap (participation and participation limitation) are particularly important. Assessment of impairment may be judged by pain intensity, disability by self-care, ambulation and endurance deficits, and handicap by deficits in vocational, social or familial roles (Patrick & D'Eon 1996).

As noted previously, a therapist will usually assess a patient's pain using the most appropriate model or frame of reference for the situation. The frame of reference focuses the assessment and in turn determines what questions must be answered through measurement. In many cases a purely biomedical approach to pain assessment may be insufficient (Vlaeyen et al 1995) because it will focus on biological measurement and exclude other psychological and environmental factors. A biopsychosocial model is often advocated (Turk 1996). This model will lead to assessment that considers interaction between biological, psychological and social components in pain experience and will determine exactly what factors within each should be measured. Gélinas et al (2008) note that the selection of a tool for pain measurement must take into account such factors as the purpose of measurement, the characteristics of the participant and the conditions of administration, along with more obvious practical considerations.

Several other factors determine which model or frame of reference is most appropriate for pain assessment. These factors include acuteness or chronicity of the pain, provision of intervention as a team member or sole pain therapist, a rehabilitation focus to the service, involvement of compensation and difficulties that might complicate assessment (such as a cognitive impairment or lack of fluency in the primary language spoken at the service). Psychological, social and demographic factors have been found to be crucial in influencing the development of chronicity of pain (Polatin & Mayer 1996) and so these areas need to be included in assessment protocols.

It is essential to remember that the information gathered in an assessment of the patient's pain must be used to the best ends. While this may sound self-evident, it is surprisingly common for the purpose of assessment information to be poorly considered. The effect is then to have not enough information, too much information for the context in which it is to be used or information that is not specific enough to the particular individual. If the information is important as an outcome measure, then it is essential that the measures used at the outset are relevant to the goals of the intervention programme and can be measured again at discharge.

In order to safeguard against these pitfalls and ensure that relevant and adequate information is obtained, the therapist needs to follow the cardinal rules of data-gathering with patients:

- Ensure there is some initial time spent to establish a collaborative relationship by getting to know the person and her or his individual situation.
- Where possible, allow for the patient to expand on formal assessment items and to elaborate on her or his responses.
- Actively listen to the patient's information and notice signals which suggest that the patient would like to talk further (e.g. hesitations, rushing over a certain aspect, comments such as 'but you don't need to hear more about that').
- Try to understand the implications for the patient's lifestyle and quality of life as much as possible.
- Remember the information.

Experienced therapists will find in the pain literature a variety of assessment models that can be used to gather information about a patient's pain. While different models will emphasize different elements of the pain experience, some factors appear consistent between a number of assessment tools. Davidson et al (2008) undertook an examination of nine established chronic pain measures and identified seven key dimensions: pain and disability, pain description, affective distress, support, positive coping strategies, negative coping strategies and activity. Previous research by Woolf & Decosterd (1999) advocated an interview-based assessment of the patient's pain that is similar to one previously advocated by physiotherapists (Maitland 1987). It comprises aspects of pain such as:

- Is the pain spontaneous or evoked?
- What is the nature and intensity of the stimulus if the pain is evoked?
- What is the quality of the pain?
- What is the pain distribution?

- Is the pain continuous or intermittent?
- What is the pain intensity?
- A clinical assessment.

Although there are important distinctions between different assessment models, in general there are three essential components of pain assessment that will need to be considered for most patients with pain. These components are description of the pain, responses to the pain and the impact of the pain on the person's life.

In the next section we will examine the various measures that can be used for each of these three components. Each component has a range of subcategories and for each subcategory there are usually a number of measurement tools or styles of measurement available. Many of these measures are summarized in the tables in this chapter.

Measurement of the description of the pain

Measures which describe pain are usually self-report in style. They are typically in the form of questionnaires, rating scales, visual analogue scales and drawings. Pain can be described in terms of its intensity (i.e. how much pain), its quality (e.g. if it is burning, aching, dull, sharp, etc.) and its location on the body.

In gathering a description of the pain from a patient, several purposes are served. A baseline description of the pain allows for comparison of changes. Ideally, pain should be monitored for some time before treatment commences, and then during treatment and at the end of treatment. The brief scales, such as the numerical rating scale, have been used daily for up to 2 weeks in chronic pain programmes and the results averaged to increase the reliability of the assessment. Although this amount of assessment will provide a baseline to truly compare to changes following intervention, it is rather more than is achievable or desirable in most clinical contexts. There is considerable evidence that self-report of pain intensity is both reliable and valid (Jamison 1996).

Numeric scales

The numeric rating scale is the most popular, but visual analogue and verbal rating scales are also well used (Jamison 1996). In a study to examine the validity of a number of commonly used measures of pain intensity, the 11-point box scale emerged as the most valid compared to a linear model of pain (Jensen et al 1989). The box scale was also accurate to score. However, this study was of patients with postoperative (i.e. acute) pain. Earlier research had suggested that the numerical rating scale was best for use with chronic pain patients (Jensen et al 1986). In Peters et al (2007) reported chronic pain patients' preference for the numerical box-21 scale for measuring pain intensity, over horizontal and vertical versions of the VAS, the box-11 scale and the verbal descriptor scale. The exception in this case was patients aged over 75 years, who were found to prefer the verbal descriptor scale. Strong et al (1991) also found the box scale to be one of two preferred pain intensity measures for use with patients with chronic low back pain, along with the VAS in a horizontal orientation. Overall, numerical scales are easy to use in clinical practice. However, unlike the VAS, they do not have ratio scale properties, i.e. a score that changes from 6 to 3 cannot be taken to represent a 50% reduction in the subjective experience of pain (Price 1999, pp 17–22). A number of assessments for use in gathering a description of the patient's pain are listed in Table 7.1, while Figure 7.1 illustrates some of these pain intensity measures.

Visual analogue scales

Visual analogue scales are simply a 10-cm line with 'stops' or 'anchors' at each end. The line may be horizontal or vertical. The patient is asked to mark the line at a point corresponding to the severity of his/her pain. End-point descriptors are 'none' and 'severe', or similar phrases. The score is the number of millimetres from the zero anchor, i.e. a figure between 0 and 100. This may present difficulties if copies do not reproduce the 100 mm line precisely. The VAS has also been shown to have good scale ratio properties, i.e. a 50% reduction in perceived pain correlates well with a similar reduction in VAS rating (Price 1999, pp 17 22).

The VAS line may be horizontal or vertical, but clinical evidence is often that the horizontal version is preferred. Patients with back pain have been known to misinterpret a vertical line as their spine and then place a mark on the line to describe the location of their pain, rather than to indicate its intensity. On the other hand, there is evidence

that the error rate for elderly patients is reduced by using a vertical scale (Gagliese & Melzack 1997).

Variations of the VAS have been developed over time. A recent example is PAULA the PAIN-METER® (PAULA) (Machata et al 2009). This visual tool was developed to accommodate patients struggling with perceptual-cognitive impairment following general anaesthesia. One side of the scale features five coloured faces with different expressions, and the patient uses a slider to place their feelings within this emotional range. The opposite side of the scale depicts a 0 100 VAS scale, which health professionals can refer to in order to correlate the visual assessment with a numeric score. Clinical trial results suggested greater reliability using the PAULA scale than using the VAS (Machata et al 2009).

The VAS and similar instruments are useful in the measurement of cancer pain because of their brevity. Measurement of cancer pain needs to be brief because tolerance of lengthy assessment may be poor in very ill people (Ahles et al 1984). The pain may change frequently, requiring measurement to be frequent. Therefore a measurement which is quick to administer but remains reliable over many applications is desirable. However, it has been observed that some patients in palliative care experience difficulty in completing the scale (Jensen 2003).

Although the VAS is easily understood even in situations of cultural or language difference (Huskisson 1983), some situations might warrant an even simpler design. For example, the full cup test (FCT; Ergün et al 2007) asks patients to draw a fill level on a picture of an empty cup, indicating how 'full' their pain feels, where an empty cup = zero pain and a full cup = total pain. This was shown to be useful for patients with low levels of education, who found the FCT easier to understand than the VAS (Ergün et al 2007). Conversely, the VAS may be considered too simplistic in other

Table 7.1 Commonly used pain evaluations for describing pain			
Assessment	**Style**	**Psychometric status**	**Utility**
Visual Analogue Scales including vertical, horizontal and numbered scales	Self report – there are a number of types, e.g. vertical, horizontal, plastic thermometer style	The accuracy of scoring on the 10-cm line is often questionable	Measure pain intensity Quick, able to be repeated regularly, and do not require complex language Useful in cancer pain
McGill Pain Questionnaire (MPQ) Also has short form (MPQ-SF)	Self-report 20 sets of adjectives to select one in each relevant category Short-form has 15-item adjective checklist and two scales for pain intensity	Total score and dimension scores Well-established reliability and validity Some problems with difficulty level of words used	Measures quality of pain – three dimensions affective, evaluative, sensory Widely used in clinical research
Pain Drawing (various protocols)	Self-report by drawing areas and types of pain with symbols on front and back outlines of the human body	Rating scales which have been developed for pain drawings have poor validity	Identifies location of pain perceived by client High face validity for patients

Visual Analogue Scale (Horizontal)

No pain ────────────────────────| Pain as bad
as it could be

Numeric Rating Scale

Please indicate on the line below the number between
0 and 100 that best describes your pain.
A zero (0) would mean 'no pain' and a one hundred (100)
would mean 'pain as bad as it could be'.

Please write only one number. _____

Box Scale

If a zero means 'no pain', and a ten (10) means 'pain as bad as it
could be', on this scale of 0Ð10,what is your level of pain?
Put an 'X' through that number.

0	1	2	3	4	5	6	7	8	9	10

Verbal Rating Scale

( ) No pain
( ) Some pain
( ) Considerable pain
( ) Pain which could not be more severe

Behavioural Rating Scale

( ) No pain
( ) Pain present, but can easily be ignored
( ) Pain present, cannot be ignored, but does not interfere with everyday activities
( ) Pain present, cannot be ignored, interferes with concentration
( ) Pain present, cannot be ignored, interferes with all tasks except taking care of
    basic needs such as toileting and eating
( ) Pain present, cannot be ignored, rest or bedrest required

Fig. 7.1 **Pain intensity measures.**

forums. Its design necessarily excludes pain descriptors, thus limiting the extent to which the nature of pain can be considered (Roden & Sturman 2009).

In 1997, Collins et al reported that a mark above 3 cm on a 10-cm scale would include 85% of patients who had rated their pain as moderate on a four-point categorical scale, and 98% of patients who reported severe pain. While this means a rating above 3 cm is going to be fairly reliable at including patients with severe pain, it will also include patients with pain that is moderate or less.

Overall, research findings suggest that while the VAS may usefully compare scores for each patient individually, it may be less reliable when used to compare individuals to each other. The aforementioned study by Peters et al (2007), comparing psychometric properties and patient preference of five different rating scales for pain intensity, also indicated that most mistakes were made on the VAS.

The pain drawing

The pain drawing has been used as a simple way to gain a graphic representation of where the patient feels pain. While this may sound like a straightforward procedure, two important aspects of the pain drawing may differ widely from setting to setting: the instructions on how to complete the pain drawing, and the scoring (if any) and interpretation of the pain drawing. A pain drawing consists of outline drawings of the human body, front and back, on which the patient indicates where the pain is by shading the painful area (Margolis et al 1986) or by indicating the type of pain (e.g. pins and needles, aching) by symbols (Ransford et al 1976). Margolis et al (1986, 1988) developed a scoring system based on the total body area in pain (see Fig. 7.2 for Margolis pain drawing and scoring system).

Ransford et al (1976) developed a detailed scoring system to screen for psychological disorders, whereby a patient's graphic representation of their pain which is physiologically impossible may indicate problems. As a result of this feature, various methods of scoring or rating pain drawings in order to suggest level of psychological distress have been attempted (Parker et al 1995; Ransford et al 1976). These rating scales have poor reliability. However, used without a scoring system, the pain drawing can be a useful tool to assist in clinical reasoning, giving as it does useful information about the location and distribution of the patient's pain.

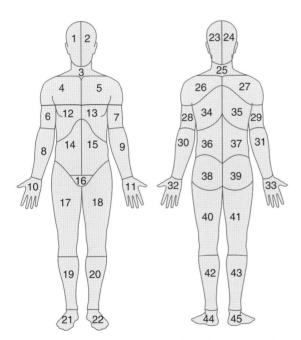

Fig. 7.2 Margolis pain drawing and scoring system. The body is divided into 45 areas. A score of 1 is assigned if the patient indicated that pain was present and a score of 0 if pain was absent, for each area. Weights are assigned to each area equal to the percentage of body surface it covers.
(Reprinted from Margolis, R.B., Tait, R.C., Krause, S.J., A rating scale for use with patient pain drawings. PAIN®, 1986, 24: 57-65. This figure has been reproduced with permission of the International Association for the Study of Pain ® (IASP). The figure may not be reproduced for any other purpose without permission).

McGill Pain Questionnaire

The MPQ (Melzack 1975) includes a numerical intensity scale, a set of descriptor words and a pain drawing. Patients are asked to indicate, from 20 groups of adjectives, descriptors of their present pain. Patients are restricted to using only one word from each group. These adjectives tap the sensory (categories 1–10), affective (categories 11–15) and evaluative (category 16) dimensions of a person's pain. A miscellaneous class (categories 17–20) of words was also described. Quantitative scores which can be derived from the MPQ are the 'number of words chosen', the 'pain rating index total', the 'pain rating index sensory', the 'pain rating index affective' and the 'pain rating index evaluative'. The MPQ is multidimensional, but its focus is still pain description. It is probably the most widely used pain evaluation measure. More recently, Melzack (1987) developed the short-form MPQ. The original MPQ adjectives and the short-form MPQ are illustrated in Figures 7.3 and 7.4.

While many researchers have utilized the MPQ in a highly quantitative way (e.g. Lowe et al 1991; Strong et al 1989), its primary value for clinicians is to identify qualitative features of a person's pain experience and to detect less than dramatic, more subtle clinical changes. From the words chosen, the therapist can also get an idea of unexpected features of a person's pain. For example, if a patient endorsed the adjective 'cold' as a descriptor of their low back pain, this would be unusual. Alternatively, for a patient with phantom limb pain to endorse the words stabbing, burning and constant is entirely expected. Jerome and his colleagues (1988) also suggest that attention be given to the specific words chosen by patients on the MPQ rather than concentrating on the total scores obtained. The reliability and validity of the MPQ are well established and are reviewed in Melzack & Katz (1994).

Comprehensive measurement of pain description, using several methods, allows the patient to feel they have fully communicated the way their pain feels to them, and so contributes to them feeling understood. A thorough evaluation can be valuable in the establishment of the therapeutic relationship. As a note of caution, there is a fine line to be negotiated between the patient feeling well-understood and feeling over-assessed and intruded upon. For this reason, measurement tools that are relatively brief yet efficient are often most suitable.

Measurement of responses to pain

A person's response to pain is very personal, based on physiology, personality, previous life experiences, family and culture. How someone responds to pain is often demonstrated by behavioural and psychological reactions or changes, and it is these features which therapists need to understand (Flaherty 1996). Aspects such as depression and illness behaviour are therefore valuable components

Name: _____ Date: _____

What does your pain feel like?

Some of the words I will read to you describe your **present** pain. Tell me which words best describe it. Leave out any word group that is not suitable. Use only a single word in each appropriate group Ð the one that applies **best**.

1	**2**	**3**	**4**
1 Flickering	1 Jumping	1 Pricking	1 Sharp
2 Quivering	2 Flashing	2 Boring	2 Cutting
3 Pulsing	3 Shooting	3 Drilling	3 Lacerating
4 Throbbing		4 Stabbing	
5 Beating		5 Lancinating	
6 Pounding			

5	**6**	**7**	**8**
1 Pinching	1 Tugging	1 Hot	1 Tingling
2 Pressing	2 Pulling	2 Burning	2 Itchy
3 Gnawing	3 Wrenching	3 Scalding	3 Smarting
4 Cramping		4 Searing	4 Stinging
5 Crushing			

9	**10**	**11**	**12**
1 Dull	1 Tender	1 Tiring	1 Sickening
2 Sore	2 Taut	2 Exhausting	2 Suffocating
3 Hurting	3 Rasping		
4 Aching	4 Splitting		
5 Heavy			

13	**14**	**15**	**16**
1 Fearful	1 Punishing	1 Wretched	1 Annoying
2 Frightful	2 Gruelling	2 Blinding	2 Troublesome
3 Terrifying	3 Cruel		3 Miserable
	4 Vicious		4 Intense
	5 Killing		5 Unbearable

17	**18**	**19**	**20**
1 Spreading	1 Tight	1 Cool	1 Nagging
2 Radiating	2 Numb	2 Cold	2 Nauseating
3 Penetrating	3 Drawing	3 Freezing	3 Agonizing
4 Piercing	4 Squeezing		4 Dreadful
	5 Tearing		5 Torturing

Fig. 7.3 The McGill Pain Questionnaire adjectives
(Copyright R. Melzack; Reprinted with permission).

of a comprehensive pain assessment. Table 7.2 lists some of the available measures in this domain.

There is some evidence that a person's fears or beliefs about the source of their pain or possibility of re-injury can influence their responses to pain and their course of recovery (Main & Watson 1996). Fear-avoidance beliefs probably arise from the patient's experience of physical activity and pain, but can be altered by cognitive and affective factors (Waddell et al 1993). In an effort to completely understand the patient's perspective, and to understand what influences their behaviour, some of these attitudes and beliefs need to be evaluated (Strong et al 1992).

There are two measures of fears or beliefs about pain that have good reliability and validity, and may be useful to

Short-Form McGill Pain Questionnaire Ronald Melzack

Patient's name: _____ Date: _____

		None	Mild	Moderate	Severe
1	Throbbing	0) ____	1) ____	2) ____	3) ____
2	Shooting	0) ____	1) ____	2) ____	3) ____
3	Stabbing	0) ____	1) ____	2) ____	3) ____
4	Sharp	0) ____	1) ____	2) ____	3) ____
5	Cramping	0) ____	1) ____	2) ____	3) ____
6	Gnawing	0) ____	1) ____	2) ____	3) ____
7	Hot-burning	0) ____	1) ____	2) ____	3) ____
8	Aching	0) ____	1) ____	2) ____	3) ____
9	Heavy	0) ____	1) ____	2) ____	3) ____
10	Tender	0) ____	1) ____	2) ____	3) ____
11	Splitting	0) ____	1) ____	2) ____	3) ____
12	Tiring-exhausting	0) ____	1) ____	2) ____	3) ____
13	Sickening	0) ____	1) ____	2) ____	3) ____
14	Fearful	0) ____	1) ____	2) ____	3) ____
15	Punishing-cruel	0) ____	1) ____	2) ____	3) ____

VAS

No pain |————————————| Worst possible pain

PPI

0 No pain ____
1 Mild ____
2 Discomforting ____
3 Distressing ____
4 Horrible ____
5 Excruciating ____

Fig. 7.4 The short-form McGill Pain Questionnaire adjectives
(Copyright R. Melzack; Reprinted with permission).

occupational therapists and physiotherapists. The Survey of Pain Attitudes (Revised) (SOPA-R) (Jensen & Karoly 1991; Jensen et al 1987), in its most recent version, assesses seven beliefs which possibly influence long-term adjustment for people with chronic pain. The subscales of the SOPA-R measure the extent to which patients believe they can control their pain: they are disabled by their pain, they are damaging themselves and should avoid exercise, their emotions affect their pain experience, medications are appropriate, others, especially family, should be solicitous, and there is a medical cure for their problem (Jensen & Karoly 1991). More recently, a further revision has been made of the SOPA-R to provide a shorter version for clinical use: the SOPA-B (brief) (Tait & Chibnall 1997). This 30-item version of the SOPA assesses the subscales of solicitude, emotionality, cure, control, harm, disability and medication.

Another tool, the Pain Beliefs and Perceptions Inventory (PBPI), examines patients' beliefs on the stability of pain over time, to what extent they see pain as a mystery and how much they are to blame for their pain (Williams & Thorn 1989). More recent work with the PBPI has supported the existence of four rather than three scales across a number of patient groups (Herda et al 1994; Morley & Wilkinson 1995; Williams et al 1994). Using the four-scaled version of the PBPI may provide a simple yet clinically useful gauge of the patient's beliefs about pain as mystery, self-blame, pain permanence and pain constancy (Williams et al 1994). A scoring key and some normative data are contained as appendices in the article by Williams et al (1994). Both the SOPA-R and the PBPI have strengths, but the psychometric properties of the SOPA-R are stronger, and it may be useful for a broader range of patients than the PBPI (Strong et al 1992).

Table 7.2 Commonly used evaluations for pain responses

Assessment	Style	Psychometric status	Utility
Fear-avoidance beliefs questionnaire	Self-report 16 items on a single page	Only the initial study so far, however this showed good test-retest reliability, and a relatively stable 2-factor structure	To measure fear-avoidance beliefs about work and physical activity, specifically for patients with low back pain
Movement and pain predictions cale (MAPPS)	10 items on a 10-point rating scale with sequential drawings of particular movements	Correlations between 7 of the self-efficacy responses and actual movement	Assesses self-efficacy expectations, pain response expectancies and the reason for not completing a movement
Survey of Pain Attitudes-Revised (SOPA-R)	Self-report (57 items) 5-point Likert scale	Internal consistency, discriminant validity, construct validity, and factor structure are all adequate	Assesses seven beliefs which may affect long-term adjustment to chronic pain is of most value for chronic low back pain
The Gauge	Self-report 27 items on a 1–10 point Likert scale	Has shown good internal consistency and test-retest reliability Convergent validity supported	Assesses the person's confidence in their ability to do a range of basic activities at home, without help
Illness Behaviour Questionnaire			Seven scales to assess abnormal illness behaviour in chronic pain and other conditions where the patient's response may appear discrepant to the physical pathology. This is widely used
Coping Strategies Questionnaire	Self-report		To determine the use of cognitive and behavioural coping strategies used to deal with pain This is widely used
Pain Beliefs and Perceptions Inventory	Self-report Has 16 items	Some debate about whether it has 3 or 4 valid sub-scales	This tool has some usage, but not as broadly as the SOPA-R
Pain Self-Efficacy Questionnaire (PSEQ)	Self-report on a 10-item questionnaire, using a 7-point scale	Internal consistency and test-retest reliability acceptable	Developed specifically for chronic pain
		Support for construct and concurrent validity	To rate confidence in performing activities despite pain

Another important concept that is related to beliefs is pain appraisal. Not all pains worry people. Some pains, such as sports-related pains, are appraised as challenging. Other pains, such as pain from a burn, are appraised as highly threatening because they cause obvious harm. Still other pains such as childbirth may be appraised as highly threatening because of the pain severity, but also as highly challenging because labour is usually perceived as normal and produces a child. The Pain Appraisal Inventory (Unruh & Ritchie 1998) is a measure of threat and challenge appraisal. The measure is applicable to many types of pain and has strong evidence of reliability and validity.

Related to attitudes and beliefs about pain is the concept of self-efficacy, or sense of confidence about ability to do certain activities. A self-efficacy expectation, combined with an outcome expectation (i.e. the belief that a particular behaviour will result in a certain outcome) may influence a person's avoidance of, or participation in, an activity (Bandura 1977). In relation to pain, it has been proposed that self-efficacy beliefs may explain in part the variability between a patient's skill level and their performance outside the treatment setting (Gage & Polatajko 1994; Strong 1995).

Several ways of measuring self-efficacy in relation to pain have been developed. The most useful are the Movement and Pain Prediction Scale (MAPPS; Council et al 1988), the Pain Self-Efficacy Questionnaire (PSEQ; Nicholas 1994) and the Self-Efficacy Gauge (Gage et al 1994).

On the MAPPS, each of 10 simple movements is shown by five sequential drawings of the movement. Patients score how far they think they could go in the movement (self-efficacy), the pain at each stage (pain-response expectancies) and the reason they couldn't complete a movement (Council et al 1988). Seven of the self-efficacy responses significantly correlated with actual movement performance. The PSEQ is a 10-item Likert-type questionnaire, designed specifically for chronic pain, where patients are asked to rate their confidence in performing activities despite pain. It has supportive validity and reliability research (Nicholas 1994). The PSEQ is shown in Figure 7.5. The Self-Efficacy Gauge (Gage et al 1994) is also a questionnaire, with 27 items. Patients rate their degree of confidence to complete certain activities without help. See Figure 7.6 for the Self-Efficacy Gauge. It was developed by an occupational therapist for use with patients with a variety of disorders, including pain conditions, where occupational performance was affected.

A number of assessments are commonly used to measure psychological aspects of a person that may arise from, or help stimulate, certain responses to pain. The Beck Depression Inventory (Beck et al 1961) is widely used to evaluate the level of depression associated with chronic pain. It is considered extremely reliable for both clinical and research use. Its use, however, is restricted, and so it is not useful for occupational and physical therapists, although therapists need to understand its value and the information it provides about patients.

The Minnesota Multiphasic Personality Inventory (MMPI; Hathaway & McKinley 1942) has also been used to gain a picture of the personality profile of the patient with chronic pain. Different profiles have been associated with different patterns of pain responses (Keefe 1982). Chronic pain patients may exhibit certain personality traits, but they are rarely significantly psychopathological, therefore tests such as the Rorschach (which can tease out personality structure) are usually not appropriate. Measures of 'reactive emotional stress' are more suitable (Jamison 1996). The MMPI is never used by physiotherapists or occupational therapists, but may be a component of the complete pain assessment battery used by the team. Main et al (1991) and Main & Spanswick (1995a) have suggested that there exist other more focused measures to assess psychological functioning and responses to pain than the MMPI. For example, Etscheidt et al (1995) have shown that the West-Haven Yale Multidimensional Pain Inventory can provide information about chronic pain patients who might require further psychological assessment, and it is a much briefer assessment than the MMPI.

The adjustment of the patient with chronic pain, or ability to manage with pain, may be measured using such measures as the Coping Strategies Questionnaire (Robinson et al 1997a; Rosenstiel & Keefe 1983) or the Illness Behaviour Questionnaire (IBQ) (Pilowsky & Spence 1983). These measures concern cognitive and behavioural coping strategies that patients can use to help them manage their pain. Both positive and negative adjustment strategies are covered. For example, two strategies assessed in the Coping Strategies Questionnaire are diverting attention and catastrophizing. The Pain Catastrophizing Scale (Sullivan et al 1995) measures catastrophizing in more depth and may be particularly useful to gain more information about coping for patients who are having substantial difficulty managing pain. Catastrophizing is linked with disability and depression. At present it is unknown whether catastrophizing can be changed to more positive coping. However, positive coping strategies are unlikely to be effective in improving coping with chronic pain without the support of a coping-skills training programme (Rosenstiel & Keefe 1983). The case example in Box 7.3 illustrates the coping strategies a patient with low back pain following a work injury may exhibit.

Recently, the clear demonstration of bias effects in some of these self-report measures has called into question their reliability when used in cases where over-reporting of poor adjustment may affect financial decisions (Robinson et al 1997b). The same study highlighted the difficulty for clinicians and researchers in interpreting results because many of these self-report scales used for chronic pain have no in-built mechanisms for identifying faking or social desirability responses. However, there is potential clinical value in having illness behaviour defined by the presence of psychological symptoms rather than the absence of physical symptoms (Main & Spanswick 1995b). Main & Spanswick (1995b) have also reported that the IBQ may differentiate neurosis from conscious exaggeration.

Clinical observations of responses to pain are also valid methods of assessment. These are typically taken while the patient is involved in assessment or treatment activities. Pain behaviours that may have been initiated by nociception may persist long after the time of healing because of the positive consequences of these behaviours (Keefe & Dolan 1986). Fordyce (1976) has described pain behaviours as comprising both verbal and non-verbal methods of communication. They include such behaviours as grimacing, moaning, bracing, total body stiffness and verbal complaints (Fordyce 1976). All formal assessment is supplemented by clinical observation and to a certain extent interpretation is based on experience. The aim is to establish a realistic level of distress, which may not be simply related to numbers of obvious pain behaviours. Patients with chronic pain may, unintentionally, use a lot of learned pain behaviours to signal their pain. However, the distress may actually be psychological at the predicament in which they find themselves, rather than a direct function of presently-felt pain. A number of scoring systems can be used, including from the original system developed by Keefe & Block (1982) and the Pain Behavior Checklist (Kerns et al 1991).

Keefe & Block (1982) developed a behavioural observation system for use with patients with chronic low back pain. The tool requires the patient to sit, stand, walk and/or recline for a number of short periods, during which

Name: _____ Date: _____

Please rate how **confident** you are that you can do the following things **at present** despite the pain. To indicate your answer circle one of the numbers on the scale under each item, where 0 = not at all confident and 6 = completely confident.
For example:

Not at   0   1   2   (3)   4   5   6 Completely
all confident   confident

Remember, this questionnaire is not asking whether or not you have been doing these things, but rather how confident you can do them at present, **despite the pain.**

1.   I can enjoy things, despite the pain

      Not at   0   1   2   3   4   5   6 Completely
      all confident   confident

2.   I can do most of the household chores (e.g. tidying up, washing dishes, etc.) despite the pain.

      Not at   0   1   2   3   4   5   6 Completely
      all confident   confident

3.   I can socialize with my friends or family members as often as I used to do, despite the pain.

      Not at   0   1   2   3   4   5   6 Completely
      all confident   confident

4.   I can cope with my pain in most situations.

      Not at   0   1   2   3   4   5   6 Completely
      all confident   confident

5.   I can do some form of work, despite the pain.
      (Work includes housework, paid and unpaid work.)

      Not at   0   1   2   3   4   5   6 Completely
      all confident   confident

6.   I can still do many of the things I enjoy doing, such as hobbies or leisure activity, despite the pain.

      Not at   0   1   2   3   4   5   6 Completely
      all confident   confident

7.   I can cope with my pain without medication.

      Not at   0   1   2   3   4   5   6 Completely
      all confident   confident

8.   I can still accomplish most of my goals in life, despite the pain.

      Not at   0   1   2   3   4   5   6 Completely
      all confident   confident

9.   I can live a normal lifestyle, despite the pain.

      Not at   0   1   2   3   4   5   6 Completely
      all confident   confident

10.   I can gradually become more active, despite the pain.

      Not at   0   1   2   3   4   5   6 Completely
      all confident   confident

Fig. 7.5 Pain self-efficacy questionnaire
(Reprinted with kind permission of Professor Michael K. Nicholas, Director, Pain Education and ADAPT Pain Management Program, Sydney Medical School).

I'd like to know whether you can do everyday activities without the help of another person. It is **okay** if you carry out an activity with the use of something such as a cane or a wheelchair. Please read each question carefully. Circle the number that is closest to your level of confidence (sureness) that you can do the activity. 1 means that you are not at all confident (sure) that you can do the activity without the help of someone else. 10 means that you are completely confident (sure) that you can do the activity without the help of another person.

While it is important for us to know the answer to as many questions as possible please feel free to skip a question if answering it would make you feel uncomfortable.

How confident (sure) am I that I can:	Not at all confident (sure)								Completely confident (sure)	
1. Walk one block?	1	2	3	4	5	6	7	8	9	10
2. Write?	1	2	3	4	5	6	7	8	9	10
3. Feed myself?	1	2	3	4	5	6	7	8	9	10
4. Look after my family?	1	2	3	4	5	6	7	8	9	10
5. Wash myself?	1	2	3	4	5	6	7	8	9	10
6. Climb a flight of stairs?	1	2	3	4	5	6	7	8	9	10
7. Remember the things that I need to remember?	1	2	3	4	5	6	7	8	9	10
8. Get to the bathroom in time?	1	2	3	4	5	6	7	8	9	10
9. Concentrate on something difficult?	1	2	3	4	5	6	7	8	9	10
10. Walk up or down a hill?	1	2	3	4	5	6	7	8	9	10
11. Stand for 5 minutes?	1	2	3	4	5	6	7	8	9	10
12. Dress myself?	1	2	3	4	5	6	7	8	9	10
13. Sign my name?	1	2	3	4	5	6	7	8	9	10
14. Drink from a cup?	1	2	3	4	5	6	7	8	9	10
15. Do the things I like to do?	1	2	3	4	5	6	7	8	9	10
16. Enjoy myself?	1	2	3	4	5	6	7	8	9	10
17. Make my needs known to others?	1	2	3	4	5	6	7	8	9	10
18. Get out of bed?	1	2	3	4	5	6	7	8	9	10
19. Make it through the day without a nap?	1	2	3	4	5	6	7	8	9	10
20. Do the things I usually do with other people?	1	2	3	4	5	6	7	8	9	10
21. Do my usual share of household jobs?	1	2	3	4	5	6	7	8	9	10
22. Get into a car?	1	2	3	4	5	6	7	8	9	10
23. Move around my home safely?	1	2	3	4	5	6	7	8	9	10
24. Have enough energy to do things I like to do?	1	2	3	4	5	6	7	8	9	10
25. Get into the bathtub?	1	2	3	4	5	6	7	8	9	10
26. Walk one mile?	1	2	3	4	5	6	7	8	9	10
27. Have sex?	1	2	3	4	5	6	7	8	9	10

Fig. 7.6 Self-efficacy gauge

Reprinted from Gage M, Noh S, Polatajko HJ, et al, 1994, Measuring perceived self-efficacy in occupational therapy. Am J Occup Ther 48(9); 783–790, with permission of the American Occupational Therapy Association.

Box 7.3 **Case example**

Mr B was a 52-year-old man who sustained a work injury when he fell 5 feet from a ladder in the storeroom and landed on the concrete floor below. He immediately went home to bed. The next day he visited his GP, reporting that he was in agony.

Plain X-rays revealed no significant findings, and his GP prescribed him bed-rest and regular panadol. Two weeks later he was still unable to work and the GP sent him to a physiotherapist. Had he been asked to complete the Coping Strategies Questionnaire, his results at this stage might have been:

- diverting attention from pain: 4/36
- reinterpreting pain sensations: 0/36
- catastrophizing: 28/36
- ignoring pain sensations: 0/36
- praying/hoping: 14/36
- coping self-statements: 8/36
- using behavioural coping: 8/36

Such a profile is not inconsistent in an acute-injury pain situation, where the anticipated outcome is pain resolution. The pain can seem an awful, overwhelming thing, but the person will have faith in the doctor or physiotherapist to give pain relief and cure the pain. At this stage, it would be highly unlikely that the patient would be diverting attention from his pain problem. Should the pain continue and the individual be one of the 10% of the population to develop a chronic pain problem, the persistence of the coping strategies mentioned above may make rehabilitation difficult. This makes it clear that a pain assessment should be multidimensional, taking into account not only the level and distribution of the pain but also the patient's subjective and behavioural response to it.

time the patient is videotaped. The videotape is then analysed for the frequency with which the patient uses guarding, bracing, rubbing, grimacing and sighing pain behaviours. Development work with the tool pointed to the validity of this system for measuring a patient's pain. In the clinical setting, more unstructured observations of pain behaviours may be utilized.

Measurement of the impact of pain

Both occupational therapists and physiotherapists have an all-encompassing interest in the patient's best function, whether that is the greatest possible range and strength of high-quality movement or the ability to manage as large a proportion as possible of the daily tasks that the patient wishes to perform. It follows, therefore, that the third level of pain evaluation commonly carried out is to measure functional status, level of activity, disability and other similar constructs.

A patient's function can be assessed in many different ways. The choice of assessment method will depend on such factors as the age of the patient (an 80-year-old man is unlikely to be assessed for return to work), the extent to which the pain has impacted to date (a patient who was bedridden and is now mobilizing will require a different measure to one who has always been mobile but limited in full range) and whether the assessment is occurring in a hospital, a clinic or home environment. There are eight potentially sequential steps which can be used in part or in full to assess function (Strong et al 1994a):

1. Ask the patient to tell you about their activities.
2. Complete an activities of daily living checklist.
3. Observe performance on tasks.
4. Have the patient complete an activity diary.
5. Staff observe the activity level of the patient.
6. Use of an automated measure of activity time.
7. Measurement of physical capacity.
8. A functional capacity evaluation.

There is considerable evidence that a daily activity diary is both reliable and valid when assessing daily activity patterns (e.g. uptime/downtime, pill-taking, mood, pain) for chronic pain patients in their home environment (Follick et al 1984). However, when self-report of uptime (i.e. time spent upright and moving rather than resting) is compared to that report by an automated measuring device, there has been a significant under-report of uptime by patients (White & Strong 1992). Abdel-Moty et al (1996) observed that both patients with chronic low back pain and healthy volunteers, when asked to self-predict their ability to stair-climb and squat and then to do the activities, showed significant under-reporting of their physical abilities. They recommended the use of both self-report and actual functional performance. The authors of this chapter also advocate such a combined approach. Keeping a diary of activity can be useful if a structured recording system is used and if patients are instructed to make entries relatively frequently throughout the day. Memory factors may impinge on accuracy. Some clinicians feel that such a focus on activities and pain is not particularly helpful. It is, however, a frequent practice in many chronic pain facilities.

A number of measures to ask patients how pain is affecting their lifestyle have been devised. Table 7.3 lists many of these. The way lifestyle is affected may also be measured by the number of activities that are still able to be enacted and enjoyed, which might be measured by something such as the Human Activity Profile (Fix & Daughton 1988). The Oswestry Low Back Pain Disability Questionnaire (ODQ) (Fairbank et al 1980) is one of the most frequently used. There are ten sections in which the patient marks one category which most accurately describes his limitations in sitting, standing, walking, lifting, having sex, socializing, sleeping, doing personal care and travelling. One item gauges pain intensity. A possible score out of 50 is obtained, and this is converted to a percentage (Fairbank et al 1980). Recent

Table 7.3 Commonly used evaluations for impact of pain			
Assessment	**Style**	**Psychometric status**	**Utility**
Short-Form health survey (SF-36)	Self-report	This has excellent validity and reliability	Designed to measure health status Has eight scales: limitations in physical activities, limitations in social activities, limitations in usual role activities, bodily pain, mental health, limitations in roles due to emotional problems, vitality, general health perceptions
Daily Activity Diary	Self-report	There is some support for reliability and validity of the diary for chronic pain patients at home	Monitors activity type and duration for each hour or 1/2 hour Also monitors pain intensity and medication intake Creates a structured record
Human Activity Profile (HAP)	Self-report, up to 94 items	Included a chronic pain sample in normative sample Norms are provided for different age and gender groups	Can be used to help determine the effect of physical impairment on human daily activity

review of the ODQ has shown it to have good face validity, some evidence of factorial and criterion-related validity, and some sensitivity to change (Fisher & Johnston 1997). These features, combined with its brevity, make it a very usable assessment of lifestyle effects for patients with low back pain.

The Sickness Impact Profile (SIP) (Bergner et al 1981) is a questionnaire with 136 items to be self-completed or administered by interview. It was designed to provide a measure of health status that is behaviourally based (Bergner et al 1981). The SIP was designed to be used with various populations, not only those in chronic pain, and is able to demonstrate change in health status over time and between groups. There have been some recent developments in trying to select items for specific use with low back pain patients, and thus create a shorter questionnaire specifically for this population (Stratford et al 1993).

Disability, as defined earlier in this chapter, is difficult to measure. The Pain Disability Index (PDI) (Tait et al 1987, 1990) is a self-report measure that asks patients to rate how much the pain prevents them from doing, or doing as well as previously, in seven areas of functioning. It measures voluntary (work, social) activities and obligatory (self-care) activities. The PDI is a valid and reliable tool, with a high internal consistency and valid factor structure (Grönblad et al 1993, 1994; Strong et al 1994b). It can be used with all types of pain and is quick to administer. Studies are still needed to ascertain its sensitivity to clinical change.

The impact of pain on a person's life can also be assessed by behavioural assessment, by measuring the patient's ability to perform actual tasks that are the same as or related to everyday life tasks. Harding et al (1994), for example, developed a battery of measures for assessing the physical functioning of patients with chronic pain. These types of assessment can be expensive and have in the past been relatively unreliable. However, more recent measurements have become more reliable. For example, Harding et al (1994)

found that a 5-minute walking test, 1-minute standing-up test, 1-minute stair-climbing test and endurance for holding the arms horizontal test were reliable, valid and useful.

Multidimensional assessment of pain

In keeping with the approaches which stress a holistic view of patients, and of management techniques for pain, there are also some assessments that are multidimensional in nature. These assessments have been designed to gather as much data as possible in the one evaluation, although different professionals may be responsible for actually conducting various parts of the assessment procedure. Such assessments have the advantage of keeping a primary focus on the whole of the patient, rather than medical or therapy subspecialties.

There are a number of multidimensional pain assessments, each of which is somewhat different in approach and style (see Table 7.4). The most well-known is probably the MPQ, through which the patient quantifies pain in three dimensions: sensory, affective and evaluative. While the MPQ gives a useful breakdown of sensory and affective components of pain, it may not be a true multidimensional assessment. It was reported earlier in this chapter as a tool to measure the description of a person's pain.

The West Haven-Yale Multidimensional Pain Inventory (WHYMPI), or the MPI as it is more commonly known, was developed from a cognitive–behavioural viewpoint to:

'Examine the impact of pain on the patients' lives, the responses of others to the patients' communications of pain, and the extent to which patients participate in common daily activities.'

(Kerns et al 1985, p. 345)

The three parts to the inventory are nevertheless quite brief to administer, and are psychometrically sound.

Table 7.4 Multidimensional pain evaluations

Assessment	Style	Psychometric status	Utility
Integrated Psychosocial Assessment Model (IPAM)	Self-report	Preliminary support	This is a set of six tools, which in combination evaluate pain intensity, disability, coping strategies, depression, attitudes to pain, and illness behaviour It provides an overall picture of psychosocial adjustment in relation to chronic pain
McGill Pain Questionnaire	Self-report 20 sets of words describing pain experience from which client selects those relevant	Considerable support for basic structure, reliability, and validity	Used to assess the quality of pain in three dimensions: affective, evaluative, sensory
Multidimensional Pain Inventory (WHYMPI)	Self-report 61 items in three scales	This is well tested for reliability and is psychometrically strong Items fall into 12 subscales	Measures interference with activity, social support, pain severity, self-control, negative mood, response of significant others, ability to engage in activities, e.g. chores, social activity
Multiperspective Multidimensional Pain Assessment Protocol (MMPAP)	Physical examinations by two physicians plus client's subjective self-report	Has been shown to be reliable and valid in initial studies Test–retest reliability is acceptable Is a standardized protocol	Used mostly for assessing patients with chronic pain for treatment and to measure outcomes Can predict future employment of disability applicants

It contains 12 scales. The MPI is designed to be used with behavioural and psychological assessment strategies. Although it is multidimensional, this is only in relation to the patient's subjective pain experience in a range of contexts. Clinically, it is useful to gain the patient's view of her or his pain feeling, how supportive their spouse is and how limited in activity the patient is. The MPI is sensitive to change following treatment.

The Integrated Psychosocial Assessment Model was developed by Strong (1992) for use with chronic pain patients in a clinical setting. This tool relates to a model of pain evaluation. Rather than designing a new assessment, Strong has used a complementary range of existing measures, which cover various aspects of the psychosocial experience of pain. This array of measurement tools, which cover pain intensity, pain disability, coping strategies, depression, attitudes to pain and illness behaviour, provides an integrated picture of patients, with similar profiles emerging in both Australia and New Zealand (Strong et al 1995). However, more work on the clinical utility of the assessment model is currently ongoing.

The fourth multidimensional assessment tool is the Multiperspective Multidimensional Pain Assessment Protocol (MMPAP; Rucker & Metzler 1995). It is a combination of physical examinations by physicians and self-report by the patient with pain. The MMPAP was designed to be of value for assessing applicants for disability pensions and has been shown to successfully predict employment status

(Rucker & Metzler 1995; Rucker et al 1996). The major domains assessed by the MMPAP are pain dimensions, medical information, mental health status, social support networks, functional limitations and abilities, and rehabilitation potential.

Further progress in the field of multidimensional pain assessment has occurred in recent years. For instance, development and initial trialling of the Richards Assessment of Pain (RAP) yielded positive results in the assessment of heterogeneous pain, warranting further research (Richards 2008). Müller et al (2008) developed a multidimensional musculoskeletal pain assessment tool, the Pain Standard Evaluation Questionnaire (SEQ Pain), as part of a broader population-based study of musculoskeletal health in Switzerland. In addition, the successful testing of the multidimensional three-item PEG scale (pain intensity (P), interference with enjoyment of life (E), and interference with general activity (G), Krebs et al. 2009), adapted and condensed from the BPI, has been noted previously in this chapter.

Advances in technology for pain assessment and measurement

As time goes on, focus on the possibilities of computerized pain assessment increases. Prototypic systems programmed to screen video images of facial expressions for established pain signals have yielded generally positive results (Prkachin 2009). Trial studies of CHRONIC PAIN-CAT, an efficient computerized assessment tool combining item response theory with computerized adaptive testing, have met with favourable patient evaluations (Anatchkova et al 2009). A study of 200 patients attending a single physician's practice found VAS pain assessments completed on a handheld electronic device to be equally as reliable as paper-based assessments using a numeric rating scale (Junker et al 2008). Furthermore, computerized assessment devices to distinguish between pain conditions based on the input of self-reporting patients have been successfully prototypically tested, although the field of application for these is currently limited (Provenzano et al 2007). In addition, Hjermstad and colleagues (2008) have attempted to create a computer-based universal assessment tool for cancer pain, as no currently available tools were found to address all relevant elements identified by experts in palliative care. In light of these innovations, it seems likely that computer-based programming will have a significant and increasing presence in the future of pain assessment and measurement.

Assessment and measurement of pain in patients from special populations

While pain is something which affects individuals in an idiosyncratic way, there are some populations of people with special features as a whole who must be considered when evaluating pain. Infants and children, older people and people with cognitive or physical impairments or other special needs often have more difficulty communicating about pain. The difficulty in communicating about pain places these individuals at greater risk for problems in pain management. We examined some of these issues in Chapters 18 and 19 provided suggestions about assessment and measurement for these special populations.

FACTORS THAT MAY INFLUENCE ASSESSMENT AND MEASUREMENT OUTCOMES

Social desirability

Social desirability is the need to obtain approval by responding in a way that is culturally acceptable, and is recognized as a factor that may affect the quality of information provided by a patient during many types of assessment. Social desirability factors may affect self-report of pain dimensions. Deshields et al (1995) found that patients with chronic pain who are more sensitive to social desirability report less psychological distress, but greater pain, than patients who were less sensitive to social desirability. That is, they seem to respond to a set which says it is acceptable to acknowledge physical pain, but not psychological distress.

Therapists need to be sensitive to the possibility of patients giving answers they see as socially desirable. The development of a good therapeutic relationship with the patient, which promotes honest communication, is invaluable. Being able to let patients know that you can see their strengths and capabilities, despite their physical or psychological distress, will encourage them to report accurately. At the same time, being able to accept that the patient's pain is real and distressing will help to minimize the patient's need to exaggerate pain. An overall demeanour from the therapist which suggests that the pain is a real problem, but that there is likely to be a future time when pain will be more manageable and less disabling, may also encourage more hopefulness.

Compensation

There is a tendency to assume that patients who stand to be compensated for their trauma and pain will be less accurate in their self-report of pain and disability, and more extreme in their demonstrated pain behaviours. To what extent compensation complicates pain assessment and intervention is a vexing question, and research in the area has, in the past, produced equivocal results. This important issue was considered more fully in Chapter 24.

Memory problems

Patients with chronic pain often report memory problems, and various reports in the literature support this clinical impression. It has sometimes been assumed that the memory difficulties are related to medication patients may be taking. However, Schnurr & MacDonald (1995) found that memory complaints were not related to medication, and that, even though memory complaints were associated with depression in chronic pain patients, depression was not a full explanation.

In assessing patients' pain profiles it may therefore be worthwhile to keep in mind the possibility of disturbances in memory. Patients may under- or over-report their pain, or be unreliable recorders within a diary. Any memory disturbance can create a feeling of anxiety, and an assessment that is structured to minimize the need for memory will be less anxiety-provoking.

Therapist attitudes

The appraisals and attitudes of the therapist to pain in general, and pain in a particular patient, can be very influential on the quality of therapy provided. Attitudes held by a therapist may be predominantly unconscious, and therefore the therapist will not be aware of acting from a basis that may compromise a patient's treatment. As noted in Chapters 3, 11 and 12, gender, culture, age, etc. may influence the patient's experience of pain; these factors may also impact upon the therapist and their attitudes and behaviours.

It would seem that being female, older of a non-Anglo-Saxon background and/or of a lower socioeconomic class may place a patient at a disadvantage in seeking management of pain, probably because of unconscious attitudes and beliefs held by health professionals. However, it is possible, as a therapist, to adapt aspects of your clinical practice to counteract the possibility of unwitting bias. Rainville et al (1995) published a survey of health professionals' attitudes towards people with pain. It is a useful examination of one's own stereotypes and prejudices.

Acknowledging that there can be a problem goes a long way towards reducing the problem. Reviewing your own attitudes will be helpful. This can be achieved by reflection, considering your personal experience of pain prior to working as a therapist, seeking feedback from a trusted colleague or establishing guidelines for practice and comparing your performance across different patients. For each patient, the assessment must be thorough and the patient's view considered as the primary source of information. Use of an interpreter, of the appropriate gender if sensitive areas are to be discussed, may be needed. All assessments chosen should be age and culture appropriate wherever possible.

CONCLUSION

In this chapter we have discussed the many issues that a physiotherapist or occupational therapist needs to consider in the assessment and measurement of a patient's pain. The underlying premise is that some sort of formal evaluation should be made of the patient's pain. The selection of appropriate measurement tools, while far from an easy task, can be guided by using an assessment model that considers a description of the patient's pain, the responses of that person to the pain and the impact of the pain on a person's life.

Therapists should choose measures which have acceptable validity and reliability and are manageable in the clinical setting. Therapists need to be attentive to patients, to listen to their words, to observe their behaviours and abilities, and to integrate such information to help with clinical decision making.

ACKNOWLEDGEMENTS

Part of this chapter was published in Manual Therapy 1999, 4:216–220 (Strong 1999).

Q Study questions/questions for revision

1. What dimensions of the patient's pain problem should be measured by the occupational therapist and the physiotherapist?
2. What are the differences between pain assessment and pain measurement?
3. Name one measure of pain quality and describe the type of data it yields about the patient's pain.
4. Identify three reasons why therapists need to obtain self-report data on a patient's pain.
5. What is a reliable measure of a patient's pain intensity?
6. How would you measure the functional implications of a patient's pain?

REFERENCES

Abdel-Moty, A.R., Maguire, G.W., Kaplan, S.H., et al., 1996. Stated versus observed performance levels in patients with chronic low back pain. Occupational Therapy in Health Care 10 (1), 3–23.

Ahlers, S.J.G.M., van Gulik, L., van der Veen, A.M., et al., 2008. Comparison of different pain scoring systems in critically ill patients in a general ICU. Critical Care 12, R15. http://dx.doi.org/10.1186/cc6789.

Ahles, T.A., Ruckdeschel, J.C., Blanchard, E.B., 1984. Cancer-related pain: II. Assessment with visual analogue scales. J. Psychosom. Res. 28 (2), 121–124.

Anatchkova, M.D., Saris-Baglama, R.N., Kosinski, M., et al., 2009. Development and preliminary testing of a computerized adaptive assessment of chronic pain. J. Pain 10 (9), 932–943.

Bandura, A., 1977. Self-efficacy: Toward a unifying theory of behavioral change. Psychol. Rev. 84 (2), 191–215.

Beck, A.T., Ward, C.H., Mendelson, M., et al., 1961. An inventory for measuring depression. Arch. Gen. Psychiatry 4 (6), 561–571.

Bergner, M., Bobbitt, R.A., Carter, W.B., et al., 1981. The Sickness Impact Profile: development and final revision of a health status measure. Med. Care 19 (8), 787–805.

Collins, S.L., Moore, R.A., McQuay, H.J., 1997. The visual analogue pain intensity scale: What is moderate pain in millimetres? Pain 72 (1,2), 95–97.

Council, J.R., Ahern, D.K., Follick, M.J., et al., 1988. Expectancies and functional impairment in chronic low back pain. Pain 33 (3), 323–331.

Davidson, M.A., Tripp, D.A., Fabrigar, L.R., et al., 2008. Chronic pain assessment: A seven-factor model. Pain Res. Manag. 13 (4), 299–308.

Deshields, T.L., Tait, R.C., Gfeller, J.D., et al., 1995. Relationship between social desirability and self-report in chronic pain patients. Clin. J. Pain 11 (3), 189–193.

Dworkin, R., Turk, D., Farrar, J., et al., 2005. Core outcomes for chronic pain clinical trials: IMMPACT recommendations. Pain 113 (1,2), 9–19.

Ergün, U., Say, B., Ozer, G., et al., 2007. Trial of a new pain assessment tool in patients with low education: The full cup test. Int. J. Clin. Pract. 61 (10), 1692–1696.

Etscheidt, M.A., Steger, H.G., Braverman, B., 1995. Multidimensional pain inventory profile classifications and psychopathology. J. Clin. Psychol. 51 (1), 29–36.

Fabrega, H.J., Tyma, S., 1976. Culture, language and the shaping of illness: an illustration based on pain. J. Psychosom. Res. 20 (4), 323–337.

Fairbank, J.C.T., Couper, J., Davies, J.B., et al., 1980. The Oswestry Low Back Disability Questionnaire. Physiotherapy 66 (8), 271–273.

Fernandez, E., Boyle, G.J., 2001. Affective and evaluative descriptors of pain in the McGill Pain Questionnaire: reduction and reorganization. J. Pain 2 (6), 318–325.

Fisher, K., Johnston, M., 1997. Validation of the Oswestry Low Back Pain Disability Questionnaire, its sensitivity as a measure of changes following treatment and its relationship with other aspects of the chronic pain experience. Physiother. Theory Pract. 13 (1), 67–80.

Fix, A.J., Daughton, D.M., 1988. Human Activity Profile: Professional Manual. Psychological Assessment Resources Inc, Odessa, FL.

Flaherty, S.A., 1996. Pain measurement tools for clinical practice and research. J. Am. Assoc. Nurse Anesth. 64, 133–140.

Follick, M.J., Ahern, D.K., Laster-Wolston, N., 1984. Evaluation of a daily activity diary for chronic pain patients. Pain 19 (4), 373–382.

Fordyce, W.E., 1976. Behavioural Methods for Chronic Pain and Illness. Mosby, St Louis, MO.

Gage, M., Polatajko, H.J., 1994. Enhancing occupational performance through an understanding of perceived self-efficacy. Am. J. Occup. Ther. 48 (5), 452–461.

Gage, M., Noh, S., Polatajko, H.J., et al., 1994. Measuring perceived self-efficacy in occupational therapy. Am. J. Occup. Ther. 48 (9), 783–790.

Gagliese, L., Melzack, R., 1997. Chronic pain in elderly people. Pain 70 (1), 3–14.

Gélinas, C., Loiselle, C.G., LeMay, S., et al., 2008. Theoretical, psychometric, and pragmatic issues in pain measurement. Pain Manag. Nurs. 9 (3), 120–130.

Gélinas, C., Fillion, L., Puntillo, K.A., 2009. Item selection and content validity of the Critical-Care Pain Observation Tool for non-verbal adults. J. Adv. Nurs. 65 (1), 203–216.

Grönblad, M., Napli, M., Wennerstrand, P., et al., 1993. Intercorrelation and test–retest reliability of the Pain Disability Index (PDI) and the Oswestry Disability Questionnaire (ODQ) and their correlation with pain intensity in low back pain patients. Clin. J. Pain 9 (3), 189–195.

Grönblad, M., Jarvinen, E., Hurri, H., et al., 1994. Relationship of the Pain Disability Index (PDI) and the Oswestry Disability Questionnaire (ODQ) with three dynamic physical tests in a group of patients with chronic low-back and leg pain. Clin. J. Pain 10 (3), 197–203.

Guyatt, G., Walter, S., Norman, G., 1987. Measuring change over time: Assessing the usefulness of evaluative instruments. J. Chronic Dis. 40 (2), 171–178.

Harding, V.R., Williams, A.C., de, C., et al., 1994. The development of a battery of measures for assessing physical functioning of chronic pain patients. Pain 58 (3), 367–375.

Harper, A.C., Harper, D.A., Lambert, L.J., et al., 1992. Symptoms of impairment, disability and handicap in low back pain: A taxonomy. Pain 50 (2), 189–195.

Hathaway, S.R., McKinley, J.C., 1942. A multiphasic personality schedule (Minnesota): III The measurement of symptomatic depression. J. Psychol. 14, 73–84.

Herda, C.A., Siegerisk, K., Basler, H.D., 1994. The Pain Beliefs and Perceptions Inventory: Further evidence for a 4-factor structure. Pain 57 (1), 85–90.

Hjermstad, M.J., Gibbins, J., Haugen, D.F., et al., 2008. Pain assessment tools in palliative care: An urgent need for consensus. Palliat. Med. 22 (8), 895–903.

Huskisson, E.C., 1983. Visual analogue scales. In: Melzack, R. (Ed.), Pain Measurement and Assessment. Raven Press, New York.

Jamison, R.N., 1996. Psychological factors in chronic pain: Assessment and treatment issues. Journal of Back & Musculoskeletal Rehabilitation 7 (2), 79–95.

Jensen, M.P., 2003. The validity and reliability of pain measures in adults with cancer. J. Pain 4 (1), 2–21.

Jensen, M.P., Karoly, P., 1991. Control beliefs, coping efforts, and adjustment to chronic pain. J. Consult. Clin. Psychol. 59 (3), 431–438.

Jensen, M.P., Karoly, P., Braver, S., 1986. The measurement of clinical pain intensity: A comparison of six methods. Pain 27 (1), 117–126.

Jensen, M.P., Karoly, P., Huger, R., 1987. The development and preliminary validation of an instrument to assess patients' attitudes towards pain. J. Psychosom. Res. 31 (3), 393–400.

Jensen, M.P., Karoly, P., O'Riordan, E.F., et al., 1989. The subjective experience of acute pain. Clin. J. Pain 5 (2), 153–159.

Jensen, M.P., Turner, J.A., Romano, J.M., 1991. Self-efficacy and outcome expectancies: Relationship to chronic pain coping strategies and adjustment. Pain 44 (3), 263–269.

Jensen, M.P., Turner, J.A., Romano, J.M., et al., 1999. Comparative reliability and validity of chronic pain intensity measures. Pain 83 (2), 157–162.

Jerome, A., Holroyd, K.A., Theofanous, A.G., et al., 1988. Cluster headache pain vs other vascular headache pain: Differences revealed with two approaches to the McGill Pain Questionnaire. Pain 34 (1), 35–42.

Junker, U., Freynhagen, R., Längler, K., et al., 2008. Paper versus electronic rating scales for pain assessment: A prospective, randomized, cross-over validation study with 200 chronic pain patients. Curr. Med. Res. Opin. 24 (6), 1797–1806.

Keefe, F.J., 1982. Behavioral assessment and treatment of chronic pain: Current status and future directions. J. Consult. Clin. Psychol. 50 (6), 896–911.

Keefe, F.J., Block, A.R., 1982. Development of an observation method for assessing pain behaviour in chronic low back pain patients. Behav. Ther. 13 (4), 363–375.

Keefe, F.J., Dolan, E., 1986. Pain behavior and pain coping strategies in low back pain and myofascial pain dysfunction syndrome patients. Pain 24 (1), 49–56.

Kerns, R.D., Turk, D.C., Rudy, T.E., 1985. The West Haven-Yale Multidimensional Pain Inventory (WHYMPI). Pain 23 (2), 145–156.

Kerns, R.D., Haythornthwaite, J., Rosenberg, R., et al., 1991. The Pain Behaviors Checklist (PBCL): Factor structure and psychometric properties. J. Behav. Med. 14 (2), 155–167.

Krebs, E.E., Lorenz, K.A., Bair, M.J., et al., 2009. Development and initial validity of the PEG, a three-item scale assessing pain intensity and interference. J. Gen. Intern. Med. 24 (6), 733–738.

Lowe, N.K., Walker, S.N., MacCallum, R.C., 1991. Confirming the theoretical structure of the McGill Pain Questionnaire in acute clinical pain. Pain 46 (1), 57–62.

Machata, A.M., Kabon, B., Willschke, H., et al., 2009. A new instrument for pain assessment in the immediate post-operative period. Anaesthesia 64 (4), 392–398.

Main, C.J., Spanswick, C.C., 1995a. Personality assessment and the MMPI. 50 years on: Do we still need our security blanket? Pain Forum 4, 90–96.

Main, C.J., Spanswick, C.C., 1995b. 'Functional overlay' and illness behaviour in chronic pain: Distress or malingering? Conceptual difficulties in medico-legal assessment of personal injury claims. J. Psychosom. Res. 39 (6), 737–753.

Main, C.J., Watson, P.J., 1996. Guarded movements: Development of chronicity. Journal of Musculoskeletal Pain 4 (4), 163–170.

Main, C.J., Evans, P.J.D., Whitehead, R.C., 1991. An investigation of personality structure and other psychological features in patients presenting with low back pain: A critique of the MMPI. In: Bond, M.R., Charlton, J.E., Woolf, C.J. (Eds.), Proceedings of the VIth World Congress on Pain. Pain Research and Clinical Management. Elsevier, Amsterdam, pp. 207–217.

Maitland, G., 1987. The Maitland concept: Assessment, examination and treatment by passive movement. In: Twomey, L., Taylor, J. (Eds.), Physical Therapy of the Low Back. Churchill Livingstone, New York.

Margolis, R.B., Tait, R.C., Krause, S.J., 1986. A rating system for use with patient pain drawings. Pain 24 (1), 57–65.

Margolis, R.B., Chibnall, J.T., Tait, R.C., 1988. Test–retest reliability of the pain drawing instrument. Pain 33 (1), 49–51.

McGrath, P.J., Unruh, A.M., 1999. Measurement of paediatric pain. In: Wall, P.D., Melzack, R. (Eds.), Textbook of Pain. fourth ed Churchill Livingstone, New York, pp. 371–384.

Melzack, R., 1975. The McGill Pain Questionnaire: Major properties and scoring methods. Pain 1 (3), 277–299.

Melzack, R., 1987. The short-form McGill Pain Questionnaire. Pain 30 (2), 191–197.

Melzack, R., Katz, J., 1994. Pain measurement in persons in pain. In: Wall, P.D., Melzack, R. (Eds.), Textbook of Pain. third ed Churchill Livingstone, New York, pp. 337–351.

Morley, S., Wilkinson, L., 1995. The pain beliefs and perceptions inventory: A British replication. Pain 61 (3), 427–433.

Müller, U., Tänzler, K., Bürger, A., et al., 2008. A pain assessment scale for population-based studies: Development and validation of the Pain Module of the Standard Evaluation Questionnaire. Pain 136 (1,2), 62–74.

Nicholas, M., 1994. Pain self-efficacy questionnaire (PSEQ): Preliminary report. Unpublished paper. University of Sydney Pain Management and Research Centre, St Leonards.

Nicholas, M.K., Asghari, A., Blyth, F.M., 2008. What do the numbers mean? Normative data in chronic pain measures. Pain 134 (1,2), 158–173.

Parker, H., Wood, R.L.R., Main, C.J., 1995. The use of the pain drawing as a screening measure to predict psychological distress in chronic low back pain. Spine 20 (2), 236–243.

Patrick, L., D'Eon, J., 1996. Social support and functional status in chronic pain patients. Canadian Journal of Rehabilitation 9, 195–201.

Payen, J.F., Bru, O., Bosson, J.L., et al., 2001. Assessing pain in critically ill sedated patients by using a behavioral pain scale. Crit. Care Med. 29 (12), 2258–2263.

Peters, M.L., Patijn, J., Lamé, I., 2007. Pain assessment in younger and older pain patients: Psychometric properties and patient preference of five commonly used measures of pain intensity. Pain Med. 8 (7), 601–610.

Pilowsky, I., Spence, N.D., 1983. Manual for the Illness Behaviour Questionnaire, second ed University of Adelaide Department of Psychiatry, Adelaide.

Polatin, P.B., Mayer, T.G., 1996. Occupational disorders and the management of chronic pain. Orthop. Clin. North Am. 27 (4), 881–890.

Price, D., 1999. Psychological mechanisms of pain and analgesia. IASP Press, Seattle.

Prkachin, K.M., 2009. Assessing pain by facial expression: Facial expression as nexus. Pain Res. Manag. 14 (1), 53–58.

Provenzano, D.A., Fanciullo, G.J., Jamison, R.N., et al., 2007. Computer assessment and diagnostic classification of chronic pain patients. Pain Med. Suppl 3, S167–S175.

Rainville, J., Bagnall, D., Phalen, L., 1995. Health care providers' attitudes and beliefs about functional impairments and chronic pain. Clin. J. Pain 11 (4), 287–295.

Ransford, A.O., Cairns, D., Mooney, V., 1976. The Pain Drawing as an aid to the psychologic evaluation of patients with low-back pain. Spine 1 (2), 127–134.

Richards, K.M., 2008. RAP project: An instrument development study to determine common attributes for pain assessment among men and women who represent multiple pain-related diagnoses. Pain Manag. Nurs. 9 (1), 33–43.

Robinson, M.E., Riley III, J.L., Myers, C.D., et al., 1997a. The Coping Strategies Questionnaire: A large sample, item level factor analysis. Clin. J. Pain 13, 43–49.

Robinson, M.E., Myers, C.D., Sadler, I.J., et al., 1997b. Bias effects in three common self-report pain assessment measures. Clin. J. Pain 13 (1), 74–81.

Roden, A., Sturman, E., 2009. Assessment and management of patients with wound-related pain. Nursing Standard 23 (45), 53–62.

Rosenstiel, A.K., Keefe, F.J., 1983. The use of coping strategies in chronic low back pain patients: Relationship to patient characteristics and current adjustment. Pain 17 (1), 33–44.

Rucker, K.S., Metzler, H.M., 1995. Predicting subsequent employment status of SSA disability applicants with chronic pain. Clin. J. Pain 11 (1), 22–35.

Rucker, K.S., Metzler, H.M., Kregel, J., 1996. Standardization of chronic pain assessment: A multiperspective approach. Clin. J. Pain 12 (2), 94–110.

Schnurr, R.F., MacDonald, M.R., 1995. Memory complaints in chronic pain. Clin. J. Pain 11 (2), 103–111.

Stratford, P., Solomon, P., Binkley, J., et al., 1993. Sensitivity of Sickness Impact Profile items to measure change over time in a low-back pain patient group. Spine 18 (13), 1723–1727.

Strong, J., 1992. Chronic low back pain: Towards an integrated psychosocial assessment model. Unpublished PhD thesis. University of Queensland, Brisbane, Australia.

Strong, J., 1995. Self-efficacy and the patient with chronic pain. In: Schacklock, M. (Ed.), Moving in on Pain. Butterworth- Heinemann, Melbourne.

Strong, J., 1999. Assessment of pain perception in clinical practice. Man. Ther. 4, 216–220.

Strong, J., Cramond, T., Maas, F., 1989. The effectiveness of relaxation techniques with patients who have chronic low back pain. Occupational Therapy Journal of Research 9, 184–192.

Strong, J., Ashton, R., Chant, D., 1991. Pain intensity measurement in chronic low back pain. Clin. J. Pain 7 (3), 209–218.

Strong, J., Ashton, R., Chant, D., 1992. The measurement of attitudes towards and beliefs about pain. Pain 48 (2), 227–236.

Strong, J., Ashton, R., Large, R.G., 1994a. Function and the patient with chronic low back pain. Clin. J. Pain 10 (3), 191–196.

Strong, J., Ashton, R., Stewart, A., 1994b. Chronic low back pain: Toward an integrated psychosocial assessment model. J. Consult. Clin. Psychol. 62 (5), 1058–1063.

Strong, J., Large, R.G., Ashton, R., et al., 1995. A New Zealand replication of the IPAM clustering model. Clin. J. Pain 11 (4), 296–306.

Strong, J., Mathews, T., Sussex, R., et al., 2009. Pain language and gender differences when describing a past pain event. Pain 145 (1–2), 86–95.

Sullivan, M.J.L., Bishop, S.R., Pivik, J., 1995. The Pain Catastrophizing Scale: Development and validation. Psychol. Assess. 7 (4), 524–532.

Tait, R.C., Chibnall, J.T., 1997. Development of a brief version of the Survey of Pain Attitudes. Pain 70 (2,3), 229–235.

Tait, R.C., Pollard, A., Margolis, R.B., et al., 1987. The Pain Disability Index: Psychometric and validity data. Arch. Phys. Med. Rehabil. 68 (7), 438–441.

Tait, R.C., Chibnall, J.T., Krause, S., 1990. The Pain Disability Index: Psychometric properties. Pain 40 (2), 171–182.

Turk, D.C., 1996. Biopsychosocial perspective on chronic pain. In: Gatchel, R.J., Turk, D.C. (Eds.), Psychosocial Approaches to Pain Management: A Practitioner's Handbook. Guilford Press, New York, pp. 3–32.

Turk, D.C., Okifuji, A., 1999. Assessment of patients' reporting of pain: An integrated perspective. Lancet 353 (9166), 1784–1788.

Turk, D., Dworkin, R., Revicki, D., et al., 2008. Identifying important outcome domains for chronic pain clinical trials: an IMMPACT survey of people with pain. Pain 137 (2), 276–285.

Unruh, A.M., Ritchie, J.A., 1998. Development of the Pain Appraisal Inventory: Psychometric properties. Pain Res. Manag. 3 (2), 105–110.

Vasuderan, S.V., 1989. Clinical perspectives on the relationship between pain and disability. Neurological Clinics 7, 429–439.

Verbrugge, L.M., 1990. Disability. Rheumatic Disease Clinics of North America 16, 741–761.

Vlaeyen, J.W.S., Kote-Snijders, A.M.K., Boeren, R.G.V., et al., 1995. Fear of movement/(re)injury in chronic low back pain and its relation to behavioural performance. Pain 62 (3), 363–372.

Voepel-Lewis, T., Zanotti, J., Dammeyer, J.A., et al., 2010. Reliability and validity of the Face, Legs, Activity, Cry, Consolability behavioral tool in assessing acute pain in critically ill patients. American Journal of Critical Care 19 (1), 55–61.

Waddell, G., 2004. The Back Pain Revolution. Churchill Livingstone, Edinburgh.

Waddell, G., Main, C.J., 1984. Assessment of severity in low-back disorders. Spine 9 (2), 204–208.

Waddell, G., Newton, M., Henderson, I., et al., 1993. A fear avoidance beliefs questionnaire (FABQ) and the role of fear-avoidance in chronic low back pain and disability. Pain 52 (2), 157–168.

White, J., Strong, J., 1992. Measurement of activity levels in patients with chronic low back pain. Occupational Therapy Journal of Research 12, 217–228.

Williams, D.A., Thorn, B.E., 1989. An empirical assessment of pain beliefs. Pain 36 (3), 351–358.

Williams, D.A., Robinson, M.E., Geisser, M.E., 1994. Pain beliefs: Assessment and utility. Pain 59 (1), 71–78.

Woolf, C.J., Decosterd, I., 1999. Implications of recent advances in the understanding of pain pathophysiology for the assessment of pain in patients. Pain 82 (Suppl. 1), S141–S147.

World Health Organization, 1980. International Classification of Impairments. Disabilities and Handicaps, WHO, Geneva.

World Health Organization, 1999. ICIDH-2 International Classification of Functioning and Disability Beta-2 Draft Full Version. WHO, Geneva.

Chapter | 8 |

Psychological interventions: a conceptual perspective

Michael J.L. Sullivan and Tsipora Mankovsky-Arnold

LEARNING OBJECTIVES

On completing this chapter, readers will have an understanding of the following psychological interventions and for whom they are intended:

1. Historical evolution of psychological treatments for pain
2. Behavioural/operant programmes
3. Back schools
4. Cognitive-behavioural therapy
5. Stress management
6. Acceptance and commitment therapy
7. Risk-targeted interventions
8. Progressive goal attainment
9. Graded activity and exposure.

The crossroads of pain, psychology and intervention have a long history. Paradoxically, interventions of antiquity for psychological problems were more concerned with the infliction of pain than its alleviation. Archaeological records suggests that shaman of the Stone Age bored holes in the skulls of 'affected' individuals, an intervention now referred to as trepanation, in order to provide an escape route for evil spirits (Selling 1943). The practice of trepanation endured well into the Middle Ages, with priests using metal implements to drill holes in individuals' skulls to rid the body of the evil spirits that possessed it (White 1896). Torturous techniques such as immersion in cold water, flogging, starving and burning were later adopted by medical practitioners of mental institutions as techniques to calm or control agitated patients.

There remain vestiges of the conceptual models of antiquity in current models of the psychology of chronic pain. The notion that some form of noxious agent is locked within the individual with chronic pain and must be released in order to bring about a cure continues to find expression in many domains of mental health practice associated with chronic pain (Blumer & Heilbronn 1982; Sternbach 1974). For example, Freudian theory suggests that certain psychological conflicts suppressed from consciousness can be converted into physical symptoms such as pain and disability. Unfortunately, many of the psychodynamic variables implicated as causative of chronic pain have been poorly defined, impossible to measure or couched within theoretical frameworks that have minimal value for either conceptualizing or treating chronic pain (Ferrari & Russell 1997; Sternbach 1974; Weintraub 1988).

Despite a century of clinical, empirical and theoretical discussions on the causes and treatment of chronic pain there is a sense that advance, considered in terms of either

© 2014 Elsevier Ltd.

conceptual understanding or treatment effectiveness, has been modest. The prevalence of pain-related disability has been increasing steadily in spite of numerous prevention and intervention initiatives that have been launched to date (Gosselin 2004; Waddell 1998). Persistent musculoskeletal pain continues to be the most costly non-malignant health condition affecting the working-age population in most industrialized countries (Cats-Baril & Frymoyer 1991; Fordyce 1995; Kuorinka & Forcier 1995; Sullivan & Frank 2000).

The lack of progress in effective management of chronic pain can be attributed to a number of factors. A central issue concerns the lack of consensus on how chronic pain should be conceptualized. In current literature, there is still debate about whether chronic pain is a legitimate physical condition or represents the expression of some form of psychological dysfunction (Abbass 2008; Blumer & Heilbronn 1982). Faced with a situation where patients present with physical symptoms with no discernible organic pathology to the medical practitioner, the 'leap to the head' might appear like a reasonable approach to managing the pain patient. Even today, it is not uncommon in medical reports to see reference to terms such as 'symptom amplification', 'pain magnification' or 'functional overlay'. These terms are pejorative, place blame on the patient for lack of treatment response and are more likely to impede than foster effective clinical management of a chronic pain condition.

According to the DSM IV, most chronic pain conditions would meet the criteria for a diagnosis of 'Pain disorder associated with a medical condition' (American Psychiatric Association Press 1994). Pain disorder is classified as one of the somatoform disorders. The essential feature of somatoform disorders is that psychological conflicts have been transformed into physical symptoms (Ford 1995). The inclusion of chronic pain phenomena within the taxonomy of psychiatric disorders perpetuates the view that mental health issues are at the root of, as opposed to the consequence of, chronic pain and encourages the undesirable clinical practice of diagnosis by exclusion (Weintraub 1988).

In many domains of intervention, there is an increasing call for the application of evidence-based principles in clinical practice (Fordyce et al 1985). It has been argued that the clinician has an ethical responsibility to provide treatments that have been shown to be effective and not to provide treatments that have been shown to be ineffective. However, a quick glance at the interventions used in typical pain treatment centres reveals all too clearly that many of the interventions are not evidence-based, and many interventions continue to be used even though they have been shown to be clearly ineffective (Fordyce et al 1982; Forrest 2002; Fullop-Miller 1938).

It has been suggested that in pain treatment centres many of the interventions used might be more aptly described as compassion-driven as opposed to evidence-driven. Clinicians intervene because they do not want to see their patients suffer. The problem with compassion-based

medicine is that it frequently proceeds in the absence of supporting evidence of efficacy and, in the case of chronic conditions, might persist indefinitely.

This chapter briefly reviews psychological approaches to the management of pain-related health conditions and pain-related disability. The review is selective as opposed to exhaustive, with emphasis on interventions that have been systematically evaluated. An attempt is also made to describe different psychological interventions for pain from a historical perspective in order to sketch the evolution of psychological perspectives on the treatment of pain over time. Where possible, references to clinical manuals are provided for readers who are interested in learning more about the specific intervention techniques described.

PSYCHOLOGICAL TREATMENT OF PAIN

Perhaps one of the earliest persuasive demonstrations of the role of psychosocial factors in pain perception came from the work of Anton Mesmer in the late 1700s (Forrest 2002; Fullop-Miller 1938). Mesmer found that magnets applied to the body of an ailing person appeared to alleviate pain and suffering. Later, Mesmer believed that the 'vital magnetism' emanated not from within the magnets, but from within his own body (Fullop-Miller 1938). He claimed he was able to alleviate pain and suffering simply by passing his hands over ailing persons.

Mesmer's treatment became so popular that he was unable to treat all the patients who sought his help. The demand for his treatment led him to develop ways of treating many individuals at once. Mesmer built 'baquets' to facilitate the treatment of several individuals at once. The baquet was a large tub built of wood and filled with water and pieces of glass and metal. Once the baquet had been infused with Mesmer's healing magnetism, patients would gather around it, place large metal rods into it and touch one end of the rod to the part of their body that was in pain. The healing forces of vital magnetism flowed up the metal rod and into the body of the ailing person, thus curing them of their affliction (Forrest 2002).

Anecdotal reports make reference to hundreds of patients who were 'cured' with Mesmer's treatment (Forrest 2002). In the days of Mesmer, it was believed that magnetism was the essential ingredient of these cures. Today, most would consider that psychological factors such as beliefs or expectancies were the essential ingredients of the cures Mesmer was able to achieve with his treatment.

Beecher's (1946) naturalistic observations of war casualties are often cited as a catalyst for the development of contemporary models of the psychology of pain. Working as a military physician, Beecher was struck by the wide range of soldiers' responses to injury and pain. He provided vivid descriptions of soldiers who had sustained severe wounds in combat yet did not request narcotics to alleviate their pain. He suggested that for many soldiers, the wounds may have represented their 'ticket to safety' and that their pain experience may have been lessened by this positive reinterpretation.

By the mid 1960s, mounting clinical and scientific evidence was calling for a model of pain that would consider both the physiological and psychological mechanisms involved in pain perception. The call was most compellingly answered by Melzack and Wall's Gate Control Theory of Pain (Melzack & Wall 1965). From an applied perspective, the work of Melzack and Wall evolved into behavioural conceptualizations of pain (Fordyce 1976), contributing ultimately to the development of biopsychosocial models of pain (Gatchel et al 2007; Turk 2002). Biopsychosocial models propose that a complete understanding of pain experience and pain-related outcomes requires consideration of physical, psychological and social factors (Gatchel et al 2007; Keefe & France 1999; Turk 1996; Waddell 1998).

BEHAVIOURAL/OPERANT PROGRAMMES

The first programmes that specifically targeted the psychological aspects of pain-related disability were based on the view that pain-related disability was a form of 'behaviour' that was maintained by reinforcement contingencies. In the 1960s and 1970s, William Fordyce and his colleagues applied the concepts of learning theory to the problem of chronic pain (Fordyce et al 1968, 1976). The focus of Fordyce's approach to treatment was not on reducing the experience of pain, but on reducing the overt display of pain. The targets selected for treatment were pain behaviours such as distress vocalizations, facial grimacing, limping, guarding, medication intake, activity withdrawal and activity avoidance (Fordyce et al 1982).

The first behavioural approaches to the management of pain and disability were conducted within inpatient settings that permitted systematic observation of pain behaviours, as well control over environmental contingencies influencing pain behaviour (Fordyce 1976). Staff were trained to monitor pain behaviour and to selectively reinforce 'well behaviours' and selectively ignore 'pain behaviours' (Fordyce et al 1982). The results of several studies revealed that the manipulation of reinforcement contingencies could exert a powerful influence on the frequency of display of pain behaviours (Fordyce et al 1985). The manipulation of reinforcement contingencies was also applied to other domains of pain-related behaviour and shown to be effective in reducing medication intake, reducing downtime and maximizing participation in goal-directed activity.

A number of clinical trials on the efficacy of behavioural treatments for the reduction of pain and disability yielded positive findings (Sanders 1996). However, given the significant resources required to implement contingency management interventions, issues concerning the cost-efficacy of behavioural therapy for pain and disability were raised. Concern was also raised over the maintenance of treatment gains since reinforcement contingencies outside the clinic setting could not be readily controlled. In order to increase access and reduce costs, behavioural treatments were modified to permit their administration on an outpatient basis. This change in delivery format compromised to some degree the control over environmental contingencies and required greater reliance on self-monitoring and self-report measures (Sanders 1996).

BACK SCHOOLS

Although back schools were first developed in the late 1960s, the first published reports of the benefits of back schools only appeared in the literature in the early 1980s (Zachrisson-Forsell 1981). The structure and content of back schools reflected the prevailing view of the time that 'information' or 'knowledge' could be powerful tools to effect change in behaviour (e.g. pain-elated disability) (Heymans et al 2005).

Back schools vary widely in terms of content, duration and the intervention disciplines used to administer the programme. The duration of back school interventions has ranged from a single information session to a 2-month inpatient programme (van Tulder et al 2000). Back school interventions have tended to use group formats with a didactic format where participants might be exposed to information about biomechanics, posture, ergonomics, exercises, nutrition, weight loss, attitudes, beliefs and coping. As a function of the type of information being provided, the interventionist might be a physician, physiotherapist, occupational therapist, nurse or psychologist (Linton & Kamwendo 1987).

The marked differences across back schools have presented significant challenges to the systematic assessment of their efficacy (van Tulder et al 2000). A recent review of randomized clinical trails of back school programmes concluded that (a) back schools yielded benefit relative to treatment-as-usual interventions, (b) the treatment effect size was small and (c) back school programmes implemented within occupational settings appeared to yield the most positive outcomes (Heymans et al 2005).

COGNITIVE-BEHAVIOURAL PROGRAMMES

Cognitive-behavioural programmes for the management of pain and pain-related disability began to appear in the 1980s (Turk et al 1983). Cognitive-behavioural programmes incorporated concepts drawn from earlier behavioural approaches as well as information-based approaches used in back schools. The objective of many cognitive-behavioural programmes is to equip individuals with the psychological tools necessary to adequately meet the challenges of persistent pain (Linton & Ryberg 2001; Linton et al 1989; Turk et al 1983).

Cognitive-behavioural interventions are currently considered the psychological treatment of choice for individuals coping with chronic pain and disability (Gatchel et al 2007; Linton 2000; Turk 2002). A number of clinical trials have demonstrated that these types of interventions can assist individuals in learning to manage or control their pain symptoms and lead to clinically significant decreases in emotional distress (Linton 2000; Linton & Ryberg 2001; Turk 2002; Williams et al 1996). There is evidence to suggest that cognitive-behavioural interventions can also impact on indices of disability such as physical tolerance and return to work rates but observed effects have been modest and less consistent (Morley et al 1999).

It is important to note that the term 'cognitive-behavioural' does not refer to a specific intervention, but rather to a class of intervention strategies. The strategies included under the heading of cognitive-behavioural interventions vary widely and may include self-instruction (e.g. motivational self-talk), relaxation or biofeedback, developing coping strategies (e.g. distraction, imagery), increasing assertiveness, minimizing negative or self-defeating thoughts, changing maladaptive beliefs about pain and goal setting (Turk et al 1983). A client referred for cognitive-behavioural intervention may be exposed to varying selections of these strategies. The goals of cognitive-behavioural programmes might also differ across settings and may include pain reduction, distress reduction, increased activity involvement or return to work (Gatchel et al 2007; Linton & Ryberg 2001).

STRESS MANAGEMENT PROGRAMMES

Stress management programmes represent a special case of cognitive-behavioural intervention. Stress management programmes proceed from the view that, unless properly managed, chronic stresses can lead to a depletion of the individual's physical and psychological resources and in turn increase the individual's susceptibility to physical or psychological dysfunction (Lazarus & Folkman 1984). Stress management approaches are considered separately from cognitive-behavioural pain management programmes since the focus of stress management programmes is not necessarily on managing pain symptoms or disability. Furthermore, while cognitive-behavioural programmes are typically used for individuals who are work-disabled due to their pain condition, stress management programmes have been used as preventive interventions for

individuals who are experiencing symptoms of persistent pain but are still working. The primary focus of stress management interventions might be on stresses within the workplace or the individual's personal stresses (Feuerstein et al 2000, 2004). There is considerable variability in the duration of stress management programmes, ranging from two sessions to 8-week programmes (Pransky et al 2002). There are indications that shorter duration stress management programmes might have negligible impact on outcomes (Feuerstein et al 2004).

Problem-solving therapy is a variant of stress management programmes that has recently been applied to individuals who are work-disabled due to musculoskeletal pain conditions (D'Zurilla 1990; Smeets et al 2008; van den Hout et al 2003). Problem-solving therapy proceeds from the view that life stresses can be minimized if the individual is able to use appropriate problem-solving strategies to deal with difficult situations that might be encountered in the work place or in daily life (D'Zurilla 1971; Nezu & Perri 1989). Problem-solving intervention programmes will typically span several weeks (8–10) and might involve didactic lectures, group discussion and homework assignments (Gallagher 2006). The limited research that has addressed the efficacy of this form of intervention indicates that the addition of problem-solving solving therapy to usual treatment might improve return to work outcomes in individuals with disabling musculoskeletal pain (Smeets et al 2008; van den Hout et al 2003).

ACCEPTANCE AND COMMITMENT THERAPY

Acceptance and commitment therapy (ACT), also referred to as contextually-based cognitive-behaviour therapy, is a type of cognitive therapy that has evolved from Stephen Hayes' work on acceptance and adaptation (Hayes et al 1999; McCracken 2005). Interestingly, ACT has its philosophical roots in religious traditions, such as Christianity and Buddhism, which view suffering as a ubiquitous element of human existence. According to Hayes and his colleagues, the medicalization of suffering and persistent and ineffective efforts to rid individuals of suffering are factors that have contributed inadvertently to the persistence and exacerbation of the suffering associated with many health and mental health conditions (Hayes et al 1999).

Proponents of ACT emphasize that they do not use the term acceptance to refer to resignation, but rather as a term to refer to the process of ceasing to struggle ineffectively against that which cannot be changed (Hayes et al 1999). In the case of chronic pain, acceptance is viewed as a first step toward successful adaptation (McCracken 2005). Acceptance is said to occur when the individual with chronic pain is willing to experience his or her pain without attempting to control it. Through treatment individuals with chronic pain are taught to acknowledge their pain, observe it as a sensation and then accept it as part of their reality without judgment. Through treatment, individuals are also encouraged to focus on their values and to commit to activities consistent with their values, in spite of ongoing pain. The individual is assisted in moving away from a focus on pain and pain control to a focus on themes or activities of greater value.

Several investigations have shown that ACT is effective in reducing pain intensity and self-reported disability (McCracken & Eccleston 2006; McCracken et al 2005; Vowles & McCracken 2008). To date, ACT has only been used with individuals with long-standing chronic pain where the prospect of significant pain alleviation is realistic low. When symptom-focused treatment of the pain condition is unlikely to yield positive outcomes, acceptance-based interventions might represent a useful option for improving the quality of life of individuals with chronic pain. It is not clear whether ACT would be effective, or even appropriate, for individuals with recent onset pain where a certain proportion of individuals would be expected to show significant recovery from their pain condition.

RISK-FACTOR TARGETED INTERVENTIONS

Recent research on risk factors for prolonged pain and disability has prompted the development of risk-factor-targeted intervention programmes (Gauthier et al 2006; Sullivan et al 2005b; Thorn et al 2002; Vlaeyen & Linton 2000; Vlaeyen et al 2001). These programmes differ from traditional cognitive-behavioural programmes with their focus on a limited set of psychological factors that have been shown to increase the risk of problematic recovery following the onset of a pain condition (Leeuw et al 2007a; Severeijns et al 2001; Sullivan 2003; Swinkels-Meewisse et al 2006). Pain catastrophizing and fear of movement have received the most attention in research examining psychological risk for chronic pain and disability (Buer & Linton 2002; Jensen et al 2001). Pain catastrophizing has been broadly defined as an exaggerated negative orientation toward actual or anticipated pain comprising elements of rumination, magnification and helplessness (Sullivan et al 1995). Pain-related fear has been defined as a negative emotional experience associated with pain, characterized by escape or avoidance behaviour (McNeil et al 2000). More than 600 papers have been published documenting a relation between catastrophizing and adverse pain outcomes, with many investigators calling for the development of interventions specifically designed to reduce catastrophic thinking associated with pain (Keefe et al 2010; Quartana et al 2009; Sullivan et al 2005a). Similarly, hundreds of investigations have documented a relation between fear of movement and adverse pain outcomes (Leeuw et al 2007a; Vlaeyen & Linton 2000).

PROGRESSIVE GOAL ATTAINMENT

The Progressive Goal Attainment Programme (PGAP) was designed as a risk factor-targeted intervention for individuals suffering from debilitating pain conditions (Sullivan et al 2006a). The primary goals of PGAP are to reduce catastrophic thinking and fear of movement in order to promote reintegration to life-role activities, increase quality of life and facilitate return-to-work. Although PGAP was designed to target psychological risk factors for pain and disability, the intervention need not be delivered by a mental health professional. The intervention is typically delivered by occupational therapists, physiotherapists or psychologists. Rehabilitation professionals attend a 2-day workshop to develop the skill set required to deliver the intervention.

Since PGAP is a risk-factor-targeted intervention, clients are only considered as potential candidates for the intervention if they obtain scores in the risk range on measures of catastrophic thinking, fear of movement or disability beliefs. In the initial weeks of the programme, the focus is on the establishment of a strong therapeutic relationship and the development of a structured activity schedule. The client is provided with a client workbook that serves as the platform for activity scheduling and contains the forms for various exercises that will be used through the treatment. Each session begins with a review of the previous week's activities and ends with planning activities for the coming week. Activity goals are established in order to promote resumption of family, social and occupational roles. Intervention techniques are invoked to target specific obstacles to rehabilitation progress (e.g. catastrophic thinking, fear of movement and disability beliefs). In the final stages of the programme, the intervention focuses on activities that will facilitate reintegration to the workplace (Sullivan et al 2006a).

PGAP has been shown to be effective in reducing catastrophic thinking, fear of movement and disability beliefs in individuals with whiplash injuries and work-related musculoskeletal injuries (Adams et al 2007; Sullivan & Adams 2010; Sullivan et al 2006a). Research has supported the view that reductions in catastrophizing are significant determinants of treatment-related improvements in depressive symptoms, physical function and return to work (Spinhoven et al 2004; Sullivan et al 2005a, 2006a, 2007a). PGAP has been implemented country-wide in New Zealand as part of a national strategy for the prevention of chronic pain and disability consequent to musculoskeletal injury. A telephonic version of PGAP is currently being tested by the Social Security Administration of the USA as a means of reducing disability and improving quality of life in individuals with long-standing disability associated with pain-related health conditions.

GRADED ACTIVITY AND EXPOSURE

The premise underlying graded activity or exposure inter-ventions is that disability can be construed as a type of phobic orientation toward activity (Vlaeyen & Linton 2000). According to the Fear-Avoidance Model, individuals will differ in the degree to which they interpret their pain symptoms in a 'catastrophic' or 'alarmist' manner. The model predicts that catastrophic thinking following the onset of pain will contribute to heightened fears of move-ment. In turn, fear is expected to lead to avoidance of activity that might be associated with pain (Vlaeyen & Linton 2000). Prolonged inactivity is expected to contribute to depression and disability (Sullivan et al 2006b). The model is recursive such that increased pain symptoms, distress and disability become the input for further catastrophic or alarmist think-ing (Vlaeyen & Linton 2000). According to the Fear-Avoidance Model, reducing fear of movement is a critical component of successful rehabilitation of individuals with debilitating pain conditions (Vlaeyen & Linton 2000). Cli-ents are typically only considered for exposure interventions if they obtain high scores on measures of fear of movement.

Graded activity or exposure to feared activities are treat-ment approaches that involve systematic exposure or engagement in activities that individuals avoid due to fears that they might experience an exacerbation of their symp-toms. Feared activities are initially identified and ranked hierarchically, from least to most feared activities. Begin-ning with the least feared activities, clients are systemati-cally exposed to movements that comprise the activities that clients are currently avoiding. Clients are repeatedly exposed to specific movements until their fear of activity subsides. As clients overcome their fears associated with the least feared activities in their feared activities hierarchy, the exposure techniques are used on activities associated with higher levels of fear (Leeuw et al 2007b).

While graded exposure has been shown to be an effective intervention for reducing the fear of specific movements, its effects do not seem to generalize to untargeted activities (Crombez et al 2002; Goubert et al 2002). As such, the clin-ical significance of the intervention might depend on the degree to which important activities of daily living or occu-pational activities can be targeted. Graded activity and exposure interventions aimed at reducing fear of move-ment have been shown to be effective in reducing disabil-ity, reducing absenteeism and facilitating return to work (Bailey et al 2010; de Jong et al 2012).

CHOOSING AMONG DIFFERENT PSYCHOLOGICAL INTERVENTIONS

The intervention approaches described in this chapter dif-fer in terms of their focus, structure, content and objectives.

With the range of potential intervention avenues currently available, the clinician might reflect on the question of which intervention approach might be most suitable for a particular client. Since little research has been conducted on matching client profiles to specific interventions, this question unfortunately cannot be addressed from an empirical standpoint. There are, however, various points of consideration that might assist the clinician in determin-ing the most appropriate intervention for his or her client.

Few would question the importance of information pro-vision in the management of chronic pain and disability. The more that clients understand about the nature of their pain condition, the more they will be able to play an active role in the management of their condition. As such, information-based approaches such as back schools might be an important element in the management of chronic pain. However, for most clients with chronic pain condi-tions, information alone is unlikely to yield clinically sig-nificant improvements in mood, suffering or disability. Information-based techniques might best be viewed as important elements of a more comprehensive approach to treatment as opposed to stand-alone interventions.

For the greater part of the last two decades, psychosocial interventions were included primarily as part of tertiary care treatment for clients with long-standing chronic pain and disability (Gatchel 2004). With little expectancy of clinical improvement of clients' pain conditions, the focus of many treatment programmes was primarily on the alle-viation of suffering. Cognitive-behavioural interventions that used distress reduction techniques such as relaxation, reappraisal and cognitive restructuring were ideally suited to achieve reductions in suffering in clients with long-standing chronic pain (Morley et al 1999).

As research accumulated showing that psychological interventions yielded significant reductions in pain and emotional distress, there was greater interest in using psy-chological interventions for clients who were at earlier stages of chronicity (Gatchel 2004; Sullivan 2003). The term 'secondary prevention' is used to describe interven-tions that are implemented for individuals considered to have 'at risk' condition or chronic pain and disability, but whose condition has not yet become chronic. With a less chronic population, the treatment objectives of psy-chological interventions changed. Since many clients still have an employment-relevant skill set, and some might also have a job to return to, there is an increased focus on return-to-function as a central objective of treatment, as opposed to a primary focus on reduction of suffering. Return to function is a central objective of interventions such as PGAP or graded exposure.

When treatment is initiated after a long period of chro-nicity, intervention strategies are more likely to address the consequences of pain and disability (e.g. affective dis-orders, drug/alcohol overuse, family dysfunction) as opposed to risk factors for pain and disability. It is impor-tant for professionals working with clients with long-standing chronic pain and disability to have a background in mental health in order to be able to intervene on psychological conditions that might be compounding the client's pain condition. However, risk factors for chronicity are not necessarily psychological disorders nor would they necessarily be considered indices of dysfunction (in the absence of a pain condition). Nevertheless, their presence contributes to a higher probability that a pain condition will persist or worsen over time. The challenge to effective secondary prevention lies not only in the development of risk-factor-targeted interventions, but in developing mechanisms by which individuals at risk can be identified. Perhaps more so than is the case for psychological disorders, risk factors for chronicity may be particularly likely to go undetected during routine primary care. Treating physicians often become aware of psychological factors in pain and disability only once chronicity has developed and the client has become treatment resistant.

Since psychological risk factors for chronic pain and disability are not mental health conditions, the development of secondary prevention interventions opened the door for using professionals who were not mental health professionals to deliver psychological interventions for pain. Intervention programmes like PGAP or graded exposure are more likely to use occupational therapists, physiotherapists or kinesiologists as interventionists than psychologists. This should be viewed as a positive change since the shortage of psychologists involved in the treatment of pain severely limits access to psychological services for individuals with debilitating pain conditions.

Thus, chronicity and clinical complexity are two factors that will influence the type of psychological intervention that will be considered, the objectives of the intervention and the training background of the professional that will be used to deliver the intervention. Undoubtedly, other psychological interventions will be added to the repertoire of psychological services offered to clients with debilitating pan conditions. It is paramount to consider the evidence base for psychological interventions for pain-related difficulties before offering them to clients with debilitating pain conditions. Offering interventions that are not evidence-based increases the probability of treatment failure and is likely to contribute to further demoralization of a client already struggling with a heavy burden of distress and disability.

REFERENCES

American Psychiatric Association Press, 1994. DSM IV. Diagnostic and Statistical Manual of Mental Disorders. American Psychiatric Association Press, Washington, DC.

Abbass, A., 2008. Short-term psychodynamic psychotherapies for chronic pain. Canadian Journal of Psychiatry 53, 710.

Adams, H., Ellis, T., Stanish, W.D., et al., 2007. Psychosocial factors related to return to work following rehabilitation of whiplash injuries. J. Occup. Rehabil. 17, 305–315.

Bailey, K., Carleton, N., Vlaeyen, J.W.S., et al., 2010. Treatments addressing pain-related fear and anxiety in patients with chronic musculoskeletal pain: a preliminary review. Cogn. Behav. Ther. 39, 46–63.

Beecher, H.K., 1946. Pain in men wounded in battle. Ann. Surg. 23, 96–106.

Blumer, D., Heilbronn, M., 1982. Chronic pain as a variant of depressive disease: the pain-prone disorder. J. Nerv. Ment. Dis. 170, 381–394.

Buer, N., Linton, S.J., 2002. Fear-avoidance beliefs and catastrophizing: occurrence and risk factor in back pain

and ADL in the general population. Pain. 99, 485–491.

Cats-Baril, W., Frymoyer, J., 1991. Identifying patients at risk of becoming disabled due to low back pain. Spine. 16, 605–607.

Crombez, G., Eccleston, C., Vlaeyen, J.W., et al., 2002. Exposure to physical movements in low back pain patients: restricted effects of generalization. Health Psychology 21, 573–578.

D'Zurilla, T., 1971. Problem-solving and behavior modification. J. Abnorm. Psychol. 78, 107–126.

D'Zurilla, T., 1990. Problem-solving training for effective stress management and prevention. Journal of Cognitive Psychotherapy 4, 327–355.

Ferrari, R., Russell, A., 1997. The whiplash syndrome – common sense revisisted. J. Rheumatol. 24, 618–622.

Feuerstein, M., Huang, G., Shaheen, M., et al., 2000. Ergo-Stress Management for Your Health: managing Job Stress and Reducing Ergonomic Risk. Monograph, Washington, DC.

Feuerstein, M., Nicholas, R., Huang, G., et al., 2004. Job stress management

and ergonomic intervention for work-related upper extremity symptoms. Appl. Ergon. 35, 565–574.

Ford, C.V., 1995. Dimensions of somatization and hypochondriasis. Neurol. Clin. 13, 241–253.

Fordyce, W.E., 1976. Behavioral Methods for Chronic Pain and Illness. Mosby, St Louis.

Fordyce, W.E., 1995. Back Pain in the Workplace. IASP Press, Seattle.

Fordyce, W., Fowler, R., Lehmann, J., et al., 1968. Some implications of learning in problems of chronic pain. J. Chronic Dis. 21, 179–190.

Fordyce, W.E., Shelton, J.L., Dundore, D.E., 1982. The modification of avoidance learning pain behaviors. J. Behav. Med. 5, 405–414.

Fordyce, W.E., Roberts, A.H., Sternbach, R.A., 1985. The behavioral management of chronic pain: a response to critics. Pain. 22, 113–125.

Forrest, D., 2002. Mesmer. Journal of Clinical and Experimental Hypnosis 50, 295–308.

Fullop-Miller, R., 1938. Triumph over pain. Literary Guild of America, New York.

Gallagher, R.M., 2006. Problem-solving therapy for pain in the older adult. Pain Med. 7, 369.

Gatchel, R., 2004. Musculoskeletal disorders: primary and secondary interventions. J. Electromyogr. Kinesiol. 14, 161–170.

Gatchel, R., Peng, Y.B., Peters, M.L., et al., 2007. The biopsychosocial approach to chronic pain: scientific advances and future directions. Psychol. Bull. 133, 581–624.

Gauthier, N., Sullivan, M.J., Adams, H., et al., 2006. Investigating risk factors for chronicity: the importance of distinguishing between return-to-work status and self-report measures of disability. J. Occup. Environ. Med. 48, 312–318.

Gosselin, M., 2004. Analyse des avantages et des couts de la sante et de la securite au travail en entreprise. IRSST, Montreal.

Goubert, L., Francken, G., Crombez, G., et al., 2002. Exposure to physical movement in chronic back pain patients: no evidence for generalization across different movements. Behav. Res. Ther. 40, 415–429.

Hayes, S.C., Strosahl, K.D., Wilson, K.G., 1999. Acceptance and commitment therapy: an experiential approach to behavior change. Guilford Press, New York.

Heymans, M.W., van Tulder, M.W., Esmail, R., et al., 2005. Back schools for nonspecific low back pain: a systematic review within the framework of the Cochrane Collaboration Back Review Group. Spine. 30, 2153–2163.

Jensen, M.P., Turner, J.A., Romano, J.M., 2001. Changes in beliefs, catastrophizing, and coping are associated with improvement in multidisciplinary pain treatment. J. Consult. Clin. Psychol. 69, 655–662.

Keefe, F.J., Francis, C., 1999. Pain: biopsychosocial mechanisms and management. Current Directions in Psychological Science 8, 137–141.

Keefe, F.J., Shelby, R.A., Somers, T.J., 2010. Catastrophizing and pain coping: moving forward. Pain 149, 165–166.

Kuorinka, I., Forcier, L., 1995. Les lesions attribuables au travail repetitifs. Editions Multimondes, Montreal.

Lazarus, R., Folkman, S., 1984. Stress, appraisal and coping. Springer, New York.

Leeuw, M., Goossens, M.E., Linton, S.J., et al., 2007a. The fear-avoidance model of musculoskeletal pain: current state of scientific evidence. J. Behav. Med. 30, 77–94.

Leeuw, M., Houben, R.M., Severeijns, R., et al., 2007b. Pain-related fear in low back pain: a prospective study in the general population. Eur. J. Pain 11, 256–262.

Linton, S., 2000. Utility of cognitive-behavioral psychological treatments. In: Nachemson, A., Jonsson, E. (Eds.), Neck and Back Pain: The Scientific Evidence of Causes, Diagnosis, and Treatment. Lippincott, Williams & Wilkins, Philadelphia, pp. 57–78.

Linton, S.J., Kamwendo, K., 1987. Low back schools. A critical review. Phys. Ther. 67, 1375–1383.

Linton, S., Ryberg, M., 2001. A cognitive-behavioral group intervention as prevention for persistent neck and back pain in a non-patient population: A randomized controlled trial. Pain. 90, 83–90.

Linton, S., Bradley, L., Jensen, I., et al., 1989. The secondary prevention of low back pain: A controlled study with follow-up. Pain. 36, 197–207.

McCracken, L.M., 2005. Contextual Cognitive Therapy for Chronic Pain. IASP Press, Seattle.

McCracken, L.M., Eccleston, C., 2006. A comparison of the relative utility of coping and acceptance-based measures in a sample of chronic pain sufferers. Eur. J. Pain. 10, 23–29.

McCracken, L.M., Vowles, K.E., Eccleston, C., 2005. Acceptance-based treatment for persons with complex, long standing chronic pain: a preliminary analysis of treatment outcome in comparison to a waiting phase. Behav. Res. Ther. 43, 1335–1346.

McNeil, D., Au, A., Zvolensky, M., et al., 2000. Fear of pain in orofacial pain patients. Pain 89, 245–252.

Melzack, R., Wall, P., 1965. Pain mechanisms: a new theory. Science. 150, 971–979.

Morley, S., Eccleston, C., Williams, A., 1999. Systematic review and meta-analysis of randomized controlled trials of cognitive-behavior therapy and behavior therapy for chronic pain in adults, excluding headache. Pain 80, 1–13.

Nezu, A., Perri, M., 1989. Social problem-solving therapy for unipolar depression: An initial dismantling investigation. J. Consult. Clin. Psychol. 57, 408–413.

Pransky, G., Robertson, M., Moon, S., 2002. Stress and work-related upper-extremity disorders: implications for prevention and management. Am. J. Ind. Med. 41, 443–455.

Quartana, P.J., Campbell, C.M., Edwards, R.R., 2009. Pain catastrophizing: a critical review. Expert Rev. Neurother. 9, 745–758.

Sanders, S.H., 1996. Operant conditioning of chronic pain: back to basics. In: Gatchel, R., Turk, D.C. (Eds.), Psychological approaches to pain management. Guilford, New York, pp. 112–130.

Selling, L.S., 1943. Men against madness. Greenberg, New York.

Severeijns, R., Vlaeyen, J.W., van den Hout, M.A., et al., 2001. Pain catastrophizing predicts pain intensity, disability, and psychological distress independent of the level of physical impairment. Clin. J. Pain. 17, 165–172.

Smeets, R.J., Vlaeyen, J.W., Hidding, A., et al., 2008. Chronic low back pain: physical training, graded activity with problem solving training, or both? The one-year post-treatment results of a randomized controlled trial. Pain 134, 263–276.

Spinhoven, P., Ter Kuile, M., Kole-Snijders, A.M., et al., 2004. Catastrophizing and internal pain control as mediators of outcome in the multidisciplinary treatment of chronic low back pain. Eur. J. Pain 8, 211–219.

Sternbach, R.A., 1974. Pain patients: Traits and treatments. Academic Press, New York.

Sullivan, M.J.L., 2003. Emerging trends in secondary prevention of pain-related disability. Clin. J. Pain 19, 77–79.

Sullivan, M.J.L., Adams, H., 2010. Psychosocial techniques to augment the impact of physical therapy interventions for low back pain. Physiother. Can. 62, 180–189.

Sullivan, T., Frank, J., 2000. Restating disability or disabling the state: four challenges. In: Sullivan, T. (Ed.), Injury and the New World of Work. UBC Press, Vancouver, pp. 3–24.

Sullivan, M., Bishop, S., Pivik, J., 1995. The Pain Catastrophizing Scale: development and validation. Psychol. Assess. 7, 524–532.

Sullivan, M., Feuerstein, M., Gatchel, R.J., et al., 2005a. Integrating psychological and behavioral interventions to achieve optimal rehabilitation outcomes. J. Occup. Rehabil. 15, 475–489.

Sullivan, M.J.L., Ward, L.C., Tripp, D., et al., 2005b. Secondary prevention of work disability: community-based psychosocial intervention for musculoskeletal disorders. J. Occup. Rehabil. 15, 377–392.

Sullivan, M.J.L., Adams, A., Rhodenizer, T., et al., 2006a. A psychosocial risk factor targeted intervention for the prevention of chronic pain and disability following whiplash injury. Phys. Ther. 86, 8–18.

Sullivan, M.J.L., Adams, H., Thibault, P., et al., 2006b. Initial depression severity and the trajectory of recovery following cognitive-behavioral intervention for work disability. J. Occup. Rehabil. 16, 63–74.

Sullivan, M.J.L., Adams, A., Tripp, D., et al., 2007. Stage of chronicity and treatment response in patients with musculoskeletal injuries and concurrent symptoms of depression. Pain 135, 151–159.

Swinkels-Meewisse, I.E., Roelofs, J., Schouten, E.G., et al., 2006. Fear of movement/(re)injury predicting chronic disabling low back pain: a prospective inception cohort study. Spine 31, 658–664.

Thorn, B., Boothy, J., Sullivan, M., 2002. Targeted treatment of catastrophizing for the management of chronic pain. Cogn. Behav. Pract. 9, 127–138.

Turk, D., 1996. Biopsychosocial perspective on chronic pain. In: Gatchel, R., Turk, D. (Eds.), Psychological Approaches to Pain Management. Guilford, New York, pp. 3–32.

Turk, D., 2002. Clinical effectiveness and cost-effectiveness of treatments for patients with chronic pain. Clin. J. Pain. 18, 355–365.

Turk, D., Meichenbaum, D., Genest, M., 1983. Pain and Behavioral Medicine: a Cognitive-Behavioral Perspective. Guilford, New York.

van den Hout, J., Vlaeyen, J., Heuts, P., et al., 2003. Secondary prevention of work-related disability in non-specific low back pain: does problem-solving therapy help? A randomized clinical trial. Clin. J. Pain. 19, 87–96.

van Tulder, M.W., Esmail, R., Bombardier, C., et al., 2000. Back schools for non-specific low back pain. Cochrane Database Syst. Rev. 2, CD000261.

Vlaeyen, J.W., Linton, S.J., 2000. Fear-avoidance and its consequences in chronic musculoskeletal pain: a state of the art. Pain 85, 317–332.

Vlaeyen, J.W., de Jong, J., Geilen, M., et al., 2001. Graded exposure in vivo in the treatment of pain-related fear: a replicated single-case experimental design in four patients with chronic low back pain. Behav. Res. Ther. 39, 151–166.

Vowles, K.E., McCracken, L.M., 2008. Acceptance and values-based action in chronic pain: a study of treatment effectiveness and process. J. Consult. Clin. Psychol. 76, 397–407.

Waddell, G., 1998. The Back Pain Revolution. Churchill Livingstone, London.

Weintraub, M., 1988. Regional pain is usually hysterical. Arch. Neurol. 44, 914–915.

White, A.D., 1896. A History of the Warfare of Science with Theology in Christendom. Appleton and Company, New York.

Williams, A.C., Pither, C.E., Richardson, P.H., et al., 1996. The effects of cognitive-behavioural therapy in chronic pain. Pain 65, 282–284.

Zachrisson-Forsell, M., 1981. The back school. Spine 6, 104–106.

Chapter | 9 |

Psychological interventions: application to management of pain

Patrick J. McGrath, Jill M. Chorney, Anna Huguet and Anita M. Unruh

LEARNING OBJECTIVES

On completing this chapter readers will have an understanding of the application of the following psychological interventions for a person living with chronic pain:

1. Patient education.
2. Operant conditioning methods.
3. Cognitive–behavioural therapy.
4. Distraction.
5. Classical conditioning methods.
6. Social support.
7. Relaxation methods.
8. Hypnosis.
9. Biofeedback.
10. Acceptance and commitment therapy.

OVERVIEW

There is excellent evidence for the use of psychological methods to treat and manage chronic pain (Eccleston et al 2009; Palermo et al 2010). However, most scientific articles or chapters do not describe methods very well. Many methods have not been individually assessed as they often form part of the package of psychological intervention. Chapter 4 provided an overview of the psychology of pain. Chapter 8 introduced the conceptual framework of the most common psychological interventions used in pain management. In this chapter, we discuss the practical application of psychological methods. We focus on interventions that have been shown to be effective either individually or in combination with other methods to familiarize those who do not have extensive training in these methods. This short chapter is not meant to replace the years of training and supervision that a psychologist may have taken in psychological methods but to give an understanding of the specific methods that are widely used as part of an evidence-based approach to chronic pain.

The development of psychological methods has been driven by theoretical models and by clinical insight. As a result, many methods have overlapping components. Although there is an emphasis on specific techniques, it is critical to understand that good clinical practice requires several non-specific elements. The three major elements include developing a patient-oriented rather than a provider-oriented approach where the needs of the patient take precedence, developing a supportive therapeutic relationship and evaluating all interventions to ensure that more good than harm is being done.

This chapter is an applied chapter of psychological interventions. We will refer from time to time to two case

© 2014 Elsevier Ltd.

scenarios. Jeremy has chronic low back pain that resulted from a fall from a ladder on a construction site. Alice has fibromyalgia that took many years to diagnose. Each section will identify resources for more information.

PATIENT EDUCATION

Description

Education, or teaching patients about chronic pain and the typical reactions to pain, is the scaffolding upon which psychological interventions depend. The purposes of education are to ensure that patients have basic knowledge about pain, to understand the diseases and disorders causing their pain, to have a shared vocabulary about pain and to correct factual errors that patients may have. Unfortunately, the content of education for pain is often not even mentioned in research reports of psychological interventions. Consequently, there is little information as to what is an appropriate type or level of educational information. In addition, education about pain is seldom a sole treatment and there are only a few studies of its specific effects. One recent study (Barsky et al 2010) found that education was as effective as cognitive–behavioural therapy or a relaxation-based intervention for pain in rheumatoid arthritis. Udermann et al (2004) found that a personalized book on chronic low back pain was able to significantly reduce symptoms in a cohort of patients. Jeremy and Alice, our fictitious patients, are likely to participate in pain education as part of their treatment in a pain clinic and will likely benefit by correcting false beliefs and gaining a helpful way of thinking about their pain.

The first element that is often included in patient education is an explanation of the physiology and anatomy of pain. Perhaps most important for the person with chronic pain is to understand the reasons why their pain acts in such a perplexing way. It is important to address the frequent lack of a direct connection between the severity of pain and the severity of known physiological damage, and the multiple complex causes of chronic pain. This discussion may include an overview of the gate control theory. Although the gate control theory (Melzack & Wall 1965) is a somewhat dated and very general theory, it provides a useful and easily understood way for patients to understand some of the most puzzling aspects of their pain. Two examples provide a good illustration for patients of the complex physiology and anatomy of pain. One example is referred pain (Murray 2009), where a pain originating in one location is felt in another. The second example is phantom limb pain (Wilkins et al 1998), where a pain is felt in a limb in the absence of that limb. These examples highlight the lack of direct connection between pain and the normal, expected relationships that are common in the healthy, intact nervous system. The role of peripheral and central sensitization (Woolf 2007) in causing the brain, the spinal cord and the peripheral nerve structures to become more sensitive in response to ongoing pain should also be discussed. Sensitization is used to explain allodynia (pain response in the absence of typically painful stimulation) and hyperaesthesia (increased sensitivity to painful stimulation).

Fear of pain and avoidance of activity or situations that may be associated with pain (see Chapter 4) cause significant problems for many people (Bailey et al 2010). For example, Jeremy may find that he is more anxious about using a ladder since his fall and may be avoiding using one on the construction site when he can. Alice may be anxious and avoidant of health professionals because she was met with so much scepticism about whether her pain was real. Alice avoids health professionals who may be recommended to her because she is anxious about being disbelieved. The pain and avoidance model is often used to highlight the differences between activity that may cause pain but will not cause harm. The model provides a framework for later strategies used to encourage activity and successful coping, and overcome debilitating patterns of thinking.

Many people who have chronic pain alternate between long periods of very little exercise and infrequent bouts of intense exercise when they recognize that they are out of shape due to prolonged inactivity. The dangers of a cycle of chronic deconditioning interspersed with intense attempts to overcome it are included in the general education about pain. The need for activity is balanced with the need to pace oneself, so as not to cause severe pain that then triggers more disability and exacerbates avoidance.

Patients are do not have sufficient understanding of the medications that they take. Both over-the-counter drugs such as acetaminophen and ibuprofen (Forward et al 1996) and prescription drugs (Banta-Green et al 2010) can be misused by underuse, overuse or failure to use the right schedule for taking the medications. Many patients have misinformation about drugs and addiction that have been fuelled by the media. As a result, knowledge of pain medications and how to use them is often a component of patient education. Sometimes, procedures and surgical approaches may also be discussed.

Patient education may include an introduction to non-medical approaches to pain management, including psychological interventions, which are discussed in this chapter, and complementary and alternative medical approaches. Patient education is often conducted early in treatment but may also be interspersed with teaching of specific skills. Patient education corrects misinformation and provides a basis for later therapeutic interventions.

Sources of more information

- Butler & Moseley (2003)
- McGrath et al (2003)
- McGrath et al (1992)

OPERANT CONDITIONING APPROACHES

Description

Operant conditioning approaches are firmly based on the operant approach developed by Skinner (1938) and elaborated over the last 50 years by others. Their use in chronic pain was popularized by Fordyce in his very well known classic work at the University of Washington (Fordyce 1976). At its simplest, pain expression is conceptualized as a behaviour much like any other behaviour, and behaviours are controlled by the antecedents and consequences of the behaviour. Functional behavioural analysis is required to pinpoint what is controlling the behaviour in each individual. Pain behaviours may include facial responses such as grimacing or avoidance behaviours such as staying in bed instead of getting up and going for a walk.

A functional analysis of pain is based on an analysis of antecedents, behaviours and consequences (ABC analysis) utilizing self-report and observation of what happened before the incident or exacerbation of pain, the antecedent (Sanders 2002). The consequences, or what happened after the incident or exacerbation of pain, would also be determined. For example, a grimace or groan might be preceded by a request to do something and followed by the withdrawal of the request. Several different patterns might be shown from a careful functional analysis. Hypotheses about functional relationships between pain, antecedents and consequences would be generated and then tested before any intervention could occur.

Operant methods include positive reinforcement, negative reinforcement, punishment, extinction and differential reinforcement. Reinforcement increases behaviour. Positive reinforcement occurs when a behaviour is followed by a pleasant or positive event. Attention to complaints is frequent positive reinforcement that increases pain behaviour. For example, if a parent pays attention to every ache and pain that a child reports and the child increases his or her report of pain, attention would be considered a positive reinforcement. Negative reinforcement involves the removal of something that increases the behaviour that is reinforced. For example, Mark, Alice's husband, might complain about Alice's pain, until Alice does household chores that have been bothering Mark. In this case, the Mark is negatively reinforcing Alice for doing chores.

Extinction is the withdrawal of reinforcement for a behaviour. Attempts at extinction are usually accompanied by an initial increase in the behaviour. For example, if Jeremy has been reinforced for being unable to do things because of pain by Susan's (his partner) attention, and this reinforcement (attention) is withdrawn, Jeremy will likely become more disabled before being able to do more independently. Extinction should usually be accompanied by differential reinforcement of other, alternative, appropriate behaviour.

Punishment is an unpleasant or negative event that follows a behaviour. A supervisor who docked pay for a worker who was impaired in job functions because of pain would be attempting punishment. Operant practitioners rarely use punishment or negative reinforcement as a treatment of pain because these negative techniques lead to withdrawal, avoidance of the punisher or aggressive responses. For example, the relationship between Alice and Mark, who is complaining about household chores, will probably deteriorate; Alice will likely avoid Mark and may start complaining about Mark's shortcomings.

Operant practitioners believe that operant methods are effective because of operant conditioning, the strengthening of patterns of behaviour because of their effects. This is described as the law of effect. Behaviours followed by positive events increase and behaviours consequated with negative events decrease.

Operant procedures seem so simple: reinforce the good, punish the bad. Nevertheless, operant strategies require careful analysis of the individual case. One event may be reinforcing for one person, but punishing for another. Moreover, complex learning histories may have developed with specific settings acting as cues for different behaviours. In addition, operant techniques such as extinction of pain complaints, if not done skilfully, can lead to unwanted results such as engendering feelings of resentment. As a result, skilled use of operant techniques is not simple.

Operant techniques are sometimes used in combination with other interventions. For example, Allen & Shriver (1997) showed that operant techniques implemented by parents significantly improved the results obtained from biofeedback treatment of headache in children.

Sources of more information

- Dahlquist (1999)
- Fordyce (1984)

COGNITIVE–BEHAVIOURAL THERAPY

Description

Cognitive–behavioural therapy (CBT) is the dominant evidence-based approach used in clinical psychology (Morley et al 1999). CBT focuses on interaction between thoughts, feelings and behaviours. Because of its broad nature, it is difficult to say which therapeutic strategies are included or omitted in CBT. It may include operant techniques and the use of relaxation or biofeedback.

The hallmark of CBT is the attempt to directly alter thoughts or cognitions. Keefe (1996) outlined a three-stage process. The first stage is patient education focused on the role that thoughts and behaviours play in pain, emphasizing that patients can have a major impact on their pain. The second stage is coping skills training. The various skills can include relaxation and cue-controlled relaxation, distraction, activity pacing, introduction of pleasant activities and cognitive restructuring. The third stage is the application of the techniques learned to the real world and the maintenance of these strategies over time. Application to the real-world environment usually involves problem solving, self-monitoring and behavioural contracting and scheduling. Maintenance is may include booster sessions. Marlatt & George (1984) provided a model for maintenance called relapse prevention. The essence of this model is to anticipate the immediate and long-term antecedents to relapse and to programme for them. Although originally developed for treatment of alcoholism, relapse prevention can also be applied to pain management to maintain learned strategies.

CBT was originally developed to treat depression and anxiety by clinician researchers such as Aaron Beck (e.g. Beck 1997) and Albert Ellis (e.g. Ellis 1998). These methods have been adapted for pain and become widespread in the treatment of chronic pain. Fundamental to CBT is the tenet that events may trigger thoughts, beliefs and evaluations that, depending on one's proclivity, may be negative and destructive or more neutral and problem solving. For example, if Jeremy wakes up with a headache in addition to his chronic low back pain, he might interpret this event as: 'Oh no, now I have headaches as well. Nothing ever goes right for me. I can't have more pain. I can't cope with this.' Or perhaps Jeremy may say, 'I am always going to be unhappy. Everything I do ends up awful. What have I done to make such a mess of everything?' This pattern of thinking becomes a spiral of negative thinking that aggravates pain and interferes with coping.

Several different approaches have been explicated to interrupt negative thinking. One of the first methods and one that is still widely used is by Albert Ellis. He popularized rational emotive therapy, now known as rational emotive behaviour therapy (http://www.rebt.org/). Ellis developed a system to recognize and dispute irrational beliefs. Ellis' ABCD method consists of recognizing that **activating events** are interpreted by people's **beliefs**, resulting in **consequences**, or ABC. **Disputing** of the beliefs as fallacious breaks the linkage between behaviour and irrational beliefs.

According to rational emotive behaviour therapy, the irrational beliefs or dysfunctional attitudes that cause people the most difficulty have two major qualities. The first is that under the surface they have powerful demands often expressed as 'must', 'should' or 'ought to'. Second, these irrational beliefs have derivatives that imply an extreme outcome. Jeremy's irrational belief might be 'People who have chronic pain cannot lead a productive life' and 'Because I have a headache today, I will always be having headaches.' The derivative from these irrational beliefs might be 'There is nothing I can do' or 'My life is miserable and without any positive aspects' or 'I am a victim of events I cannot control.'

Disputing the false beliefs and their derivatives might take the form of 'Just because I have a headache now, doesn't mean it will last forever. What can I do to help the headache?' Or Jeremy might say, 'In spite of my pain, I am doing well with my job and my friends. I have a loving family who support me.' Another alternative is, 'Having a headache is not the end of the world, I have managed headaches well in the past.' These modes of thinking would lead to more rational approaches such as problem solving to ensure that the headache does not interfere with Jeremy's life.

The tendency to assume the worst in pain situations has been aptly termed pain catastrophizing. Sullivan et al (1995) developed the Pain Catastrophizing Scale and extensively investigated the role of catastrophic thinking in pain. Catastrophic thinking in relation to pain tends to be ruminative, e.g. I keep thinking about how much it hurts, involve magnification of the impact, e.g. I wonder whether something serious may happen, and portrays the sufferer as helpless, e.g. there is nothing I can do to reduce the intensity of the pain. Pain catastrophizing is related to levels of chronic pain, disability from pain and failure to recover. Higher levels of pain catastrophizing have also been linked to difficulty in using distraction effectively.

Somewhat different approaches have been used by other cognitive–behavioural therapists. Don Meichenbaum (1977) emphasized the role of anticipation of difficult situations, monitoring inner speech and self–instruction, and developing new styles of inner speech in reaction to pain and other situations. Turk et al's text (1983) provides detailed descriptions of CBT applied to pain. Cognitive strategies are generally combined into treatment packages with behavioural techniques such as operant or classical conditioning, distraction and relaxation. Other related strategies such as problem solving, sleep hygiene and communication or assertiveness training are often included in CBT programmes for chronic pain.

Theoretical rationale

The theoretical rationale for CBT lies in the nexus among thoughts, feelings and behaviour. CBT therapists believe that changing thoughts in a deliberate and planned way will change feelings and behaviour. Trying to change behaviour alone without examination of thoughts and feelings is likely to maintain behaviour change only in the context of external factors. To change behaviour over the long term from an internal perspective, one must examine the thoughts and feelings that drive behaviour in combination with external reinforcers.

Sources of more information

- Ellis (1994) – this is an updated edition of Albert Ellis's classic text
- Turk et al (1983) – this classic text is still well worth reading

DISTRACTION

Description

Distraction has been widely studied in acute pain, especially in procedure pain. A recent Cochrane Review (Uman et al 2009) has shown that distraction is quite effective in reducing pain from needle procedures.

The evidence for effectiveness of distraction in long-term pain comes mostly from correlation studies. People who report more ability to distract themselves have better outcome in their chronic pain. The exact nature of the relationship has been hard to document (Roelofs et al 2006). Most interventions promoting distraction in chronic pain are part of comprehensive interventions, thus hindering the capacity to demonstrate the long-term effects of distraction in chronic pain. Chronic pain decreases the ability to focus attention (Dick & Rashiq 2007). Thus, it is not entirely clear if the failure to distract oneself is the cause of persistent pain or the result of chronic pain. The likelihood is that both processes are active.

There is some evidence that active distraction that engages a person's attention is more effective than less engaging distraction. For example, virtual reality strategies that draw attention into a virtual world and provide opportunities to interact with action in it have been effective in reducing pain due to burn procedures (Hoffman et al 2008). Active distraction involves the person doing something engaging rather than passively participating in a distraction.

Alice always enjoyed painting but gave it up when her children were young. She has recently started painting again. Although her pain is much the same, she has noticed that while she is painting she is absorbed in the work and when she has finished doing some part of the painting she feels happier, although her fibromyalgia is still present.

Theoretical rationale

Distraction is thought to operate because distraction occupies attention, thus diverting attention from pain and decreasing the perception of pain partially or even completely (Eccleston & Crombez 1999). Pain patients can become hypervigilant to noxious stimuli and distraction may reduce this hypervigilance (Sharpe et al 2010).

Sources of more information

- Eccleston & Crombez (1999)
- Fernandez & Turk (1989)

CLASSICAL CONDITIONING APPROACHES

Description

The classical conditioning paradigm, first described by Ivan Pavlov (1927), can also be applied to explain the aetiology of chronic pain and to change chronic pain behaviours. Pavlov's dogs, after some training, learned to salivate (conditioned response) to the ringing of a bell, since the bell (conditioned stimulus) was previously paired with a dish of food (unconditioned stimulus). The same mechanism can be involved in the acquisition of chronic pain behaviours. For example, Alice has fibromyalgia. Alice may have tried, during periods of decreased pain, to do household chores (e.g. ironing, cleaning), which triggered worse pain (unconditioned response). Over time, through this continued association and the process of generalization to the stimulus, certain physical movements, physical activity and circumstances surrounding physical activity (conditioned stimulus) have elicited a similar response to the unconditioned response for Alice. Muscular tension as a result of the anticipatory fear of pain and anxiety becomes associated with the activity followed by more pain. As a consequence, Alice may have progressively decreased her activity levels and mobility, and increased her levels of pain.

There are two behavioural techniques, systematic desensitization and therapeutic graded exposure, which are used most frequently to treat chronic pain behaviours based on the classical conditioning paradigm. We will apply each of these to Alice's pain problem.

Systematic desensitization (SD) is a classical conditioning procedure that reverses classical conditioning (associative learning) by pairing the conditioned object or situation with either pleasant or neutral events. This technique was originally developed by Wolpe for anxiety (Wolpe 1958). It is used for chronic pain patients who have high levels of fear. This approach uses a stimulus hierarchy. Graded sequences of approximations to the conditioned stimulus (the feared event) are used to gradually introduce the person to the conditioned stimulus moving through the sequence from the least fearful to the most fearful situations. The procedure consists of three steps:

Step 1 Relaxation training: Alice is first taught relaxation, using any type of relaxation technique (e.g. progressive muscle relaxation, relaxation without tension).
Step 2 Hierarchy construction: Alice constructs a list of the least fearful to most fearful situations of the conditioned stimulus (approximately 10–15).
Step 3 Applying the technique: Alice practises relaxing, with each situation in the hierarchy sequence confronted sequentially. The aim for Alice is to overcome the fear

behaviours that occur when she confronts a stimulus that provokes anxiety or fear. Alice applies the relaxation technique with each situation to once again become calm. Once relaxation is reached, the next fearful situation in the hierarchy is introduced.

Therapeutic graded exposure is similar to systematic desensitization in that Alice is gradually introduced to the conditioned stimulus (the situation that Alice fears and avoids). The procedure is different from systematic desensitization in that Alice is exposed to the situation in real life without learning relaxation. Again, a hierarchy of situations is created by Alice that increases in difficulty with each activity (without going beyond what most people can do on a daily basis). Gradually, Alice is brought into physical contact with each feared activity on the hierarchy to learn that expected and feared dangerous consequences will not occur. Exposure to various activities (e.g. lifting, bending, performing a movement, etc.) is effective in reducing fear and avoidance associated with beliefs that activity will trigger pain (Boersma et al 2004; Woods & Asmundson 2008). Exposure will also increase daily function through the reduced association of fear and anxiety with pain.

These techniques are usually integrated as components into behavioural or CBT treatment programmes. In part due to this, the effect of some these techniques by themselves has rarely been explored.

Theoretical rationale

Systematic desensitization and therapeutic graded exposure are thought to operate by the uncoupling of a specific conditioned stimulus with fear or anxiety by deliberate coupling of the conditioned stimulus with relaxation (systematic desensitizations) or through graded exposure.

Sources of more information

- Bailey et al (2010)
- Vlaeyen et al (2002)

SOCIAL SUPPORT METHODS

Description

Social support has been offered in group-based (Sancisi et al 2009) or electronic formats (Poloman et al 2007) for individuals with chronic or recurrent pain. Although the form of social support may vary, the underlying goal is to increase an individual's adaptive coping with pain by providing an outlet for emotional expression, peer modelling and reinforcement of successful coping efforts. Social support has been an area of interest in other health conditions, especially in cancer (Nausheen et al 2009).

Support groups may be led by participants or co-led with a health professional. They often have a less formal structure than other group-based psychological interventions (e.g. group-based CBT). This flexible approach can empower participants, but it can be problematic if participants focus only on negative aspects of their functioning or on maladaptive coping strategies. To avoid these potential pitfalls, some groups aim for participants to share both negative and positive experiences (Subramaniam et al 1999). Positive experiences that are given attention and acknowledged by other participants in the group are reinforced and remembered as success experience.

While support groups and social networking may be primary sources of support, more structured interventions such as group-based CBT often also provide individuals with opportunities for social support. Group-based CBT interventions are as effective as individual interventions, and the group setting may lead to quicker improvement (Turner-Stokes et al 2003).

Theoretical rationale

Social support may be protective against the negative effect associated with stressful life experiences such as chronic pain. In particular, strong social support may buffer the negative effects associated with catastrophizing and bolster coping that has more positive outcomes. There is some evidence that spousal support, for example, decreases the negative effects of catastrophizing (Holtzman & Delongis 2007).

Sources of more information

- Holtzman et al (2004)
- Holtzman & Delongis (2007)

RELAXATION METHODS

Several different approaches to relaxation have been developed, including tension–relaxation, suggestion and breathing approaches. Combinations and variations on these strategies are often used. Tension–relaxation methods were developed by Edmund Jacobsen in the 1920s and 1930s. His progressive relaxation method was employed to treat a wide variety of disorders. Luthe & Schultz (1969) developed autogenic training focusing on suggestion and body positioning. Benson (1975) popularized breathing techniques as a method of relaxation training.

Description

The evidence for the effectiveness of relaxation methods has been well established in the headache literature (Buse & Andrasik 2009) and has been generalized to chronic pain. There are several methods of relaxation and none have been shown to be more effective than others.

Tension–relaxation methods (Jacobson 1938) have been simplified since the time of Jacobsen. Bernstein & Borkovec's (1973) manual was devoted to this approach. Typically, the patient sits in a comfortable chair or lies down. Fifteen or 20 muscle groups are sequentially tensed for 5–15 seconds and then relaxed. The tension phase serves as a contrast to the relaxation and there is also a rebound effect inducing relaxation. The instruction to relax is often accompanied by suggestions or images of calmness and relaxation. Different muscle groups are used.

Suggestion methods were developed by Johannes Schulz in the 1930s and called autogenic training or autogenic therapy (Luthe & Schultz 1969). The method uses self-suggestions of heaviness, warmth and relaxation for different body parts, e.g. legs, arms and hands, accompanied by deep slow breathing. Many variations are used.

The breathing methods of relaxation were borrowed from Eastern practices but made popular by Benson (Benson 1975). Benson emphasizes focusing attention and deep slow breathing.

These methods have much in common. They involve self-statements to focus attention on calming the body. Most involve deep and slow breathing. Many variations have been developed. The initial investment in learning to relax has been modified from the early practitioners who considered 30 or more sessions the norm. Currently, a course of relaxation training is usually about 8–10 weekly training sessions, with daily practice of 30 minutes or so by the patient on their own. Relaxation may be taught individually or in groups. Daily practice of full relaxation may be augmented with mini relaxation sessions interspersed throughout the day. Sometimes audiotapes are used to help with daily practice. Once learned, a maintenance programme is often sufficient for many patients.

Patients may find that a combination of relaxation methods may help for pain in different situations. For example, Alice may use a short relaxation of five deep 'belly breaths' before she goes to meet with a health professional to help calm herself and prepare. She may use tension and relaxation of different muscle groups at bedtime to help her fall asleep.

Theoretical rationale

Although theories vary, relaxation may have its effect by:

- reducing muscle tension and subsequent ischaemic pain
- changing brain chemistry, especially serotonin, and thus altering pain perception
- altering sense of control and self-efficacy
- modulating autonomic arousal, thus dampening response to stress
- distracting from pain.

Sources of more information

- Benson (1975)
- Bernstein & Borkovec (1973)
- Luthe & Schultz (1969)

ACCEPTANCE AND COMMITMENT THERAPY

Description

Acceptance and commitment therapy (ACT) is a relatively recent approach that was developed by Hayes et al during the 1990s (Hayes et al 1999) and has been applied to chronic pain (see also Chapter 4). The originators of these methods and some other theorists and clinicians believe ACT to be significantly different from CBT but others argue that they are similar in drawing on the cognitions and emotions that are the underpinning of behaviour (see discussion in Hofmann & Asmundson 2008).

The goal of ACT is to help Jeremy or Alice to accept their pain and other associated issues such as fatigue or fear or anxiety of pain as they are – sensations and thoughts. To illustrate, Jeremy would be taught to view the pain and associated personal, internal experiences without judgment as they are very difficult to control or reduce. ACT helps Jeremy to commit to actions that are guided by his personal values in an attempt to improve and enrich his life despite his pain.

The following components of ACT (Hayes et al 2006) would be used with Jeremy during treatment:

1. *Confronting the system*: Jeremy is encouraged to first think about the strategies that he has used in the past to try to reduce his pain and then examine whether these strategies have worked. Jeremy is facing situations where attempts to reduce and control his pain have failed.
2. *Acceptance*: Jeremy is encouraged to stop trying to control the pain.
3. *Cognitive de-fusion*: Jeremy is taught that thoughts are just thoughts and they do not need to be believed nor need to be a reason to move away from actions that are personally meaningful.
4. *Present focus (mindfulness)*: Jeremy is taught to increase awareness as best as he can of his thoughts, feelings, sensations and any other private events as they occur, and see them as they are, without any judgment.
5. *Self-as context*: Jeremy is taught to be aware of and observe his own thoughts from the perspective of a constant observer.
6. *Values-based process*: Jeremy is encouraged to choose his life values in different domains (i.e. social life, work

131

life) and set concrete realistic goals in accordance to these values.

7. *Committed action*: Jeremy is encouraged to take actions linked to his chosen values.

Recent studies on ACT show that ACT is effective in treating chronic pain patients in both adult and child populations (Johnston et al 2010; Vowles & McCracken 2008; Wicksell et al 2007, 2008). However, there is not enough research to conclude that ACT is superior to other active treatments.

Sources of more information

- Dahl & Lundgren (2006)
- Dahl et al (2005)
- McCracken (2005)

HYPNOSIS

Hypnosis has a long history in the treatment of pain. It has been commonly used in the management of acute pain, especially in children (Liossi & Hatira 1999), but has also been used in recurrent and chronic pain. In a recent review of 19 controlled trials of hypnosis, Jensen & Patterson (2006) found that interventions using hypnotic suggestion were significantly more effective than no treatment in reducing pain. There is limited additional evidence that hypnosis may be superior to physical therapy or medication management in some chronic pain conditions (Hannen et al 1991). A meta-analysis review of hypnosis for acute pain in adults is in progress through the Cochrane Collaboration (Hallquist et al 2009).

Description

Definitions of hypnosis vary, but central to the technique is the use of suggestion to modify subjective experiences.

There are generally three stages in the use of hypnosis: induction, suggestion and awakening. The first stage is termed 'induction' and is the phase in which the individual transitions from the typical awake state to an altered level of consciousness or trance state. Methods of induction vary widely, with many including some form of counting (downwards from 10) or visualization (being in an elevator going down). Physical positions can also be used for induction (fingers crossed and resisting index fingers from touching). In children, storytelling is often used as an induction technique (Kuttner 1988). Once a trance is induced, the second phase of hypnosis involves using language to suggest desired altered experiences. Suggestions for pain management may include phrases such as 'you might be surprised at how comfortable you can be' or 'notice how

your sensations change, maybe becoming less intense or less bothersome'. Several suggestions are generally used in one hypnosis session. In the final stage of hypnosis, the individual is brought back to the awake and alert state of consciousness in a gradual and self-regulated way. Counting or visualizing (in the opposite direction from induction) are typically used.

Despite what is portrayed in popular media, hypnosis is generally self-directed and requires openness to the strategy on the part of the individual using the strategy. Individuals cannot be 'hypnotized' (for therapeutic purposes) to engage in a behaviour that they are not willing to do. Hypnosis is not effective for all individuals and suggestibility appears to be related to treatment effect (Milling et al 2006).

Theoretical rationale

There are two major theoretical approaches to hypnosis. One approach suggests that hypnosis is an altered state of consciousness (Hilgard 1971) whereas the second sees hypnosis as a combination of focused attention and suggestion (e.g. Spanos 1996). Recent neuroimaging studies have supported the effect of hypnosis on pain.

Sources of more information

- Syrjala & Abrams (2002)

BIOFEEDBACK

Biofeedback involves the acquisition of a physiological measurement signal, display of that signal to the patient and learning how to modify the physiological response being monitored. For example, electrical potentials from muscles that vary with tension in a muscle group can be monitored from surface electrodes. The electromyographic (EMG) signal can be transformed into a sound whose pitch varies with the tension in the muscle. A patient can try different ways to change the pitch of the signal and learn to lower their muscle tension in the muscles being monitored.

Description

EMG for tension headache and finger temperature biofeedback have been most frequently used and validated as effective treatments (references) for tension and migraine headache, respectively. Other signals that have been used in biofeedback include skin temperature, brain waves or electroencephalograph (EEG), heart rate, sweating (galvanic skin response, GSR) and pulse volume. Because of advances in technology, biofeedback equipment has become simpler and more available.

Theoretical rationale

The most straightforward rationale for biofeedback is that the patient learns to control physiological responses that subserve pain. However, this is very difficult to understand when one takes the example of some forms of biofeedback, such as finger temperature biofeedback, as cool hands do not cause migraine headache. Some assert that the major impact of biofeedback is a general relaxation response or an increase in perceived self-efficacy.

Sources of more information

- Schwartz & Andrasik (2003)

CONCLUSION

There has been extensive evaluation of psychological methods in chronic pain, but often there is limited description of these methods. In this chapter, we provide a description and recommend references to obtain more detailed information. Although we provide descriptions and rationales on each treatment strategy separately, these strategies are commonly used in combination with each other and with other related strategies (e.g. activity pacing, medication management). For Jeremy and Alice, there would be options to determine which of these strategies might fit best with the type of pain they are experiencing and their specific needs.

REFERENCES

Allen, K.D., Shriver, M.D., 1997. Enhanced performance feedback to strengthen biofeedback treatment outcome with childhood migraine. Headache 37, 169–173.

Bailey, K., Carleton, N., Vlaeyen, J.W.S., et al., 2010. Treatments addressing pain-related fear and anxiety in patients with chronic musculoskeletal pain: a preliminary review. Cognitive Behavior Therapy 39, 46–63.

Banta-Green, C.J., Von Korff, M., Sullivan, M.D., et al., 2010. The Prescribed Opioids Difficulties Scale: a patient-centered assessment of problems and concerns. Clin. J. Pain 26, 489–497.

Barsky, A.J., Ahern, D.K., Orav, E.J., et al., 2010. A randomized trial of three psychosocial treatments for the symptoms of rheumatoid arthritis. Seminars in Arthritis Rheumatism 40, 222–232.

Beck, A., 1997. The past and the future of cognitive therapy. J. Psychother. Pract. Res. 6, 276–284.

Benson, H., 1975. The relaxation response. Morrow and Company, New York.

Bernstein, D.A., Borkovec, T.D., 1973. Progressive relaxation training: a manual for the helping profession. Research Press, Champaign, IL.

Boersma, K., Linton, S., Overmeer, T., et al., 2004. Lowering fear-avoidance and enhancing function through exposure in vivo: a multiple baseline study across six patients with back pain. Pain 108, 8–16.

Buse, D.C., Andrasik, F., 2009. Behavioral medicine for migraine. Neurol. Clin. 27, 445–465.

Butler, D., Moseley, L., 2003. Explain Pain. Noigroup Publications, Adelaide.

Dahl, J.C., Lundgren, T.L., 2006. Living beyond your pain: using acceptance and commitment therapy to ease chronic pain. New Harbinger, Oakland, CA.

Dahl, J., Wilson, K.G., Luciano, C., et al., 2005. Acceptance and commitment therapy for chronic pain. Context Press, Reno, NV.

Dahlquist, L.M., 1999. Pediatric Pain Management. Plenum Publishers, New York.

Dick, B.D., Rashiq, S., 2007. Disruption of attention and working memory traces in individuals with chronic pain. Anesth. Analg. 104, 1223–1229.

Eccleston, C., Crombez, G., 1999. Pain demands attention: a cognitive-affective model of the interruptive function of pain. Psychol. Bull. 125, 356–366.

Eccleston, C., Williams, A.C., Morley, S., 2009. Psychological therapies for the management of chronic pain (excluding headache) in adults. Cochrane Database Syst. Rev. 15 (2), CD007407.

Ellis, A., 1994. Reason and emotion in psychotherapy: comprehensive method of treating human disturbances; revised and updated. Citadel Press, New York.

Ellis, A., 1998. How to control your anxiety before it controls you. Kensington Publishing Group, New York.

Fernandez, E., Turk, D.C., 1989. The utility of cognitive coping strategies for altering pain perception: a meta-analysis. Pain 38, 123–135.

Fordyce, W.E., 1976. Behavioral methods in chronic pain and illness. Mosby, St Louis.

Fordyce, W., 1984. Behavioral science and chronic pain. Postgrad. Med. J. 60, 865–868.

Forward, S.P., Brown, T.L., McGrath, P.J., 1996. Mothers' attitudes and behavior toward medicating children's pain. Pain 69, 469–474.

Hallquist, M.N., Jensen, M.P., Patterson, D.R., et al., 2009. Clinical hypnosis for acute pain in adults (Protocol). Cochrane Database Syst. Rev. 3, CD006599. http://dx.doi.org/10.1002/14651858.CD006599.

Hannen, H.C., Hoenderos, H.T., van Romunde, L.K., et al., 1991. Controlled trial of hypnotherapy in the treatment of refractory fibromyalgia. J. Rheumatol. 18, 72–75.

Hayes, S.C., Strosahl, K.D., Wilson, K.G., 1999. Acceptance and commitment therapy: an experiential approach to behavior change. Guilford Press, New York.

Hayes, S.C., Luoma, J.B., Bond, F.W., et al., 2006. Acceptance and commitment therapy: model, processes and outcomes. Behav. Res. Ther. 44, 1–25.

Hilgard, E., 1971. Hypnotic phenomena: the struggle for scientific acceptance. Am. Sci. 59, 567–577.

Hoffman, H.G., Patterson, D.R., Seibel, E., et al., 2008. Virtual reality pain control during burn would debridement in the hydrotank. Clin. J. Pain 24, 299–304.

Hofmann, S.G., Asmundson, G.J., 2008. Acceptance and mindfulness-based therapy: new wave or old hat? Clin. Psychol. Rev. 28, 1–16.

Holtzman, S., Delongis, A., 2007. One day at a time: the impact of daily satisfaction with spouse response on pain, negative affect and catastrophizing among individuals with rheumatoid arthritis. Pain 131, 202–213.

Holtzman, S., Newth, S., Delongis, A., 2004. The role of social support in coping with daily pain among patients with rheumatoid arthritis. J. Health Psychol. 9, 677–695.

Jacobson, E., 1938. Progressive relaxation. University of Chicago Press, Chicago.

Jensen, M., Patterson, D.R., 2006. Hypnotic treatment of chronic pain. J. Behav. Med. 29, 95–124.

Johnston, M., Foster, M., Shennan, J., et al., 2010. The effectiveness of an acceptance and commitment therapy self-help intervention for chronic pain. Clin. J. Pain 26, 393–402.

Keefe, F.J., 1996. Cognitive behavioral therapy for managing pain. Clin. Psychol. 49, 4–5.

Kuttner, L., 1988. Favorite stories: a hypnotic pain-reduction technique for children in acute pain. Am. J. Clin. Hypn. 30, 289–295.

Liossi, C., Hatira, P., 1999. Clinical hypnosis versus cognitive behavioral training for pain management with paediatric cancer patients undergoing bone marrow aspirations. Int. J. Clin. Exp. Hypn. 47, 104–116.

Luthe, W., Schultz, J.H., 1969. Autogenic Therapy. Grune and Stratton, Inc, New York.

Marlatt, G.A., George, W.H., 1984. Relapse prevention: introduction and overview of the model. Br. J. Addict. 79, 261–273.

McCracken, L.M., 2005. Contextual cognitive-behavioral therapy for chronic pain. International Association for the Study of Pain, Seattle.

McGrath, P.J., Finley, G.A., Turner, C.J., 1992. Making Cancer Less Painful. http://pediatric-pain.ca/content/Families.

McGrath, P.J., Finley, G.A., Ritchie, J., et al., 2003. Pain Pain Go Away, second ed. http://pediatric-pain.ca/content/Families.

Meichenbaum, D., 1977. Cognitive behavior modification: an integrative approach. Plenum Press, New York.

Melzack, R., Wall, P.D., 1965. Pain mechanisms: a new theory. Science 19, 971–979.

Milling, L.S., Reardon, J.M., Carosella, G.M., 2006. Mediation and moderation of psychological pain treatments: response expectancies and hypnotic suggestibility. J. Consult. Clin. Psychol. 74, 253–262.

Morley, S., Eccleston, C., Williams, A., 1999. Systematic review and meta-analysis of randomized controlled trials of cognitive-behavior therapy and behavior therapy for chronic pain in adults, excluding headache. Pain 80, 1–13.

Murray, G., 2009. Referred pain, allodynia and hyperalgesia. J. Am. Dent. Assoc. 140, 1122–1124.

Nausheen, B., Gidron, Y., Peveler, R., et al., 2009. Social support and cancer progression: a systematic review. J. Psychosom. Res. 67, 403–415.

Palermo, T.M., Eccleston, C., Lewandowski, A.S., et al., 2010. Randomized controlled trials of psychological therapies for management of chronic pain in children and adolescents: an updated meta-analytic review. Pain 148, 387–397.

Pavlov, I.P., 1927. Conditioned reflexes: an investigation of the physiological activity of the cerebral cortex. translated and edited by Anrep G V. Oxford University Press, London.

Poloman, R.C., Droog, N., Purinton, M., et al., 2007. Social support web-based resources for patients with chronic pain. Journal of Pain and Palliative Care Pharmacotherapy 21, 49–55.

Roelofs, J., Peters, M.L., Patijn, J., et al., 2006. An electronic diary assessment of the effects of distraction and attentional focusing on pain intensity in chronic low back pain patients. Br. J. Health Psychol. 11, 595–606.

Sancisi, E., Rausa, M., Zanigni, S., et al., 2009. Self-help group and medication overuse headache: preliminary data. Neurol. Sci. 30, 459–463.

Sanders, S.H., 2002. Operant conditioning of chronic pain: back to basics. In: Turk, D.C., Gatchel, R.J. (Eds.), Psychological approaches to pain management, second ed. Guilford Press, New York, pp. 128–137.

Schwartz, M.S., Andrasik, F. (Eds.), 2003. Biofeedback: a practioner's guide. third ed. Guilford Press, New York.

Sharpe, L., Nicholson Perry, K., Rogers, P., et al., 2010. A comparison of the effect of attention training and relaxation on responses to pain. Pain 150, 469–476.

Skinner, B.F., 1938. The behavior of organisms: an experimental analysis. Appleton-Century, Oxford.

Spanos, N.P., 1996. Multiple identities & false memories: a sociocognitive perspective. American Psychological Association, Washington, DC.

Subramaniam, V., Stewart, M.W., Smith, J.F., 1999. The development and impact of a chronic pain support group: a qualitative and quantitative study. J. Pain Symptom Manage. 17, 376–383.

Sullivan, M.J.L., Bishop, S.R., Pivikm, J., 1995. The Pain Catastrophizing Scale: Development and Validation. Psychol. Assess. 7, 524–532.

Syrjala, K.L., Abrams, J.R., 2002. Hypnosis and imagery in the treatment of pain. In: Turk, D., Gatchel, R.J. (Eds.), Psychological Approaches to Pain Management: A Practitioner's Handbook, second ed. Guilford Press, New York, pp. 187–209.

Turk, D.C., Meichenbaum, D., Genest, M., 1983. Pain and behavioral medicine: a cognitive-behavioral perspective. Guilford Press, New York.

Turner-Stokes, L., Erkeller-Yuksel, F., Miles, A., et al., 2003. Outpatient cognitive behavioral pain management programs: a randomized comparison of a group-based multidisciplinary versus an individual therapy model. Arch. Phys. Med. Rehabil. 84, 781–788.

Udermann, B.E., Spratt, K.F., Donelson, R.G., et al., 2004. Can a patient educational book change behavior and reduce pain in chronic low back pain patients? Spine 4, 425–435.

Uman, L.S., Chambers, C.T., McGrath, P.J., et al., 2009. Psychological interventions for needle-related procedural pain and distress in children and adolescents. http://dx.doi.org/10.1002/14651858. CD005179.pub2.

Vlaeyen, J.W.S., de Jong, J., Sieben, J., et al., 2002. Graded Exposure in vivo for pain-related fear. In: Turk, D.C., Gatchel, R.J. (Eds.), Psychological Approaches to Pain Management: A Practitioner's Handbook, second ed. Guilford Press, New York, pp. 210–233.

Vowles, K.E., McCracken, L.M., 2008. Acceptance and values-based action in chronic pain: a study of treatment effectiveness and process. J. Consult. Clin. Psychol. 76, 397–407.

Wicksell, R.K., Melin, L., Olsson, G.L., 2007. Exposure and acceptance in the rehabilitation of adolescents with idiopathic chronic pain – a pilot study. Eur. J. Pain 11, 267–274.

Wicksell, R.K., Ahlqvist, J., Bring, A., et al., 2008. Can exposure and acceptance strategies improve functioning and life satisfaction in people with chronic pain and whiplash-associated disorders (WAD)? A randomized controlled trial. Cogn. Behav. Ther. 37, 169–182.

Wilkins, K.L., McGrath, P.J., Finley, G.A., et al., 1998. Phantom limb sensations and phantom limb pain in child and adolescent amputees. Pain 78, 7–12.

Wolpe, J., 1958. Psychotherapy through Reciprocal Inhibition. Stanford University Press, Palo Alto, CA.

Wolpe, J., 1985. Psychotherapy by reciprocal inhibition. Stanford University Press, Stanford.

Woods, M.P., Asmundson, G.J.G., 2008. Evaluating the efficacy of graded in vivo exposure for the treatment of fear in patients with chronic back pain: a randomized controlled clinical trial. Pain 136, 271–280.

Woolf, C.J., 2007. Central sensitization: uncovering the relation between pain and plasticity. Anesthesiology 106, 864–867.

Chapter 10

Neuropathic pain and complex regional pain syndrome

Nicola U. Cook and Hubert van Griensven

CHAPTER CONTENTS

LEARNING OBJECTIVES

By the end of this chapter the reader should have an understanding of:

1. Pathophysiological mechanisms underlying neuropathic pain and complex regional pain syndrome.
2. Symptoms that alert the clinician to the possible presence of these conditions.
3. Current diagnostic criteria and their limitations.
4. A methodical approach to examination and treatment, based on current international evidence and guidelines.

OVERVIEW

This chapter covers two types of pain which have confused and frustrated patients and clinicians alike. In neurogenic or neuropathic pain the confusion can be attributed to the tendency of this pain to present with symptoms which normally do not go together, such as sensitivity to one type of stimulation with insensitivity to another. Neurogenic or neuropathic pain can mimic other pain conditions, but frequently lacks any response to normal pain-relieving modalities. Complex regional pain syndrome (CRPS) is equally enigmatic in its often violent response to what seems to be a minor injury of a limb. It is called type 2 if it coincides with neuropathy and type 1 if it does not. CRPS often involves swelling and discolouration of the affected limb, and is always painful.

This chapter was written with particular attention to information that is relevant to the clinician. It first discusses neuropathic and neurogenic pain, starting with clinical characteristics, examination techniques and clinical reasoning. It ends with a review of therapeutic recommendations and practical advice. The second part of the chapter is devoted to CRPS. It discusses modern diagnostic criteria and their application in the examination and diagnosis of CRPS, followed by detailed recommendations for treatment and management.

Part 1: Neuropathic pain

INTRODUCTION

Neuropathic pain is defined by the International Association for the Study of Pain (IASP) as 'pain caused by a

© 2014 Elsevier Ltd.

Box 10.1 Conditions possibly associated with neuropathy (based on Hansson et al 2002; Ross 2004)

Central

Stroke

Multiple sclerosis

Spinal cord injury

Syringomyelia or syringobulbia

Epilepsy

Space-occupying lesions

Peripheral

Mononeuropathies

Trauma, including surgery

Nerve entrapment (see Table 10.1)

Post-herpetic neuralgia

Trigeminal and glossopharyngeal neuralgia

Ischaemia

Inflammation or infection

Spinal nerve root pathology, e.g. as a result of a intervertebral disc lesion

Plexus injury, e.g. brachial plexus avulsion

Other plexopathy, e.g. following viral syndrome

Tumour

Nerve damage induced by radiation or chemotherapy

Polyneuropathies

Metabolic, e.g. diabetic

Toxic, e.g. misuse of alcohol or other drugs

Nutritional, e.g. vitamin B deficiency

Amyloidosis

Vasculitis

Note: Phantom pain is not included here because of its complex pain genesis.

lesion or disease of the somatosensory nervous system' (International Association for the Study of Pain, 2011). The IASP no longer lists the term *neurogenic pain*, although in practice the two terms are often used interchangeably.

Neuropathic pain can have its origin in either the central or peripheral nervous system and can have a number of causes (Box 10.1). The diagnosis of neuropathic pain is not straightforward because it can mimic other painful conditions and present with seemingly contradictory signs and symptoms. This is further complicated by the fact that pain may have a nociceptive as well as a neurogenic component, requiring careful examination and possibly multimodal treatment.

Selecting the most efficient treatment can be even more difficult, as presentation and responses are extremely variable, even within one type of neuropathic pain. This has led to the suggestion that treatments should aim to address underlying mechanisms instead of aetiological categories (Woolf & Max 2001). A herculean effort by a German team has now established that instead patients can be grouped according to their responses to sensory testing, which is moving us closer to achieving this (Maier et al 2010).

MECHANISMS OF NEUROPATHIC PAIN

A few basic concepts are essential for the understanding of neuropathic pain. The first is the concept of *projection*: the intact sensory nervous system projects information to the cortex and other cerebral structures, where awareness arises. Signals coming in via nociceptive pathways are typically interpreted by the brain as pain stemming from a somatic problem. Damage anywhere along the sensory pathway alters nerve function and may lead to pain, which is erroneously interpreted by the brain as coming from the tissues at the peripheral end of the sensory line. The patient will therefore describe abnormal sensations in the body, and it is the task of the clinician to find out which ones are indeed coming from the body and which ones are generated from within the nervous system. For an overview of projection pathways, please refer to Chapter 5.

The second concept is that damage to sensory nerves does not simply lead to negative symptoms like numbness and hypoaesthesia, but often creates positive phenomena such as hyperaesthesia and allodynia. This is because neurones change in response to damage, unlike the passive wiring systems with which they are often compared. The main neural changes responsible for these phenomena are as follows.

Neuronal function relies on *ion channels*, which are protein structures that cross the cell membrane and on opening allow specific ions (e.g. calcium, sodium or potassium) to flow either in or out. For example, once an action potential is generated, the change in voltage opens adjacent *voltage-gated* ion channels, which in turn leads to a voltage change further along, etc. This is how impulses are conducted. In myelinated neurones these ion channels are concentrated around nodes of Ranvier, and the impulses seemingly skip from one node to the next (saltatory conduction). Other types of ion channels may be opened by either mechanical forces or specific chemicals, including neurotransmitters (*ligands*).

Any changes in the distribution or type of ion channel along the neuron, or degeneration of the myelin sheath, alters neuronal function and may cause neuropathic pain. For example, damage to peripheral nerves leads to dense concentrations of sodium channels along the axon (Devor et al 1994). This can produce ectopic impulse-generating sites that make the neurons depolarize spontaneously. Additionally it produces mechanosensitivity, which is demonstrated with Tinel's test, for example for carpal or tarsal tunnel syndrome. This may be a risk particularly where nerves run close to tight or firm musculoskeletal structures (Devor 2006).

In relation to alterations in ion channel distribution, chemicals called *neurotrophic factors* are important. During prenatal development and after birth the tissues produce these *neurotrophins*, which draw the developing neurones towards them (Baccei & Fitzgerald 2006; Jessell & Sanes 2000). These factors either bind with tyrosine kinases (trk) receptors on the neural terminal, leading to the production of chemical messengers inside the neuron, or they are absorbed into the neural terminal. Messengers are constantly transported back to the cell body, where they affect protein synthesis, thereby determining the structures produced to make up the neuron, including the ion channels. Once the nervous system has stopped developing, the tissues' neurotrophins continue to maintain the structure and function of the neurones that innervate them. Changes in this communication between tissue and neuron, for instance because of nerve compression, can alter the neuronal make-up and cause neurogenic pain.

Neurotrophic factors are also released by Schwann cells, macrophages and other cells as part of Wallerian degeneration, along with other inflammatory mediators (Devor 2006; Marchand et al 2005). This promotes sprouting of the proximal stump. As some sprouts connect with and grow into the original endoneuriums, the remaining ones die back. However, if growth is blocked (for instance by scar tissue) the sprouts may form a *neuroma*, which can be extremely sensitive. Sprouting has also been observed in adjacent uninjured neurones (*collateral sprouting*).

Axonal damage may lead to a loss of insulation of individual neurones within a nerve. Activity in an axon can now produce excitation of adjacent fibres, making it possible for pain to develop in the absence of local stimulation. This is known as *crosstalk* (Devor 2006). Additionally, coupling between sympathetic neurons and afferents has been described. This is the result of the formation of noradrenaline receptors along damaged afferent axons (Jänig & Baron 2002). It has the potential to increase a patient's pain in response to sympathetic activity, for instance with mental and emotional stress, physical exertion or feeling unwell. If this mechanism is suspected, it is important to reassure the patient that their symptoms are not psychogenic.

Finally, central changes may contribute to neuropathic pain, as described in Chapter 6. Neuropathy can lead to the development of central sensitization, heightening the response to sensory stimulation and recruiting Aβ fibres into the generation on pain. Moreover, this is reinforced by reduced spinal and descending control (Dickenson & Bee 2008).

EXAMINATION

The clinical characteristics of neuropathy affect any or all components of a nerve and may therefore include sensory, autonomic or motor changes. Sensory changes may be wide ranging and include increased or decreased sensation or pain, allodynia, paraesthesia, dysaesthesia, spatial changes and temporal changes such as latency, aftersensation and summation (Hansson & Kinnman 1996). Neuropathies may present with different combinations of signs and symptoms, with large variations between individuals and conditions. Classic descriptions include burning and electrical pains as well as paraesthesia and numbness, but these symptoms are not always present, nor does their absence exclude neuropathy. Signs may well be paradoxical, such as intense pain felt in a cutaneous region that is numb to the touch. Finally, neuropathies may mimic, and occur alongside, other conditions (Table 10.1). It is for these reasons that careful subjective and objective clinical examination is essential. If there is any doubt about the diagnosis, a referral should be made to a neurologist or pain specialist (Dworkin et al 2007).

Careful history taking is the cornerstone of every examination. This may start with filling in a body chart, and it may be advantageous to ask the patient to do this. The exact signs and symptoms and the way they developed can suggest what the pathology and aetiology are. Concomitant diseases can also give an indication (see Box 10.1) and may require their own tests. Spontaneous as well as evoked signs and symptoms must be explored, as well as their exact localization on the body. Patients may be concerned that they may not believed because of the potentially contradictory nature of the symptoms, so it is essential to reassure them that what they report is not uncommon/understandable. Neuropathic symptoms and the way they behave are often strange to patients, so it is recommended that clinicians give patients a chance to formulate their own descriptions of symptoms without attempting to step in. At the end of history taking, the clinician should have at least one hypothesis regarding the underlying pathology.

A number of validated screening tools based on common features can aid the diagnosis (Table 10.2). The Leeds Assessment of Neuropathic Symptoms and Signs (LANSS), Neuropathic Pain Questionnaire (NPQ), Douleur Neuropathique en 4 (DN4), painDETECT and ID-Pain all include questions about the most common neuropathic symptoms, such as tingling, electrical and burning sensations. The inclusion of other sensations or numbness varies by questionnaire. The LANSS and DN4 have the advantage of including a few basic sensory tests. The complexity of neuropathic presentation means that these tests can be used to assess the likely presence of neuropathy, but not to diagnose or evaluate treatment. A recent development is the use of the McGill questionnaire, which at present requires further evaluation (Dworkin et al 2009).

In most cases the distribution of signs and symptoms follows a distribution that is anatomically consistent with a peripheral nerve, spinal nerve root or plexus, or a structure

Table 10.1 Entrapment neuropathies of the extremities

Nerve	Entrapment site	Symptoms	May masquerade as
Radial	Lateral elbow	Pain and sensory changes, radial distribution	Tennis elbow, De Quervain's
Radial	Wartenberg's point, under brachioradialis	Pain and sensory changes, radial distribution	De Quervain's
Median	Carpal tunnel	Paraesthesia and pain in hand	
Median	Pronator teres	Pain in median distribution	Carpal tunnel syndrome
Ulnar	Cubital tunnel	Pain and sensory changes in ulnar distribution	
	Tunnel of Guyon	Pain and sensory changes in ulnar distribution	
Lateral femoral cutaneous	Inguinal ligament	Pain and sensory changes in antero-lateral thigh	L3 nerve root entrapment
Saphenus	Medial knee	Medial knee and calf pain	
Common peroneal	Proximal fibular head	Pain and sensory changes in antero-lateral lower leg and dorsum foot	L4–5 nerve root entrapment
Superficial peroneal	Lateral lower leg	Pain and sensory changes in dorsum foot and first four toes	L5 nerve root entrapment
Deep peroneal	Metatarsal 1	Pain in first and second toes	
Tibial	Medial ankle (tarsal tunnel)	Pain in heel, sole and toes	Plantar faciitis, tibialis posterior tendonitis, tarsal tunnel syndrome
Medial and lateral plantar	Medial calcaneum	Pain in sole and toes	Plantar faciitis, tibialis posterior tendonitis, tarsal tunnel syndrome
Digital pedal	Between metatarsal heads	Pain in toe, typically third or fourth	

Adapted from van Griensven, H. 2005, Pain in practice. Theory and treatment strategies for manual therapists. Butterworth Heinemann, with permission of Elsevier.

in spinal cord, brain stem or higher. The objective examination is aimed at testing the hypothetical cause of the symptoms. If pain is a prominent feature, the clinician is advised to test modalities such as motor function and reflexes first in order not to sensitize the nervous system.

Sensory testing is the final part of the examination and aims to map out the exact distribution of sensory changes (for specific examples and potential difficulties see Hansson 1994). Ideally a number of tests are done because neuropathies do not always affect all sensory modalities, but basic tests include light touch, pinprick and proprioception. Sensory tests are briefly summarized in Box 10.2; for further reading refer to MacDermid (2005). In the case of positive features such

as hyperaesthesia and allodynia, testing from outside the affected area towards its perimeter is recommended. However, negative features, i.e. reduced sensation, may be best tested from inside the zone going outwards.

Once a diagnosis of neuropathy has been established, a clear explanation of signs and symptoms to the patient is required. In some cases a treatment strategy can be discussed, although often the aim of further action is management and not a cure (British Pain Society 2008). If diagnosis or further management cannot be determined from the examination, specialized diagnostic techniques such as imaging, neurophysiological testing, quantitative sensory testing, thermography or diagnostic nerve block may be required (Hansson et al 2002, 2007).

Table 10.2 Neuropathic screening tools (Bennett et al 2007)

Comparison of items within five neuropathic pain screening tools *(shaded boxes highlight features shared by two or more tools)*

	LANSS[a]	DN4[a]	NPQ	pain*DETECT*	ID Pain
Symptoms					
Pricking, tingling, pins and needles	•	•	•	•	•
Electric shocks or shooting	•	•	•	•	•
Hot or burning	•	•	•	•	•
Numbness		•	•	•	•
Pain evoked by light touching	•		•	•	•
Painful cold or freezing pain		•	•		
Pain evoked by mild pressure				•	
Pain evoked by heat or cold				•	
Pain evoked by changes in weather			•		
Pain limited to joints[b]					○
Itching		•			
Temporal patterns				•	
Radiation of pain				•	
Autonomic changes	•				
Clinical examination					
Brush allodynia	•	•			
Raised soft touch threshold	•	•			
Raised pin prick threshold	•	•			

Bennett, M., Attal, N., Backonja, M., Baron, R., Bouhassira, D., Freynhagen, R., Scholz, J., Tölle, T., Wittchen, H., & Jensen, T., Using screening tools to identify neuropathic pain. *PAIN*, 2007, 127(3); 199-203. This table has been reproduced with permission of the International Association for the Study of Pain® (IASP). This table may not be reproduced for any other purpose without permission.
[a] Tools that involve clinical examination.
[b] Used to identify non-neuropathic pain.

Box 10.2 Sensory modalities and testing methods

Threshold sensation	Semmes-Weinstein monofilaments
Vibration threshold	Tuning fork
Tactile discrimination	Two-point discrimination (2PD) Diskcriminator
Sensory function of the hand	STI and Sollerman hand test
Cold intolerance	Self-report or cold stress test

TREATMENT AND MANAGEMENT OF NEUROPATHIC PAIN

There is little correspondence between disease or injury on one hand and specific mechanisms of neuropathy on the other. Efforts to identify which mechanisms play a role in each individual patient, and therefore which drugs have the best chance of success, are currently underway (Baron 2006b). Novel drug targets and other developments are reviewed in Dray (2008).

Treatment recommendations based on the available evidence are summarized in the section below; for a full review of mechanisms see Dworkin et al (2007) and Baron (2006b). Treatment objectives can be summarized as follows (Jensen 2008):

- Reduce peripheral sensitization.
- Reduce ectopic activity.
- Decrease central sensitization.
- Reduce central facilitation and increase central inhibition.

Note that the latter has physiological as well as psychological components.

Overall approach

First, it is essential to establish a diagnosis and treat the cause of the neuropathic pain. Refer to a specialist if there are doubts about diagnosis or treatment. Take into account any comorbidities, and explain the diagnosis and plan to the patient along with realistic expectations.

Second, treatment must be started. Any underlying disease must be treated and neuropathic symptom management should start with at least one of the following:

- A secondary amine tricyclic antidepressant TCA (nortriptyline, desipramine) or a selective serotonin and noreprinephrine reuptake inhibitor SSNRI (duloxetine, venlafaxine) (Kingery 1997). Explain to the patient that the treatment is not for depression.
- A ligand to voltage-gated calcium channel (gabapentin, pregabalin).
- For localized peripheral neuropathy, a lidocaine patch to target voltage-gated sodium channels (Black et al 2002; Galer et al 2002).
- For acute neuropathic pain, neuropathic cancer pain or severe episodic exacerbations, opioid medication or tramadol.

It must be noted that only partial pain relief can be expected in only half of the patients, and that side effects can form a significant prohibitive factor (O'Connor 2009). It is therefore important to also start non-pharmacological treatment as appropriate. There is low-level evidence for the use of transcutaneous electrical nerve stimulation (TENS; see Chapter 14) and spinal cord stimulation (SCS; Jensen 2008). Therapy intervention needs to be directed to address the key treatment objectives (Jensen 2008), with modalities chosen as appropriate to the patient. As with all forms of persistent pain, realistic understanding, coping strategies and family involvement are essential. Anxiety, depression and problems sleeping must be addressed as applicable.

Third, the clinician should reassess the pain and associated quality of life regularly and for a sufficiently long period of time – this varies per drug but is at least 3–4 weeks. Continuation of treatment is recommended if the pain drops to manageable levels and side effects are tolerable. If relief is less marked, a further component of the treatment options outlined above can be added (Rhodes 2011). On the other hand, if relief is only minor or non-existent try another form of treatment altogether.

Finally, if single and combined treatments fail, other forms of medication or referral to a specialist pain service must be considered. Second-line treatments are opioids and tramadol, while third-line include antiepileptics such as carbamazepine and lamotrigine, antidepressants like citalopram and paroxetine, mexilitine, N-methyl-D-aspartate (NMDA) receptor antagonists such as ketamine, and capsaicin cream. Unfortunately no treatments have been proved effective for lumbosacral radiculopathy, which is perhaps the most common form of neuropathic pain (Dworkin et al 2007).

Desensitization

This is a process of reducing hypersensitivity in an area by sensory bombardment of the nerve endings in order to decrease touch-evoked pain and discomfort (Waylett-Rendall 1995). For suggested mediums of treatment see Box 10.3.

It is imperative to reassure the patient that touch is something not to be scared of, even though it may cause a temporary increase in pain and feel damaging. The exception is in the presence of a neuroma, in which pain is worsened by desensitization, even when applied carefully.

Desensitization is broadly carried out in one of two ways. *Graded exposure* involves a gradual increase in sensory stimulation from tolerated to non-tolerated, with progression through each treatment or home exercise session. The more pain-provocative method is to alternate between tolerated and non-tolerated stimulation activities, allowing rapid adaptation of the tissue to the stimulus.

Desensitization should be carried out for 5–10 minutes, a minimum of three or four times a day, but up to six times a day. To read further regarding desensitization, and for specific examples of desensitization protocols, see Waylett-Rendall (1995).

Sensory re-education

The patient can be given exercise tasks involving touch and recognition of textures, patterns and objects whilst using the assistance of visual feedback. This process uses activities where vision guides touch, in an attempt to reprogramme the brain after an insult to the nervous system. The earliest published sensory re-education programme was set out by

---

Box 10.3 Items to use for desensitization

Textures can be used for light touch or light massage. Examples are cotton wool, terry towelling, wool, soft Velcro, felt, foam, hard Velcro, leather, carpet, plastic and silk.

Particles such as rice, pasta, sand, foam pieces, popcorn, beans, lentils and sago can be used for immersion of the body part.

Other modalities are flowing air from a fan, running water, percussion/tapping, vibration and functional tasks. Vibration is often the form of stimulation that is tolerated earliest in this process.

Box 10.4 **Sensory re-education**

1. Touch the body part or hold an object with eyes open.
2. Aim to identify the surface/texture/object.
3. Compare these feelings to the normal side.
4. Concentrate thoughts on the shape, texture and temperature of the item, e.g. a marble table is flat, smooth, shiny and cold, a tennis ball is fuzzy/soft, warm to touch, round and slightly rough.
5. Once the patient can achieve the above with eyes open, progress to repeating all steps with eyes closed.

Wynn-Parry in 1966 and used localization of touch and recognition of shapes and textures (Rosen et al 2003).

The basis of the exercises is to perform simple repetitive tasks with the aim of re-educating both the peripheral and central nervous systems (Box 10.4), relating the tasks to the function of the affected body part. In upper limb dexterity, stereognosis, manipulation etc. are especially important, while the lower limb requires tolerance to weight-bearing and a variety of different afferent inputs. See Wynn-Parry (1980, p. 226) for a more detailed description of training programmes for the upper limb.

All textures and particles used for desensitization can be used for sensory re-education, as well as small and large everyday objects and different surfaces. Using sensory re-education in isolation has shown disappointing results (Rosen et al 2003), so Lundborg and Rosen (2007) have proposed a two-phase approach. Phase 1 addresses cortical reorganization of the somatosensory cortex and aims to maintain the cortical hand representation. Phase 2 explores novel principles to enhance the effects of sensory training, using selective deafferentiation.

Phase 1 uses visuo-tactile and audio-tactile interaction and can be used either when complete paraesthesia is present or if there is any type of altered sensory feedback. This phase should be used for all patients who have a possibility of cortical reorganization. Phase 1 activities include:

- imagined movements
- observed movements, either of the contralateral side or another individual's body part
- reading or listening to 'action words' relating to activities involving the body part
- mirror therapy (see Part 2 for more detail)
- use of a sensor glove (a glove that gives auditory feedback) or texture rods that are rubbed whilst being held close to the ear, such that the sound of touch can be heard.

Functional Magnetic Resonance Imaging (fMRI) has demonstrated that observing hands being touched activates visual as well as somatosensory areas in the brain cortex (Lundborg 2008). Activation of the somatosensory cortex by visual observation of touch has also been demonstrated in the lower extremity (Keysers et al 2004). Empirically, sensory re-education procedures can stimulate recovery of sensation and normalize sensory feedback in neuropathic pain that presents as altered sensations such as allodynia, hyperaesthesia and dysaesthesia amongst others.

Phase 2 involves the use of Eutectic Mixture of Local Anesthetics (EMLA) anaesthetic cream (liaise with the Multi-disciplinary team (MDT) if required) and uses the principle of brain plasticity to enhance traditional sensory re-education activities. The EMLA cream is applied to the area of the body adjacent to the deafferented area. This is thought to allow expansion of the adjacent cortical representation, increasing the effectiveness of sensory re-education to this area. In a double-blind, randomized clinical trial, the EMLA group showed a significantly improved tactile discrimination when compared with the control group (Rosen et al 2006).

Cortical remapping

Changes in the somatosensory cortex of the brain have been determined in response to both ongoing pain (Flor et al 1997) and injury to peripheral nerves (Jensen 2002; Lundborg & Rosen 2007; Rosen et al 2003). In order to address these cortical changes the principles used in Phase 1 of Lundborg & Rosen's sensory re-education may be used (Lundborg & Rosen 2007). The graded motor imagery programme and mirror therapy can also be used (see Part 2).

Aids and adaptations

Maintaining the function of the affected body part and ideally functional independence is an important component of treatment. To optimize function of the lower limb, it should be considered whether walking aids or orthoses may help to improve gait quality and ability to continue weight bearing. Any aid has the potential to be exceptionally helpful as long as the patient is be monitored to prevent dependence, which may hinder timely recovery. Upper limb aides are many and varied, and can assist with personal or domestic activities of daily living. Examples include adapted knives, can and jar openers, aides to assist with fastening clothes or shoes and many more. It is worthwhile liaising with the local occupational therapy department for details of suppliers or local shops who stock this type of equipment, or for a more comprehensive assessment of the patient's needs.

Part 2: Complex regional pain syndrome

INTRODUCTION

The characteristics of CRPS were described in 1872 by S Weir Mitchell, and years of hypotheses and names for the condition followed (Box 10.5). CRPS often develops in response to minor trauma to the limbs (Box 10.6). The term CRPS was introduced in 1994 by the IASP in order

Box 10.5 **Terms used for CRPS (after Abram 1990; Wilson 1990)**

The length of the list reflects the confusion over the interpretation of CRPS.

Algo(neuro)dystrophy
Causalgia
Chronic traumatic oedema
Complex regional pain disorder
Neurodystrophy
Pain-dysfunction syndrome
Post-traumatic oedema
Post-traumatic osteoporosis
Post-traumatic pain syndrome
Post-traumatic spreading neuralgia
Reflex (sympathetic) dystrophy
Shoulder-hand syndrome
Südeck's atrophy
Sympathalgia
Sympathetic overdrive syndrome
Traumatic arthritis

Box 10.6 **Initiating events of CRPS**

The results of four studies have been pooled for a total of 778 patients (Abram 1990).

Trauma

Blunt   32%
Laceration   11%
Fracture   21%
Sprain   2%
Nerve injury   1%
Total trauma   67%

Postoperative

Carpal tunnel   6%
Dupuytren's   4%
Ganglion cyst   2%
Other   2%
Unspecified   5%
Total postoperative   21%

Burns

Thermal   1%
Electrical   1%
Total burns   2%

Other

Myocardial infarction (MI)   2%
Cerebral disease   1%
Spinal cord injury   <1%
Other/unknown   5%

to provide clarity of diagnosis and treatment (Merskey et al 1994; Stanton-Hicks et al 1995). It was chosen for the following reasons:

- *complex* expresses the varying clinical features (Hayek & Mekhail 2004; Stanton-Hicks et al 1995, 1998)
- *regional* emphasizes that in the majority of cases it involves a region of the body, usually an extremity (Hayek & Mekhail 2004; Stanton-Hicks et al 1998)
- *pain* is the sine qua non for diagnosis (Hayek & Mekhail 2004; Stanton-Hicks et al 1995) – in rare conditions that otherwise resemble CRPS, pain may be minimal or absent.

A set of consensus-based diagnostic criteria was created for CRPS (Table 10.3) which have since been shown to have high sensitivity but low specificity, i.e. the criteria would rarely miss a case of CRPS, but over-diagnosis is likely (Bruehl et al 1999; Galer et al 1998; Harden et al 1999). In order to overcome this shortcoming, an alternative set of improved diagnostic criteria were developed using four clinical subgroups (sensory, motor/trophic, sudomotor/oedema and vasomotor) (Bruehl et al 1999; Harden & Bruehl 2005; Harden et al 1999) (Table 10.4). For clinical work the final *Budapest criteria* provide excellent sensitivity (0.99) and greatly improved specificity (0.68) (Harden et al 2010). These criteria have been incorporated in recent guidelines (Goebel et al 2012).

CLINICAL CHARACTERISTICS OF CRPS

Clinicians may first suspect CRPS from their initial observation. Application of the four subgroups described by Harden and Bruehl (2005) is strongly recommended to maximize the chance of correct diagnosis and treatment. For more detailed information about CRPS clinical characteristics, refer to van de Vusse et al (2003) and Stanton-Hicks et al (1995, 1998, 2002).

Pain and sensory changes

In CRPS these are characterized by hyperpathia, allodynia, hyperalgesia and hyperaesthesia (see Appendix Glossary). Typical descriptors used by patients include aching, burning, pricking or shooting, deep, spontaneous, superficial, throbbing and sharp. Sensory changes may include decreased temperature sensation and decreased sensitivity to pin-prick.

Allodynia may present in response to one or a number of different stimuli, including temperature and mechanical, vibration and spatial stimuli. Temperature allodynia is produced in response to cold or hot stimuli. Mechanical allodynia may be either static (sensitivity to light touch or pressure) or dynamic (sensitivity to brushing or stroking of the skin). Vibration allodynia may be provoked by activities such as travelling in a car or touching anything with

Table 10.3 Current IASP CRPS criteria (Stanton-Hicks 1995)

Complex regional pain syndrome (CRPS)

A term describing a variety of painful conditions following injury which appears regionally having a distal predominance of abnormal findings, exceeding in both magnitude and duration the expected clinical course of the inciting event often resulting in significant impairment of motor function, and showing variable progression over time.

CRPS type 1 (RSD)

1. Type I is a syndrome that develops after an initiating noxious event.
2. Spontaneous pain or allodynia/hyperalgesia occurs, is not limited to the territory of a single peripheral nerve, and is disproportionate to the inciting event.
3. There is or has been evidence of oedema, skin blood flow abnormality, or abnormal sudomotor activity in the region of the pain since the inciting event.
4. This diagnosis is excluded by the existence of conditions that would otherwise account for the degree of pain and dysfunction.

CRPS type II (causalgia)

1. Type II is a syndrome that develops after a nerve injury.
2. Spontaneous pain or allodynia occurs and is not necessarily limited to the territory of the injured nerve.
3. There is or has been evidence of oedema, skin blood flow abnormality, or abnormal sudomotor activity in the region of the pain since the inciting event.
4. This diagnosis is excluded by the existence of conditions that would otherwise account for the degree of pain or dysfunction.

Reprinted from Stanton-Hicks M, Jaenig W, Hassenbusch S, et al. Reflex sympathetic dystrophy: changing concepts and taxonomy. PAIN 1995, Oct; 63(1): 127–133. This table has been reproduced with permission of the International Association for the Study of Pain®(IASP®). The table may not be reproduced for any other purpose without permission.

Table 10.4 Proposed changes to the diagnostic criteria (Harden & Bruehl 2005)

General definition of the syndrome

CRPS describes an array of painful conditions that are characterized by a continuing (spontaneous and/or evoked) regional pain that is seemingly disproportional in time or degree to the usual course of any known trauma or other lesion. The pain is regional (not in a specific nerve territory or dermatome) an usually has a distal predominance of abnormal sensory, motor, sudomotor, vasomotor, and/or trophic findings. The syndrome shows variable progression over time.

There are two versions of the proposed diagnostic criteria: a clinical version meant to maximise diagnostic sensitivity with adequate specificity, and a research version meant to more equally balance optimal sensitivity and specificity.

Proposed modified clinical diagnostic criteria for CRPS

1. Continuing pain, which is disproportionate to any inciting event.
2. Must report at least one symptom in three of the four following categories:
   Sensory: Reports of hyperaesthesia and/or allodynia.
   Vasomotor: Reports of temperature asymmetry and/or skin colour changes and/or skin colour asymmetry.
   Sudomotor/oedema: Reports of oedema and/or sweating changes and/or sweating asymmetry.
   Motor/trophic: Reports of decreased range of motion and/or motor dysfunction (weakness, tremor, dystonia) and/or trophic changes (hair, nails, skin).
3. Must display at least one sign* at time of evaluation in two or more of the following categories:
   Sensory: Evidence of hyperalgesia (to pinprick) and/or allodynia (to light touch and/or deep somatic pressure and/or joint movement).
   Vasomotor: Evidence of temperature asymmetry and/or skin colour changes and/or asymmetry.
   Sudomotor/oedema: Evidence of oedema and/or sweating changes and/or sweating asymmetry.
   Motor/trophic: Evidence of decreased range of motion and/or motor dysfunction (weakness, tremor, dystonia) and/or trophic changes (hair, nails, skin).
4. There is no other diagnosis that better explains the signs and symptoms.

Continued

Table 10.4   Proposed changes to the diagnostic criteria (Harden & Bruehl 2005)—cont'd

Proposed modified research diagnostic criteria for CRPS

1. Continuing pain, which is disproportionate to any inciting event.
2. Must report at least one symptom in each of the four following categories:
   Sensory: Reports of hyperesthesia and/or allodynia.
   Vasomotor: Reports of temperature asymmetry and/or skin colour changes and/or skin colour asymmetry.
   Sudomotor/oedema: Reports of oedema and/or sweating changes and/or sweating asymmetry.
   Motor/trophic: Reports of decreased range of motion and/or motor dysfunction. (weakness, tremor, dystonia) and/or trophic changes (hair, nails, skin).
3. Must display at least one sign* a the time of evaluation in two or more of the following categories:
   Sensory: Evidence of hyperalgesia (to pinprick) and/or allodynia (to light touch and/or deep somatic pressure and/or joint movement).
   Vasomotor: Evidence of temperature asymmetry and/or skin colour changes and/or asymmetry.
   Sudomotor/oedema: Evidence of oedema and/or sweating changes and/or sweating asymmetry.
   Motor/trophic: Evidence of decreased range of motion and/or motor dysfunction (weakness, tremor, dystonia) and/or trophic changes (hair, nails, skin).
4. There is no other diagnosis that better explains the signs and symptoms.

*A sign is counted only if observed at the time of diagnosis.

Summary of sensitivity and specificity of the proposed clinical and research criteria

Criterion type	Symptoms required for diagnosis	Signs required for diagnosis	Sensitivity	Specificity
Clinical	3	2	0.85	0.69
Research	4	2	0.70	0.96

Reprinted from Harden RN, Bruehl S. Diagnostic criteria: The statistical deviation of the four criterion factors. In Wilson PR, Stanton-Hicks M, Harden RN, editors of CRPS: Current Diagnosis and Therapy. IASP Press ©, Seattle, 1995. This table has been reproduced with permission of the International Association for the Study of Pain®(IASP®). The table may not be reproduced for any other purpose without permission.

mild vibration. Spatial allodynia is under-reported but commonly experienced; some patients describe an increase in pain when someone or something approaches the affected area. It is worth asking patients about this because they may be reluctant to report symptoms without physical cause.

Motor and trophic changes

These changes were grouped together because of statistical significance. Motor changes include motor neglect, limitation of range of movement, weakness, tremor, dystonia, motor dysfunction, myoclonus and reduced or altered muscle power. Patients may not use the affected limb in daily tasks, feel that it is not readily available for use or describe lack of coordination.

Trophic changes affect the appearance of skin, hair and nails. They can be observed during assessment (sign) or be intermittent (symptom). Skin changes are typically fibrosis, hyperkeratosis and thin glossy skin (Stanton-Hicks et al 2002). Patients will present with or describe skin that is flaky, thick, thin, fragile or shiny. Hair can sometimes be absent, but most frequently grows thicker

and darker, which can be distressing. Nails may grow thick and strong or become flaky and brittle. These signs must be different from the norm for that individual to be significant.

Vasomotor changes

Patients may present with changes or asymmetry in temperature and skin colour. These are often intermittent and substantially noticeable when they occur. Patients may have skin that is very red or very pale, or mottled (blotchy purple and white). Temperature can be either very hot or very cold, and may fluctuate between the two. In winter, CRPS patients often need to wear gloves when outdoors.

Sudomotor changes and oedema

These signs and symptoms include changes or asymmetries in sweating and swelling or oedema. Oedema is common after trauma, but excessively so in CRPS. The swelling often fluctuates and may be exacerbated by simple function or even imagined movements (Moseley 2004a). Changes in sweating can present as hyperhydrosis or anhydrosis (Stanton-Hicks et al 2002). Excessive sweating may present in response to activities and is often embarrassing. Functionally anhydrosis is most limiting though, especially in the hand, as the fine layer of moisture on the palms gives significant assistance to grip.

MECHANISMS OF CRPS

Despite many years of research, the understanding of what causes or maintains the diverse range of signs and symptoms associated with CRPS is still far from complete. One of the confounding issues is that there are no absolute diagnostic tests. Research studies may therefore include participants who present with similar signs and symptoms, but who have different underlying pathologies. A unifying theory continues to elude scientists and clinicians alike. This section discusses aspects of the syndrome that have been identified.

Inflammation

Clinically, limbs with CRPS display the classic characteristics of inflammation such as *rubor*, *calor* and *dolor*, especially in the acute phase. The origin of this inflammation may be at least partially neurogenic, i.e. facilitated by the release of neuropeptides from the terminals of nociceptive fibres (see Basbaum & Jessell 2000 for a description of the process). Substance P (SP) causes extravasation of plasma and release of histamine from mast cells, which in turn leads to local sensitization and vasodilation. Calcitonin gene-related peptide (CGRP) also dilates the blood vessels in the region. This mechanism has been demonstrated by subjecting CRPS patients and healthy controls to strong transcutaneous nerve stimulation (Weber et al 2001). The patients showed a much stronger vasodilation response and enhanced protein extravasation. There is further support from the observation that the administration of a SP receptor antagonist may reduce CRPS-like signs in a nerve injury model of the rat (Kingery et al 2003). It must be remembered, however, that it is plausible yet uncertain whether underlying mechanisms are the same in patients. It is also not clear whether the release of noradrenaline by local sympathetic neurons plays a role (Baron 2006a).

Pain and sensory changes

Pain, the cardinal feature of CRPS, is likely to be the result of both peripheral and central sensitization (see Chapter 6). The local processes discussed above account for local pain and sensitization. However, sensory changes may spread beyond the affected tissues and even to the contralateral side, which suggests alterations of sensory processing in the central nervous system. Rommel et al (1999) applied sensory tests to 24 patients with CRPS, of whom 20 had sensory changes beyond the affected area, including 16 with changes beyond the affected limb. Eight patients had hemisensory changes and in four the upper quadrant was affected. Interestingly, the most common general changes were *hypo*aesthesia and *hypo*algesia, while mechanical hyperalgesia was found in the affected limb of 10 patients. A further study expanded on the range of sensory modalities affected and established that psychological disorders could not account for changes beyond the affected area (Rommel et al 2001). A heightened cortical response to mechanical stimulation and altered cortical representation have also been demonstrated in patients with CRPS (Juottonen et al 2002).

Hypothetically, CRPS type 1 resulting from trauma, including surgery, may be the result of minor local nerve damage. Indeed, evidence of local damage to small diameter cutaneous nerves (C and Aδ) has been found in some studies (Oaklander & Fields 2009; Oaklander et al 2006). This might account for the fact that the majority of patients experience negative sensory changes such as hypoaesthesia (Veldman et al 1993). The relevance of these neuropathies is disputed, however, and they may be little more than a consequence of trophic changes in the local tissues (Jänig & Baron 2006).

Autonomic involvement

The sympathetic division of the autonomic nervous system regulates a wide range of functions. Unlike the parasympathetic nervous system, it affects somatic tissues such as cutaneous and musculoskeletal structures. Sympathetic output is regulated on a segmental level via somato-sympathetic reflexes, and centrally by the hypothalamus. It is influenced by both homeostatic requirements and emotional state.

One of the now superseded terms for CRPS is reflex sympathetic dystrophy (RSD), reflecting the assumption that it was a disorder of the sympathetic nervous system. This was reasonable given that this autonomic division controls vascular and sudomotor responses. The sympathetic overdrive theory suggested that persistent nociceptive input might drive increases in sympathetic activity on a spinal segmental level, with the resultant tissue effects maintaining nociception (Abram 1990). However, this theory could not account for the range of sensory changes associated with CRPS because the sympathetic system is purely efferent.

It has since become clear that an individual's pain may or may not have a sympathetically maintained component, which may explain why only a percentage of patients will benefit from sympathetic blockade (Harden & Bruehl 2005). CRPS patients are now subcategorized as having sympathetically maintained or sympathetically independent pain (SMP or SIP; Harden & Bruehl 2005). Some of these changes are local, but central sympathetic regulation may also be altered (Jänig & Baron 2003).

Vasomotor and sudomotor changes

Circulation in the somatic tissues is affected by local chemicals, including inflammatory mediators, which may be released by damaged or inflamed tissues. As discussed above they may be released from the local terminals of nociceptive fibres, creating Lewis' classic triple response of reddening, wheal and spreading flare (de Morree 1989). Finally, sympathetic fibres control circulation through the release of noradrenaline (NA).

Based on studies involving warming and cooling of the body along with measurement of factors such as blood flow and plasma levels of NA, the following hypothesis has been produced (see Wasner & Baron 2005 for a review). Normally there is tonic activity of the sympathetic nervous system regulating the release of NA. In the skin NA binds with the α-adrenoreceptors of the blood vessels and maintains relative vasoconstriction. Acute CRPS is associated with a central reduction of sympathetic tone, leading to a reduction in vasoconstriction and therefore reddening and warming. However, there is evidence that as CRPS persists the vessels develop higher concentrations of α-adrenoreceptors, leading to increased sensitivity to NA but also circulating adrenaline, known as *supersensitivity*. On the other hand, changes to the number of capillaries and their quality have also been observed (see Groeneweg et al 2009 for a review). The overall result is vasoconstriction, coldness and secondary hypotrophic changes.

Hyperhydrosis has been found in over 50% of patients with CRPS (Veldman et al 1993). Sudomotor response to changes in body temperature and axon reflexis increased in the affected limb (Birklein et al 1997). Sweat glands do not develop adrenergic supersensitivity, so their altered activity has been attributed to changes in the central regulation of the sympathetic nervous system (Jänig & Baron 2003). The mechanisms underlying these changes are as yet unclear (Jänig & Baron 2003).

Motor changes

Tremor and lack of coordination may be found in around 50% of CRPS patients, while muscle spasm may develop in 25% of long-term sufferers (Veldman et al 1993). The exact reasons for these symptoms are yet to be explained and are likely to vary between individuals (see van Hilten et al 2005 for a review). A period of immobility, for instance after an injury or operation, may itself engender a lack of motor control. Tissue swelling is likely to make a limb more difficult to control as well, similar to wearing a boxing glove. This and other tissue changes are likely to distort proprioceptive feedback, joint and muscle contractures potentially playing a role in both cause and effect.

Pain and other sensory changes can interfere with proprioception and coordination. Central control may be affected: CRPS patients may have an altered response of the motor cortex (Juottonen et al 2002). This may explain the success of motor imagery strategies in some cases (Moseley 2004b; Moseley et al 2008a).

Psychological factors

Anecdotally, clinicians have reported that some patients display a 'CRPS personality'. To date, the weight of evidence is against such a claim. For example, Ciccone et al (1997) compared a group of CRPS sufferers with patients with either low back pain or local neuropathic pain. A range of measures assessing symptom reporting, illness behaviour and psychological distress failed to find a significant difference between the groups. There was also no greater incidence of childhood trauma. Similarly, a review of the literature found no evidence of CRPS as a psychogenic disorder (Covington 1996). Patients who develop CRPS following a wrist fracture are psychologically indistinguishable from those who do not (Puchalski & Zyluk 2005). Even patients with severe CRPS and dystonia do not have a distinct psychological profile (Reedijk et al 2008).

Covington (1996) suggests that severe pain may be the cause of suffering rather than vice versa, and that pain-related behaviour such as disuse may affect the progression of the condition. In this sense CRPS is no different from other painful conditions. Psychological factors must therefore be addressed along with other signs and symptoms, but they should never be a reason to dismiss a patient's presentation or exclude them from treatment.

CLINICAL EXAMINATION

A positive diagnosis of CRPS requires that at the time of clinical assessment the patient has a reported symptom in *three* of the four categories and a displayed physical sign in *two* of the four categories. There must also be no other diagnosis that better explains the signs and symptoms. There is consensus that the diagnosis should be established as soon as possible, in order to start interdisciplinary treatment in the early phases (Atkins 2003; Rho et al 2002; Stanton-Hicks et al 2002; Thomas & Degnan 2005; Zhongyu et al 2005).

Subjective assessment

This is no different from the assessment of other painful conditions, and should include a body chart filled out by the patient and at least the 11-point numerical pain scale to assess intensity (Bear-Lehman & Abreu 1989; Glassey 2001).

CRPS patients are often embarrassed about their symptoms and may feel that they are too 'odd' to report. Even with only a mild suspicion of CRPS, it is worth asking specific questions to elicit a full subjective history. Clinicians should systematically ask about each of the diagnostic criteria.

Objective assessment

This part of the examination is guided by an accurate subjective history. Not all aspects have to be completed during the initial consultation and it may take several sessions to assess all aspects fully. The clinician should ensure that at least one assessment measure has been taken from each of the four diagnostic subsections. Harden et al (2010) demonstrated that each individual diagnostic component is reasonably sensitive, but not as specific as the combination of all components. Early instigation of treatment is essential so the initial consult should always include some treatment, typically at least patient education and a home exercise programme.

Sensory changes. Particular attention should be paid to allodynia and hyperalgesia. Threshold sensation and mechanical allodynia may be measured by Semmes-Weinstein monofilaments (Bear-Lehman & Abreu 1989; Li et al 2005; Prosser & Conolly 2003) or von Frey hairs (Tichelaar et al 2006). Light palpation of the affected limb (Li et al 2005; Prosser & Conolly 2003) should be carried out to assess hyperalgesia or hyperpathia (Atkins 2003). Vibration and weight bearing (ideally using a force-plate) may be included in a comprehensive assessment. It may be useful to determine a subjective rating of the pain elicited by each type of physical stimulation.

Vasomotor changes. Temperature changes are assessed through palpation. Thermography gives greater objectivity (Bruehl et al 1996; Uematsu et al 1981), but tends to be reserved for research. Colour changes are determined as part of detailed clinical observation.

Sudomotor changes and oedema. Oedema can be measured using a volumeter (Bear-Lehman & Abreu 1989; Li et al 2005; Prosser & Conolly 2003) or using a tape measure and referring to anatomical landmarks (Bear-Lehman & Abreu 1989; Hunter et al 1995; Li et al 2005; Prosser & Conolly 2003). Note that atrophy on the affected side can skew the accuracy of circumferential measurements. Changes or asymmetry in sweat production are determined through palpation.

Motor and trophic changes. It is essential to measure range of motion (ROM) using goniometry. The reliability and validity of goniometry are greatest when using an agreed standardized protocol (Bear-Lehman & Abreu 1989; Burr et al 2003; Pratt & Burr 2001). The quality of the movement and any motor dysfunction must also be noted. Assessment of strength may be limited by pain and should be judged per individual, but a baseline strength measurement using the Medical Research Council standards (MacAvoy & Green 2007) or with dynamometry for grip strength (Coldham et al 2006; Massy-Westropp et al 2004) is preferable, but strength assessment is best deferred if it is likely to significantly increase symptoms.

Changes to skin, hair and nails are assessed through both observation and palpation. Skin quality should be recorded, as well as hair and nail changes.

THE TREATMENT OF CRPS

The overall aims for treatment of CRPS are to:

- maximize function
- relieve pain
- improve quality of life.

Because of the complex nature of CRPS, multifaceted and usually multidisciplinary care is essential. As such therapy intervention should be part of a well-structured integrated clinical pathway (Krakousky 2005; Rho et al 2002; Stanton-Hicks et al 1998, 2002). The primary goal of treatment is functional restoration (Stanton-Hicks et al 2002). Invasive therapies such as regional sympathetic blocks or sympathetic blocks may be considered in extreme cases, but are not discussed here (refer to Baron 2006a or Wilson et al 2005 for discussions).

Therapy intervention for CRPS

Therapy intervention is the mainstay of CRPS treatment (Rho et al 2002; Stanton-Hicks et al 2002) and may be provided by physical therapists and/or occupational therapists. Disappointingly, however, there is a serious lack of clinical trials on physical therapy management of CRPS and no RCTs (Dommerholt 2004), although there are consensus-based therapy guidelines from expert panels (Stanton-Hicks et al 1998, 2002) and a systematic review (Daly & Bialocerkowski 2008). Figure 10.1 shows the IASP treatment algorithm for CRPS (Stanton-Hicks et al 2002). Experts agree that patients who do not respond to treatment by 12–16 weeks should be given a trial of more interventional therapies (Stanton-Hicks et al 2002).

It is imperative to create specific, measureable, achievable, realistic and time-related (SMART) goals with the patient and use improvements in functional ability as a measure of progress. Therapy should be based on best practice *and* tailored to the individual patient by thorough clinical assessment. Stanton-Hicks et al (1998) suggest that 'the dynamic and unique nature of this disease entity must allow for individual flexibility and application of treatment protocols and the variable use of exercise therapy'. Therapy interventions, whilst challenging the patient's abilities, should *not* cause an exacerbation of their signs or symptoms, and need to be graded to prevent this.

Education

Adequate analgesia, encouragement and education are essential (Stanton-Hicks et al 2002). Symptoms are wide-ranging, often distressing and disproportionate to the initiating event. Although the mechanisms are not fully understood, it is important to explain that the signs and symptoms all come under one umbrella of CRPS.

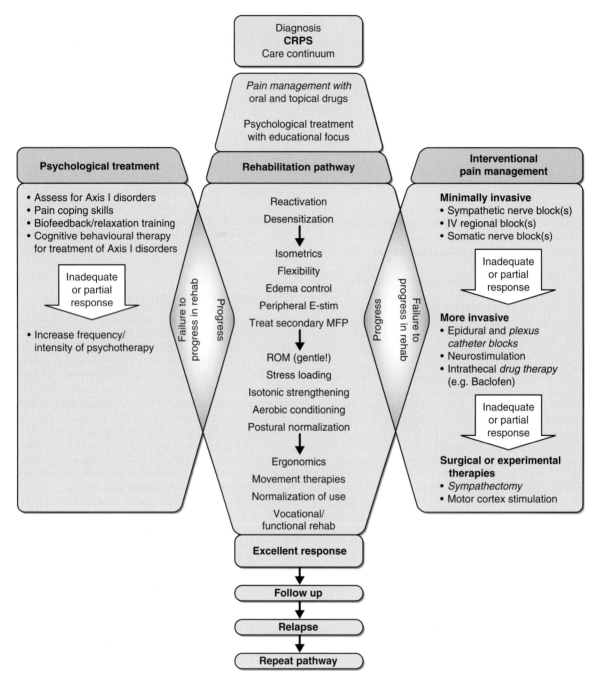

Fig. 10.1 IASP treatment algorithm for CRPS.
Stanton-Hicks, M.D., Burton, A.W., Bruehl, S.P., et al, 2002, An updated interdisciplinary clinical pathway for CRPS: report of an expert panel, 2002 World Institute of Pain, Pain Prac.,2, 1–16 with permission of John Wiley & Sons, © World Institute of Pain.

It is also important to empathize with the patient and reassure them that their symptoms are not imagined and can be treated. Education about the importance of full participation in therapy alongside pain management and possibly psychological treatments is essential to facilitate optimal recovery. Time spent educating is valuable to engage and motivate, to counter fear-avoidance and to develop a therapeutic alliance and rapport (Stanton-Hicks et al 1998). The patient should be encouraged to continue to engage the body part in normal functional activities where possible, whilst avoiding exacerbation of symptoms. Pacing of activities should be discussed.

Motivation is an integral part of the recovery process and an important component of the therapist's role. It is achieved through positive reinforcement, encouragement, education and SMART goal setting, working with the patient to pick appropriate short- and long-term goals, and breaking goals down into smaller subsections as required.

Management of pain

It is essential to explain that concurrent medication, taken regularly and not as needed, facilitates rehabilitation and recovery. The exact methods will differ depending on whether the patient has acute or chronic CRPS. If there is any doubt, liaison with the treating doctor or pain management team is recommended, especially if the therapist is the first-line practitioner. In some areas there will be locally agreed pathways of care.

TENS can be a useful pain-relieving adjunct to therapy (see Chapter 14). It can be used by the patient and may reduce treatment dependency. The use of TENS is advised by Stanton-Hicks et al (1998, 2002) based on consensus, but Daly and Bialocerkowski (2008) state that there is no evidence to support the effectiveness of TENS. Empirically, some patients gain great benefit from its application.

Medication

The following review is based on evidence-based guidelines drawn up by a multidisciplinary task force (Perez et al 2010) unless stated otherwise. The use of specialist medications and invasive methods of drug delivery fall outside the scope of this text.

The evidence for paracetamol, NSAIDs and opioids was either absent or insufficient, but it should be noted that empirical reports from experts suggests that NSAIDs and opioids can be effective to control pain (Baron 2006a). Six hundred to 1800 mg of gabapentin taken daily for the first 8 weeks was shown to reduce pain, and gabapentin might also reduce sensory abnormalities. Unfortunately no evidence was found for the use of other anticonvulsants such as pregabalin and carbamazepine. Although tricyclic antidepressants may be used for the neuropathic component of CRPS, the task force found no studies to justify its use.

Corticosteroids have been reported as effective in reducing symptoms. It is unclear how to determine dosage and duration of treatment in chronic cases, but 10 mg of oral prednisolone three times a day has been shown to help CRPS of up to 13 weeks' duration (Christensen et al 1982). Bisphosphonates can reduce inflammatory signs and pain in CRPS, especially in the early phases (Oaklander 2005). Dimethylsulphoxide cream (50%) has a beneficial effect on symptoms, especially CRPS that is mainly warm, while *N*-acetylcysteine appears to be more effective for CRPS that is mainly cold.

The treatment of motor symptoms with oral muscle relaxants has been reported as beneficial in a few patients, but the numbers are insufficient to be able to make recommendations. Botox injections have often been reported to be ineffective.

Finally, there is some indication that vitamin C may be effective in preventing CRPS (Besse et al 2009; Zolinger et al 2007). While most clinicians are presented with CRPS when it is already established, vitamin C may be introduced as a prophylactic measure in future.

Desensitization

Desensitization can use any form of non-noxious sensory stimulation, but its effectiveness is specific to the somatosensory modality used (Allen et al 2004). The aim is to help restore normal sensory processing (Stanton-Hicks et al 1998) and the process was described in Part 1. *Graded exposure* is a form of functional desensitization that has been used in the treatment of chronic CRPS.

Oedema management

Oedema can be managed in a number of ways, often using a range of modalities (Boscheinen-Morrin & Conolly 2001; Clemens & Foss-Campbell 1993; Hunter et al 1995; Li et al 2005; Palmada et al 1999; Prosser & Conolly 2003; Rho et al 2002; Stanton-Hicks et al 2002):

- *Elevation* reduces oedema by increasing venous and lymphatic flow.
- *Retrograde massage* increases venous and lymphatic return. The massage must be applied gently, in order not to shut down venous and lymphatic drainage.
- *Compression* can be provided in the form of gloves or bandages. It works by reinforcing body tissue hydrostatic pressure (HP) and facilitating venous and lymphatic flow.
- *Active exercise* stimulates the muscle pump and increases blood flow, thus reducing oedema.
- *Contrast baths*. The application of alternating hot and cold therapy alters afferent input, resulting in a decrease in pain and an increase in HP. Caution must be exercised if the patient has thermal allodynia.
- *Splinting* can aid reduction of oedema in the hand through optimal placement of joints and soft tissues. Position of safe immobilization (POSI) splinting maintains soft tissue length and can prevent or help treatment of joint contractures. If the patient is at risk of developing contractures, splinting can be used prophylactically.

Range of movement and exercise

Stanton-Hicks et al (2002) emphasize the importance of starting with adequate analgesia then working on flexibility with active exercise. The efficacy of active range of motion (AROM) exercises has been well documented

(Boscheinen-Morrin & Conolly 2001; Hunter et al 1995; Li et al 2005; Prosser & Conolly 2003). AROM exercises are performed to maintain tendon gliding and supple joints, and to minimize adhesions (Clemens & Foss-Campbell 1993). It is important that the exercise programme is tailored to the individual and does not exacerbate pain (Atkins 2003; Li et al 2005). Stanton-Hicks et al (1998, 2002) and Rho et al (2002) also suggest introducing isometric exercises alongside AROM in the early stages. It is important to avoid aggressive or passive ROM treatment (Stanton-Hicks et al 1998).

The consensus guidelines (Rho et al 2002; Stanton-Hicks et al 1998, 2002) describe a gradual progression of AROM and isotonic strengthening, followed by stretching, stress loading (see below), postural normalization and general aerobic conditioning. The exercise programme provided should address all joints with active or passive limitation, whilst maintaining a focus on functional movements. Progression should occur when the patient can comfortably achieve exercise tasks at their current level. When trauma is the initiating event, the exercises initiated should be appropriate for the stage of healing.

Muscle strengthening starts with isometric exercises. When progressing to isotonic exercise, traditional equipment for strengthening can be used. Functional strengthening tasks and vocationally related training activities should not be overlooked as they facilitate an increase in strength and function concurrently, and can be very motivating. Aerobic conditioning and core muscle training can promote general well-being and function, assist with feelings of low mood, and promote strength and stability.

Hydrotherapy can be very useful. In the early stages water can assist exercise and promote weightbearing, whilst also acting to reduce oedema. Later water can be used to resist movement, to exercise aerobically and to promote strength and stability.

Stress loading, also known as *scrub and carry*, is a process of 'active traction and compression exercises that provide stressful stimuli to the extremity without joint motion' (Watson & Carlson 1987). The stress-loading programme was developed through clinical experience and was designed to be used in isolation, before other therapies. Watson and Carlson (1987) describe a regime of *scrubbing* plywood with a bristle brush for 3 minutes, three times a day in four-point kneeling or on a table with the shoulder directly above the hand and *carrying* a purse or briefcase of 1–5 lb in weight (as tolerated by the patient) 'whenever standing or walking'. The authors describe improvement of symptoms in 5 days for the average patient, although they explain to patients that symptoms may increase at first. To progress the treatment, duration of scrubbing and the weight being carried are gradually increased. Other modalities are introduced as the pain subsides (Watson & Carlson 1987).

The stress-loading regime tends to be used as an adjunct to other therapies, especially when CRPS develops early after a traumatic injury when the tissue does not have sufficient tensile strength to safely load and traction it. In this case active exercise is more likely to be safe. Stress loading is recommended as part of the package of care available to a patient with CRPS and as a progression of treatment rather than a starting point (Rho et al 2002; Stanton-Hicks et al 2002).

Addressing cortical changes

The techniques available to specifically address cortical changes associated with CRPS are based mainly on mirror therapy, the graded motor imagery (GMI) programme and observed tactile discrimination.

Mirror therapy

This approach was developed by Ramachandran (1998) in the treatment of phantom limb pain and first used for

---

Box 10.7 Key principles of mirror therapy

In practice mirror therapy involves placing the affected limb behind a mirror that is freestanding and large enough to obscure the affected body part, or inside a mirror box. The unaffected limb is placed in front of the mirror, creating an image of the other limb as the reflection. Once this position has been assumed, the patient is asked to concentrate fully on the reflection in the mirror and to perform active range of movement exercises, rehabilitation activities or functional tasks. Any activity is possible with the mirror, but it is recommended that activities are based on the patient's individual needs, their interests and their capabilities at the time.

General principles are as follows.

- Use of the mirror must not provoke pain.
- It is alright to use unilateral movements of the unaffected limb (with the affected limb staying completely at rest).
- Bilateral movements, rehabilitation activities or functional tasks performed using the mirror *must* be symmetrical.
- Mirror exercises need focused concentration from the individual.
- Exercises of short duration performed frequently throughout the day are more effective. Research protocols that have been used vary from 5 to 15 minutes' duration, three to nine times a day (Grunert-Pluss et al 2008; McCabe et al 2003; Moseley 2004b, 2005; Selles et al 2008; Tichelaar et al 2006).
- It is best to agree a treatment regime with the patient: 5–10 minutes five times a day is likely to have great benefit.
- Full concentration from the patient during each session is important, and frequency not duration gains the best results.

CRPS by McCabe et al (2003). The focus was on correcting a presumed disruption of normal interaction between motor intention and sensory feedback (McCabe et al 2003). Mirror therapy was found to be effective only in the treatment of acute CRPS (McCabe et al 2003). Mirror movements (see below) may work by reconciling sensory feedback with motor output (Moseley 2005). Visual feedback of the affected hand is replaced with that of the (reflected) unaffected hand (Moseley 2004b). Mirror therapy as a treatment modality for pain reduction and in CRPS has been further investigated by many authors, with work by McCabe et al (2003) and Moseley (2004 a,b, 2005) being most robust.

When using mirror therapy in isolation, the patient must be assessed fully with the mirror to ensure no exacerbation of pain (see Box 10.7). If any pain is elicited, unilateral unaffected limb activities can be tried. If this still causes pain or an increase in other signs or symptoms of CRPS, the GMI should be used. Moseley et al (2008a) state that mirror therapy is more likely to be effective as part of GMI than in isolation. For an appraisal of research of mirror therapy and its theoretical underpinning see Moseley et al (2008a).

Graded motor imagery

GMI is a specific programme for the cortical retraining of rehabilitation activities (Box 10.8). The order in which the activities are performed to obtain pain relief has been researched by Moseley et al (2004b). The mechanism is thought to be the sequential activation of pre-motor and motor networks, followed by reconciliation of sensory feedback and motor output through mirror movements (Moseley et al 2008b).

Moseley (2005) researched the components in varying orders and reached the following conclusions:

- Laterality decreases neuropathic pain scale scores irrespective of its order in GMI.
- The order of mirror therapy and imagined movements was found to be important.
- Imagined movements only imparted an effect when they followed laterality.
- Mirror therapy only imparted an effect when it followed imagined movements.
- Results are consistent with sequential activation of cortical motor networks.

For further reading on GMI the reader is directed to Moseley (2004b, 2006) and www.gradedmotorimagery.com.

In CRPS the extent of primary somatosensory reorganization correlates with the magnitude of pain (Moseley 2005). Although pain and swelling caused by imagined movement alone has been described, extensive pilot work was unable to confirm this (Moseley 2004a). Recognizing right/left hand activates pre-motor cortices (Moseley 2004a). The neurones associated with movement preparation are

---

> **Box 10.8 Practical application of graded motor imagery**
>
> GMI consists of three stages (Moseley 2004b, 2005). In studies each stage has been performed for 2 weeks before progressing to the next stage, but the optimal frequency and duration for clinical practice have not been established.
>
> 1. Recognition of hand laterality, shown to activate the pre-motor cortices. The patient uses a pack of 56 cards (see www.noigroup.com) showing hands in random orientations. They look at each card and put it on the left or right according to the hand shown. The time taken to complete the task and the number of cards placed incorrectly are recorded to chart progress.
> 2. Imagined hand movements, shown to activate the primary motor cortex. The patient is shown a picture of a hand and has to imagine adopting the position shown.
> 3. Mirror movements. The patient uses the mirror box to perform bilateral tasks according to the hand position shown in pictures. They adopt the postures on each picture slowly and smoothly. In clinical practice mirror movements are used as described in the mirror therapy section.
>
> The clinician is advised to agree a programme with the patient, emphasizing the importance of frequency of activity. As with mirror therapy a treatment regime of 5–10 minutes five times a day is likely to have great benefit.

---

activated *before* those associated with movement execution and this is the basis of the GMI sequencing.

GMI has been shown to reduce pain and swelling in subjects with long-standing CRPS, using a homogeneous wrist fracture group (Moseley 2004b). The results of a randomized controlled trial showed that GMI reduced pain and disability in patients with CRPS type 1 and phantom limb pain (Moseley 2006).

In summary, the efficacy of mirror therapy in isolation has been demonstrated in the treatment of acute CRPS. In the treatment of chronic conditions its use is supported only as part of a graded motor imagery programme.

Observed tactile discrimination

In CRPS decreased tactile acuity is related to reorganization of the primary sensory cortex and to pain (Moseley & Weich 2009), while tactile training may increase tactile acuity and reduce pain (Moseley et al 2008a). Moseley et al (2008a) demonstrated that discrimination of the location and diameter of tactile stimuli applied to the affected limb of patients with unilateral CRPS can decrease pain and the two-point discrimination (TPD) threshold, whereas tactile stimulation alone cannot. Focusing one's attention on the stimulated area increased S1 response to touch and improved tactile performance (Moseley et al 2008a). Moseley and Weich (2009) further demonstrated that a single 30-minute tactile discrimination session led to a sustained improvement in tactile acuity if the CRPS patients looked towards the affected limb during the training, while watching the skin of the opposite body part in a mirror.

Functional tasks and workshop activities

A functional activity programme aids return to work, sport or simple domestic tasks (Prosser & Conolly 2003). Functional, goal-orientated tasks increase motivation and can enhance self-esteem (Palmada et al 1999). The clinician is advised to agree functional SMART goals with the patient, and grade them as appropriate.

Aids and adaptations, used with due consideration, can be helpful to promote independence (see Part 1). Workshop activities can engage a patient and promote functional use of the affected limb. Activities relating to a patient's hobbies or work tasks should be a priority. Stanton-Hicks et al (1998) emphasize the importance of vocational rehabilitation with work hardening. It is valuable to liaise with the individual's workplace to discuss appropriate tasks.

CONCLUSION

Neuropathic pain and CRPS can be difficult to diagnose and even harder to treat. Armed with an understanding of possible underlying mechanisms and a systematic approach to assessment and reasoning, clinicians can avoid some of the pitfalls of diagnosing these conditions. The diagnosis, a range of therapeutic options and a flexible mind can make a real difference to patients.

Q Self-test questions

1. Why could the presentation of neuropathy be paradoxical?
2. Name three ways to clinically decide whether a pain is likely to be nociceptive or neuropathic.
3. Name three ways to manage or treat neuropathic pain.
4. Are CRPS symptoms considered proportionate to the inciting event?
5. What are the four main subgroups for diagnosis of CRPS?
6. Describe two forms of objective assessment for each of the four subgroups.
7. Name three types of motor or trophic changes in CRPS.

REFERENCES

Abram, S., 1990. Incidence-hypothesis-epidemiology. In: Stanton-Hicks, M. (Ed.), Pain and the sympathetic nervous system. Kluwer Academic Publishers, Boston, pp. 1–16.

Allen, R.J., Wu, C., Horiuchi, G., et al., 2004. Pressure desensitization effects on pressure tolerance and function in patients with complex regional pain syndrome. Orthopaedic Physical Therapy Practice 16 (4), 13–16.

Atkins, R.M., 2003. Aspects of current management: complex regional pain syndrome. J. Bone Joint Surg. 85 (B), 1100–1106.

Baccei, M., Fitzgerald, M., 2006. Development of pain pathways and mechanisms. In: McMahon, S., Koltzenburg, M. (Eds.), Wall and Melzack's Textbook of Pain, fifth ed. Churchill Livingstone, Edinburgh, pp. 143–158.

Baron, R., 2006a. Complex regional pain syndromes. In: McMahon, S.,

Koltzenburg, M. (Eds.), Wall and Melzack's Textbook of Pain, fifth ed. Churchill Livingstone, Edinburgh, pp. 1011–1027.

Baron, R., 2006b. Mechanisms of disease: neuropathic pain – a clinical perspective. Nat. Rev. Neurosci. 2 (2), 95–106.

Basbaum, A., Jessell, T., 2000. The perception of pain. In: Kandel, E., Schwartz, J., Jessell, T. (Eds.), Principles of neural science, fourth ed. McGraw-Hill, New York, pp. 472–491.

Bear-Lehman, J., Abreu, B.C., 1989. Evaluating the hand: Issues in reliability and validity. Phys. Ther. 69, 1025–1033.

Bennett, M., Attal, N., Backonja, M., et al., 2007. Using screening tools to identify neuropathic pain. Pain 127 (3), 199–203.

Besse, J.L., Gadeyne, S., Galand-Desme, S., et al., 2009. Effect of vitamin C on prevention of CRPS

type 1 in foot and ankle surgery. Foot and Ankle Surgery 15, 179–182.

Birklein, F., Skumavc, M., Spitzer, A., et al., 1997. Sudomotor function in sympathetic reflex dystrophy. Pain 69 (1), 49–54.

Black, J., Dib-Hajj, S., Cummins, T., et al., 2002. Sodium channels as therapeutic targets in neuropathic pain. In: Hansson, P.T., Fields, H.L., Hill, R.G., Marchettini, P. et al., (Eds.), Neuropathic Pain: Pathophysiology and Treatment. IASP Press, Seattle, pp. 19–36.

Boscheinen-Morrin, J., Conolly, W.B., 2001. The hand: Fundamentals of therapy, third ed. Butterworth-Heinemann, Oxford.

British Pain Society, 2008. A case of neuropathic pain. British Pain Society, Royal College of General Practitioners, London.

Bruehl, S., Lubenow, T.R., Nath, H., et al., 1996. Validation of thermography in the diagnosis of reflex sympathetic dystrophy. Clin. J. Pain 12, 316–325.

Bruehl, S., Harden, R.N., Galer, B.S., et al., 1999. External validation of IASP diagnostic criteria for Complex Regional Pain Syndrome and proposed research diagnostic criteria. Pain 81, 147–154.

Burr, N., Pratt, A.L., Stott, D., 2003. Inter-rater and intra-rater reliability when measuring interphalangeal joints: comparison between three hand-held goniometers. Physiotherapy 89 (11), 641–652.

Christensen, K., Jensen, E.M., Noer, I., 1982. The reflex dystrophy syndrome response to treatment with systemic corticosteroids. Acta Chirurgica Scand. 148, 653–655.

Ciccone, D., Bandilla, E., Wu, W., 1997. Psychological dysfunction in patients with reflex sympathetic dystrophy. Pain 71 (3), 323–333.

Clemens, S., Foss-Campbell, B., 1993. Rehabilitation following traumatic hand injury: Hand therapist's perspective. Part 1: Acute phase of hand rehabilitation. Plast. Surg. Nurs. 13 (3), 129–134.

Coldham, F., Lewis, J., Lee, H., 2006. The reliability of one vs. three grip trials in symptomatic and asymptomatic subjects. J Hand Ther. 19 (3), 318–327.

Covington, E., 1996. Psychological issues in reflex sympathetic dystrophy. In: Stanton-Hicks, M., Jänig, W. (Eds.), Reflex Sympathetic Dystrophy: A Reappraisal, vol. 6. IASP Press, Seattle, pp. 191–216.

Daly, A.E., Bialocerkowski, A.E., 2008. Does evidence support physiotherapy management of adult complex regional pain syndrome type one? A systematic review. Eur. J. Pain 13, 339–353.

de Morree, J., 1989. Dynamiek van het menselijk bindweefsel. Functie, beschadiging en herstel. Bohn, Scheltema & Holkema, Utrecht.

Devor, M., 2006. Response of nerves to injury in relation to neuropathic pain. In: McMahon, S., Koltzenburg, M. (Eds.), Wall and Melzack's Textbook of Pain, fifth ed. Churchill Livingstone, Edinburgh, pp. 905–928.

Devor, M., Lomazov, P., Matzner, O., 1994. Sodium channel accumulation in injured axons as a substrate for neuropathic pain. In: Boivie, J., Hansson, P., Lindblom, U. (Eds.),

Touch, temperature, and pain in health and disease:mechanisms and assessment. IASP Press, Seattle, pp. 207–230.

Dickenson, A., Bee, L., 2008. Neurobiological mechanisms of neuropathic pain and its treatment. In: Castro-Lopes, J., Raja, S., Schmelz, M. (Eds.), Pain 2008. An updated review. IASP Press, Seattle, pp. 277–286.

Dommerholt, J., 2004. Clinical management: CRPS. Complex regional pain syndrome – 2: Physical Therapy Management. Journal of Bodywork and Movement Therapies 8 (4), 241–248.

Dray, A., 2008. Neuropathic pain: emerging treatments. Br. J. Anaesth. 101, 48–58.

Dworkin, R., O'Connor, A., Backonja, M., et al., 2007. Pharmacologic management of neuropathic pain: evidence based recommendations. Pain 132, 237–251.

Dworkin, R., Turk, D., Revicki, D., et al., 2009. Development and initial validation of an expanded and revised version of the Short-form McFill Pain Questionnaire (SF-MPQ-2). Pain 144 (1,2), 35–42.

Flor, H., Braun, C., Elbert, T., et al., 1997. Extensive reorganisation of primary somatosensory cortex in chronic back pain patients. Neurosci. Lett. 224, 5–8.

Galer, B.S., Bruehl, S., Harden, N., 1998. IASP diagnostic criteria for Complex Regional Pain Syndrome: A preliminary empirical validation study (review article). Clin. J. Pain 14 (1), 48–54.

Galer, B., Jensen, M., Ma, T., et al., 2002. The lidocaine patch 5% effectively treats all neuropathic pain qualities: results of a randomized, double-blind, vehicle-controlled, 3-week efficacy study with use of the Neuropathic Pain Scale. Clin. J. Pain 18, 297–301.

Glassey, N., 2001. A study of the effect of night extension splintage on post-fasceictomy Dupuytren's patients. British Journal of Hand Therapy. 6 (3), 89–94.

Goebel, A., Barker, C., Turner-Stokes, L., et al., 2012. Complex regional pain syndrome in adults: UK guidelines for diagnosis, referral and management in primary and secondary care. Royal College of Physicians, London.

Groeneweg, G., Huygen, F., Coderre, T., et al., 2009. Regulation of peripheral blood flow in Complex Regional Pain Syndrome: clinical implication for symptomatic relief and pain management. BMC Musculoskelet. Disord. 10, 116.

Grunert-Pluss, N., Hufschmid, U., Santschi, L., et al., 2008. Mirror therapy in hand rehabilitation: A review of the literature, the St Gallen protocol for mirror therapy and evaluation of a case series of 52 patients. British Journal of Hand Therapy 13 (1), 4–9.

Hansson, P., 1994. Possibilities and potential pitfalls of combined bedside and quantitative somatosensory analysis in pain patients. In: Boivie, J., Hansson, P., Lindblom, U. (Eds.), Touch, temperature, and pain in health and disease: mechanisms and assessments. IASP Press, Seattle, pp. 113–132.

Hansson, P., Kinnman, E., 1996. Unmasking mechanisms of peripheral neuropathic pain in a clinical perspective. Pain Reviews. 3 (4), 272–292.

Hansson, P., Lacerenza, M., Marchettini, P., 2002. Aspects of clinical and experimental neuropathic pain: the clinical perspective. In: Hansson, P.T., Fields, H.L., Hill, R.G., Marchettini, P. et al. (Eds.), Neuropathic Pain: Pathophysiology and Treatment. IASP Press, Seattle, pp. 1–18.

Hansson, P., Backonja, M., Bouhassira, D., 2007. Usefulness and limitations of quantitative sensory testing: Clinical and research application in neuropathic pain states. Pain 129 (3), 256–259.

Harden, R., Bruehl, S., 2005. Diagnostic criteria: the statistical derivation of the four criterion factors. In: Wilson, P., Stanton-Hicks, M., Harden, R. (Eds.), CRPS: current diagnosis and therapy. IASP Press, Seattle, pp. 45–58.

Harden, R.N., Bruehl, S., Galer, B.S., et al., 1999. Complex Regional Pain Syndrome: Are the diagnostic criteria valid and sufficiently comprehensive? Pain 83, 211–219.

Harden, R., Bruehl, S., Perez, R., et al., 2010. Validation of proposed diagnostic criteria (the 'Budapest Criteria') for Complex Regional

Pain Syndrome. Pain 150 (2), 268–274.

Hayek, S.M., Mekhail, N.A., 2004. Complex regional pain syndrome: redefining reflex sympathetic dystrophy and causalgia. The Physician and Sportsmedicine 32, 5.

Hunter, J.M., Mackin, E.J., Callahan, A.D., 1995. Rehabilitation of the hand: Surgery and therapy, fourth ed. Mosby, St Louis.

International Association for the Study of Pain, 2011. IASP Taxonomy. http://www.iasp-pain.org/Content/NavigationMenu/GeneralResourceLinks/PainDefinitions/default.htm.

Jänig, W., Baron, R., 2002. The role of the sympathetic nervous system in neuropathic pain: clinical observations and animal models. In: Hansson, P.T., Fields, H.L., Hill, R.G., Marchettini, P. et al. (Eds.), Neuropathic Pain: Pathophysiology and Treatment. IASP Press, Seattle, pp. 125–149.

Jänig, W., Baron, R., 2003. Complex regional pain syndrome: mystery explained? Lancet Neurol. 2, 687–697.

Jänig, W., Baron, R., 2006. Is CRPS 1 a neuropathic pain syndrome? Pain 120 (3), 227–229.

Jensen, T.S., 2002. An improved understanding of neuropathic pain. Eur. J. Pain 6 (Suppl. B), 3–11.

Jensen, T., 2008. Management of neuropathic pain. In: Castro-Lopes, J., Raja, S., Schmelz, M. (Eds.), Pain 2008. An updated review. IASP Press, Seattle, pp. 287–295.

Jessell, T., Sanes, J., 2000. The generation and survival of nerve cells. In: Kandel, E., Schwartz, J., Jessell, T. (Eds.), Principles of neural science, fourth ed. McGraw-Hill, New York, pp. 1041–1062.

Juottonen, K., Gockel, M., Silen, T., et al., 2002. Altered central sensorimotor processing in patients with complex regional pain syndrome. Pain 98 (3), 315–323.

Keysers, C., Wicker, B., Gazzola, V., et al., 2004. A touching sight: SII/PV activation during the observation and experience of touch. Neuron 42, 335–346.

Kingery, W., 1997. A critical review of controlled clinical trials for peripheral neuropathic pain and complex regional pain syndromes. Pain 73 (2), 123–139.

Kingery, W., Davies, M., Clark, J., 2003. A substance P receptor (NK1) antagonist can reverse vascular and nociceptive abnormalities in a rat model of complex regional pain syndrome type II. Pain 104 (1), 75–84.

Krakousky, A., 2005. Complex pain syndrome and functional rehabilitation. Acta Physcologia. 19 (4), 390.

Li, Z., Paterson-Smith, B., Smith, T.L., et al., 2005. Diagnosis and management of complex regional pain syndrome complicating upper extremity recovery. J. Hand Ther. 18 (2), 270–277.

Lundborg, G., 2008. Lund University Faculty of Medicine. http://www.med.lu.se/klinvetmalmo/hand_surgery/clinical_projects/enhanced_sensory_relearning (accessed 04.02.10).

Lundborg, G., Rosen, B., 2007. Hand function after nerve repair. Acta Physiol. 189, 207–217.

MacAvoy, M.C., Green, D.P., 2007. Critical reappraisal of Medical Research Council muscle testing for elbow flexion. J. Hand Surg. 32A, 149–153.

Maier, C., Baron, R., Tölle, T., et al., 2010. Quantitative sensory testing in the German Research Network on Neuropathic Pain (DNFS): somatosensory abnormalities in 1236 patients with different neuropathic pain syndromes. Pain 150 (3), 439–450.

Marchand, F., Perretti, M., McMahon, S., 2005. Role of the immune system in chronic pain. Nat. Rev. Neurosci. 6, 521–532.

Massy-Westropp, N., Rankin, W., Ahern, M., et al., 2004. Measuring grip strength in normal adults: reference ranges and a comparison of electronic and hydraulic instruments. J. Hand Surg. 29 (3), 514–519.

McCabe, C.S., Haigh, R.C., Ring, E.F.J., et al., 2003. A controlled pilot study of the utility of visual feedback in the treatment of complex regional pain syndrome (type 1). Rheumatology 42, 97–101.

MacDermid, J., 2005. Measurement of health outcomes following tendon and nerve repair. J. Hand Ther. 18 (2), 297–312.

Merskey, H., Lindblom, U., Mumford, J., et al., 1994. Pain terms, a current list with definitions and notes on usage. In: Merskey, H., Bogduk, N. (Eds.),

Classification of chronic pain. IASP Press, Seattle, pp. 207–214.

Moseley, G.L., 2004a. Imagined movements cause pain and swelling in a patient with complex regional pain syndrome. Neurology 62, 1644.

Moseley, G.L., 2004b. Graded motor imagery is effective for long-standing complex regional pain syndrome: a randomized controlled trial. Pain 108 (1,2), 192–198.

Moseley, G.L., 2005. Is successful rehabilitation of complex regional pain syndrome due to sustained attention to the affected limb? A randomised clinical trial. Pain 114, 54–61.

Moseley, G.L., 2006. Graded motor imagery for pathologic pain: a randomized controlled trial. Neurology 67 (12), 2129–2134.

Moseley, G.L., Weich, K., 2009. The effect of tactile discrimination training is enhanced when patients watch the reflected image of their unaffected limb during training. Pain 144, 314–319.

Moseley, G., Gallace, A., Spence, C., 2008a. Is mirror therapy all it is cracked up to be? Current evidence and future directions. Pain 138 (1), 7–10.

Moseley, G.L., Zalucki, N.M., Wiech, K., 2008b. Tactile discrimination, but not tactile stimulation alone, reduces chronic limb pain. Pain 137, 600–608.

Oaklander, A.L., 2005. Evidence-based pharmacotherapy for CRPS and related conditions. In: Wilson, P.R., Stanton-Hicks, M., Harden, R.N. (Eds.), CRPS: current diagnosis and therapy. IASP Press, Seattle.

Oaklander, A., Fields, H., 2009. Is reflex sympathetic dystrophy/complex regional pain syndrome type I a small-fibre neuropathy? Ann. Neurol. 65, 629–638.

Oaklander, A., Rissmiller, J., Gelman, L., et al., 2006. Evidence of focal small-fibre axonal degeneration in complex regional pain syndrome-I (reflex sympathetic dystrophy). Pain 120 (3), 235–243.

O'Connor, A., 2009. Neuropathic pain: a review of the quality of life impact, costs, and cost-effectiveness of therapy. Pharmacoeconomics 27 (2), 95–112.

Palmada, M., Shah, S., O'Hare, K., 1999. Hand oedema: Pathophysiology and treatment. British Journal of Hand Therapy 4 (1), 26–32.

Perez, R., Zollinger, P., Dijkstra, P., et al., CRPS1 Task Force, 2010. Evidence based guidelines for complex regional pain syndrome type 1. BMC Neurol. 10, 20.

Pratt, A.L., Burr, N., 2001. A review of goniometry use within current hand therapy practice. British Journal of Hand Therapy 6 (2), 45–49.

Prosser, R., Conolly, W.B., 2003. Rehabilitation of the Hand and Upper Limb. Butterworth-Heinemann, Oxford.

Puchalski, P., Zyluk, A., 2005. Complex regional pain syndrome type 1 after fractures of the distal radius: A prospective study of the role of psychological factors. J. Hand Surg. 30 (6), 574–580.

Ramachandran, V., 1998. Phantoms in the brain. Fourth Estate Limited, London.

Reedijk, W., van Rijn, M., Roelofs, K., et al., 2008. Psychological features of patients with complex regional pain syndrome type I related dystonia. Mov. Disord. 23 (11), 1551–1559.

Rho, R.H., Brewer, R.P., Lamer, T.J., et al., 2002. Complex regional pain syndrome. Mayo Clin. Proc. 77, 174–180.

Rhodes, C., 2011. Update on therapies for neuropathic pain. The Pain Practitioner Fall Issue 44–47.

Rommel, O., Gehling, M., Dertwinkel, R., et al., 1999. Hemisensory impairment in patients with complex regional pain syndrome. Pain 80 (1,2), 95–101.

Rommel, O., Malin, J., Zenz, M., et al., 2001. Quantitative sensory testing, neurophysiological and psychological examination in patients with complex regional pain syndrome and hemisensory deficits. Pain 8 (1), 279–293.

Rosen, B., Balkenius, C., Lundborg, G., 2003. Sensory re-education today and tomorrow: A review of evolving concepts. British Journal of Hand Therapy 8 (2), 48–56.

Rosen, B., Bjorkman, A., Lundborg, G., 2006. Improved sensory relearning after nerve repair induced by selective temporary anaesthesia – a new concept in hand rehabilitation. J. Hand Surg. 31B, 126–132.

Ross, E., 2004. Peripheral neuropathy. In: Ross, E. (Ed.), Pain management. Hanley & Belfus, Philadelphia, pp. 81–89.

Selles, R.W., Schreuders, T.A.R., Stam, H.J., 2008. Mirror therapy in

patients with causalgia (complex regional pain syndrome type II) following peripheral nerve injury: two cases. J. Rehabil. Med. 40, 312–314.

Stanton-Hicks, M., Janig, W., Hassenbuch, S., et al., 1995. Reflex Sympathetic Dystrophy: Changing concepts and taxonomy. Pain 63, 127–133.

Stanton-Hicks, M.D., Baron, R., Boas, R., et al., 1998. Complex Regional Pain Syndromes: Guidelines for therapy (consensus report). Clin. J. Pain 14 (2), 155–166.

Stanton-Hicks, M.D., Burton, A.W., Bruehl, S.P., et al., 2002. An updated interdisciplinary clinical pathway for CRPS: Report of an expert panel. Pain Pract. 2 (1), 1–16.

Thomas, R.J., Degnan, G.G., 2005. Managing complex regional pain syndrome. Journal of Musculoskeletal Medicine 22, 514–526.

Tichelaar, Y.I.G.V., Geertzen, J.H.B., Keizer, D., et al., 2006. Mirror box therapy added to cognitive behavioural therapy in three chronic complex regional pain syndrome type I patients: a pilot study. Int. J. Rehabil. Res. 30, 181–188.

Uematsu, S., Hendler, N., Hungerford, D., et al., 1981. Thermography and electromyography in the differential diagnosis of chronic pain syndromes and reflex sympathetic dystrophy. Electromyogr. Clin. Neurophysiol. 2, 165–182.

Van de Vusse, A.C., Stomp-van den Berg, S.G.M., de Vet, H.C.W., et al., 2003. Interobserver reliability of diagnosis in patients with Complex Regional Pain Syndrome. Eur. J. Pain 7, 259–265.

van Griensven, H., 2005. Pain in practice. Theory and treatment strategies for manual therapists. Butterworth Heinemann, Oxford, p. 49.

van Hilten, J., Blumberg, H., Schwartzman, R., 2005. Factor IV: movement disorders and dystrophy – pathophysiology and measurement. In: Wilson, P., Stanton-Hicks, M., Harden, R. (Eds.), CRPS: current diagnosis and therapy. IASP Press, Seattle, pp. 119–137.

Veldman, P., Reynen, H., Arntz, I., et al., 1993. Signs and symptoms of reflex sympathetic dystrophy: prospective

study of 829 patients. Lancet 342 (8878), 1012–1016.

Wasner, G., Baron, R., 2005. Factor II: vasomotor changes – pathophysiology and measurement. In: Wilson, P., Stanton-Hicks, M., Harden, R. (Eds.), CRPS: current diagnosis and therapy. IASP Press, Seattle, pp. 81–106.

Watson, H., Carlson, L., 1987. Treatment of reflex sympathetic dystrophy of the hand with an active "stress loading" program. J. Hand Sung. 12A (2pt1), 779–785.

Waylett-Rendall, J., 1995. Desensitisation of the traumatised hand. In: Hunter, J., Mackin, E., Callahan, A. (Eds.), Rehabilitation of the Hand: Surgery and Therapy, fourth ed. Moseby, St Louis, pp. 693–700.

Weber, M., Birklein, F., Neundorfer, B., et al., 2001. Facilitated neurogenic inflammation in complex regional pain syndrome. Pain 91 (3), 251–257.

Weir Mitchell, S., 1872. Gunshot wounds and other injuries of nerves. Lippincott, Philadelphia.

Wilson, P., 1990. Sympathetically maintained pain: diagnosis, measurement, and efficacy of treatment. In: Stanton-Hicks, M. (Ed.), Pain and the sympathetic nervous system. Kluwer Academic Publishers, Boston, pp. 91–123.

Wilson, P.R., Stanton-Hicks, M., Harden, R.N. (Eds.), 2005. CRPS: current diagnosis and therapy. IASP Press, Seattle.

Woolf, C., Max, M., 2001. Mechanism-based pain diagnosis: issues for analgesic drug development. Anesthesiology 95 (1), 241–249.

Wynn-Parry, C.B., 1980. Sensory rehabilitation of the hand. Aust. N. Z. J. Surg. 50 (3), 224–227.

Zhongyu, L., Paterson-Smith, B., Smith, T.L., et al., 2005. Diagnosis and management of complex regional pain syndrome complicating upper extremity recovery. J. Hand Ther. 18, 270–277.

Zolinger, P., Tuinebreijer, W., Breederveld, R., et al., 2007. Can vitamin C prevent complex regional pain syndrome in patients with wrist fracture? J. Bone Joint Surg. 89, 1424–1431.

Chapter | **11** |

Pain pharmacology and the pharmacological management of pain

Maree T. Smith and Arjun Muralidharan

OVERVIEW

In the general population, the sensation of pain is generally perceived in a negative connotation because of its association with physical damage to the body and its unpleasant affective quality (Apkarian 2008). This perception is reinforced by the International Association for the Study of Pain (IASP) definition of pain as 'an unpleasant sensory and emotional experience associated with actual or potential tissue damage, or is described in terms of such damage' (Merskey & Bogduk 1994).

Pain detection and signalling involve a complex cascade of events. Nociceptors are free nerve endings that detect potentially damaging mechanical, electrical, thermal and chemical stimuli, resulting in the generation of action potentials (Woolf & Ma 2007). These action potentials are transmitted predominantly via first-order neurons (Aδ and C fibres) to laminae I and II of the dorsal horn of the spinal cord, from where they are relayed by second-order neurons via spinothalamic tracts to higher centres in the brain (Sherrington 1906). This nociceptive input may in turn activate descending inhibitory pathways to reduce the severity of the perceived pain (Sherrington 1906). Levels of pain reported by patients comprise nociception and interpretation of its emotional significance by the anterior cingulate cortex (Rainville et al 1997).

It is well understood that the pathobiology of human pain encompasses a mosaic of biological and psychological phenotypes that are underpinned by multiple contributing factors (Diatchenko et al 2006). However, despite great advances in our collective understanding of the neurobiology of chronic pain over the last two decades, with the identification of a vast array of receptors, ion channels and enzymes as potential novel drug targets, translation of this knowledge into new pain medicines for clinical use has been painstakingly slow. For this reason, the medications currently available for prescribing by frontline clinicians for the pharmacological treatment of pain in patients are similar to those available a decade ago.

Hence, in the following sections of this chapter we provide a brief overview of receptors, ion channels and enzymes identified over the past two decades as potential novel targets for the development of the next generation of pain therapeutics. This is followed by a description of analgesic and adjuvant agents that are currently used in the clinical setting for the pharmacological treatment of pain.

Pain classification

Pain may be classified according to a number of different criteria, including duration (acute and chronic), type (nociceptive, inflammatory and neuropathic) and severity (mild, moderate and severe); the corresponding definitions are given in Table 11.1.

© 2014 Elsevier Ltd.

Table 11.1 Pain classifications and definitions

Based on duration	Based on type	Based on severity
Acute pain The IASP has defined acute pain as 'pain of recent onset and probable limited duration; it usually has an identifiable temporal and causal relationship to injury or disease' (Merskey & Bogduk 1994) Acute pain generally comprises two phases: the first phase alerts the individual to potentially dangerous stimuli and the second phase is regarded as a 'protective' mechanism characterized by 'guarding' of the injured tissue as a means of promoting healing and recovery (Merskey & Bogduk 1994) Chronic pain Chronic pain is defined as pain lasting for a long period of time It commonly persists beyond the time of healing of an injury (Merskey & Bogduk 1994) Persistent pain is often regarded as a maladaptive response that confers no physiological advantage, such that the pain state itself has become the 'disease' requiring treatment (Cousins 2007)	Nociceptive pain Nociceptive pain is caused by ongoing activation of Aδ and C nociceptors in response to a noxious stimulation of somatic or visceral structures such as that associated with trauma, surgery or heart attack Inflammatory pain Inflammatory pain is that associated with chronic inflammation such as occurs in patients with arthritis, chronic visceral pain or temporomandibular joint disorders Neuropathic pain Neuropathic pain is pain initiated or caused by a primary lesion or dysfunction in the nervous system (Merskey & Bogduk 1994) Recently, a redefinition of neuropathic pain has been proposed (Treede et al 2008), whereby neuropathic pain is defined as 'pain arising as a direct consequence of a lesion or disease affecting the somatosensory system'	1. Mild pain 2. Moderate pain 3. Severe pain Using the pain numeric rating scale (NRS), patients report their pain intensity on a 10-point scale: from 0 (no pain) to 10 (worst possible pain) On basis of pain NRS scores, pain has been categorized as mild, moderate or severe pain for score range 1–3, 4–6 and 7–10. respectively (Serlin et al 1995)

Nociceptive pain

Physiological or nociceptive pain is part of an early warning system that has evolved to instruct motor neurons of the central nervous system to produce actions that minimize further injury after detection of physical harm (Zhuo 2007). Examples of acute nociceptive pain include postoperative pain and pain following trauma with pain resolving as healing takes place.

Inflammatory pain

Inflammatory pain occurs in response to tissue injury and sensitization of nociceptors by a range of pro-inflammatory mediators that are released at the injury site. For acute inflammatory conditions, inflammatory pain resolves once the initial tissue injury heals (Reichling & Levine 2009). However, in chronic inflammatory disorders such as rheumatoid arthritis and visceral pain conditions such as chronic pancreatitis, the pain persists while inflammation is active (Michaud et al 2007).

Neuropathic pain

Neuropathic pain is a type of pain that occurs after injury to either peripheral nerves or the sensory pathways in the spinal cord or brain. It resembles inflammatory pain in that spontaneous pain and hypersensitivity are usually present,

but the underlying disease pathology is in the nervous tissue (Jensen & Finnerup 2009).

Put simply, acute nociceptive and inflammatory pains may be considered part of an alarm system warning of injury to limit movement that would otherwise exacerbate the injury and delay healing. By contrast, persistent neuropathic pain could be considered as having a defective alarm system, resulting in the sending of false alerts that are nevertheless interpreted as painful signals.

Peripheral sensitization

Following tissue and/or peripheral nerve injury, multiple chemical mediators are released, forming an 'inflammatory soup' comprising cytokines, growth factors, kinins, hydrogen ions, ATP, serotonin, histamine, neuropeptides and prostaglandins. This results in an inflammatory response and sensitization of various components of the somatosensory system (Fig. 11.1) (Thacker et al 2007). Following peripheral sensitization, there is neuronal hyperexcitability, resulting in ectopic discharge of primary afferents and the development of so-called 'central sensitization' in the spinal cord. The net result is that innocuous stimuli are detected as painful (allodynia) and/or there is a heightened response to painful stimuli either at the site of injury (primary hyperalgesia) or extending into the surrounding uninjured tissue (secondary hyperalgesia) (Vanderah 2007).

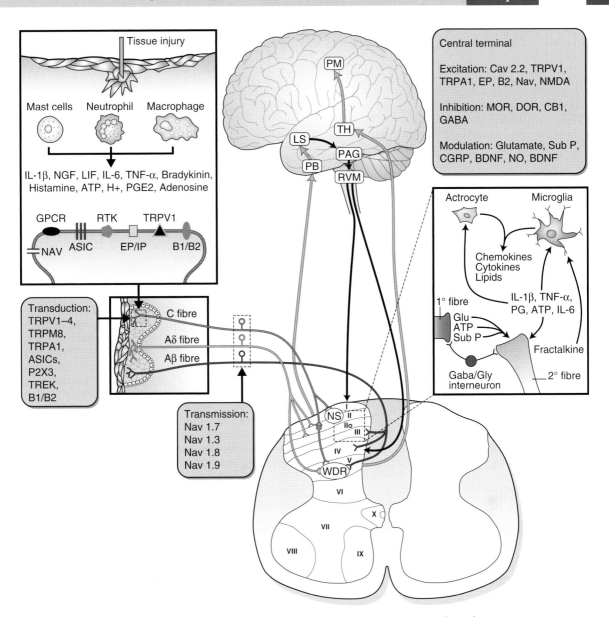

Fig. 11.1 Schematic diagram summarizing neuronal and non-neuronal mechanisms implicated in the pathobiology of chronic pain.

Multiple receptors and ion channels have been identified on the peripheral terminals of primary afferent nerve fibres, including receptors for serotonin (5-HT), bradykinin (B1 and B2), histamine, nerve growth factor (TrK_A), ATP (purinergic), epinephrine, prostaglandin E_2 (PGE_2), tumour necrosis factor alpha (TNF-α) and interleukins (IL) as well as sodium channels, acid-sensing ion channels (ASIC) and vanilloid (TRPV1) receptors (Basbaum et al 2009; Coggeshall & Carlton 1997; Sato et al 1993; Woolf & Mannion 1999). Nociceptor hyperexcitability develops after exposure to the 'proinflammatory soup' of chemical mediators released from damaged blood vessels, nerve terminals and immune cells that accumulate at the site of injury. This in turn results in activation of multiple receptors and ion channels to induce and maintain peripheral sensitization (Reichling & Levine 2009). Enhanced excitability of peripheral nerves with lowered activation thresholds and/or increased action potential frequency secondary to inflammation-induced peripheral sensitization is transduced intracellularly by kinase pathways including mitogen activated protein kinase (MAPK) such as p38 MAPK and extracellular signal related kinase (ERK) (Crown et al 2008;

Ji 2004; Zhuang et al 2005), protein kinase A (PKA) (Bhave et al 2002) and protein kinase C (PKC) (Bhave et al 2003). Activated kinases contribute to peripheral sensitization through phosphorylation and activation of multiple receptors and ion channels (Reichling & Levine 2009).

As neuropathic pain persists after ganglionectomy involving removal of the injured afferent soma, it is clear that maintenance of neuropathic pain is not dependent solely on changes that occur in injured afferents (Sheth et al 2002). A hallmark of neuropathic pain is ectopic activity in damaged primary afferents underpinned by accumulation and dysregulated function of voltage-gated sodium channels after peripheral nerve injury (Costigan et al 2009). This aberrant activity spreads rapidly to the cell bodies in the dorsal root ganglia to generate ectopic activity in adjacent undamaged sensory afferents (ephaptic transmission), which in turn leads to an expansion of the perceived painful area (receptive field). Furthermore, sympathetic efferents have been shown to activate sensory afferents via α-adrenoceptors, with these interactions between adjacent sensory and autonomic afferents and ganglion cells providing a mechanism for the spread of ectopic discharge between nerve fibre types (Zhang & Strong 2008).

More recently, satellite glial cells (SGCs), which form complete sheath-like structures around sensory neurones in the DRG, have been shown to respond to pro-inflammatory agents including ATP, nitric oxide and bradykinin (Hanani 2005). SGCs are implicated in nociceptive signalling as they express a broad range of transmitter molecules (e.g. somatostatin, NGF, BDNF, GDNF and IL-6), as well as receptors (e.g. trkA, bradykinin B2 receptors, orexin-1, somatostatin, TNF-α type-1, IL-1 and peripheral benzodiazepine receptor) and ion channels (e.g. inwardly rectifying K^+ channels) (Takeda et al 2009). Hence, SGCs are proposed to have a chemosensory role and contribute to sensory neurotransmission after tissue or peripheral nerve injury (Hanani 2005; Ohara et al 2009; Takeda et al 2009).

Central sensitization

So-called central sensitization that develops at spinal and supraspinal levels of the central nervous system (CNS) secondary to persistent inflammation or nerve injury is underpinned by multiple factors (Latremoliere & Woolf 2009). These include increased responsiveness of nociceptive neurons to normal or subthreshold afferent input, changes in the expression of receptors, ion channels and enzymes, changes in the properties of inhibitory interneurons, and activation of descending inhibitory as well as opposing descending facilitatory mechanisms (Fig. 11.1; Latremoliere & Woolf 2009; Urban et al 1999; Vanegas & Schaible 2004). Furthermore, recent research implicates activated non-neuronal cells in the development and maintenance of the central sensitization of neurons in the CNS (Vallejo et al 2010; Watkins et al 2007).

Mechanisms underpinning central sensitization include persistent activation of the N-methyl-D-aspartate (NMDA)-nitric oxide synthase (NOS)-nitric oxide (NO) signalling cascade, upregulation of sodium channels and acid-sensing ion channels, as well as TRPV1, TRPM8 and α-receptors (Baron 2009; Costigan et al 2009; Harvey & Dickenson 2008). Other mechanisms include enhanced dynorphin signalling at supraspinal levels of the CNS (Lai et al 2001) as well as degeneration of inhibitory GABAergic interneurons in the spinal cord to cause disinhibition and increase sensitivity (Scholz et al 2005).

Under normal homeostatic conditions, non-neuronal cells such as microglia and astrocytes have important 'house-keeper' roles to support the ongoing function and survival of neurons in the CNS. Microglia comprise 5–10% of glia in the CNS (Watkins et al 2007) and their major function is immune surveillance (Raivich 2005). Astrocytes comprise 40–50% of all glial cells in the CNS to provide trophic support, energy and neurotransmitter precursors to neurons, regulation of extracellular concentrations of various ions and neurotransmitters, as well as neurite outgrowth, formation of synapses, neuronal differentiation and survival (Perea & Araque 2005). However, following activation, microglia and astrocytes release a range of pronociceptive substances, including cytokines, chemokines, neurotrophic factors, ATP, excitatory amino acids and nitric oxide, that enhance pain by increasing the excitability of nearby neurons (Fig. 11.1) (Vallejo et al 2010). Recent studies also implicate a role for activated microglia and astrocytes in the development of analgesic tolerance and opioid-induced hyperalgesia that may develop following chronic morphine administration (Wang et al 2010).

Bearing in mind the contribution of non-neuronal cells to central sensitization, it follows that the optimal pharmacological management of chronic pain may require pharmacotherapeutic agents directed at both neuronal and non-neuronal targets at spinal and supraspinal sites of the CNS.

Nociceptive neurotransmitters and their target receptors

Factors contributing to the pathophysiology of persistent pain include pro-inflammatory mediators released in response to nerve injury, transcriptional changes at the level of the dorsal root ganglia, phenotypic changes in neural pathways, activation of glial cells in the nervous system, structural modifications including nerve sprouting and neurodegeneration of GABAergic neurons in the CNS, resulting in a hyperexcitable nervous system (Basbaum et al 2009). Specific molecular interactions that drive the aforementioned changes in neuronal excitability may differ according to the specific injury and the consequent chemical environments that are created (Basbaum et al 2009). The molecular interactions involve all major families of regulatory proteins, including G-protein coupled receptors (GPCRs), ion channels, enzymes, neurotrophins and kinases, thereby offering an abundance of potential analgesic targets and therapeutic opportunities (Stone & Molliver 2009). Examples include glutamate (Mayer 2005), GABAergic (Goudet et al 2009), neurokinin (Seybold 2009), calcitonin gene-related peptide (Seybold 2009), bradykinin (Dray 1997), prostanoid (Zeilhofer 2007), purinergic (Teixeira et al 2010), protease (Vergnolle et al 2003), neurotrophin (Hefti 1997), opioid (Snyder & Pasternak 2003), cannabinoid (Brown 2007), cytokine (Uceyler et al 2009), chemokine (Abbadie et al 2009) and transient receptor potential vanilloid receptors (Broad et al 2009), as well as sodium (Bhattacharya et al 2009), calcium (Yaksh 2006) and acid-sensing ion channels (Sluka et al 2009).

Despite the aforementioned large number of receptors and ion channels serving as potential targets for the development of a range of novel pain therapeutics, these are yet to reach the clinic. Hence, pain will continue to be managed with the currently available medications according to the principles succinctly encapsulated by the World Health Organization's three-step Analgesic Ladder (World Health Organization 1986).

MAJOR GOALS FOR THE PHARMACOLOGICAL TREATMENT OF CLINICAL PAIN

1. Increase inhibitory neurotransmission to provide analgesia by decoupling the response between an acute noxious stimulus (e.g. post-surgery or trauma) and the painful sensation that would normally be evoked (Doubell et al 1999).
2. Prevent development of peripheral or central sensitization under circumstances where this would normally occur (Doubell et al 1999).
3. Restore the normal responsiveness of the nociceptive signalling system in patients suffering from states of either hypo- or hypersensitivity so that responses to defined low- or high-intensity stimuli are perceived correctly as innocuous or painful sensations, respectively (Doubell et al 1999).

PHARMACOLOGICAL TREATMENT OF PAIN

WHO analgesic ladder

Almost a quarter of a century after its introduction in 1986 to guide the pharmacological management of chronic cancer pain, the WHO three-step analgesic ladder (Fig. 11.2) is now widely used to more broadly guide the pharmacological treatment of both acute and chronic pain.

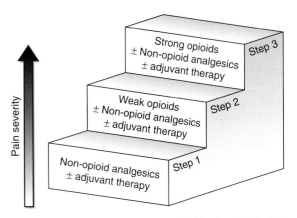

Fig. 11.2 WHO three-step analgesic ladder (World Health Organization 1986).

According to step 1 of the analgesic ladder, non-opioid analgesics, including paracetamol (acetaminophen), non-steroidal anti-inflammatory drugs (NSAIDs, e.g. aspirin and ibuprofen) and coxibs (e.g. celecoxib), are recommended for the treatment of mild pain. Adjuvants (e.g. tricyclic antidepressants, anticonvulsants and antiarrhythmics) may be co-administered if pain has a neuropathic component. When mild pain progresses to moderate pain (step 2), weak opioid analgesics such as codeine, tramadol and dextropropoxyphene are added to non-opioids with adjuvants co-administered for pain with a neuropathic component. For moderate to severe pain (step 3), strong opioid analgesics, including morphine, oxycodone, hydromorphone and fentanyl, are recommended. Morphine is recommended by the WHO as the strong opioid analgesic of choice due to its worldwide availability at low cost. Strong opioid analgesics may be co-administered with non-opioids and/or adjuvants, as required (World Health Organization 1986).

The WHO guidelines also recommend that patients receive individualized dose titration to ensure an adequate dosage of the selected analgesic and/or adjuvant with drug treatment administered on a scheduled 'round the clock' basis rather than 'as required' (World Health Organization 1986). Controlled-release and sustained-release formulations of opioid analgesics allow the convenience of once or twice-daily dosing, which improves patient compliance and analgesic outcomes. For the treatment of breakthrough pain, such as that which occurs during dressing changes or due to incident pain upon mobilization, additional bolus doses of immediate-release opioid analgesic formulations may be administered on an 'as required' basis.

Whilst the oral dosing route is preferred for most patients, it is not practical during labour or in the immediate post-operative period due to impaired gastrointestinal transit. In circumstances where more rapid pain relief is required or there is inadequate pain relief and intolerable side effects, such as severe vomiting, severe dysphagia or

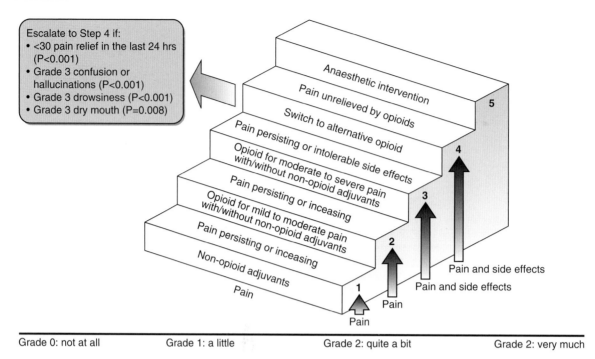

Escalate to Step 4 if:
• <30 pain relief in the last 24 hrs (P<0.001)
• Grade 3 confusion or hallucinations (P<0.001)
• Grade 3 drowsiness (P<0.001)
• Grade 3 dry mouth (P=0.008)

Anaesthetic intervention
Pain unrelieved by opioids — 5

Switch to alternative opioid
Pain persisting or intolerable side effects — 4

Opioid for moderate to severe pain with/without non-opioid adjuvants
Pain persisting or increasing — 3

Opioid for mild to moderate pain with/without non-opioid adjuvants
Pain persisting or increasing — 2

Non-opioid adjuvants
Pain — 1

Pain and side effects
Pain and side effects
Pain
Pain

Grade 0: not at all   Grade 1: a little   Grade 2: quite a bit   Grade 2: very much

Fig. 11.3 Overview of proposed five-step WHO analgesic and side-effect ladder.
Reprinted from Riley J, Ross J R, Gretton S K, A'hern R, Du Bois R, Welsh K, Thick M 2007 Proposed 5-step World Health Organization analgesic and side effect ladder. European Journal of Pain Supplements 1:23–30, with permission of John Wiley & Sons.

bowel obstruction, changing the route of administration to parenteral (e.g. intravenous, subcutaneous, intramuscular), rectal, buccal, sublingual, transdermal or spinal (epidural, intrathecal) may restore adequate analgesia with tolerable adverse effects (Walsh 2005). Another strategy for restoring satisfactory analgesia with tolerable side effects involves 'opioid rotation' by switching from the first opioid to another (Walsh 2005).

Recently, modifications to the original WHO analgesic ladder have been proposed. For example, Eisenberg et al suggested that invasive procedures such as neurolytic blocks should be considered for patients experiencing inadequate pain relief or intolerable side effects as an adjunct or alternative to pharmacotherapy (Eisenberg et al 2005). More recently, Riley et al proposed the addition of two steps to the original WHO three-step analgesic ladder (Fig. 11.3), with the fourth step recommending use of 'opioid rotation' for patients experiencing inadequate pain relief and intolerable side effects; if opioid rotation fails, progress to a fifth step involving use of anaesthetic intervention is recommended (Riley et al 2007).

ANALGESIC AGENTS

Pharmacotherapy with analgesic and adjuvant agents underpins the pharmacological management of pain across all age groups from neonates to older persons. An overview of currently available analgesic agents for clinical use is provided in the following sections.

Non-opioid analgesics

A summary of commonly used non-opioid analgesics and their dosing schedules is provided in Table 11.2.

Paracetamol

Paracetamol (acetaminophen) is a non-opioid analgesic that is widely utilized for the symptomatic relief of fever, headaches and minor aches and pains (Remy et al 2006). Paracetamol is an active ingredient in a large number of pharmaceutical preparations, including over-the-counter cold and flu products as well as prescription medicines (Munir et al 2007). Paracetamol produces pain relief and antipyretic actions after oral administration of usual adult doses of 1 g three or four times daily but not exceeding a total daily dose of 4 g (Myers & LaPorte 2009). In contrast to NSAIDs, paracetamol does not inhibit platelet aggregation and does not damage the gastric mucosa (Munir et al 2007; Remy et al 2006). A recent systematic review concluded that single 1 g doses of paracetamol provide effective analgesia for up to 4 hours in ~50% of patients with acute post-operative pain. In addition, patients

Table 11.2 Clinically available non-opioid analgesics and their dosing schedules

Drug name	Brand name	Dose/formulation available
Paracetamol (acetaminophen)	Tylenol®, Panadol®	325 mg, 500 mg
Oral NSAIDs (non-prescription)		
Aspirin	Bayer® Ecotrin®	325 mg 325 mg EC
Ibuprofen	Advil®, Motrin®	200 mg
Naproxen	Aleve®	220 mg
Topical agents (non-prescription)		
Capsaicin	Theragen® Zostrix®	60 g tube (0.025%) 60 g tube (0.075%)
Traditional NSAIDs (prescription)		
Diclofenac	Cataflam® Voltaren®	75 mg bid 50 mg bid, 100 mg ER daily
Etodolac	Lodine®	400 mg bid, 400 mg tid
Ibuprofen	Motrin®	400 mg tid, 800 mg tid
Indometacin	Indocin®	50 mg tid, 75 mg SR bid
Ketoprofen	Oruvail®	75 mg tid, 200 mg ER daily
Melocixam	Mobic®	7.5 mg daily, 15 mg daily
Nabumetone	Relafen®	1000 mg daily, 1500 mg daily
Naproxen	Anaprox® Naprelan® Naprosyn®	250 mg tid 500 mg bid 500 mg tid
Piroxicam	Feldene®	20 mg daily
COX-2 inhibitor (coxib)		
Celecoxib	Celebrex®	100 mg bid, 200 mg bid, 400 mg bid

(adapted from (AHRQ 2009)
EC, enteric coated; ER, extended release; SR, sustained release; bid, twice a day; tid, three times a day.

reported few, mainly mild, adverse effects whose severity and frequency were similar to those reported by patients administered placebo (Toms et al 2008).

Although paracetamol readily crosses the blood–brain barrier, the mechanism through which it produces its analgesic and antipyretic effects is unclear. Proposed mechanisms include modulation of serotoninergic signalling, a central cyclooxygenase-3 (COX-3) mechanism and even a cannabinoid-mediated mechanism (Bonnefont et al 2003; Myers & LaPorte 2009; Pickering et al 2006). The poor ability of paracetamol to inhibit COX-1 and COX-2 and its central model of action likely underpins its lack of anti-inflammatory efficacy (Lee et al 2004; Shamoon & Hochberg 2000).

Paracetamol adverse effects

The most serious adverse effect of paracetamol is potentially fatal liver toxicity, which may occur if therapeutic doses are exceeded. Hepatotoxicity is mediated by a reactive metabolite, N-acetyl-p-benzoquinoneimine (NAPQI), which normally accounts for only 5–8% of a therapeutic dose of paracetamol and is detoxified by conjugation with glutathione in the liver (Larson et al 2005; Whitcomb & Block 1994). However, if the amount of NAPQI formed exceeds liver stores of glutathione, then hepatotoxicity will occur, potentially resulting in liver failure. In the presence of glutathione depletion due to starvation, alcohol abuse or impaired liver function, the daily dosage of paracetamol should not exceed 3 g due to the increased risk of hepatotoxicity (Food and Drug Administration 1999; Larson et al 2005; Remy et al 2006; Whitcomb & Block 1994).

If a patient seeks medical attention soon after paracetamol overdose, activated charcoal can be used to decrease paracetamol absorption. The mainstay of treatment involves administration of acetylcysteine, a precursor for glutathione in an endeavour to increase glutathione production sufficiently to prevent liver failure. However, if liver damage is severe, then a liver transplant will be required. In the USA alone, almost half of the acute liver failure cases and a third of deaths are due to paracetamol overdose induced liver toxicity (Larson et al 2005).

Oral non-steroidal anti-inflammatory drugs

NSAIDs are chemically diverse compounds that have analgesic, antipyretic and anti-inflammatory properties, and are amongst the most widely prescribed drug products globally (Dugowson & Gnanashanmugam 2006). There are multiple chemical classes of NSAIDs, including salicylates (aspirin, methyl salicylate, diflunisal), arylalkanoic acids (indometacin, sulindac, diclofenac), the 'profens' or 2-arylpropionic acids (ibuprofen, naproxen, ketoprofen, ketorolac) and oxicams (piroxicam, meloxicam).

NSAIDs inhibit the synthesis of prostaglandins, endogenous molecules that have diverse paracrine effects, including pronociceptive signalling, as well as modulation of inflammation and temperature regulation in the hypothalamus (Zeilhofer 2007). With the exception of aspirin, NSAIDs produce their anti-inflammatory and analgesic effects by competitive inhibition of the two isoforms of the enzyme cyclooxygenase, COX-1 and COX-2, to inhibit formation of prostaglandins and thromboxane from arachidonic acid (Vane 1971).

COX-1 is constitutively expressed in platelets, the gastrointestinal tract and the kidneys, whereas COX-2 is inducible and found in the kidneys and the CNS (Zeilhofer 2007). The desired anti-inflammatory action of NSAIDs is largely due to inhibition of COX-2, whereas aspirin irreversibly acylates both COX-1 and COX-2 (Dugowson & Gnanashanmugam 2006). Although classified as mild analgesics, NSAIDs are effective for the treatment of pain involving peripheral tissue sensitization (Burke & Fitzgerald 2006) and they have opioid-sparing effects to reduce post-operative opioid consumption, resulting in reduced opioid-related adverse events (Marret et al 2005).

PGE2 release in the hypothalamus is responsible for triggering an increase in body temperature during inflammation (Zeilhofer 2007) and so NSAIDs produce their antipyretic effects secondary to inhibition of PGE2 formation in the hypothalamus. At doses as low as 30 mg/day, aspirin irreversibly inhibits COX-1-dependent formation of thromboxane A2 in platelets to inhibit platelet aggregation with an 8–12 day duration of action, i.e. the turnover time of platelets; it is this action that underpins the cardioprotective effects of aspirin (Munir et al 2007).

Adverse effects of NSAIDs

The most common adverse effects of NSAIDs are gastrointestinal, renal and respiratory. All NSAIDs, including coxibs, can cause or aggravate hypertension, congestive heart failure, edema and kidney problems (Agency for Healthcare Research and Quality 2009).

Prostaglandins, whose synthesis is catalysed by COX-1, have a cytoprotective effect in the gastric mucosa and so NSAID-induced inhibition of COX-1 may result in dyspepsia, gastric irritation, ulceration and bleeding as well as diarrhoea (AHRQ 2009). Although most NSAIDs show little selectivity between COX-1 and COX-2, selectivity is seen at low doses for some agents. For example, at relatively low doses such as 7.5 mg daily, meloxicam is a preferential inhibitor of COX-2 (Munir et al 2007).

Prostaglandins have an important role in maintaining normal glomerular perfusion and filtration rates through their vasodilatory effects on *afferent arterioles* of the *glomeruli* (AHRQ 2009). In renal failure, where the kidney is trying to maintain renal perfusion pressure by elevated angiotensin II levels that constrict the afferent arteriole into the glomerulus in addition to the efferent arteriole, prostaglandins have a protective affect on the afferent arteriole (AHRQ 2009). If this is blocked by NSAID administration, there is decreased renal perfusion pressure, resulting in renal toxicity (AHRQ 2009).

It is important to also be aware that aspirin-exacerbated respiratory disease presenting as rhinitis and asthma occurs in ~10% of the general population and in ~21%

of adults when determined by an oral provocation testing (Dugowson & Gnanashanmugam 2006). Hence, NSAIDs should be avoided in patients with known aspirin sensitivity.

In terms of NSAID-induced adverse effects, it is important to recognize the following (AHRQ 2009):

1. NSAIDs increase the risk of gastrointestinal bleeding at higher doses; people older than 75 years have the highest risk.
2. NSAIDs should be avoided in people receiving anticoagulant therapy.
3. Consider using paracetamol instead as it is associated with a lower risk of gastrointestinal bleeding.
4. Co-administration of the PGE_1 analogue misoprostol or proton pump inhibitors in conjunction with NSAIDs can prevent duodenal and gastric ulceration (Rostom et al 2002).
5. Celecoxib, ibuprofen at doses of 800 mg three times a day and diclofenac (75 mg twice a day) have increased risk of myocardial infarction. Naproxen does not increase the risk of myocardial infarction even at a dose of 500 mg twice a day.

Topical NSAIDs

Topical NSAIDs are often used to treat acute musculoskeletal conditions due to the potential of this delivery route to provide pain relief whilst minimizing the incidence of systemic adverse events (Massey et al 2010). Clinical trials show that topical NSAIDs are effective and relatively safe for the treatment of osteoarthritic pain, with fewer systemic side effects compared with oral NSAIDs (Altman et al 2009; Barthel et al 2009; Simon et al 2009). In a recent systematic review of 47 clinical studies that compared various topical NSAIDs in a range of formulations, including sprays, gels and creams, for the treatment of acute pain relative to the corresponding placebo preparations, the number needed to treat for clinical success (50% pain relief) was 4.5 for treatment periods in the range 6 to 14 days (Massey et al 2010). Topical preparations of ibuprofen, diclofenac, ketoprofen and prioxicam were of similar efficacy but indometacin and benzydamine were not significantly better than placebo. There were very few systemic adverse events and adverse-event-related withdrawals (Massey et al 2010).

Coxibs

Coxibs are selective COX-2 inhibitors that were developed to avoid the gastric irritation of NSAIDs due to their COX-1 inhibitory effects, whilst retaining equivalent analgesic properties to NSAIDs (Dugowson & Gnanashanmugam 2006). In 1999, celecoxib was the first coxib to be approved for the relief of pain and inflammation in patients with osteoarthritis, rheumatoid arthritis and primary dysmenorrhoea (Patrono et al 2001). It was quickly followed by rofecoxib, etoricoxib, valdecoxib, parecoxib and lumiracoxib (Capone et al 2005; Cheer & Goa 2001;

Table 11.3 Opioid receptor types, effects transduced and endogenous ligands

Opioid receptor types[1]		Effects[2]	Endogenous ligands[3]
μ, mu or MOP	μ1	Supraspinal analgesia, dependence, withdrawal, analgesic tolerance, euphoria, emesis, sedation, prolactin release, increased feeding behaviour, immune suppression, possibly pruritus	β-endorphin (non-selective) Enkephalins (non-selective) Endomorphin-1 Endomorphin-2
	μ2	Spinal analgesia, respiratory depression, decreased gastrointestinal motility, decreased growth hormone release	
δ, delta or DOP	δ1	Supraspinal analgesia, stimulates feeding, growth hormone release	Enkephalins (non-selective) β-endorphin (non-selective)
	δ2	Supraspinal and spinal analgesia	
κ, kappa or KOP	κ1	Dysphoric responses	Dynorphin A Dynorphin B α-neoendorphin
	κ2	Decreased gastrointestinal transit, sedation, feeding behaviour	
	κ3	Supraspinal analgesia	
NOP		Analgesia and morphine tolerance	Nociception/orphanin FQ (N/OFQ)

[1] Names per current NC-IUPHAR recommended nomenclature.
[2] Adapted from Maher and Chaiyakul (2003).
[3] Adapted from IUPHAR database.

Fenton et al 2004; Wittenberg et al 2006). However, after chronic administration for longer than 12 months, the selective COX-2 inhibitors rofecoxib and valdecoxib were shown to significantly increase the risk of untoward cardiovascular events and so these agents were withdrawn from the market (Munir et al 2007).

OPIOID ANALGESICS

Opioid analgesics may be classified on the basis of their (i) WHO Analgesic Ladder classification as 'weak' or 'strong', (ii) chemical structure or (iii) pharmacodynamic profiles as agonists, partial agonists or antagonists at opioid receptors (Krenzischek et al 2008; Trescot et al 2008). The various opioid receptor types/subtypes, the effects transduced and their respective endogenous ligands are summarized in Table 11.3.

Strong opioid analgesics are recommend by the WHO as the drugs of choice for the management of moderate to severe pain whereas weak opioid analgesics are used in patients with mild to moderate pain, particularly when there are contradictions for NSAID usage (Krenzischek et al 2008). A comparison of equi-analgesic doses of clinically ultilized opioid analgesics is shown in Table 11.4 and common starting doses for a range of orally administered opioids are listed in Table 11.5.

Apart from pain relief, opioid analgesics produce a range of adverse effects, including nausea, vomiting, sedation, pruritis, respiratory depression, constipation, thermoregulatory effects, immunomodulation, tolerance and physical

Table 11.4 Total daily oral morphine equivalent conversion table (Nissen et al 2001)

Opioid analgesic	Conversion factor
Pethidine (oral)	× 0.125
Pethidine (IV)	× 0.4
Methadone	× 1.5
Oxycodone	× 1.5
Buprenorphine	× 50
Codeine	× 0.16
Dextropropoxyphene	× 0.1
Morphine (IV)	× 3
Morphine (oral)	× 1

IV, intravenous.

dependence (Zollner & Stein 2007). Although it is widely believed that the analgesic and other effects produced by opioid analgesics are evoked by activation of the μ-opioid receptor, it is widely appreciated by frontline clinicians that there are intra-individual between-opioid differences in terms of both analgesic and tolerability profiles (Smith 2008). However, the precise mechanistic basis underpinning these observations is poorly understood at present.

Strategies recommended by the American Pain Society and the American Academy of Pain Medicine (Chou et al., 2009) to minimize opioid-related adverse effects include:

1. pro-active preventive treatment, especially for constipation and nausea

Table 11.5 Starting doses of selected opioids (Argoff $ Silvershein 2009)

| Opioid | Oral administration | | Duration of effect (h) | Plasma half-life (h) |
	Dose	Frequency (h)		
Codeine	15–60 mg	3–6	4–6	3
Fentanyl	100–200 µg	6a	0.5–1 (IV), 72 (TD), 2–4 (TM)	3.7
Hydrocodone	2.5–10 mg	3–6	4–8	2.5–4
Hydromorphone	2–4 mg	3–4	4–5	2–3
Levorphanol	2–4 mg	6–8	6–8	12–16
Methadone	5–10 mg	6–8	4–6	24
Morphine	15–30 mg (IR)	3–4 (IR)	3–6	2–3.5
Oxycodone	10 mg (CR), 5–10 mg (IR)	12 (CR), 3–6 (IR)	8–12 (CR), 3–4 (IR)	2.5–3
Oxymorphone	10 mg (IR), 5–10 mg (ER)	4–6 (IR), 12 (ER)	3–6	7–9.5
Propoxyphene	65–100 mg	4	4–6	6–12
Tramadol	50–100 mg (IR), 100 mg (ER)	4–6 (IR), 24 (ER)	4–6 (IR), 24 (ER)	5–7

IV, intravenous; TD, transdermal; TM, transmucosal; IR, immediate-release; CR, controlled-release; ER, extended-release.

[a] Not more than four doses per day.

2. titrating opioid doses slowly
3. verifying that adverse effects are genuinely opioid-related rather than due to another problem
4. possibly changing the dosing regimen or route of administration to obtain relatively constant blood levels, if adverse effects are a problem
5. addition of, or increasing, non-opioid or adjuvant analgesic doses for an opioid sparing effect
6. addition of another drug to counteract the adverse effect
7. frequent reassessment.

Weak opioid analgesics

Codeine

Codeine is a weak opioid analgesic that has low affinity for the µ-opioid receptor. It is generally considered to be a prodrug for morphine, with approximately 5–10% of an orally administered dose being metabolized to morphine (Zollner & Stein 2007). Codeine is susceptible to metabolic drug–drug interactions via either inhibition (e.g. buproprion, celecoxib, cimetidine) or induction (e.g. dexamethasone, rifampin) of its metabolism. Codeine may be administered as an oral tablet or intramuscularly or coformulated with paracetamol or an NSAID in tablet form. Doses of codeine generally do not exceed 60 mg (Trescot et al 2008).

Meperidine

Meperidine (also known as pethidine), is a weak µ-opioid agonist whose analgesic potency is ~10% that of morphine. Meperidine is metabolized to normeperidine

(Gilman et al 1980), which may accumulate in patients with decreased renal function and in those receiving multiple doses, resulting in myoclonus (Marinella 1997). The consensus is that use of meperidine should be discouraged in favour of other opioids (Latta et al 2002).

Tramadol

Tramadol has been used for the treatment of mild to moderate pain in Germany for the past three decades and in the UK, USA and elsewhere since the mid 1990s (Grond & Sablotzki 2004). After i.v. administration, the potency of tramadol is similar to that of meperidine, i.e. ~10% that of morphine (Grond & Sablotzki 2004). After oral administration, the bioavailability of tramadol is high, approximately 70% (Grond & Sablotzki 2004). The starting dose of tramadol is 50 mg once or twice daily, which may be increased gradually to a maximum of 400 mg/day (100 mg, four times daily) in patients without renal or hepatic dysfunction or 300 mg/day in older patients (>75 years) (O'Connor & Dworkin 2009). For the treatment of neuropathic pain, tramadol has an Number Needed to Treat (NNT) of 3.8 (Hollingshead et al 2006).

The analgesic effects of tramadol are mediated via multiple mechanisms in the CNS, including activation of the descending noradrenergic and serotoninergic inhibitory system as well as weak µ-opioid agonist activity (Grond & Sablotzki 2004). Tramadol is metabolized in the liver to a potent µ-opioid agonist metabolite known as M1, which also contributes to its analgesic actions. Because of the complexity of its analgesic profile, the Food and Drug Administration has classified tramadol as a non-traditional, centrally acting analgesic (Grond & Sablotzki 2004).

Tramadol has a low incidence of adverse effects, particularly respiratory depression, constipation and abuse potential (Grond & Sablotzki 2004). However, convulsions have been reported when doses of tramadol exceed the recommended limits. In addition, the risk of seizures in patients taking other medications that lower the seizure threshold, such as selective serotonin reuptake inhibitors, tricyclic antidepressants and antipsychotic drugs, is potentially increased by tramadol (Gardner et al 2000).

Strong opioid analgesics

Morphine

Morphine is an opioid alkaloid found in high abundance in opium, the dried exudate of the unripe seed capsule of the opium poppy, *Papaver somniferum* (Boerner 1975). It was first isolated by the German pharmacist Freidrich Serturner, and named 'morphium' after Morpheus the Greek God of Dreams (Milne et al 1996). Morphine remains the 'gold standard' opioid analgesic recommended by the WHO (1986) for the relief of moderate to severe chronic cancer pain. Morphine is also widely utilized for the management of acute moderate to severe pain such as that which occurs following trauma or heart attack and post-operatively (Bovill 1987).

The oral bioavailability of morphine is low at ∼20% due to extensive first-pass metabolism in the gastrointestinal mucosa and the liver to form two major active metabolites, namely the analgesically active morphine-6-glucuronide (M6G) and the analgesically inactive morphine-3-glucuronide (M3G), which account for ∼10% and >50% of the dose, respectively (Smith 2000). In patients with renal impairment, these two glucuronide metabolites may accumulate, resulting in respiratory depression and/or neuro-excitation (Smith 2000).

Morphine is available in a range of formulations, including oral tablets, capsules and mixtures, rectal suppositories and parenteral formulations for administration by the intramuscular, intravenous, subcutaneous, epidural and intrathecal routes. Oral morphine dosage forms include both immediate-release and sustained-release formulations, with the latter enabling the convenience of once or twice daily dosing (Argoff & Silvershein 2009). There is also an extended-release epidural formulation of morphine available for use in the USA which utilizes a proprietary liposomal carrier, DepoFoam, to provide prolonged analgesia (up to 48 hours) without the need for an indwelling catheter (Viscusi et al 2005).

Oxycodone

Oxycodone is a semi-synthetic derivative of thebaine, a naturally occurring alkaloid in the opium poppy (Kalso 2005). The analgesic potency of oxycodone is ∼1.5 times that of morphine following intravenous injection for the relief of post-operative pain (Lenz et al 2009) and after administration of oral controlled-release tablet formulations for the management of cancer-related pain (Bruera et al 1998).

The oral bioavailability of oxycodone is high at 60–87% in healthy subjects and patients with cancer (Leow et al 1992). In humans, oxycodone is principally metabolized to its analgesically inactive, N-demethylated metabolite, noroxycodone (Lalovic et al 2006; Poyhia et al 1992). Although up to 10% of an oxycodone dose is metabolized to its O-demethylated metabolite oxymorphone, a potent µ-opioid agonist, it is rapidly further metabolized to its glucuronide metabolite, resulting in very low circulating plasma concentrations of oxymorphone (Lalovic et al 2006; Poyhia et al 1991; 1992). Hence, the pharmacodynamic effects of oxycodone are generally attributed to the parent drug alone (Lalovic et al 2006).

Like morphine, oxycodone is available in a range of formulations, including oral tablets, capsules and mixtures, rectal suppositories and parenteral formulations for intravenous administration. Oral oxycodone dosage forms include oral mixture, immediate-release tablets and controlled-release tablets that allow twice daily dosing (Argoff & Silvershein 2009).

Although oxycodone produces its analgesic effects via activation of opioid receptors (Leow & Smith 1994), it interacts with a different population of opioid receptors (putative κ₂) to morphine (Nielsen et al 2007), which probably underpins the low extent of cross-tolerance between these two opioids in animal studies (Nielsen et al 2000) and the success of opioid rotation from morphine to oxycodone in humans (Narabayashi et al 2008).

Methadone

Methadone is a synthetic µ-opioid agonist that is a racemic mixture of two enantiomers, the dextrorotatory (S-methadone) and levorotatory (R-methadone) stereoisomers. S-methadone produces analgesia via activation of descending serotoninergic and noradrenergic inhibitory mechanisms and it also has antitussive activity (Codd et al 1995). R-methadone produces analgesia through its activity as an agonist at µ-opioid receptors (Leppert 2009). Both enantiomers also have antagonist activity at NMDA receptors (Gorman et al 1997). Methadone is available in oral and rectal preparations and in ampoules for parenteral administration (Manfredi et al 2003). For patients with an addiction to opioids, methadone is commonly utilized as maintenance treatment and it is also used in patients with chronic pain (Lugo et al 2005).

Following administration of high doses of methadone (> 60 mg per day) in combination with tricyclic antidepressants or other drugs that inhibit its metabolism, there is a lengthening of the QTc interval, thereby initiating torsades de pointes (Ehret et al 2007; Krantz et al 2002). Unfortunately, a lack of awareness of the long and highly variable elimination half-life (12–150 hours) of methadone and its many metabolic drug–drug interactions has led to a dramatic increase in deaths associated with this opioid (Trescot et al 2008).

Hydromorphone

Hydromorphone is a semi-synthetic morphine analogue that is a μ-opioid agonist with a parenteral potency approximately five times that of morphine for the relief of moderate to severe acute pain (Horn & Nesbit 2004; Quigley 2002). For the relief of chronic cancer pain, hydromorphone is equivalent to morphine in terms of pain relief and adverse event profiles (Murray & Hagen 2005). After oral administration, hydromorphone undergoes extensive first-pass metabolism with more than 50% of every dose metabolized to hydromorphone-3-glucuronide (H3G). Hydromorphone is available in immediate-release and controlled-release oral formulations as well as parenteral preparations that can be administered by either the epidural or intrathecal routes (Hagen et al 1995; Hays et al 1994).

Although H3G is an analgesically inactive metabolite, it can accumulate in renal failure and produce neuro-excitatory side effects (Davison & Mayo 2008; Smith 2000).

Buprenorphine

Buprenorphine is semi-synthetic derivative of thebaine that is a partial μ-opioid agonist, a κ-opioid antagonist and also binds to the nociceptin (ORL-1) receptor (Johnson et al 2005; Pick et al 1997). It is thought that the slow dissociation of buprenorphine from the μ-opioid receptor is responsible for its slow onset and long duration of action whereas its κ-opioid antagonist properties are thought to underpin its limited spinal analgesia, dysphoria and psychotomimetic effects (Johnson et al 2005). Buprenorphine is ~25–50 times more potent than morphine (Evans & Easthope 2003) with a ceiling effect for analgesia thought to be related to its partial μ-opioid agonist activity (Davis 2005).

Following oral administration, the bioavailability of buprenorphine is low at ~14% due to extensive first-pass metabolism (Picard et al 2005) whereas after buccal, sublingual, intranasal and transdermal administration the bioavailability of buprenorphine is increased to 30–60% as these dosing routes avoid first-pass metabolism (Davis 2005; Evans & Easthope 2003; Johnson et al 2005). Because of its long half-life (~26 hours), buprenorphine is a suitable alternative to methadone for opioid maintenance therapy in opioid-dependent individuals (Johnson et al 2005; Robinson 2002). A combination product containing buprenorphine and the opioid antagonist naloxone in a 4:1 ratio, respectively, has been developed to deter illicit conversion of buprenorphine tablets to parenteral routes (Harris et al 2004).

Fentanyl

Fentanyl is semi-synthetic μ-opioid agonist that has a rapid onset of action (1–5 minutes) but short duration (<1 hour) (Stanley 2005). Although fentanyl is structurally related to meperidine, it is ~80–100-fold more potent than parenteral morphine (Pasero 2005). To compensate for its short duration of action, several transdermal patch formulations of fentanyl have been developed (Davis 2006; Hair et al 2008; Heitz et al 2009; Herndon 2007; Hoy & Keating 2008; Marier et al 2006; Portenoy & Lesage 1999). Fentanyl has been used clinically for ~40 years in the field of pain management (Pasero 2005; Stanley 2005).

For post-operative pain relief, fentanyl may be administered by the intraspinal route whereas for procedural or breakthrough pain administration by the intravenous, oral transmucosal, intranasal or inhaled routes is preferred (Hair et al 2008; Peng & Sandler 1999). Fentanyl is metabolized primarily to norfentanyl, a pharmacologically inactive metabolite (Horn & Nesbit 2004).

Tapentadol

Tapentadol is a recently approved centrally acting oral analgesic whose activity is attributed to its moderate affinity at μ-opioid receptors as well as its inhibition of norepinephrine reuptake in the CNS to activate descending inhibitory mechanisms (Hartrick 2009; Wade & Spruill 2009). This latter action has been proposed to provide an 'opioid-sparing' effect resulting in an overall improvement in tolerability compared with other μ-opioid analgesics (Tzschentke et al 2006). The oral bioavailability of tapentadol is reportedly 32% due to first-pass metabolism, primarily to tapentadol-O-glucuronide (Kneip et al 2008).

At present, the immediate-release formulation (50, 75 and 100 mg tablets) of tapentadol is approved in the USA for the relief of moderate to severe acute pain in adult patients (Frampton 2010). When compared with oxycodone in a head-to-head clinical trial, tapentadol (50–100 mg every 4–6 hours) provided non-inferior analgesia to oxycodone (10 or 15 mg every 4–6 hours) with a superior gastrointestinal adverse effect profile compared with oxycodone (Hartrick 2009).

Ultra-short-acting opioid analgesics

Remifentanil

Remifentanil, a 4-anilinopiperidine derivative of fentanyl, is an ultra-short-acting μ-opioid agonist indicated for the relief of post-operative pain (Kucukemre et al 2005). The primary metabolite, remifentanil acid, has negligible activity compared with remifentanil (Battershill & Keating 2006). Parenteral remifentanil has a rapid onset of action (~1 minute) and a rapid offset of action following discontinuation (~3–10 minutes) (Battershill & Keating 2006).

Other ultra-short-acting structural analogues of fentanyl for use in anaesthesia include alfentanil, sufentanil and remifentanil. The ultra-short-acting agents are preferred in patients with cardiovascular instability (Horn & Nesbit 2004).

Opioid antagonists for improving constipation

Two peripherally selective μ-opioid receptor antagonists, alvimopan and methylnaltrexone, are approved in the USA for improving opioid-induced constipation. Oral alvimopan is approved for use in adult patients who have undergone partial small or large bowel resection (limited use: 15 doses, up to 7 days only; Rao & Go 2010). Methylnaltrexone, a quaternary derivative of naltrexone, is available for subcutaneous injection and is indicated in patients with advanced and late-stage illness requiring chronic opioid therapy but experiencing opioid-induced constipation (Rao & Go 2010). The recommended methylnaltrexone doses are based on patient weight as follows: 8 mg (for 38–62 kg), 12 mg (for 62–114 kg) and 0.15 mg/kg for patients falling outside this weight range (Wyeth Pharmaceuticals 2009).

ADJUVANT MEDICATIONS

Antidepressants

Tricyclic antidepressants (TCAs) are recommended as first-line agents for the management of neuropathic pain with an NNT of 3.6 (Dworkin et al 2010; Saarto & Wiffen 2007). TCAs produce their analgesic actions through inhibition of the re-uptake of norepinephrine to augment descending inhibition (Jann & Slade 2007). TCAs also modulate other signalling pathways, including histaminergic, cholinergic and glutaminergic neurotransmission (Sindrup et al 2005). Recent evidence suggests that they may also block Na^+ channels (Dick et al 2007).

TCAs produce numerous side effects, including CNS (sedation, tremor, insomnia, convulsion), anticholinergic (dry mouth, blurred vision, constipation) and cardiovascular (orthostatic hypotension, cardiac arrhythmias) effects (Attal et al 2006). To minimize the impact of these adverse effects, TCAs should be started at low dosages, administered at night and titrated slowly. An adequate trial of a TCA can take 6–8 weeks, including 2 weeks at the maximum tolerated dosage (Dworkin et al 2007).

Although the newer classes of antidepressants such as the selective serotonin reuptake inhibitors (SSRIs), serotonin norepinephrine reuptake inhibitors (SNRIs) and buproprion (dopamine and norepinephrine reuptake inhibitor) produce few side effects, there is variable efficacy for the relief of neuropathic pain (Saarto & Wiffen 2005). SSRIs such as citalopram and paroxetine have limited efficacy

for the treatment of neuropathic pain (Otto et al 2008). By contrast, SNRIs such as duloxetine (NNT = 5.8) and velafaxine appear to have efficacy for the relief of neuropathic pain (Dworkin et al 2007; Sultan et al 2008).

Anticonvulsants

Gabapentin and its structural analogue pregabalin are second-generation anticonvulsants that interact with the a_2d subunit of voltage-gated calcium channels to reduce Ca^{2+} influx into the presynaptic nerve terminal and reduce release of pro-nociceptive neurotransmitters such as glutamate and substance P (Dickenson & Ghandehari 2007). Multiple randomized controlled trials have shown that these agents are efficacious for the relief of a variety of neuropathic pain states, including painful diabetic neuropathy (PDN), postherpetic neuralgia, phantom limb pain and mixed neuropathic pain (Dworkin et al 2007; Finnerup et al 2005).

After oral dosing, pregabalin exhibits dose-dependent pharmacokinetics and its oral bioavailability decreases as the dose increases across the therapeutic dose range, commencing at 900 mg per day in three divided doses up to a maximum dose of 3600 mg per day (McLean 1994). The more recently developed pregabalin is an improvement on gabapentin in that it exhibits linear pharmacokinetics and it is approximately six times more potent than gabapentin (Gidal 2006). Starting doses of pregabalin are 150 mg per day administered in two or three divided doses with up-titration to 300 mg per day after 1–2 weeks (O'Connor & Dworkin 2009). The dosages of gabapentin and pregabalin should be reduced in patients with significant renal impairment as these agents are eliminated by renal mechanisms (Tassone et al 2007). The most commonly reported adverse events for gabapentin and pregabalin are dizziness, somnolence and peripheral oedema. Although gabapentin/pregabalin and the TCAs appear to have similar efficacy for the alleviation of PDN, gabapentin/pregabalin have a superior safety profile (Gidal 2006; Tassone et al 2007).

Lamotrigine is a sodium channel blocker and inhibitor of Na^+ influx-mediated release of excitatory neurotransmitters. Although it appeared to show efficacy in small cross-over clinical trials for the in treatment of trigeminal neuralgia, PDN and post-stroke pain at doses exceeding 200 mg per day (Finnerup et al 2005), more recently conducted large, parallel group, double-blind, placebo-controlled studies failed to show efficacy (Rao et al 2008; Vinik et al 2007).

Phenytoin and carbamazepine were the first anticonvulsants shown to have efficacy for the alleviation of neuropathic pain (Gilron et al 2006; Jensen 2002). However, as these agents have a significant spectrum of unpleasant side effects, their use is limited. Although carbamazepine is an effective and commonly prescribed agent for the relief of trigeminal neuralgia (Wiffen et al 2005), its more widespread use for the alleviation of neuropathic pain is restricted by adverse effects, including dyslipidaemia, decreased serum sodium levels, changes in sex hormone concentrations, increased body weight and multiple metabolic drug–drug interactions as it is a potent inducer of hepatic cytochrome P450 enzymes (Gilron et al 2006; McCleane 2003). Additionally, carbamazepine has been linked to rare cases of liver toxicity, necessitating regular blood tests to monitor liver enzymes (Wiffen et al 2005). Carbamazepine can also lead to reversible decreases in white cell count distinct from aplastic anaemia that require monitoring (Wiffen et al 2005).

NMDA receptor antagonists

The role of NMDA receptors in the induction and maintenance of central sensitization is well documented (D'Mello & Dickenson 2008). Although considerable research effort has been focused on the development of novel NMDA receptor antagonists for the relief of neuropathic pain, this has been largely unsuccessful to date. Hence, a number of studies have investigated the potential efficacy of clinically available NMDA receptor antagonists such as ketamine, memantine and dextromethorphan for the relief of neuropathic pain and/or for potential opioid-sparing effects.

Ketamine, an analogue of phencyclidine, is a non-competitive NMDA receptor antagonist with a history of use as a general dissociative anaesthetic (Chizh & Headley 2005). A significant drawback of ketamine is that it produces hallucinations and ataxia at doses only slightly larger than those needed to produce analgesia (Childers & Baudy 2007). However, in subanaesthetic doses, ketamine has been shown to have analgesic properties (Kronenberg 2002). Ketamine may be used as a co-analgesic for its opioid-sparing effects (Bell et al 2006; Kronenberg 2002). When ketamine is administered in subanaesthetic doses most reports are of no or mild psychotomimetic effects (Kronenberg 2002).

Dextromethorphan, a non-competitive NMDA receptor antagonist and an antagonist at a3β4 neuronal nicotinic receptors, is found in many over-the-counter cough and cold preparations as an antitussive agent (Damaj et al 2005). Its lack of efficacy for the relief of neuropathic pain is generally thought to be due to its low affinity antagonism at NMDA receptors (Chizh & Headley 2005).

Cannabinoids

Evidence from animal studies and clinical observations indicate that cannabinoids have some analgesic properties. However, CNS depression seems to be the predominant limiting adverse effect. In chronic neuropathic pain, 10,10-dimethylheptyl-D8-tetrahydrocannabinol-11-oic acid (CT-3), at a dose of 40 mg/day was more effective than placebo, without major side effects (Karst et al 2003). Sativex (GW Pharmaceuticals, Salisbury,

Wiltshire, UK), a cannabis plant-based prescription pharmaceutical product administered as an oromucosal spray delivering a fixed dose of 2.7 mg tetrahydrocannabinol (THC) and 2.5 mg cannabidiol (CBD), has been approved in Canada for multiple sclerosis-related central neuropathic pain.

Local anaesthetics

Lidocaine (lignocaine) and mexiletine are widely used local anaesthetics that are generally considered to be third-line agents for the management of neuropathic pain when administered by systemic routes (Vadalouca et al 2006). This is because these agents not only block sodium channels on sensory nerves but also block sodium channels in cardiac tissue and the brain, potentially resulting in cardiac conduction block and neurotoxicity, respectively (Vadalouca et al 2006).

Hence, to mitigate the systemic side effects of local anaesthetics, the lidocaine patch 5% may be used for the relief of neuropathic pain in patients with postherpetic neuralgia and peripheral neuropathic pain (Khaliq et al 2007; Meier et al 2003). Randomized controlled trials show that the lidocaine patch 5% is well tolerated and systemic side effects are unusual (Heitz et al 2009).

Capsaicin patch

Capsaicin is a hydrophobic, colourless and odourless chemical irritant that is the pungent component of the red chilli pepper (Sawynok 2005). Capsaicin binds selectively to the TRPV1 receptor on C fibres, resulting in initial excitation of neurons followed by a period of prolonged desensitization and pain relief subsequent to depletion of substance P from presynaptic nerve terminals (Veronesi & Oortgiesen 2006). Topically applied capsaicin at a low concentration (0.075%) lacked efficacy for the alleviation of PDN, postherpetic neuralgia, HIV neuropathic pain or postsurgical neuropathic pain (Mason et al 2004). However, when used at high concentration (8%), topically applied capsaicin produced long-lasting pain relief in HIV neuropathic pain (Simpson et al 2008) and in postherpetic neuralgia (Backonja et al 2008).

α_2-adrenergic receptor agonists

After intrathecal administration, clonidine, an α_2-adrenoceptor agonist, evokes analgesia and has opioid sparing effects (Smith & Elliott 2001). Opioid sparing effects of α_2-agonists such as clonidine and dexmedetomidine were also evident after systemic dosing routes in the post-operative setting (Arain et al 2004; Jalonen et al 1997; Park et al 1996).

Glucocorticoids

Glucocorticoids have potent anti-inflammatory effects involving suppression of immune responses as well as the production of prostaglandins and leukotrienes (Goppelt-Struebe et al 1989). In the post-operative setting, several randomized controlled trials have shown that addition of glucocorticoids to analgesic regimens improves post-operative pain relief whilst reducing analgesic consumption and reducing post-operative nausea, vomiting and fatigue (Kehlet 2007; Romundstad et al 2006). However, they are generally considered to be of limited value in the management of chronic pain due to their severe adverse effect profile involving the CNS, musculoskeletal, endocrine, cardiovascular and gastrointestinal systems with bone loss being one of the most serious side effects (Moghadam-Kia & Werth 2010). For short-term intra-articular use, corticosteroids such as triamcinolone, methylprednisolone and betamethasone show benefit for increasing joint mobility and for providing pain relief (Habib et al 2010; Hepper et al 2009).

INVASIVE PROCEDURES

Invasive procedures including reversible blockade with local anaesthetics, augmentation with spinal cord stimulation, ablation with neurolytic agents and intraspinal routes of delivery to improve an effective drug's therapeutic index are warranted for the treatment of chronic cancer and non-cancer pain when conventional pharmacological therapies are unsuccessful due to either inadequate pain relief and/or intolerable side effects (Eisenberg et al 2005; Markman & Philip 2007). Invasive interventions such as intrathecal opioids, neurolytic coeliac plexus blockade and spinal cord stimulation have been shown to be not only efficacious but also to reduce exposure to the side effects of systemically administered analgesic agents. These techniques need to be tailored to the individual patient and they complement, rather than replace, pharmacological and non-pharmacological treatments for the management of chronic pain (Markman & Philip 2007).

Neurolytic celiac plexus blockade

Neurolytic coeliac plexus blockade using agents such as alcohol (50–100%) or phenol is the most extensively utilized ablative procedure for the treatment of cancer pain, particularly intra-abdominal cancer pain. This type of block has a duration of analgesia in the order of months (Markman & Philip 2007; Miguel 2000).

Implantable intrathecal drug delivery

Patients with non-cancer pain experiencing inadequate pain relief and/or intolerable side effects with conventional pharmacotherapy may be considered for an implanted intrathecal drug delivery device (Markman & Philip 2007). Indications include failed back syndrome, neuropathic pain, axial spinal pain, complex regional pain syndrome, diffuse pain, brachial plexitis, central pain, failed spinal cord stimulation (SCS) therapy, arachnoiditis, post-stroke pain, spinal cord injury pain and peripheral neuropathy (Markman & Philip 2007).

Devices used to deliver analgesic agents into the epidural and intrathecal spaces include programmable implantable pumps, implanted accessible reservoir systems and tunnelled exteriorized catheters. A major benefit of intraspinal delivery systems is that they allow logarithmic scale reductions in the dosage requirements of analgesic agents relative to systemic routes of administration, but close monitoring of patients is essential, particularly during the initial dose titration phase (Markman & Philip 2007). Medications that have been given spinally include opioids, local anaesthetics, spasmolytics (e.g. baclofen), α_2-agonists (e.g. clonidine) and ziconotide (Markman & Philip 2007; Miguel 2000).

Following insertion of a small catheter into the cerebrospinal fluid in the intrathecal space, the catheter is attached to a small, subcutaneously implanted, battery-powered programmable pump, which is refilled at 1–3 monthly intervals (Markman & Philip 2007). This mode of delivery bypasses systemic metabolism and ensures that the administered medications are delivered in close proximity to target receptors. The net result is a longer duration of action and a reduced rate of systemic side effects relative to more conventional dosing routes. Before definitive pump implantation, selected patients undergo psychological profiling and the potential therapeutic benefit of intrathecal drug delivery is tested via an external pump (Markman & Philip 2007).

Catheter-related problems that commonly occur in up to 25% of patients include kinking, disconnection, blockage and granuloma formation at the catheter tip as a result of prolonged high-rate infusion (Markman & Philip 2007).

Spinal cord stimulation

For the treatment of chronic radicular pain after lumbar and cervical spine surgery, spinal cord stimulation is commonly used as a late-stage therapy supported by the outcomes of randomized controlled trials showing superior outcomes relative to lumbar re-operation (Markman & Philip 2007). For spinal cord stimulation, cylindrical catheter-like leads or flat, paddle-shaped leads are positioned in the dorsal epidural space and an electrical field is generated via connection of the stimulating metal contacts with a programmable pulse generator (Markman & Philip 2007). The resulting electrical field stimulates the axons of the dorsal root and dorsal column fibres, resulting in activation of descending inhibition and blockade of activity in the lateral spinothalamic tract (Markman & Philip 2007). The battery, similar in size to a cardiac pacemaker, is implanted subcutaneously and connected to the leads via a subcutaneous tunnel (Markman & Philip 2007).

CONCLUSIONS

Considerable research over the last two decades has shown that the neurobiology of pain is highly complex, with multiple concurrent changes in expression levels of a broad array of receptors and ion channels that represent potential novel targets for the development of the next generation of pain therapeutics. Although several potential new pain therapeutics are in preclinical or clinical development, these are yet to reach the market. Hence, the currently available analgesic and adjuvant medications will continue to be utilized for the foreseeable future to manage clinical pain, according to the principles succinctly summarized by the WHO three-step analgesic ladder (World Health Organization 1986). Briefly, this involves use of non-opioid analgesics for the relief of mild pain, with adjuvants added when pain has a neuropathic component. When mild pain progresses to moderate pain weak opioid analgesics are added to non-opioids and/or adjuvants as required. For moderate to severe pain, strong opioid analgesics are prescribed, often in combination with non-opioids and/or adjuvants as required. More invasive interventions are recommended for the 10–30% of patients whose pain is not relieved by conventional pharmacotherapy.

Given the complexity of the pathobiology underpinning chronic pain revealed by research to date, it is difficult to conceive how there could ever be a single 'gold-standard' drug treatment for the optimal management of all types of pain. Development of methods to enable mechanism-based pharmacotherapy of pain is required to improve our ability to individualize the pharmacological management of pain within a multidisciplinary approach that includes non-pharmacological and psychosocial interventions.

REFERENCES

Abbadie, C., Bhangoo, S., De Koninck, Y., et al., 2009. Chemokines and pain mechanisms. Brain Res. Rev. 60, 125–134

Agency for Healthcare Research and Quality, U.S. Department of Health and Human Services, 2009. Choosing nonopioid analgesics for osteoarthritis: clinician summary guide. J. Pain Palliat. Care Pharmacother. 23, 433–457.

Altman, R.D., Dreiser, R.L., Fisher, C.L., et al., 2009. Diclofenac sodium gel in patients with primary hand osteoarthritis: a randomized, double-blind, placebo-controlled trial. J. Rheumatol. 36, 1991–1999.

Apkarian, A.V., 2008. Pain perception in relation to emotional learning. Curr. Opin. Neurobiol. 18, 464–468.

Arain, S.R., Ruehlow, R.M., Uhrich, T.D., et al., 2004. The efficacy of dexmedetomidine versus morphine for postoperative analgesia after major inpatient surgery. Anesth. Analg. 98, 153–158.

Argoff, C.E., Silvershein, D.I., 2009. A comparison of long- and short-acting opioids for the treatment of chronic noncancer pain: tailoring therapy to meet patient needs. Mayo Clin. Proc. 84, 602–612.

Attal, N., Cruccu, G., Haanpaa, M., et al., 2006. EFNS guidelines on pharmacological treatment of neuropathic pain. Eur. J. Neurol. 13, 1153–1169.

Backonja, M., Wallace, M.S., Blonsky, E.R., et al., 2008. NGX-4010, a high-concentration capsaicin patch, for the treatment of postherpetic neuralgia: a randomised, double-blind study. Lancet Neurol. 7, 1106–1112.

Baron, R., 2009. Neuropathic pain: a clinical perspective. Handb. Exp. Pharmacol. 3–30.

Barthel, H.R., Haselwood, D., Longley 3rd., S., et al., 2009. Randomized controlled trial of diclofenac sodium gel in knee osteoarthritis. Semin. Arthritis Rheum. 39, 203–212.

Basbaum, A.I., Bautista, D.M., Scherrer, G., et al., 2009. Cellular and molecular mechanisms of pain. Cell 139, 267–284.

Battershill, A.J., Keating, G.M., 2006. Remifentanil: a review of its analgesic and sedative use in the intensive care unit. Drugs 66, 365–385.

Bell, R.F., Dahl, J.B., Moore, R.A., et al., 2006. Perioperative ketamine for acute postoperative pain. Cochrane Database Syst. Rev. CD004603.

Bhattacharya, A., Wickenden, A.D., Chaplan, S.R., 2009. Sodium channel blockers for the treatment of neuropathic pain. Neurotherapeutics 6, 663–678.

Bhave, G., Zhu, W., Wang, H., et al., 2002. cAMP-dependent protein kinase regulates desensitization of the capsaicin receptor (VR1) by direct phosphorylation. Neuron. 35, 721–731.

Bhave, G., Hu, H.J., Glauner, K.S., et al., 2003. Protein kinase C phosphorylation sensitizes but does not activate the capsaicin receptor transient receptor potential vanilloid 1 (TRPV1). Proc. Natl. Acad. Sci. U. S. A. 100, 12480–12485.

Boerner, U., 1975. The metabolism of morphine and heroin in man. Drug Metab. Rev. 4, 39–73.

Bonnefont, J., Alloui, A., Chapuy, E., et al., 2003. Orally administered paracetamol does not act locally in the rat formalin test: evidence for a supraspinal, serotonin-dependent antinociceptive mechanism. Anesthesiology 99, 976–981.

Bovill, J.G., 1987. Which potent opioid? Important criteria for selection. Drugs 33, 520–530.

Broad, L.M., Mogg, A.J., Beattie, R.E., et al., 2009. TRP channels as emerging targets for pain therapeutics. Expert Opin. Ther. Targets 13, 69–81.

Brown, A.J., 2007. Novel cannabinoid receptors. Br. J. Pharmacol. 152, 567–575.

Bruera, E., Belzile, M., Pituskin, E., et al., 1998. Randomized, double-blind, cross-over trial comparing safety and efficacy of oral controlled-release oxycodone with controlled-release morphine in patients with cancer pain. J. Clin. Oncol. 16, 3222–3229.

Burke, A.S.E., Fitzgerald, G.A., 2006. Analgesic-antipyretic agents. McGraw-Hill, New York.

Capone, M.L., Tacconelli, S., Patrignani, P., 2005. Clinical pharmacology of etoricoxib. Expert Opin. Drug Metab. Toxicol. 1, 269–282.

Cheer, S.M., Goa, K.L., 2001. Parecoxib (parecoxib sodium). Drugs. 61, 1133–1141; discussion 1142–1143.

Childers, Jr., W.E., Baudy, R.B., 2007. N-methyl-D-aspartate antagonists and neuropathic pain: the search for relief. J. Med. Chem. 50, 2557–2562.

Chizh, B.A., Headley, P.M., 2005. NMDA antagonists and neuropathic pain – multiple drug targets and multiple uses. Curr. Pharm. Des. 11, 2977–2994.

Chou, R., Fanciullo, G.J., Fine, P.G., et al., 2009. Clinical Guidelines for the Use of Chronic Opioid Therapy in Chronic Noncancer Pain. J. Pain 10, 113–130.e22.

Codd, E.E., Shank, R.P., Schupsky, J.J., et al., 1995. Serotonin and norepinephrine uptake inhibiting activity of centrally acting analgesics: structural determinants and role in antinociception. J. Pharmacol. Exp. Ther. 274, 1263–1270.

Coggeshall, R.E., Carlton, S.M., 1997. Receptor localization in the mammalian dorsal horn and primary afferent neurons. Brain Res. Brain Res. Rev. 24, 28–66.

Costigan, M., Scholz, J., Woolf, C.J., 2009. Neuropathic pain: a maladaptive response of the nervous system to damage. Annu. Rev. Neurosci. 32, 1–32.

Cousins, M.J., 2007. Persistent pain: A disease entity. J. Pain Symptom Manage. 33, S4–S10.

Crown, E.D., Gwak, Y.S., Ye, Z., et al., 2008. Activation of p38 MAP kinase is involved in central neuropathic pain following spinal cord injury. Exp. Neurol. 213, 257–267.

Damaj, M.I., Flood, P., Ho, K.K., et al., 2005. Effect of dextrometorphan and dextrorphan on nicotine and neuronal nicotinic receptors: in vitro and in vivo selectivity. J. Pharmacol. Exp. Ther. 312, 780–785.

Davis, M.P., 2005. Buprenorphine in cancer pain. Support. Care Cancer 13, 878–887.

Davis, M.P., 2006. Management of cancer pain: focus on new opioid analgesic formulations. Am. J. Cancer 5, 171–182.

Davison, S.N., Mayo, P.R., 2008. Pain management in chronic kidney disease: the pharmacokinetics and pharmacodynamics of hydromorphone and hydromorphone-3-glucuronide in hemodialysis patients. J. Opioid Manag. 4, 335–336, 339–344.

Diatchenko, L., Nackley, A.G., Slade, G.D., et al., 2006. Idiopathic pain disorders – pathways of vulnerability. Pain 123, 226–230.

Dick, I.E., Brochu, R.M., Purohit, Y., et al., 2007. Sodium channel blockade may contribute to the analgesic efficacy of antidepressants. J. Pain 8, 315–324.

Dickenson, A.H., Ghandehari, J., 2007. Anti-convulsants and anti-depressants. Handb. Exp. Pharmacol. 177, 145–177.

D'Mello, R., Dickenson, A.H., 2008. Spinal cord mechanisms of pain. Br. J. Anaesth. 101, 8–16.

Doubell, T.P., Mannion, R.H., Woolf, C.J., 1999. The dorsal horn: state-dependent sensory processing, plasticity and the generation of pain. In: Wall, P.D., Melzack, R. (Eds.), Textbook of Pain, fourth ed. Churchill Livingstone, London.

Dray, A., 1997. Kinins and their receptors in hyperalgesia. Can. J. Physiol. Pharmacol. 75, 704–712.

Dugowson, C.E., Gnanashanmugam, P., 2006. Nonsteroidal anti-inflammatory drugs. Phys. Med. Rehabil. Clin. N. Am. 17, 347–354, vi.

Dworkin, R.H., O'Connor, A.B., Backonja, M., et al., 2007. Pharmacologic management of neuropathic pain: evidence-based recommendations. Pain 132, 237–251.

Dworkin, R.H., O'Connor, A.B., Audette, J., et al., 2010. Recommendations for the pharmacological management of neuropathic pain: an overview and literature update. Mayo Clin. Proc. 85, S3–14.

Ehret, G.B., Desmeules, J.A., Broers, B., 2007. Methadone-associated long QT syndrome: improving pharmacotherapy for dependence on illegal opioids and lessons learned for pharmacology. Expert Opin. Drug Saf. 6, 289–303.

Eisenberg, E., Marinangeli, F., Birkhahn, J., et al., 2005. Time to modify the analgesic ladder? Pain: Clinical Updates XIII (5), 1–4.

Evans, H.C., Easthope, S.E., 2003. Transdermal buprenorphine. Drugs 63, 1999–2010; discussion 2011–2012.

Fenton, C., Keating, G.M., Wagstaff, A.J., 2004. Valdecoxib: a review of its use in the management of osteoarthritis, rheumatoid arthritis, dysmenorrhoea and acute pain. Drugs 64, 1231–1261.

Finnerup, N.B., Otto, M., McQuay, H.J., et al., 2005. Algorithm for neuropathic pain treatment: an evidence based proposal. Pain. 118, 289–305.

Food and Drug Administration, 1999. Over-the-counter drug products containing analgesic/antipyretic active ingredients for internal use; required alcohol warning; final rule; compliance date. Food and Drug Administration, HHS. Fed. Regist. 64, 13066–13067.

Frampton, J.E., 2010. Tapentadol immediate release: a review of its use in the treatment of moderate to severe acute pain. Drugs 70, 1719–1743.

Gardner, J.S., Blough, D., Drinkard, C.R., et al., 2000. Tramadol and seizures: a surveillance study in a managed care population. Pharmacotherapy 20, 1423–1431.

Gidal, B.E., 2006. New and emerging treatment options for neuropathic pain. Am. J. Manag. Care 12, S269–S278.

Gilman, A.G., Goodman, L.S., Gilman, A., 1980. Opioid Analgesics and Antagonists. Macmillan, New York.

Gilron, I., Watson, C.P., Cahill, C.M., et al., 2006. Neuropathic pain: a practical guide for the clinician. CMAJ 175, 265–275.

Goppelt-Struebe, M., Wolter, D., Resch, K., 1989. Glucocorticoids inhibit prostaglandin synthesis not only at the level of phospholipase A2 but also at the level of cyclo-oxygenase/PGE isomerase. Br. J. Pharmacol. 98, 1287–1295.

Gorman, A.L., Elliott, K.J., Inturrisi, C.E., 1997. The d- and l-isomers of methadone bind to the non-competitive site on the N-methyl-D-aspartate (NMDA) receptor in rat forebrain and spinal cord. Neurosci. Lett. 223, 5–8.

Goudet, C., Magnaghi, V., Landry, M., et al., 2009. Metabotropic receptors for glutamate and GABA in pain. Brain Res. Rev. 60, 43–56.

Grond, S., Sablotzki, A., 2004. Clinical pharmacology of tramadol. Clin. Pharmacokinet. 43, 879–923.

Habib, G.S., Saliba, W., Nashashibi, M., 2010. Local effects of intra-articular corticosteroids. Clin. Rheumatol. 29, 347–356.

Hagen, N., Thirlwell, M.P., Dhaliwal, H.S., et al., 1995. Steady-state pharmacokinetics of hydromorphone and hydromorphone-3-glucuronide in cancer patients after immediate and controlled-release hydromorphone. J. Clin. Pharmacol. 35, 37–44.

Hair, P.I., Keating, G.M., McKeage, K., 2008. Transdermal matrix fentanyl membrane patch (matrifen): in severe cancer-related chronic pain. Drugs 68, 2001–2009.

Hanani, M., 2005. Satellite glial cells in sensory ganglia: from form to function. Brain Res. Brain Res. Rev. 48, 457–476.

Harris, D.S., Mendelson, J.E., Lin, E.T., et al., 2004. Pharmacokinetics and subjective effects of sublingual buprenorphine, alone or in combination with naloxone: lack of dose proportionality. Clin. Pharmacokinet. 43, 329–340.

Hartrick, C.T., 2009. Tapentadol immediate release for the relief of moderate-to-severe acute pain. Expert Opin. Pharmacother. 10, 2687–2696.

Harvey, V.L., Dickenson, A.H., 2008. Mechanisms of pain in nonmalignant disease. Curr. Opin. Support. Palliat. Care 2, 133–139.

Hays, H., Hagen, N., Thirlwell, M., et al., 1994. Comparative clinical efficacy and safety of immediate release and controlled release hydromorphone for chronic severe cancer pain. Cancer 74, 1808–1816.

Hefti, F., 1997. Pharmacology of neurotrophic factors. Annu. Rev. Pharmacol. Toxicol. 37, 239–267.

Heitz, J.W., Witkowski, T.A., Viscusi, E.R., 2009. New and emerging analgesics and analgesic technologies for acute pain management. Curr. Opin. Anaesthesiol. 22, 608–617.

Hepper, C.T., Halvorson, J.J., Duncan, S.T., et al., 2009. The efficacy and duration of intra-articular corticosteroid injection for knee osteoarthritis: a systematic review of level I studies. J. Am. Acad. Orthop. Surg. 17, 638–646.

Herndon, C.M., 2007. Iontophoretic drug delivery system: focus on fentanyl. Pharmacotherapy 27, 745–754.

Hollingshead, J., Duhmke, R.M., Cornblath, D.R., 2006. Tramadol for neuropathic pain. Cochrane Database Syst. Rev. 3, CD003726.

Horn, E., Nesbit, S.A., 2004. Pharmacology and pharmacokinetics of sedatives and analgesics. Gastrointest. Endosc. Clin. N. Am. 14, 247–268.

Hoy, S.M., Keating, G.M., 2008. Fentanyl transdermal matrix patch (Durotep MT patch; Durogesic DTrans; Durogesic SMAT): in adults with cancer-related pain. Drugs 68, 1711–1721.

Jalonen, J., Hynynen, M., Kuitunen, A., et al., 1997. Dexmedetomidine as an anesthetic adjunct in coronary artery bypass grafting. Anesthesiology 86, 331–345.

Jann, M.W., Slade, J.H., 2007. Antidepressant agents for the treatment of chronic pain and depression. Pharmacotherapy 27, 1571–1587.

Jensen, T.S., 2002. Anticonvulsants in neuropathic pain: rationale and clinical evidence. Eur. J. Pain 6 (Suppl. A), 61–68.

Jensen, T.S., Finnerup, N.B., 2009. Neuropathic pain: Peripheral and central mechanisms. Eur. J. Pain Suppl. 3, 33–36

Ji, R.R., 2004. Peripheral and central mechanisms of inflammatory pain, with emphasis on MAP kinases. Curr. Drug Targets Inflamm. Allergy 3, 299–303.

Johnson, R.E., Fudala, P.J., Payne, R., 2005. Buprenorphine: considerations for pain management. J. Pain Symptom Manage. 29, 297–326.

Kalso, E., 2005. Oxycodone. J. Pain Symptom Manage. 29, S47–S56.

Karst, M., Salim, K., Burstein, S., et al., 2003. Analgesic effect of the synthetic cannabinoid CT-3 on chronic neuropathic pain: a randomized controlled trial. JAMA 290, 1757–1762.

Kehlet, H., 2007. Glucocorticoids for peri-operative analgesia: how far are we from general recommendations? Acta Anaesthesiol. Scand. 51, 1133–1135.

Khaliq, W., Alam, S., Puri, N., 2007. Topical lidocaine for the treatment of postherpetic neuralgia. Cochrane Database Syst. Rev. CD004846.

Kneip, C., Terlinden, R., Beier, H., et al., 2008. Investigations into the drug–drug interaction potential of tapentadol in human liver microsomes and fresh human hepatocytes. Drug Metab. Lett. 2, 67–75.

Krantz, M.J., Lewkowiez, L., Hays, H., et al., 2002. Torsade de pointes associated with very-high-dose methadone. Ann. Intern. Med. 137, 501–504.

Krenzischek, D.A., Dunwoody, C.J., Polomano, R.C., et al., 2008. Pharmacotherapy for acute pain: implications for practice. Pain Manag. Nurs. 9, S22–S32.

Kronenberg, R.H., 2002. Ketamine as an analgesic: parenteral, oral, rectal, subcutaneous, transdermal and intranasal administration. J. Pain Palliat. Care Pharmacother. 16, 27–35.

Kucukemre, F., Kunt, N., Kaygusuz, K., et al., 2005. Remifentanil compared with morphine for postoperative patient-controlled analgesia after major abdominal surgery: a randomized controlled trial. Eur. J. Anaesthesiol. 22, 378–385.

Lai, J., Ossipov, M.H., Vanderah, T.W., et al., 2001. Neuropathic pain: the paradox of dynorphin. Mol. Interv. 1, 160–167.

Lalovic, B., Kharasch, E., Hoffer, C., et al., 2006. Pharmacokinetics and pharmacodynamics of oral oxycodone in healthy human subjects: role of circulating active metabolites. Clin. Pharmacol. Ther. 79, 461–479.

Larson, A.M., Polson, J., Fontana, R.J., et al., 2005. Acetaminophen-induced acute liver failure: results of a United States multicenter, prospective study. Hepatology 42, 1364–1372.

Latremoliere, A., Woolf, C.J., 2009. Central sensitization: a generator of pain hypersensitivity by central neural plasticity. J. Pain 10, 895–926.

Latta, K.S., Ginsberg, B., Barkin, R.L., 2002. Meperidine: a critical review. Am. J. Ther. 9, 53–68.

Lee, C., Straus, W.L., Balshaw, R., et al., 2004. A comparison of the efficacy and safety of nonsteroidal antiinflammatory agents versus acetaminophen in the treatment of osteoarthritis: a meta-analysis. Arthritis Rheum. 51, 746–754.

Lenz, H., Sandvik, L., Qvigstad, E., et al., 2009. A comparison of intravenous oxycodone and intravenous morphine in patient-controlled postoperative analgesia after laparoscopic hysterectomy. Anesth. Analg. 109, 1279–1283.

Leow, K.P., Smith, M.T., 1994. The antinociceptive potencies of oxycodone, noroxycodone and morphine after intracerebroventricular administration to rats. Life Sci. 54, 1229–1236.

Leow, K.P., Smith, M.T., Williams, B., et al., 1992. Single-dose and steady-state pharmacokinetics and pharmacodynamics of oxycodone in patients with cancer. Clin. Pharmacol. Ther. 52, 487–495.

Leppert, W., 2009. The role of methadone in cancer pain treatment – a review. Int. J. Clin. Pract. 63, 1095–1109.

Lugo, R.A., Satterfield, K.L., Kern, S.E., 2005. Pharmacokinetics of methadone. J. Pain Palliat. Care Pharmacother. 19, 13–24.

Maher, T.J., Chaiyakul, P., 2003. Opioids (Bench). In: Smith, H.S. (Ed.), Drugs for pain. Hanley and Belfus, Philadelphia, pp. 83–96.

Manfredi, P.L., Foley, K.M., Payne, R., et al., 2003. Parenteral methadone: an essential medication for the treatment of pain. J. Pain Symptom Manage. 26, 687–688.

Marier, J.F., Lor, M., Potvin, D., et al., 2006. Pharmacokinetics, tolerability, and performance of a novel matrix transdermal delivery system of fentanyl relative to the commercially available reservoir formulation in healthy subjects. J. Clin. Pharmacol. 46, 642–653.

Marinella, M.A., 1997. Meperidine-induced generalized seizures with normal renal function. South Med. J. 90, 556–558.

Markman, J.D., Philip, A., 2007. Interventional approaches to pain management. Med. Clin. North Am. 91, 271–286.

Marret, E., Kurdi, O., Zufferey, P., et al., 2005. Effects of nonsteroidal antiinflammatory drugs on patient-controlled analgesia morphine side effects: meta-analysis of randomized controlled trials. Anesthesiology 102, 1249–1260.

Mason, L., Moore, R.A., Derry, S., et al., 2004. Systematic review of topical capsaicin for the treatment of chronic pain. BMJ. 328, 991.

Massey, T., Derry, S., Moore, R.A., et al., 2010. Topical NSAIDs for acute pain in adults. Cochrane Database Syst. Rev. 6, CD007402.

Mayer, M.L., 2005. Glutamate receptor ion channels. Curr. Opin. Neurobiol. 15, 282–288.

McCleane, G., 2003. Pharmacological management of neuropathic pain. CNS Drugs. 17, 1031–1043.

McLean, M.J., 1994. Clinical pharmacokinetics of gabapentin. Neurology 44, S17–S22; discussion S31–S32.

Meier, T., Wasner, G., Faust, M., et al., 2003. Efficacy of lidocaine patch 5% in the treatment of focal peripheral neuropathic pain syndromes: a randomized, double-blind, placebo-controlled study. Pain. 106, 151–158.

Merskey, H., Bogduk, N., 1994. Classification of chronic pain. IASP Press, Seattle.

Michaud, K., Bombardier, C., Emery, P., 2007. Quality of life in patients with rheumatoid arthritis: does abatacept make a difference? Clin. Exp. Rheumatol. 25, S35–S45.

Miguel, R., 2000. Interventional treatment of cancer pain: the fourth step in the World Health Organization analgesic ladder? Cancer Control 7, 149–156.

Milne, R.W., Nation, R.L., Somogyi, A.A., 1996. The disposition of morphine and its 3- and 6-glucuronide metabolites in humans and animals, and the importance of the metabolites to the pharmacological effects of morphine. Drug Metab. Rev. 28, 345–472.

Moghadam-Kia, S., Werth, V.P., 2010. Prevention and treatment of systemic glucocorticoid side effects. Int. J. Dermatol. 49, 239–248.

Munir, M.A., Enany, N., Zhang, J.M., 2007. Nonopioid analgesics. Anesthesiol. Clin. 25, 761–774, vi.

Murray, A., Hagen, N.A., 2005. Hydromorphone. J. Pain Symptom Manage. 29, S57–S66.

Myers, S.H., Laporte, D.M., 2009. Acetaminophen: Safe Use and Associated Risks. J. Hand Surg. 34, 1137–1139.

Narabayashi, M., Saijo, Y., Takenoshita, S., et al., 2008. Opioid rotation from oral morphine to oral oxycodone in cancer patients with intolerable adverse effects: an open-label trial. Jpn. J. Clin. Oncol. 38, 296–304.

Nielsen, C.K., Ross, F.B., Smith, M.T., 2000. Incomplete, asymmetric, and route-dependent cross-tolerance between oxycodone and morphine in the Dark Agouti rat. J. Pharmacol. Exp. Ther. 295, 91–99.

Nielsen, C.K., Ross, F.B., Lotfipour, S., et al., 2007. Oxycodone and morphine have distinctly different pharmacological profiles: radioligand binding and behavioural studies in two rat models of neuropathic pain. Pain 132, 289–300.

Nissen, L.M., Tett, S.E., Cramond, T., et al., 2001. Opioid analgesic prescribing and use – an audit of analgesic prescribing by general practitioners and The Multidisciplinary Pain Centre at Royal Brisbane Hospital. Br. J. Clin. Pharmacol. 52, 693–698.

O'Connor, A.B., Dworkin, R.H., 2009. Treatment of neuropathic pain: an overview of recent guidelines. Am. J. Med. 122, S22–S32.

Ohara, P.T., Vit, J.P., Bhargava, A., et al., 2009. Gliopathic pain: when satellite glial cells go bad. Neuroscientist 15, 450–463.

Otto, M., Bach, F.W., Jensen, T.S., et al., 2008. Escitalopram in painful polyneuropathy: a randomized, placebo-controlled, cross-over trial. Pain 139, 275–283.

Park, J., Forrest, J., Kolesar, R., et al., 1996. Oral clonidine reduces postoperative PCA morphine requirements. Can. J. Anaesth. 43, 900–906.

Pasero, C., 2005. Fentanyl for acute pain management. J. Perianesth. Nurs. 20, 279–284.

Patrono, C., Patrignani, P., Garcia Rodriguez, L.A., 2001. Cyclooxygenase-selective inhibition of prostanoid formation: transducing biochemical selectivity into clinical read-outs. J. Clin. Invest. 108, 7–13.

Peng, P.W., Sandler, A.N., 1999. A review of the use of fentanyl analgesia in the management of acute pain in adults. Anesthesiology 90, 576–599.

Perea, G., Araque, A., 2005. Properties of synaptically evoked astrocyte calcium signal reveal synaptic information processing by astrocytes. J. Neurosci. 25, 2192–2203.

Picard, N., Cresteil, T., Djebli, N., et al., 2005. In vitro metabolism study of buprenorphine: evidence for new metabolic pathways. Drug Metab. Dispos. 33, 689–695.

Pick, C.G., Peter, Y., Schreiber, S., et al., 1997. Pharmacological characterization of buprenorphine, a mixed agonist-antagonist with kappa 3 analgesia. Brain Res. 744, 41–46.

Pickering, G., Loriot, M.A., Libert, F., et al., 2006. Analgesic effect of acetaminophen in humans: first evidence of a central serotonergic mechanism. Clin. Pharmacol. Ther. 79, 371–378.

Portenoy, R.K., Lesage, P., 1999. Management of cancer pain. Lancet. 353, 1695–1700.

Poyhia, R., Olkkola, K.T., Seppala, T., et al., 1991. The pharmacokinetics of oxycodone after intravenous injection in adults. Br. J. Clin. Pharmacol. 32, 516–518.

Poyhia, R., Seppala, T., Olkkola, K.T., et al., 1992. The pharmacokinetics and metabolism of oxycodone after intramuscular and oral administration to healthy subjects. Br. J. Clin. Pharmacol. 33, 617–621.

Quigley, C., 2002. Hydromorphone for acute and chronic pain. Cochrane Database Syst. Rev. CD003447.

Rainville, P., Duncan, G.H., Price, D.D., et al., 1997. Pain affect encoded in human anterior cingulate but not somatosensory cortex. Science 277, 968–971.

Raivich, G., 2005. Like cops on the beat: the active role of resting microglia. Trends Neurosci. 28, 571–573.

Rao, S.S., Go, J.T., 2010. Update on the management of constipation in the elderly: new treatment options. Clin. Interv. Aging 5, 163–171.

Rao, R.D., Flynn, P.J., Sloan, J.A., et al., 2008. Efficacy of lamotrigine in the management of chemotherapy-induced peripheral neuropathy: a phase 3 randomized, double-blind, placebo-controlled trial, N01C3. Cancer 112, 2802–2808.

Reichling, D.B., Levine, J.D., 2009. Critical role of nociceptor plasticity in chronic pain. Trends Neurosci. 32, 611–618.

Remy, C., Marret, E., Bonnet, F., 2006. State of the art of paracetamol in acute pain therapy. Curr. Opin. Anaesthesiol. 19, 562–565.

Riley, J., Ross, J.R., Gretton, S.K., et al., 2007. Proposed 5-step World Health Organization analgesic and side effect ladder. European Journal of Pain Supplements. 1, 23–30.

Robinson, S.E., 2002. Buprenorphine: an analgesic with an expanding role in the treatment of opioid addiction. CNS Drug Rev. 8, 377–390.

Romundstad, L., Breivik, H., Roald, H., et al., 2006. Methylprednisolone reduces pain, emesis, and fatigue after breast augmentation surgery: a single-dose, randomized, parallel-group study with methylprednisolone 125 mg, parecoxib 40 mg, and placebo. Anesth. Analg. 102, 418–425.

Rostom, A., Dube, C., Wells, G., et al., 2002. Prevention of NSAID-induced gastroduodenal ulcers. Cochrane Database Syst. Rev. CD002296.

Saarto, T., Wiffen, P.J., 2005. Antidepressants for neuropathic pain. Cochrane Database Syst. Rev. CD005454.

Saarto, T., Wiffen, P.J., 2007. Antidepressants for neuropathic pain. Cochrane Database Syst. Rev. CD005454.

Sato, K., Kiyama, H., Park, H.T., et al., 1993. AMPA, KA and NMDA receptors are expressed in the rat DRG neurones. Neuroreport 4, 1263–1265.

Sawynok, J., 2005. Topical analgesics in neuropathic pain. Curr. Pharm. Des. 11, 2995–3004.

Scholz, J., Broom, D.C., Youn, D.H., et al., 2005. Blocking caspase activity prevents transsynaptic neuronal apoptosis and the loss of inhibition in lamina II of the dorsal horn after peripheral nerve injury. J. Neurosci. 25, 7317–7323.

Serlin, R.C., Mendoza, T.R., Nakamura, Y., et al., 1995. When is cancer pain mild, moderate or severe? Grading pain severity by its interference with function. Pain 61, 277–284.

Seybold, V.S., 2009. The role of peptides in central sensitization. Handb. Exp. Pharmacol. 194, 451–491.

Shamoon, M., Hochberg, M.C., 2000. Treatment of osteoarthritis with acetaminophen: efficacy, safety, and comparison with nonsteroidal anti-inflammatory drugs. Curr. Rheumatol. Rep. 2, 454–458.

Sherrington, C.S., 1906. The integrative action of the nervous system. Scribner, New York.

Sheth, R.N., Dorsi, M.J., Li, Y., et al., 2002. Mechanical hyperalgesia after an L5 ventral rhizotomy or an L5 ganglionectomy in the rat. Pain 96, 63–72.

Simon, L.S., Grierson, L.M., Naseer, Z., et al., 2009. Efficacy and safety of topical diclofenac containing dimethyl sulfoxide (DMSO) compared with those of topical placebo, DMSO vehicle and oral diclofenac for knee osteoarthritis. Pain 143, 238–245.

Simpson, D.M., Brown, S., Tobias, J., 2008. Controlled trial of high-concentration capsaicin patch for treatment of painful HIV neuropathy. Neurology. 70, 2305–2313.

Sindrup, S.H., Otto, M., Finnerup, N.B., et al., 2005. Antidepressants in the treatment of neuropathic pain. Basic Clin. Pharmacol. Toxicol. 96, 399–409.

Sluka, K.A., Winter, O.C., Wemmie, J.A., 2009. Acid-sensing ion channels: A new target for pain and CNS diseases. Curr. Opin. Drug Discov. Devel. 12, 693–704.

Smith, M.T., 2000. Neuroexcitatory effects of morphine and hydromorphone: evidence implicating the 3-glucuronide metabolites. Clin. Exp. Pharmacol. Physiol. 27, 524–528.

Smith, H.S., 2008. Peripherally-acting opioids. Pain Physician 11, S121–S132.

Smith, H., Elliott, J., 2001. Alpha(2) receptors and agonists in pain management. Curr. Opin. Anaesthesiol. 14, 513–518.

Snyder, S.H., Pasternak, G.W., 2003. Historical review: Opioid receptors. Trends Pharmacol. Sci. 24, 198–205.

Stanley, T.H., 2005. Fentanyl. J. Pain Symptom Manage. 29, S67–S71.

Stone, L.S., Molliver, D.C., 2009. In search of analgesia: emerging poles of GPCRs in pain. Mol. Interv. 9, 234–251.

Sultan, A., Gaskell, H., Derry, S., et al., 2008. Duloxetine for painful diabetic neuropathy and fibromyalgia pain: systematic review of randomised trials. BMC Neurol. 8, 29.

Takeda, M., Takahashi, M., Matsumoto, S., 2009. Contribution of the activation of satellite glia in sensory ganglia to pathological pain. Neurosci. Biobehav. Rev. 33, 784–792.

Tassone, D.M., Boyce, E., Guyer, J., et al., 2007. Pregabalin: a novel gamma-aminobutyric acid analogue in the treatment of neuropathic pain, partial-onset seizures, and anxiety disorders. Clin. Ther. 29, 26–48.

Teixeira, J.M., Oliveira, M.C., Parada, C.A., et al., 2010. Peripheral mechanisms underlying the essential role of P2X7 receptors in the development of inflammatory hyperalgesia. Eur. J. Pharmacol. 644, 55–60.

Thacker, M.A., Clark, A.K., Marchand, F., et al., 2007. Pathophysiology of peripheral neuropathic pain: immune cells and molecules. Anesth. Analg. 105, 838–847.

Toms, L., McQuay, H.J., Derry, S., et al., 2008. Single dose oral paracetamol (acetaminophen) for postoperative pain in adults. Cochrane Database Syst. Rev. CD004602.

Treede, R.D., Jensen, T.S., Campbell, J.N., et al., 2008. Neuropathic pain: redefinition and a grading system for clinical and research purposes. Neurology 70, 1630–1635.

Trescot, A.M., Datta, S., Lee, M., et al., 2008. Opioid pharmacology. Pain Physician 11, S133–153.

Tzschentke, T.M., De Vry, J., Terlinden, R., et al., 2006. Tapentadol HCl. Drugs Future. 31, 1053–1061.

Uceyler, N., Schafers, M., Sommer, C., 2009. Mode of action of cytokines on nociceptive neurons. Exp. Brain Res. 196, 67–78.

Urban, M.O., Zahn, P.K., Gebhart, G.F., 1999. Descending facilitatory influences from the rostral medial medulla mediate secondary, but not primary hyperalgesia in the rat. Neuroscience 90, 349–352.

Vadalouca, A., Siafaka, I., Argyra, E., et al., 2006. Therapeutic management of chronic neuropathic pain: an examination of pharmacologic treatment. Ann. N. Y. Acad. Sci. 1088, 164–186.

Vallejo, R., Tilley, D.M., Vogel, L., et al., 2010. The role of glia and the immune system in the development and maintenance of neuropathic pain. Pain Pract. 10.

Vanderah, T.W., 2007. Pathophysiology of pain. Med. Clin. North Am. 91, 1–12.

Vane, J.R., 1971. Inhibition of prostaglandin synthesis as a mechanism of action for aspirin-like drugs. Nat. New. Biol. 231, 232–235.

Vanegas, H., Schaible, H.G., 2004. Descending control of persistent pain: inhibitory or facilitatory? Brain Res. Brain Res. Rev. 46, 295–309.

Vergnolle, N., Ferazzini, M., D'Andrea, M.R., et al., 2003. Proteinase-activated receptors: novel signals for peripheral nerves. Trends Neurosci. 26, 496–500.

Veronesi, B., Oortgiesen, M., 2006. The TRPV1 receptor: target of toxicants and therapeutics. Toxicol. Sci. 89, 1–3.

Vinik, A.I., Tuchman, M., Safirstein, B., et al., 2007. Lamotrigine for treatment of pain associated with diabetic neuropathy: results of two randomized, double-blind, placebo-controlled studies. Pain 128, 169–179.

Viscusi, E.R., Martin, G., Hartrick, C.T., et al., 2005. Forty-eight hours of postoperative pain relief after total hip arthroplasty with a novel, extended-release epidural morphine formulation. Anesthesiology 102, 1014–1022.

Wade, W.E., Spruill, W.J., 2009. Tapentadol hydrochloride: a centrally acting oral analgesic. Clin. Ther. 31, 2804–2818.

Walsh, D., 2005. Advances in opioid therapy and formulations. Support. Care Cancer. 13, 138–144.

Wang, Z., Ma, W., Chabot, J.G., et al., 2010. Morphological evidence for the involvement of microglial p38 activation in CGRP-associated development of morphine antinociceptive tolerance. Peptides. 12, 2179–2184.

Watkins, L.R., Hutchinson, M.R., Ledeboer, A., et al., 2007. Norman Cousins Lecture. Glia as the 'bad guys': implications for improving clinical pain control and the clinical utility of opioids. Brain Behav. Immun. 21, 131–146.

Whitcomb, D.C., Block, G.D., 1994. Association of acetaminophen hepatotoxicity with fasting and ethanol use. JAMA 272, 1845–1850.

Wiffen, P., Collins, S., McQuay, H., et al., 2005. Anticonvulsant drugs for acute and chronic pain. Cochrane Database Syst. Rev. CD001133.

Wittenberg, R.H., Schell, E., Krehan, G., et al., 2006. First-dose analgesic effect of the cyclo-oxygenase-2 selective inhibitor lumiracoxib in osteoarthritis of the knee: a randomized, double-blind, placebo-controlled comparison with celecoxib [NCT00267215]. Arthritis Res. Ther. 8, R35.

Woolf, C.J., Ma, Q., 2007. Nociceptors – noxious stimulus detectors. Neuron 55, 353–364.

Woolf, C.J., Mannion, R.J., 1999. Neuropathic pain: aetiology, symptoms, mechanisms, and management. Lancet. 353, 1959–1964.

World Health Organization, 1986. Cancer pain relief. WHO, Geneva.

Wyeth Pharmaceuticals, 2009. Relistor (methylnaltrexone bromide) Prescribing Information. Philadelphia, U. S. A. Wyeth Pharmaceuticals Inc.

Yaksh, T.L., 2006. Calcium channels as therapeutic targets in neuropathic pain. J. Pain 7, S13–S30.

Zeilhofer, H.U., 2007. Prostanoids in nociception and pain. Biochem. Pharmacol. 73, 165–174.

Zhang, J.M., Strong, J.A., 2008. Recent evidence for activity-dependent initiation of sympathetic sprouting and neuropathic pain. Sheng Li Xue Bao 60, 617–627.

Zhuang, Z.Y., Gerner, P., Woolf, C.J., et al., 2005. ERK is sequentially activated in neurons, microglia, and astrocytes by spinal nerve ligation and contributes to mechanical allodynia in this neuropathic pain model. Pain 114, 149–159.

Zhuo, M., 2007. Neuronal mechanism for neuropathic pain. Mol. Pain 3, 14.

Zollner, C., Stein, C., 2007. Opioids. Handb. Exp. Pharmacol. 177, 31–63.

Chapter | 12 |

Manual therapy and influence on pain perception

Chris McCarthy

LEARNING OBJECTIVES

By the end of the chapter the reader should have an appreciation of:

- MT in the context of biopsychosocial management of MSK pain
- the effects of MT on local tissue, spinal and supraspinal pain mechanisms
- the effects of pleasant touch on pain
- the effects of treatment-related pain on pain perception
- the effects of MT on motor control
- how MT may be applied in practice.

INTRODUCTION

Manual therapy (MT) is considered to be a complex intervention from a clinical trials perspective (Dieppe 2004), so it is difficult to design methodologies that evaluate the specific effects, actions and interactions of the process. Although MT has non-specific effects, including placebo, it has a sound physiological basis to support its undoubted clinical effectiveness (Hoving et al 2006, UK BEAM 2004a). In the same way that movement is universal to the human condition, manually applied touch has an impact at every level of our physiology. Manually guided or passively produced movement influences local tissue healing, selectively influences afferent neurological stimulus, influences spinal and supraspinal moderation of afferent information, provides an experience of pain or pleasure, conveys an emotional context to physical sensation and signals actual or perceived threat. Consequently, establishing the precise elements of interventions that will target our patients' specific needs and expectations is a combination of intuition, expert knowledge and refined communication with the patient. This highly attuned work means that MT can never be applied as a 'one size fits all' approach, which may account for the varying results in research trials.

This chapter describes the underlying principles and treatment of MT for those readers who do not necessarily practice it. Some of the physiological evidence for how MT may reduce pain and improve function in musculoskeletal (MSK) pain patients will be presented and the interactions between mechanisms discussed.

THE RATIONALE OF MANUAL THERAPY

Manual therapies could conceivably boast the longest tradition in analgesic history, being reportedly undertaken in the earliest writings on medicine (Mattick & Wyatt 2000). While the magnitude of analgesic effect of MT

© 2014 Elsevier Ltd.

may be less than, for instance, surgery or pharmaceutical opiates, it is a ubiquitous approach to MSK pain that can offer immediate pain relief (Wright 1995), improvements in tissue healing (Zusman 2010), reductions in anxiety and fear of movement (Gifford 2000), pleasurable and rewarding tactile stimulation (Leknes & Tracey 2008), increased motivation to replicate pain-relieving movement (Schultz 2002), and a window of opportunity to relearn pain-free movement memories through repetition and active involvement in the rehabilitation process (Zusman 2004, 2005). MT is associated with some minor adverse events (treatment soreness, which actually may be a component of its effect), but major adverse events are rare (Carnes et al 2010), and clinical and cost effectiveness are acceptable (UK BEAM 2004b). It is not surprising that MT approaches to pain relief continue to be undertaken by therapists with large proportions of MSK pain patients.

MANUAL THERAPY IN A BIOPSYCHOSOCIAL CONTEXT

We all move and to move is to change place, position or posture. The positions we adopt to allow full function are three-dimensional and continuously adapting to the functional demands placed on us. Naturally, the body cannot always immediately change to accommodate these demands and consequently short- and long-term dysfunction can result. In a system that continuously changes position and demands the acquisition of new and challenging positions, the integrated control of movement can be compromised. When movement has become dysfunctional, the body receives prompts to that effect (pain, restriction) and a change in state is registered. We unconsciously register that we are not moving efficiently and the value of this information is assessed and we adopt strategies to address this situation (cessation, adaptation). We can learn to reduce the pain by changing some aspect of the way we move and with time new movement patterns occur. If we have been unable to improve our movement and reduce pain, we may seek assistance from an expert in movement dysfunction such as a manual therapist (McCarthy 2010).

Movement dysfunction is a complex situation that must be considered in a biopsychosocial context. Our bodies are continuously moving from one starting position of movement to another. The point at which this process is considered dysfunctional is dependent on the perception of the individual (Pincus & Morley 2001). The psychological perspective of the individual and inter-related societal influences have a huge bearing on just when function is considered to have become dysfunctional. For some the body has become dysfunctional only as they undergo anaesthesia prior to surgery, for others when they develop

an inkling that something is not quite right. Thus, the presentation of MSK dysfunction is incredibly variable.

Patients are people undertaking a therapeutic process of change to address a perceived problem. Thus, all patients have a perception that something is problematical, so we must assess them from a biopsychosocial perspective. Each patient will present with a biopsychosocial profile that will need to be carefully interpreted to allow the successful tailoring of intervention. Carefully weighted intervention, which targets important aspects of the patient profile, will optimally influence the patient's perception of their problem. In other words, we cannot afford to look at a patient from only one perspective. The ability of our clinical examination to weigh the relative value of each domain of a patient's biomechanical, physiological, psychological and social profile is vital for our practice (McCarthy 2010).

The model in Fig 12.1 shows the necessity of considering the psychological and social influences on patients attending with painful symptoms. Let us imagine a patient who has restricted movement of their L5/S1 lumbar motion segment, with this physiological impairment leading to the symptom of pain in the back. A manual therapist would quickly recognize this causal relationship, but a skilled manual therapist will evaluate the psychosocial influences

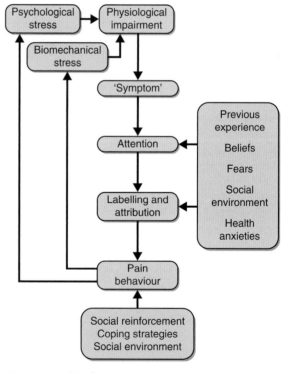

Fig. 12.1 **Model of symptom, attention and stress in MSK pain.** *Reprinted from Watson, P.J. 2002, Psychophysiological models of pain, in Placebo and nocebo. Pain management. Muscles and pain Topical Issues in Pain, 4., CNS Press, Falmouth, UK, with permission.*

on the perception, cause and maintenance of symptoms before instigating a strategy to change the symptoms. If, for example, the patient has had an excellent response to previous MT, has low levels of fear of movement and appropriate beliefs regarding causality, has a social environment encouraging recovery, and has no maladaptive coping strategies, the priority for treatment would be to address the biomechanical stressors and physiological impairment of the region. The techniques and explanations used would teach the patient that the local movement restriction was indeed minor as it responded to just a few seconds of stretching. The patient would learn that a simple stretch could reduce pain and limitation, and learn how to replicate this stretch as required. Any fear of movement would be reduced and self-efficacy facilitated, leading to reduced likelihood of reoccurrence. However, if the psychosocial influences on the patient were the opposite, treating the biomechanical stressors and physiological impairment would have an unpredictable, possibly deleterious, effect on symptoms.

The influence of the MT approach may become more predictable once maladaptive psychosocial influences have been addressed and when there is a realistic expectation that MT will be effective. Thus, addressing the physiological impairments in the absence of an appreciation of the patient's psychosocial influences on perception will lead to unpredictable responses at best. By the same token, simply addressing the psychosocial influence on symptom perception without considering the physiological impairment of MSK dysfunction can also lead to unpredictable responses. Establishing how we accurately weigh and target the predominant barriers to recovery in our patient's profile is our biggest challenge for the future of diagnostic practice (Billis et al 2007a,b, 2010, McCarthy 2003, McCarthy & Cairns 2005, McCarthy et al 2004, 2006).

There are many presentations of MSK dysfunction which suggest that a mechanically focused intervention may be the optimal strategy for treatment, for instance when the dysfunction has a strong relationship to the positions the body is held or moved into. Some of these appear to be more dominantly influenced by movement control than the psychosocial influences underpinning them. The quest to identify who is most suited to MT as opposed to other conservative therapies is currently being undertaken by researchers around the world (Childs et al 2004, Cleland et al 2010, Flynn et al 2002, Fritz et al 2007), but patients make this judgement every day, based on their perceptions and expectations.

Ultimately, we all have expectations of how our perceived symptoms should respond, based on previous experience and information from social contacts, healthcare professionals and the media. If our own strategies to reduce pain prompts have proven unsuccessful within a timescale we perceive as appropriate we may seek assistance from healthcare professionals. If we have an expectation that MT will benefit us we may proactively instigate a consultation (an active coping style as opposed to a maladaptive passive coping style). MT is therefore more than a passive treatment, and it does not foster a maladaptive passive coping style in patients. It is essential that the manual therapist recognizes maladaptive passive coping styles, reduces anxiety, fear of movement and catastrophizing, and encourages self-efficacy. If not, there is a danger that the effectiveness of MT will be poor or even counteract recovery.

Healthcare behaviour has been compared with the interaction between child and mother in response to the child hurting itself (Gifford 2000). Firstly, the child will seek help from someone trustworthy; they will then receive attention and a diagnosis (mother has a look). Subsequently, they will receive reassurance and treatment (mother explains that it is nothing serious and rub it better) and finally be distracted from the pain and reactivated (mother makes the child laugh and sends them off to fetch the sweets). This process reduces fear, provides pleasant alternative stimulus (touch), reduces attention on the pain and focuses the attention on a task that can be achieved leading to reward. It will be very familiar to manual therapists and those who have experienced MT. MT is an interaction between patient and practitioner that involves the use of touch, specific movement, learning and reward. The interpretation of its effectiveness will be wholly governed by the biopsychosocial influences on the patient and practitioner. Untangling the individual components of this complex interaction is difficult and while our understanding of some underlying mechanisms is developing, their interactions are far from fully established.

Patients seek the intervention from manual therapists when their strategies for ameliorating pain and dysfunction have not met their own expectations. Thus, patients attend some time after their painful dysfunction has first been perceived. This is more than enough time for the nervous and therefore MSK systems to have adapted physiologically to the painful afferent stimuli (DeLeo 2006, Ren & Dubner 1999). MT approaches influence physiological processes within the higher centres of the central nervous system. It can help our management of the patient when we have even a basic understanding of the mechanisms involved.

MECHANISMS OF PAIN RELIEF THROUGH MANUAL THERAPY

The underlying hypothesis of MT is that the specific position, direction and quality with which movements are performed and learned have a superior effect on reducing pain and dysfunction compared with movement in a random fashion. If a position or movement is strongly related to the patient's pain and dysfunction, then interventions are chosen which utilize these features. Specific assessment and specific correction of movement dysfunction are therefore paramount for the manual therapist.

In conjunction with a detailed examination of the specific biomechanical and physiological impairments of a MSK dysfunction, the manual therapist has several ways to alter the perception of pain at their disposal (Table 12.1).

The somatosensory system

The skin, joints and muscles are supplied with receptors to allow the interpretation of movement and nociceptive stimuli (Fig. 12.2). Skin mechanoreceptors can be categorized based on the type of stimulation to which the receptor responds, the speed with which they adapt to stimulus and the size of their field of reception (Box 12.1). The neuroanatomy of our skin, the first contact receptor for tactile stimulus, allows clear distinction between deep and superficial stimuli.

Joints and ligaments also have mechanoreceptors (Table 12.2). Type I receptors, found infrequently in ligaments, are slowly adapting receptors with a low threshold and continuous firing, even at rest. Type II receptors are dynamic with rapid adaptation and a low threshold to stimulus, thus they convey information at the beginning of joint motion. Type III receptors are also dynamic-type receptors with a high threshold and slow adaptation providing sensation at the extremes of movement. These fibres can also transmit some nociceptive stimuli at extremes of deformation (Wyke 1972). Type IV receptors are free nerve endings in the tissues and are responsible for the majority of nociceptive sensation (Michelson & Hutchins 1995). Thus, placing a joint towards the end of range of motion to conduct MT influences specific skin, joint capsule and ligament receptors that are not activated in a neutral (loose-packed) position.

Muscles are richly innervated with mechanoreceptors, classified as above (Mense 2003). Muscle spindles (Type Ia and II) are extremely sensitive to length changes in the muscle and have an efferent innervations (gamma motor neurons) in order to dynamically respond to changes in muscle length. In contrast, Golgi tendon organs are high threshold and insensitive to small muscle length changes but do respond to forceful muscle contraction and extreme stretch stimulation (Mense 2003). In a gross simplification of a very intricate process, mechanoreceptors join with nociceptors in an afferent system, transmitting information to the cerebral cortex.

Aβ afferents transmitting mechanoreceptive information terminate mainly in laminae III to V, which is projected to the primary (S1) and secondary somatosensory (S2) cortex via the dorsal-medial lemniscal pathway. In addition, pleasant touch (slow, light stroking of the skin, distinct to discriminatory touch) is transmitted in unmyelinated, slow C fibres known as *C tactile afferents* (Liu et al 2007). This afferent information projects to the limbic system. While this information does not provide discriminative information, it does facilitate the evaluation of the emotional attachment to touch (Andrew 2010). This 'valuation' of tactile afferent information occurs predominantly in the orbitofrontal cortex, an area that processes sexual

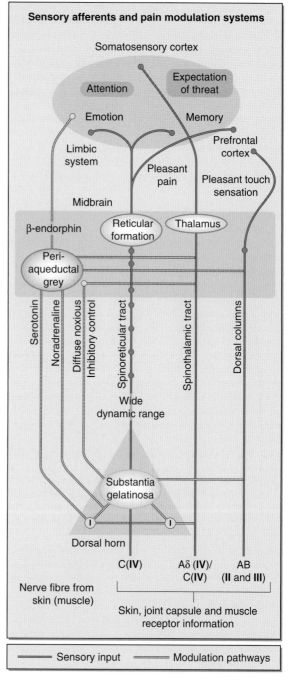

Fig. 12.2 Diagram of the somatosensory systems.

and affective components of pain/pleasure sensations (Leknes & Tracey 2008). Finally, excessive mechanical as well as chemical and thermal stimuli activate nociceptive C and Aδ fibres (for their neuroanatomy and function refer to Chapters 5 and 6).

Table 12.1 Theoretical processes in pain relief with manual therapy

Mechanism	Précis
Selective afferent stimulation	Selective stimulation of fast-adapting afferents (light touch and stroking) of the skin Selective stimulation of slow-adapting skin afferents (deep pressure/pain sensation) Stimulation of high-threshold (type III) joint and muscle afferents (stretch/pain sensation) Stimulation of C-tactile afferents with slow, light, stroking touch
Reduced local tissue afferent barrage	Reduced tonic activity in muscle, skin and joint afferents following 'lengthening' manoeuvres Mechanical perturbation inducing fibroblastic tissue healing Down-regulation of local inflammatory cytokines
Gate control	Stimulation of Aβ fibres (mechanoreceptive afferent information) modulates perception of Aδ- and C-fibre afferent information
Descending pain inhibition	Mechanoreceptive afferent (type III) stimulation of PAG–RVM centres inhibits perception of nociceptive pain Inhibition of dorsal horn sensitisation in response to type III afferent information (deep stretch, pressure stimulus)
Distant noxious inhibitory control	Pain evoked remotely reduces the relative attention to pre-existing pain
Pleasure/pain tactile mechanisms	Pleasant touch causes phasic release of dopamine to reduce attention to pain and increase motivation repeat the movement that induced the hypoalgesic reward Deep pressure/stretch and tactile pain stimulate pleasure centres in the orbitofrontal cortex that reduce the perception of pain
Ablation of painful movement memories	Reduction in pain perception facilitates the relearning of pain-free memories
Learning of pain-free movement memories	Correction of physiological impairment allows fearless, pain-free movement that facilitates the relearning of pain-free memories of movement
Distraction	Reduction in attention on the painful function to focus on other afferent information (stretch, pleasant touch, control with reward for mastery) Production of deep, pressure, stretching tactile pain averts attention from distressing pain
Habituation	Plastic changes in the central nervous system, in response to repetition of pain free stimulus, reduce the sensitivity to nociceptive afferents in a process of long-term potentiation

PAG, periaqueductal grey, RVM, rostral ventromedial medulla.

The gate control theory

The gate control theory (Melzack & Wall 1965) proposed that the information transmitted in the larger and faster Aβ afferents can reduce the passage of nociceptive information conveyed by Aδ and C fibres at the level of the dorsal horn. This mechanism was found to be mediated by inhibitory interneurons, which synapse with primary afferents and second-order wide dynamic range (WDR) neurons within the cord. They can exert a suppressing influence on the firing thresholds of post-synaptic second-order cells (Giordano 2005).

It must be noted that a significant proportion of small-diameter afferents can be excited with stimulation of Aβ receptors (Schweinhardt et al 2006), particularly in the presence of substance P and other sensitizing chemicals. For mechanisms leading to nociceptive contribution of non-noxious stimuli, refer to Chapter 6. In these circumstances, movement within the normal range of a joint or muscle can stimulate sensitized (previously silent) small-diameter joint nociceptors (Type IV) simultaneously to the higher threshold fibres (Type III) (Wright et al 2002). Thus, the gate control theory is able to explain some of the immediate pain-relieving effects from mechanoreceptor stimulation, but it does not fully cover the pain modulation that is commonly observed as an effect of MT. This is because MT does something much deeper than that.

Box 12.1 Mechanical cutaneous stimulation is detected by a combination of receptors.

- Meissner corpuscles (FA1): light stroking and fast vibration; fast acting, local specific stimulation.
- Pacinian corpuscles (FA2): deep, quick touch; fast and large field, thus poor spatial resolution.
- Ruffini endings (SA2): slow acting with a large receptive field; respond to slow direction-specific stretch; poor spacial resolution.
- Merkel cell neurite complexes (SA1): slow acting; better special resolution (Macefield 2005).
- Pleasant touch can activate receptors on C fibres (see 'The somatosensory system').

Thus, sensations on the skin are generated by distinctly different receptors, enabling us to accurately appreciate the type, depth and direction of cutaneous stimulation.

Table 12.2 Mechanoreceptors in joint capsules and ligaments (Wyke 1972)

Type	Morphology	Parent nerve	Physiology
I	Thinly encapsulated globular corpuscles in clusters of 3 to 6	Small, myelinated	Low threshold, slow adapting Static and dynamic
II	Thickly encapsulated corpuscles in clusters of 2 to 4	Medium, myelinated	Low threshold, rapidly adapting Dynamic
III	Thinly encapsulated fusiform corpuscles	Large, myelinated	High threshold, slowly adapting Dynamic
IV	Plexuses and free nerve endings	Very small, myelinated	High threshold Pain receptors

Reprinted from Wyke, B., 1972, Articular neurology, Physiotherapy, 58(3); 94–99, with permission from Elsevier.

Hypoalgesia mediated by the central inhibition

Over the last 20 years there has been significant investigation of the effects of MT-induced mechanoreceptive afferent barrage on the perception of nociceptive pain (Schmid et al 2008). A number of authors have demonstrated MT-induced hypoalgesia concurrent to up-regulation of noradrenergic *fight or flight* system responses. For example, Vicenzino et al (1998) demonstrated the excitatory effects of cervical mobilization techniques on sympathetic function (respiratory and heart rate). There has been a strong assertion that descending pain mechanisms associated with the noradrenergic/serotinergic systems result in immediate followed by longer lasting reduction in pain perception (Schmid et al 2008, Sterling et al 2001, Vicenzino et al 1998, Wright 1999).

With regard to MT-induced hypoalgesia, the periaqueductal grey (PAG) and rostroventromedial medullary (RVM) centres of the brain stem are likely to be important components of the descending pain inhibition systems (Close et al 2009, Schmid et al 2008, Sterling et al 2001, Vicenzino et al 1998, Wright 1999; see Chapter 6). There are distinct areas within the PAG that mediate transmission of nociceptive information. Afferent stimulation of the dorsal PAG elicits a fight or flight reaction, with sympatho-excitation leading to a modulation of pain that is effectively instantaneous (Wright 1995). The dorsal PAG mediates a noradrenergic mechanism, which specifically influences cortical perception of nociceptive pain and induces an inhibition of substance P release from the terminals of nociceptive fibres at the peripheral source of pain (Pertovaara 2006). The ventral PAG facilitates recuperative behaviour through an opioid/serotinergic-mediated pathway. Typically this response is observed 20–45 minutes post MT treatment (Close et al 2009, Schmid et al 2008, Sterling et al 2001, Vicenzino et al 1998, Wright 1999).

These systems have been shown to be bidirectional and thus are able to inhibit or facilitate nociception, in response to the importance of the stimuli via ON and OFF cells within the RVM (Close et al 2009, Heinricher et al 2009). For example, nocioceptive thresholds can be raised (reducing perception of pain) during feeding and micturition (via OFF cell activation) and lowered in the presence of acute inflammation (via ON cell activation) as attention is focused toward the most functionally important stimulus. The response of both OFF and ON cells, and therefore descending mediation, can be diminished in the presence of chronically painful, inflammatory conditions (Pinto-Ribeiro et al 2008).

Numerous investigators have demonstrated that high-threshold mechanoreceptive afferent barrage, be it from the spine (Bretischwerdt et al 2010, George et al 2006, Ruiz-Saez et al 2007), peripheral joints (Slater et al 2006, Vicenzino et al 2001), muscles (Bretischwerdt et al 2010) or nerves (Beneciuk et al 2009), can result in clinically meaningful reductions in nociception (Schmid et al 2008). This reduction in pain perception has been measured both locally to the site of MT and in sites distant to the areas receiving MT (Bretischwerdt et al 2010, Cleland et al 2005).

Recent work has suggested a more selective response to MT in terms of its extent of effect and its mediation of particular nociceptive afferent information (Beneciuk et al 2009, George et al 2006, Willett et al 2010). A study undertaken by George et al (2006) compared changes in thermal sensitivity at distant and local sites in response to a spinal manipulation technique, specific lumbar extension exercises and general exercise (static bicycle). The authors found that local increases in pain thresholds were observed in response to lumbar MT and lumbar extension exercise but not for general exercise. Their data suggest that local mechanoreceptive afferent information from either voluntary or passively applied movement is capable of evoking pain inhibition. Significant levels of distant hypoalgesia were not observed, leading the authors to suggest that MT may have a more local influence on pain perception. Several groups have demonstrated greater hypoalgesia closer to the site of MT stimulation than at distant sites (Perry & Green 2008, Willett et al 2010). Undoubtedly these effects are influenced by higher cortical centres, as they appear to be more pronounced in the presence of the expectation that MT will be effective (Bialosky et al 2008). The magnitude of induced hypoalgesia is influenced by expectation of effect, with negative expectations reducing hypoalgesic effects local to their application (Bialosky et al 2008).

The potential that MT selectively inhibits C-fibre afferent information has been highlighted in recent studies measuring the effect of MT on temporal summation of nociceptive stimulation. Temporal summation can be measured in the laboratory through increases in reported pain intensity as a result of repeated noxious stimulation of constant intensity at an application frequency higher than 0.3 Hz (Mendell 1966). The degree of temporal summation is thought to correlate to the extent of dorsal horn wind up (see Chapter 6). One study investigated the effect of spinal MT on asymptomatic subjects' temporal summation to repeated thermal stimulus (George et al 2006), while the other investigated the effect of upper limb neural tension testing (see Elvey 1997 for details of this test) on afferent nociception and temporal summation (Bialosky et al 2009). Both studies demonstrated a greater inhibition of temporal summation with MT than with the comparative interventions (sham MT, extension exercise or exercise bicycle), suggesting that MT may reduce dorsal horn sensitization. Aδ fibre information appeared to be less influenced by MT than that from C fibres, suggesting that the thresholds for the Aδ transportation of instantaneous 'protective' pain is less influenced by MT. This may be explained by the fact that simple deep pressure sensations mediated by Aδ fibres appear to have less limbic and cortical moderation en route to the somatosentory cortex, with less need for interpretation of its value (Rolls et al 1983).

Interestingly, previous work has demonstrated that a greater magnitude of temporal summation is evoked by frequent stimulation of deep tissue nociceptors than by stimulating receptors in the skin (Nie et al 2005). The fact that these recent studies have suggested that brief MT stimuli to the deeper tissues can reduce the magnitude of subsequent temporal summation suggests that certain sensory stimuli may be more effective than others in evoking changes in pain.

Diffuse noxious inhibitory control

Diffuse noxious inhibitory control (DNIC), the inhibition of activity in WDR spinal neurons triggered by a separate, spatially distant noxious stimulus, is considered to be the underlying mechanism of counter-irritation theory, where 'one pain masks another' (Jinks et al 2003; see Chapter 6 for a discussion of the mechanism). DNIC is thought to provide a 'surrounding inhibition' that heightens the contrast in importance between the noxious stimulation and the pre-existing pain (Pinto-Ribeiro et al 2008).

MT techniques may produce mild pain from deep pressure and stretch during application, stimulating Type III and IV fibres. A recent review of minor adverse reactions to MT treatment reveals that approximately 50% of patients report some transient treatment soreness during or posttreatment (Carnes et al 2010), thus manual therapists may have to accept, and perhaps require, that some techniques will induce a little 'therapeutic pain'. It is possible that the infliction of mild pain, in association with a therapeutic manoeuvre, is monitored and countered by our pain modulation systems without being associated with the degree of distress or sensitization of a traumatizing injury.

The pleasure and pain of manual therapy

As discussed, human neuroanatomy enables us to indentify light touch, deep pressure, stretch and high-threshold stretch and pressure, which may be perceived as pain. In addition, we have afferent nerve fibres that convey pleasant emotive stroking sensations to our brains (Olausson et al 2002). In light of this, there has been recent interest in our processing of painful and pleasant afferent information and the beginnings of an understanding of their interactions.

Avoiding pain and seeking pleasure are key concepts for survival (Leknes & Tracey 2008). Relief from severe pain will be considered more rewarding than relief when in less pain (Leknes & Tracey 2008). In Fields' motivation-decision model of pain (Fields 2007), any activity that reduces a threat to survival will exert an antinociceptive influence, more significantly than the perceived importance of the current pain. For example, a long distance runner will experience pain during the race that they perceive as being less important than the reward of completing/winning and consequently the pain is down-regulated during the race. In a similar vein, whilst the tactile stretch and pressure of some MT techniques may induce some pain, this may be seen as an acceptable pain as the post-treatment reward will be considered more important than the treatment discomfort. Thus, post-MT hypoalgesia might be considered as the reward following the uncomfortable process of generating it.

Induced hypoalgesia, particularly if the magnitude of relief is unexpectedly high, will also evoke a phasic release of the neurotransmitter dopamine (Schultz 2002). Phasic bursts of dopamine release increase the motivation to seek the reward that has just precipitated its release, but not actually the degree of enjoyment of the reward. However, dopamine release does produce corresponding increases in opiod levels, which in turn enhance the enjoyment of the reward (Leknes & Tracey 2008). The magnitude of the phasic dopamine response is related to unexpectedness and the size of the reward experienced (Schultz 2002). Responses to repeated constant stimuli will lead to a lowering of the level of phasic dopamine release and thus a reduction in the motivation to repeat the stimulus. Unexpectedly large pain relief will intensify the motivation to repeat the behaviour that caused the relief. Interestingly, chronic pain patients have been shown to have low tonic dopamine levels and correspondingly low motivation to adopt changes in pain behaviour (Wood et al 2007).

Phasic release of dopamine, in response to an unpredictably large reward (reduction in pain), motivates the adoption of the new behaviour, so MT-induced hypoalgesia may facilitate change in patients. When responses to treatment become predictable there is an associated reduction in dopamine-driven motivation and a change in eliciting stimulus is required to restore motivation to change (Schultz 2002). MT treatment progression typically involves changing intensity, position, direction, velocity and other features of stimulus to ensure that response to treatment does not plateau and become predictable. The direct impact MT techniques have on dopamine-mediated motivation to change and perception of pain may be one reason why manual therapy's approach to progression of treatment (Maitland 1966) has evolved over the years.

Not all MT treatment induces pain (Maitland 1966). Massage, gentle stretching, manually controlled muscle contractions and stroking of the skin are all pleasant tactile sensations. Human beings are very accurate in interpreting the emotional content of touch (Hertenstein et al 2006), with touch sensations being interpreted in the limbic system and in multiple centres through the cortex, particularly the orbito-frontal cortex (OFC) (Rolls et al 2003). The more affective aspects of touch (pleasant touch and distressing pain) appear to be assessed in the OFC, while more neutral pressure/stretch (Aδ afferent information) is processed more immediately in the somatosensory cortex (Rolls et al 2003).

The OFC is involved in the judgement of the value of reward and threat of stimuli, and is vital in motivation and learning (Schultz 2002). Light touch and slow stroking motions provide afferent information that is processed as conveying a pleasant emotional message (Hertenstein et al 2006). Thus, pleasant tactile sensation will be processed in areas of the brain that weigh up the value of the reward of MT against its current pain state. In response to pleasant empathetic touch that is considered pleasurable and pain relieving the reward includes supraspinal facilitation of the hypoalgesic descending pain mechanisms (Leknes & Tracey 2008). Thus one credible theory of how hypoalgesia is elicited (Fields 2007) suggests that pleasurable tactile MT can reduce pain by tipping the homeostatic pain balance from pain towards pleasure through limbic and cortical mediation in the brain. It would seem that whether MT stimulus is pleasant or uncomfortable, there are physiological mechanisms that may explain the changes in pain perception demonstrated (Schmid et al 2008). Over the coming years we will no doubt develop a better understanding of their interactions, allowing us to refine MT further.

MANUAL THERAPY AS AN AID TO MOTOR CONTROL

Restoration of movement and control of movement are key objectives of MT. Aberrant movement associated with chronic pain can be considered maladaptive, and maladaptive motor control associated with pain may in itself maintain pain. It has been suggested that pain diverts attention away from processing movement performance (Price 2000, Price & Gilden 2000), and pain has been associated with reductions in proprioceptive ability (Gill & Callaghan 1998). In addition, fear of movement associated with pain has been shown to influence the recruitment, strength and endurance of paraspinal muscles (Watson et al 1997). These findings suggest that key elements of MT treatment should be the reduction of pain and improvement of proprioception (Hodges 2003, Hodges et al 2003).

By reducing pain and subsequently encouraging patients to actively move into functional positions they could not previously achieve, these maladaptations in movement control can be corrected. The expectation is that following MT, attention to movement performance is not distracted, fear of movement is reduced, and muscles are recruited and controlled more efficiently and accurately due to improved proprioception. In addition, graded exposure to previously painful movements will lead to a reduction in postsynaptic afferent stimuli due to habituation of presynaptic nerve calcium ion channels and the neuroplastic depression of spinal neurons (Boal & Gillette 2004). Habituation has been referred to as 'pain boredom' (Gifford 2000) and may be a significant mechanism in understanding the effectiveness of techniques such as McKenzie repeated movements (McKenzie 1987) or oscillatory mobilization (Maitland 1966, Robson & Gifford 2006). Thus the learning of fearless painless movement memories (Robson & Gifford 2006) may lead to extinction of maladaptive pain memories (Zusman 2004).

EFFECTS OF MANUAL THERAPY ON LOCAL TISSUE

Over 20 years ago, Max Zusman argued that stretching joints with oscillatory mobilizations reduces intra-articular pressure and lengthens joint capsules and ligaments, leading to a temporary reduction in nociceptive afferent barrage (Zusman 1986). Zusman has now returned to this discussion and suggested that local tissue mobilization may facilitate fibroblastic and myofibroblastic tissue repair (Zusman 2010). Zusman has proposed that 'manually applied (progressive) tensile loading or stretch could provide the specific external counter force or "anchor point" needed to facilitate or enhance the structural and biochemical events associated with optimal tissue repair and growth' (Zusman 2010). Another aspect of local change in target tissues in response to MT has been highlighted in the last few years (Teodorczyk-Injeyan et al 2006). These investigators assessed levels of inflammatory cytokines in response to a single spinal manipulative thrust to a clinically dysfunctional spinal segment of the thoracic spine compared to a sham procedure and a control condition (venipuncture). They showed a systemic down-regulation of pro-inflammatory cytokines in response to the application of MT. This suggests that MT may induce a reduction in inflammatory chemicals within target tissues, leading to reduced pain, improved motor control and a rapid return to normal function.

MANUAL THERAPY CASE STUDY

The clinical reasoning behind the application of MT can be difficult to access and understand, so this chapter presents a case study of a typical MT approach to a common MSK pain syndrome. It describes a presentation, examination process and treatment following a *combined movement* paradigm (McCarthy 2001, 2010). This concept was developed by Dr Brian Edwards, a specialist manipulative physiotherapist, and has been updated and developed in subsequent years (McCarthy 2010). Combined movement theory advocates the use of specific starting positions for passive mobilization, manipulation or muscle contractions and will be familiar to those versed in the writings of Geoffrey Maitland (Maitland 1966).

Initial interview

Symptomology

A 29-year-old male presented with pain in the right lower cervical spine, referring into the right shoulder across the top of the scapula. The pain was not radicular in quality but severe (8/10). There was no suggestion of an upper motor neuron lesion and no indication of other red flags. There were no features suggestive of segmental cervical instability or shoulder derangement. There was no history of cervical locking, catching or weakness. No headache. No significant barriers to recovery in terms of attitudes to pain, pain behaviours, compensation, dilemmas over diagnosis, emotional problems, family history of pain or blue/black flags (Main & Williams 2002).

Relevant history

Symptoms developed over a 6-day period following a mild rear shunt whiplash injury 3 weeks ago.

Behaviour of symptoms

Pain was reproduced with low cervical flexion and left lateral flexion. Sitting with the neck in this position reproduced symptoms within 2 minutes. The symptoms were eased, immediately, by positioning the lower cervical spine in extension and right lateral flexion. No latent pain was exhibited. No change in pain with the application of heat.

Diurnal pattern

No stiffness in the cervical spine in the morning. Neck and shoulder pain developed in the evening. Sleep was not disturbed.

Special questions

General health was good. No weight loss, dizziness, dysphagia, dysarthria or diplopia, no raised blood pressure or symptoms of cervical artery dysfunction. Radiographs of the cervical spine were normal. The patient was not currently taking any anticoagulant or steroid therapy and had received no benefit from anti-inflammatory medication. No history of locking, clunking or giving way of the shoulder.

Clinical reasoning: The patient has a presentation suggesting a predominant pain mechanism that is driven by a nociceptive source. There is little to suggest widespread central sensitivity or a major neurogenic driver to the pain. Pain is worsened with increased afferent signal from tissues and lessened with reduced stimulus on peripheral receptors, hence the 'mechanical presentation' label often applied to this kind of presentation.

Interpretation: There is strong evidence for the hypoalgesic effect of MT on afferent nociceptive perception. The investigation of MT as a potent analgesic treatment is appropriate for this patient.

Plan of the objective examination

List your hypotheses for the nature of the condition.
1. Posterior facet capsule sprain
2. Posterior paraspinal strain
3. Posterior annual disc sprain

Which two hypotheses will you test against each other in the initial physical examination?

Primary   sensitized articular periarticualr tissue
Secondary sensitized muscle tissue

Is the nature of the condition severe?
Yes ☐   No ☐

Is the nature of the condition irritable?
Yes ☐   No ☐

To what point are you allowing movement to occur?
Before pain ☐
To pain   ☐
To limit   ☐

What is the functional demonstration/primary retest marker?
Active flexion contralateral, lateral flexion

What is the primary pain mechanism of this patient's condition?
Nociceptive   ☐
Peripheral neurogenic ☐
Central   ☐
Autonomic   ☐
Affective   ☐

To what extent will you perform a neurological exam?
None required   ☐
Local peripheral   ☐
Lower motor neuron, upper motor neuron, limbs ☐
Lower motor neuron, upper motor neuron, limbs and cranial ☐

What is the weighting of the following components of the problem (Table 12.3 and Fig. 12.3)?
Likely first treatment:
In: extension, right lateral flexion...........................
Will: Anterior capsular stretch, large amplitude movement, in resistance (Grade III)

Table 12.3 Weighting of componets of the problem

	%
ARTHROGENIC	50
MYOGENIC	40
NEUROGENIC	1
INFLAMMAGENIC	2
PSYCHOGENIC	1
SOCIOGENIC	1
PATHOGENIC	1
VISCEROGENIC	1
OSTEOGENIC	3

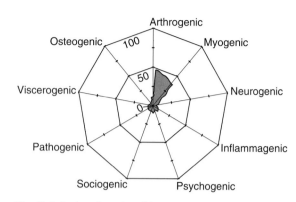

Fig. 12.3 Radar plot of problem components (%).

Comments/cautions:
Pain relief approach, progressing to a stretch of the tissues driving the nociceptive pattern of presentation.

Physical examination

Observation

No atrophy of the cervical musculature was observed. Increased muscle tone of the right sternocleidomastoid, upper fibres of trapezuis, levator scapulae and right scalenes.

Active movement

Pain reproduced earliest in range with left lateral flexion (the most most painful movement termed the "Prime Movment". Restriction to flexion apparent at the C5/6 level. Pain reproduced further into range with flexion than with left lateral flexion. Restriction to movement was most obvious in the mid-cervical region. Proprioceptive ability was reduced slightly when testing reposition of the head with eyes closed (Jull et al 2007).

Passive physiological intervertebral movement

Because of the severity, the examination was undertaken in right lateral flexion and extension (posterior structures off stretch) to establish the movement that most reduced pain and dysfunction. Right lateral flexion induced greatest increase in movement and reduction in muscle tone.

Effect of trial of brief passive treatment: Treatment using right lateral flexion of C5 on C6 reduced the pain produced by the functional demonstration by 10%.

Passive accessory intervertebral movement

Because of the severity, the examination was undertaken in right lateral flexion and extension (posterior structures off stretch) to establish the movement that most reduced pain and dysfunction. Anterior pressure (AP) on C5 induced greatest increase in movement and reduction in muscle tone (greater than induced by AP movement of C4 or C6).

Effect of trial of brief passive treatment: Treatment using this accessory movement reduced the pain produced by the functional demonstration by 40%.

Muscular assessment

In right lateral flexion and extension due to severity of pain, palpation of musculature revealed hypertonicity of deep paraspinals (C4 to C6) and hypertonicity of the region's phasic muscles. No trigger points were detected.

Effect of trial of brief passive treatment: Palpation and length assessment of sternocleidomastoid, upper fibres of trapezuis, levator scapulae and right scalenes did not alter the functional demonstration

First treatment

Position: right lateral flexion, extension
Technique: unilateral antero-posterior (AP) glide of C5 on C6, Grade III, 1×1 minute
Outcome: 40% reduction in pain

Clinical reasoning: This treatment was thought to induce the greatest change in the patient's dysfunction. The starting position for this technique allowed the production of specific passive movement at the site of pain generation. The starting position and movement induced did not stretch the posterior aspects of the motion segment. Pain relief was rapid and within seconds the therapist was be able to detect a reduction in paraspinal hypertonicity and a concurrent increase in compliance to passive movement. This occurred after 1 minute of mobilization and thus the technique was stopped to allow reassessment of the patients' demonstration of dysfunction.

Hypothetical mechanisms: In response to the stimulation of tactile C fibres with type II and III afferent fibres, a mediation of nociceptive transmission occurred at spinal and supraspinal levels. Changes in excitability at the dorsal root ganglion and dorsal horn down-regulated release of substance P and other cytokinins in local tissues, reducing motor-neuron pool activity and lessening paraspinal muscle spasm. Thus, nociceptively driven pain perception was reduced.

Immediate and unexpectedly large improvements in pain stimulated a phasic release of dopamine that facilitated opiod release and motivated the patient to repeat the process. The threat and anxiety that was associated with the painful movement was reduced and thus a stress-free, fearless environment to relearn efficient motor control was produced.

Second treatment

Position: identical starting position
Technique: identical technique
Outcome: no improvement

Clinical reasoning: As the previous treatment technique had been so beneficial it was repeated. During the technique the therapist perceived less change in muscle tone and compliance to passive movement.

Hypothetical mechanisms: The impact on pain was less because previous lengthening of the tissues had already lead to a reduction in local afferent barrage. In addition, there was less unexpected effect, which is required to stimulate phasic dopamine release. Previously experienced dramatic reductions in pain may relatively reduce the impact of smaller reductions in pain. A change in afferent stimulus was required to maintain the improvement in pain perception.

Third treatment

Position: right side flexion, flexion
Technique: unilateral PA glide of C5 on C6, Grade III, 1×1 minute
Outcome: 25% reduction in pain

Clinical reasoning: The dysfunction was now not severe and so new afferent stimulus and mechanical stretch could be introduced. This starting position induced more stretch on the posterior structures than the previous technique, but the starting position avoided the patient's prime movement. The patient's prime movement was left lateral flexion and thus the progression of stretch into flexion (counter-clockwise around the box) rather than into left-lateral flexion (clockwise around the box).

Hypothetical mechanisms: The descending inhibitory effects evoked by stimulus of the anterior tissues (structures not likely to be the nociceptive source) had plateaued and now a graded exposure to stimulus was evoked for the posterior tissues. By gradually introducing a progressive exposure to tension on the nociceptors, posterior to the spine, a process of habituation had occured (Progressive reduction in afferent barrage and hypoalgesic adaptations in the dorsal horn, spinal cord and supraspinal centres had ensued in response to repeated exposure to submaximal stimulus of the "trigger" nociceptors) (Boal & Gillette 2004).

This change of stimulus was new to the system and consequently phasic dopamine was produced in higher volumes. In addition, specific lengthening of the tissues containing the nociceptive "trigger" had increased the resting length of the tissue and thus reduced their firing (Zusman 1986).

Fourth treatment

Position: identical starting position
Technique: identical technique
Outcome: no improvement

Clinical reasoning: As the previous treatment technique had been so beneficial it was repeated. During the technique the therapist perceived less change in muscle tone and compliance to passive movement.

Hypothetical mechanisms: The level of afferent stimulus had desensitised the posterior structures maximally for that stimulus. The impact on pain was less because previous lengthening of the tissues had already lead to a reduction in local afferent barrage. In addition, there was less unexpected effect, which is required to stimulate phasic dopamine release. An increase in afferent stimulus was required to maintain the process of habituation.

Fifth treatment

Position: left lateral flexion, flexion
Technique: unilateral PA glide of C5 on C6, Grade III, 1×1 minute
Outcome: pain free, Repositioning tests improved but still impaired.

Clinical reasoning: It was necessary to progress the starting position for mobilization into the prime combination (the position of functional pain). The technique used had maximally stretched the posterior structures and evoked maximal afferent barrage from mechanoreceptors stimulated to their maximum tension. A degree of non-threatening treatment-induced 'stretch pain' was induced.

Interpretation: Habituation to the gradual exposure to tension had reduced nociceptive pain perception. The lengthening of tissues, generating nociceptive pain, reduced the afferent stimulus after stretch as tension on nociceptors had been reduced. Movement of healing tissue had facilitated mechanosensitive tissue healing processes (Zusman 2010) and reduced central sensitivity at the dorsal horn (Boal & Gillette 2004). Stimulation of mechanoreceptive afferents inhibited nociception and the "pleasantly" uncomfortable sensations of stretch evoked pleasure centres in the OFC. Subsequent phasic dopamine release facilitated the desire to repeat the movement into the previously painful space and the facilitation of pain-free movement memories had begun. Motor control strategies easier to regain now that pain has reduced, proprioceptive control improves with repetition of movement by increasing the control demands of movement tasks (Jull et al 2007).

Sixth treatment

Provision of a 'mimicking' home stretching/exercise programme

Clinical reasoning: As the dysfunction had significantly improved it was important to explain to the patient the mechanisms of this effect and to reinforce the message that

the dysfunction was a simple "mechanical fault". Emphasizing the benign mechanical aspect of the painful dysfunction reduced anxiety and fear avoidance. It was imperative that the patient was educated about the importance of a home stretching programme that mimicked what had been undertaken. This reinforced their active involvement in managing their dysfunction and ensured that they maintained the improvements in motor control they had just gained.

Interpretation: Regular movement into areas that were previously painful stimulated mechanoreceptive afferents and desensitised nociceptive pathways, leading to periods of hypoalgesia. This led to reduced fear of moving into this spatial area, reduced painful memories and the generation of pain-free memories of movement onto this area, spatially represented in the cortex. This neuroplastic change reduced central sensitivity to this movement and through habituation inhibited central sensitization. Regular perturbation and stretching of tissue will aid the mechano-sensitive aspects of the healing and tissue remodelling process over the subsequent weeks.

CONCLUSION

MT is a common approach to managing MSK pain that offers immediate pain relief (Wright 1995), improvements in tissue healing (Zusman 2010), reductions in anxiety and fear of movement (Gifford 2000), pleasurable and rewarding tactile stimulation (Leknes & Tracey 2008), increased motivation to replicate pain-relieving movement (Schultz 2002) and a window of opportunity to relearn pain-free movement memories (Zusman 2004) through repetition and active involvement in the rehabilitation process (Zusman 2002). MT is associated with some minor adverse events such as treatment soreness, which may actually be a component of its effect, but major adverse events are rare (Carnes et al 2010). The clinical and cost effectiveness of MT are considered to be acceptable to western society, so it is widely recommend in the management of MSK dysfunction (Savigny et al 2009, UK BEAM 2004a). Although MT often involves simple, specific strategies to regain normal movement it encompasses the biopsychosocial aspects of managing patients, experiencing pain, and is indeed a complex intervention. Our understanding of its impact on health will only deepen if we accept that MT needs complex, mixed-method research designs and interpretation over the coming years. MT has prevailed from the history of health care however those of us who use this approach are sure we can be more effective with the aid of sophisticated, modern research approaches.

Study questions

1. What is the biggest challenge for the future of diagnostic practice?
2. What do C tactile afferents convey?
3. What does the gate control theory propose?
4. What is dorsal horn wind-up and how does MT affect it?

5. What does the phasic release of dopamine in response to MT do?
6. How does pain reduce motor control?
7. How do local tissue changes reduce pain perception?

REFERENCES

Andrew, D., 2010. Quantitative characterization of low-threshold mechanoreceptor inputs to lamina I spinoparabrachial neurons in the rat. J. Physiol. 588 (Pt 1), 117–124.

Beneciuk, J.M., Bishop, M.D., George, S.Z., 2009. Effects of upper extremity neural mobilization on thermal pain sensitivity: a sham-controlled study in asymptomatic participants. J. Orthop. Sports Phys. Ther. 39 (6), 428–438.

Bialosky, J.E., Bishop, M.D., Robinson, M.E., et al., 2008. The influence of expectation on spinal manipulation induced hypoalgesia: an experimental study in normal subjects. BMC Musculoskelet. Disord. 9, 19.

Bialosky, J.E., Bishop, M.D., Price, D.D., et al., 2009. The mechanisms of manual therapy in the treatment of musculoskeletal pain: a comprehensive model. Man. Ther. 14 (5), 531–538.

Billis, E.V., McCarthy, C.J., Oldham, J.A., 2007a. Subclassification of low back pain: a cross-country comparison. Eur. Spine J. 16 (7), 865–879.

Billis, E.V., McCarthy, C.J., Stathopoulos, I., et al., 2007b. The clinical and cultural factors in classifying low back pain patients within Greece: a qualitative exploration of Greek health professionals. J. Eval. Clin. Pract. 13 (3), 337–345.

Billis, E., McCarthy, C.J., Gliatis, J., et al., 2010. Which are the most important discriminatory items for subclassifying non-specific low back pain? A Delphi study among Greek health professionals. J. Eval. Clin. Pract. 16 (3), 542–549.

Boal, R.W., Gillette, R.G., 2004. Central neuronal plasticity, low back pain and spinal manipulative therapy. J. Manipulative Physiol. Ther. 27, 314–326.

Bretischwerdt, C., Rivas-Cano, L., Palomeque-del-Cerro, L., et al., 2010. Immediate effects of hamstring muscle stretching on pressure pain sensitivity and active mouth opening in healthy subjects. J. Manipulative Physiol. Ther. 33 (1), 42–47.

Carnes, D., Mars, T.S., Mullinger, B., et al., 2010. Adverse events and manual therapy: a systematic review. Man. Ther. 15 (4), 355–363.

Childs, J.D., Fritz, J.M., Flynn, T.W., et al., 2004. A clinical prediction rule to identify patients with low back pain most likely to benefit from spinal manipulation: a validation study. Ann. Intern. Med. 141 (12), 920–928.

Cleland, J.A., Childs, J.D., McRae, M., et al., 2005. Immediate effects of thoracic manipulation in patients with neck pain: a randomized clinical trial. Man. Ther. 10 (2), 127–135.

Cleland, J.A., Mintken, P.E., Carpenter, K., et al., 2010. Examination of a clinical prediction rule to identify patients with neck pain likely to benefit from thoracic spine thrust manipulation and a general cervical range of motion exercise: multi-center randomized clinical trial. Phys. Ther. 90 (9), 1239–1250.

Close, L.N., Cetas, J.S., Heinricher, M.M., et al., 2009. Purinergic receptor immunoreactivity in the rostral ventromedial medulla. Neuroscience 158 (2), 915–921.

DeLeo, J.A., 2006. Basic science of pain. J. Bone Joint Surg. Am. 88 (Suppl. 2), 58–62.

Dieppe, P., 2004. Complex interventions. Musculoskeletal Care. 2 (3), 180–186.

Elvey, R.L., 1997. Physical evaluation of the peripheral nervous system in disorders of pain and dysfunction. J. Hand Ther. 10 (2), 122–129.

Fields, H.L., 2007. Understanding how opioids contribute to reward and analgesia. Reg. Anesth. Pain Med. 32 (3), 242–246.

Flynn, T., Fritz, J., Whitman, J., et al., 2002. A clinical prediction rule for classifying patients with low back pain who demonstrate short-term improvement with spinal manipulation. Spine (Phila Pa 1976). 27 (24), 2835–2843.

Fritz, J.M., Lindsay, W., Matheson, J.W., et al., 2007. Is there a subgroup of patients with low back pain likely to benefit from mechanical traction? Results of a randomized clinical trial and subgrouping analysis. Spine (Phila Pa 1976) 32 (26), E793–E800.

George, S.Z., Bishop, M.D., Bialosky, J.E., et al., 2006. Immediate effects of spinal manipulation on thermal pain sensitivity: an experimental study. BMC Musculoskelet. Disord. 7, 68.

Gifford, L., 2000. The patient in front of us: from genes to environment. In: Gifford, L. (Ed.), Biopsychosocial Assessment and Management. Relationships and Pain, Topical Issues in Pain. CNS Press.

Gill, K.P., Callaghan, M.J., 1998. The measurement of lumbar proprioception in individuals with and without low back pain. Spine 23 (3), 371–377.

Giordano, J., 2005. The neurobiology of nociceptive and anti-nociceptive systems. Pain Physician 8 (3), 277–290.

Heinricher, M.M., Tavares, I., Leith, J.L., et al., 2009. Descending control of nociception: Specificity, recruitment and plasticity. Brain Res. Rev. 60 (1), 214–225.

Hertenstein, M.J., Keltner, D., App, B., et al., 2006. Touch communicates distinct emotions. Emotion. 6 (3), 528–533.

Hodges, P.W., 2003. Core stability exercise in chronic low back pain. Orthop. Clin. North Am. 34 (2), 245–254.

Hodges, P.W., Moseley, G.L., Gabrielsson, A., et al., 2003. Experimental muscle pain changes feedforward postural responses of the trunk muscles. Exp. Brain Res. 151 (2), 262–271.

Hoving, J.L., de Vet, H.C., Koes, B.W., et al., 2006. Manual therapy, physical therapy, or continued care by the general practitioner for patients with neck pain: long-term results from a pragmatic randomized clinical trial. Clin. J. Pain 22 (4), 370–377.

Jinks, S.L., Martin, J.T., Carstens, E., et al., 2003. Peri-MAC depression of a nociceptive withdrawal reflex is accompanied by reduced dorsal horn activity with halothane but not isoflurane. Anesthesiology 98 (5), 1128–1138.

Jull, G., Falla, D., Treleaven, J., et al., 2007. Retraining cervical joint position sense: the effect of two exercise regimes. J. Orthop. Res. 25 (3), 404–412.

Leknes, S., Tracey, I., 2008. A common neurobiology for pain and pleasure. Nat. Rev. Neurosci. 9 (4), 314–320.

Liu, Q., Vrontou, S., Rice, F.L., et al., 2007. Molecular genetic visualization of a rare subset of unmyelinated sensory neurons that may detect gentle touch. Nat. Neurosci. 10 (8), 946–948.

Macefield, V.G., 2005. Physiological characteristics of low-threshold mechanoreceptors in joints, muscle and skin in human subjects. Clin. Exp. Pharmacol. Physiol. 32 (1–2), 135–144.

Main, C.J., Williams, A., 2002. Musculoskeletal Pain. BMJ 325 (7363), 534–537.

Maitland, G.D., 1966. Manipulation-mobilisation. Physiotherapy 52 (11), 382–385.

Mattick, A., Wyatt, J.P., 2000. From Hippocrates to the Eskimo – a history of techniques used to reduce anterior dislocation of the shoulder. J. R. Coll. Surg. Edinb. 45 (5), 312–316.

McCarthy, C.J., 2001. Spinal manipulative thrust technique using combined movement theory. Man. Ther. 6 (4), 197–204.

McCarthy, C.J., 2003. The specifics of lower back pain. Therapy Weekly 30 (8), 8–9.

McCarthy, C.J., 2010. Combined Movement Theory: A Rational Approach to Mobilisation and Manipulation of the Vertebral Column. Elsevier, Oxford.

McCarthy, C.J., Cairns, M.C., 2005. Why is the recent research regarding non-specific pain so non-specific? Man. Ther. 10 (4), 239–241.

McCarthy, C.J., Arnall, F.A., Strimpakos, N., et al., 2004. The bio-psycho-social classification of non-specific low back pain: A systematic review. Phys. Ther. Rev. 9, 17–30.

McCarthy, C.J., Rushton, A., Billis, V., et al., 2006. Development of a clinical examination in non-specific low back pain: a Delphi technique. J. Rehabil. Med. 38 (4), 263–267.

McKenzie, R., 1987. Low back pain. N. Z. Med. J. 100 (827), 428–429.

Melzack, R., Wall, P.D., 1965. Pain mechanisms: a new theory. Science 150 (699), 971–979.

Mendell, L.M., 1966. Physiological properties of unmyelinated fiber projection to the spinal cord. Exp. Neurol. 16 (3), 316–332.

Mense, S., 2003. The pathogenesis of muscle pain. Curr. Pain Headache Rep. 7 (6), 419–425.

Michelson, J.D., Hutchins, C., 1995. Mechanoreceptors in human ankle ligaments. J. Bone Joint Surg. Br. 77 (2), 219–224.

Nie, H., Rendt-Nielsen, L., Andersen, H., et al., 2005. Temporal summation of pain evoked by mechanical stimulation in deep and superficial tissue. J. Pain 6 (6), 348–355.

Olausson, H., Lamarre, Y., Backlund, H., et al., 2002. Unmyelinated tactile afferents signal touch and project to insular cortex. Nat. Neurosci. 5 (9), 900–904.

Perry, J., Green, A., 2008. An investigation into the effects of a unilaterally applied lumbar mobilisation technique on peripheral sympathetic nervous system activity in the lower limbs. Man. Ther. 13 (6), 492–499.

Pertovaara, A., 2006. Noradrenergic pain modulation. Prog. Neurobiol. 80 (2), 53–83.

Pincus, T., Morley, S., 2001. Cognitive-processing bias in chronic pain: a review and integration. Psychol. Bull. 127 (5), 599–617.

Pinto-Ribeiro, F., Ansah, O.B., Almeida, A., et al., 2008. Influence of arthritis on descending modulation of nociception from the paraventricular nucleus of the hypothalamus. Brain Res. 1197, 63–75.

Price, D.D., 2000. Psychological and neural mechanisms of the affective dimension of pain. Science 288 (5472), 1769–1772.

Price, C.M., Gilden, D.L., 2000. Representations of motion and direction. J. Exp. Psychol. Hum. Percept. Perform. 26 (1), 18–30.

Ren, K., Dubner, R., 1999. Central nervous system plasticity and persistent pain. J. Orofac. Pain 13 (3), 155–163.

Robson, S., Gifford, L., 2006. Manual therapy in the 21st century. In: Gifford, L. (Ed.), Treatment. Communication. Return to Work. Cognitive-behavioural. Pathophysiology, Topical Issues in Pain. CNS Press.

Rolls, E.T., Rolls, B.J., Rowe, E.A., 1983. Sensory-specific and motivation-specific satiety for the sight and taste of food and water in man. Physiol. Behav. 30 (2), 185–192.

Rolls, E.T., O'Doherty, J., Kringelbach, M.L., et al., 2003. Representations of pleasant and painful touch in the human orbitofrontal and cingulate cortices. Cereb. Cortex 13 (3), 308–317.

Ruiz-Saez, M., Fernandez-de-las-Penas, C., Blanco, C.R., et al., 2007. Changes in pressure pain sensitivity in latent myofascial trigger points in the upper trapezius muscle after a cervical spine manipulation in pain-free subjects. J. Manipulative Physiol. Ther. 30 (8), 578–583.

Savigny, P., Watson, P., Underwood, M., 2009. Early management of persistent non-specific low back pain: summary of NICE guidance. BMJ 338, b1805.

Schmid, A., Brunner, F., Wright, A., et al., 2008. Paradigm shift in manual therapy? Evidence for a central nervous system component in the response to passive cervical joint mobilisation. Man. Ther. 13 (5), 387–396.

Schultz, W., 2002. Getting formal with dopamine and reward. Neuron 36 (2), 241–263.

Schweinhardt, P., Glynn, C., Brooks, J., et al., 2006. An fMRI study of cerebral processing of brush-evoked allodynia in neuropathic pain patients. Neuroimage 32 (1), 256–265.

Slater, H., Rendt-Nielsen, L., Wright, A., et al., 2006. Effects of a manual therapy technique in experimental lateral epicondylalgia. Man. Ther. 11 (2), 107–117.

Sterling, M., Jull, G., Wright, A., 2001. Cervical mobilisation: concurrent effects on pain, sympathetic nervous system activity and motor activity. Man. Ther. 6 (2), 72–81.

Teodorczyk-Injeyan, J.A., Injeyan, H.S., Ruegg, R., 2006. Spinal manipulative therapy reduces inflammatory cytokines but not substance P production in normal subjects. J. Manipulative Physiol. Ther. 29 (1), 14–21.

Uk BEAM, 2004a. United Kingdom back pain exercise and manipulation (UK BEAM) randomised trial: effectiveness of physical treatments for back pain in primary care. BMJ. 329 (7479), 1377.

Uk BEAM, 2004b. United Kingdom back pain exercise and manipulation (UK BEAM) randomised trial: cost effectiveness of physical treatments for back pain in primary care. BMJ. 329 (7479), 1381.

Vicenzino, B., Collins, D., Benson, H., et al., 1998. An investigation of the interrelationship between manipulative therapy-induced hypoalgesia and sympathoexcitation. J. Manipulative Physiol. Ther. 21 (7), 448–453.

Vicenzino, B., Paungmali, A., Buratowski, S., et al., 2001. Specific manipulative therapy treatment for chronic lateral epicondylalgia produces uniquely characteristic hypoalgesia. Man. Ther. 6 (4), 205–212.

Watson, P.J., Booker, C.K., Main, C.J., et al., 1997. Surface electromyography in the identification of chronic low back pain patients: the development of the flexion relaxation ratio. Clin. Biomech. (Bristol, Avon). 12 (3), 165–171.

Willett, E., Hebron, C., Krouwel, O., 2010. The initial effects of different rates of lumbar mobilisations on pressure pain thresholds in asymptomatic subjects. Man. Ther. 15 (2), 173–178.

Wood, P.B., Schweinhardt, P., Jaeger, E., et al., 2007. Fibromyalgia patients show an abnormal dopamine response to pain. Eur. J. Neurosci. 25 (12), 3576–3582.

Wright, A., 1995. Hypoalgesia post-manipulative therapy: a review of a potential neurophysiological mechanism. Man. Ther. 1 (1), 11–16.

Wright, A., 1999. Recent concepts in the neurophysiology of pain. Man. Ther. 4 (4), 196–202.

Wright, A., Graven-Nielsen, T., Davies, I.I., et al., 2002. Temporal summation of pain from skin, muscle and joint following nociceptive ultrasonic stimulation in humans. Exp. Brain Res. 144 (4), 475–482.

Wyke, B., 1972. Articular neurology – a review. Physiotherapy 58 (3), 94–99.

Zusman, M., 1986. Spinal manipulative therapy: Review of some proposed mechanisms and a new hypothesis. Aus. J. Physiotherapy 32 (2), 89–99.

Zusman, M., 2002. Forebrain-mediated sensitization of central pain pathways: 'non-specific' pain and a new image for MT. Man. Ther. 7 (2), 80–88.

Zusman, M., 2004. Mechanisms of musculoskeletal physiotherapy. Phys. Ther. Rev. 9, 39–49.

Zusman, M., 2005. Cognitive-behavioural components of musculoskeletal physiotherapy: the role of control. Phys. Ther. Rev. 10, 89–98.

Zusman, M., 2010. There's something about passive movement. . .. Med. Hypotheses 75 (1), 106–110.

Chapter 13

Exercise therapy

Nadine E. Foster, Annette Bishop, Melanie A. Holden and Krysia Dziedzic

CHAPTER CONTENTS

LEARNING OBJECTIVES

At the end of this chapter readers will be able to:

1. Understand the key principles of exercise.
2. Understand the prevalence and impact of three of the most common musculoskeletal pain problems.
3. Describe the key findings from best available evidence about the role of exercise as a core treatment for persistent musculoskeletal pain.
4. Understand the importance of the key characteristics of exercise programmes that help deliver better outcomes for patients.

OVERVIEW

Chronic or persistent musculoskeletal pain is a major health problem (White & Harth 1999) treated by many different healthcare providers. The most common types of chronic musculoskeletal pain are low back pain and joint pain related to osteoarthritis (Breivik et al 2006), including knee pain and hand pain. The primary prevention of these conditions has not proved feasible and modern management approaches, following biopsychosocial principles, are thus not orientated around a cure but rather around prevention of unnecessary disability and minimizing morbidity (Jordan et al 2010). It is clear that exercise, encompassing a wide range of interventions, such as general (aerobic) exercise, specific body-region exercises for strengthening, flexibility, control and balance, continuing normal physical activities and increasing general physical activity levels, is a core treatment option for those with musculoskeletal pain. Therapeutic exercise is one of the core skills upon which the physiotherapy profession is based, although many other health professionals are involved in advising and supporting patients in exercise and physical activity. This chapter focuses on the role of exercise in the management of persistent pain and provides a summary of the physiological and psychological principles for exercise before highlighting three specific examples of low back pain, knee pain and hand pain. The chapter then considers the particular importance of exercise adherence in realizing the potential of exercise therapy for improving the longer term outcomes of those with persistent pain before concluding with key implications for both clinical practice and future research.

KEY DEFINITIONS AND PRINCIPLES

Physical activity is any bodily movement produced by the skeletal muscles that results in energy expenditure (www.cdc.gov/nccdphp/dnpa/physical/terms). In contrast,

© 2014 Elsevier Ltd.

exercise is planned, structured and repetitive movement to maintain or improve physical fitness (e.g. cardiovascular fitness, muscle strength, endurance, flexibility and body composition) and psychological well-being (ACSM 2006). Therapeutic exercise is the systematic implementation of planned physical movements, postures or activities to remediate or prevent impairments, and enhance function, fitness and well-being (APTA 2001). Whilst the focus of this chapter is therapeutic exercise for persistent musculoskeletal pain, where evidence is available to suggest that general physical activity and lifestyle changes have merit in achieving beneficial outcomes for patients these are also included.

A therapeutic exercise programme for someone with persistent musculoskeletal pain may have several different goals, for example to improve function or reduce pain, to increase muscle strength, endurance or motor control, to improve range of movement or flexibility, or to help with coordination and balance. All goals should be mutually agreed between the patient and healthcare professional, and the selection of an appropriate exercise programme is informed by a holistic assessment of the patient, not only considering relevant subjective and objective clinical findings about the present condition but also about how the problem is affecting the individual, their general health (including other co-morbidities and other musculoskeletal pain), previous exercise experience and their attitude towards exercise. A number of design variables for the exercise programme must then be considered (Fig. 13.1), including the type of exercise prescribed, the volume of exercise (e.g. number of repetitions and sets of a strength exercise or walking distance), the intensity of exercise (e.g. weight for a resistance exercise or speed of a walking programme), and the frequency and duration of exercise (i.e. number of times the programme is completed per week over a specific period of time).

These design variables should be based on key physiological principles, provided in detail elsewhere (Glynn & Fiddler 2009, Hurley & Bearne 2009, McArdle et al 1996), but summarized below.

- Specificity: Any exercise will train a system for the particular task being carried out as the training stimulus. Hence, for example, it is important that an exercise aimed at muscle strengthening targets the correct muscle, in the range and using the type of muscle work specific to the task required.

- Overload: A system must be exercised at a level beyond that to which it is normally accustomed in order to achieve a training effect. Achieving the appropriate overload for an individual requires manipulation of the exercise programme design variables such as through increasing frequency, intensity, duration and mode of exercise. The choice of whether or not to use apply the overload principle must be based on an assessment of psychological variables (Chapters 4 and 7) and evidence of sensitization (Chapter 6). Patients with persistent pain may have to exercise little and often, in a time contingent manner.

- Adaptation: The system being exercised will gradually adapt to the overload or training stimulus, and this will continue as long as the training stimulus continues to be increased until the tissue or system can no longer adapt further.

- Individuality: Different individuals will respond to a given exercise training stimulus in different ways, and many factors contribute to individual variation in this training response. Training benefits are improved if the exercise programme is designed to meet the individual's needs and capabilities.

- Reversibility: The beneficial effects of exercise are transient and reversible. They begin to be lost as soon as the exercise stimulus stops and this happens in a similar timeframe as it takes to train the system.

In addition, there are key psychological factors to take into consideration when prescribing an exercise programme for musculoskeletal pain patients, and whilst these tend to receive less attention than the physiological principles of exercise, they are important in determining whether an individual initially engages in, and continues with, exercise over time. In order to realize the benefits of exercise,

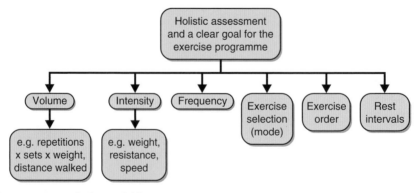

Fig. 13.1 **Exercise programme design variables.**

effort and determination on the part of the individual is needed. Key psychological factors include motivation, self-efficacy to exercise (or confidence in their ability to perform tasks like exercise) and personal or internal control (Bandura 1977, Friedrich et al 2005, Marcus et al 1992, McAuley 1992). Thus, patient education alongside the therapeutic exercise programme is important to increase their understanding of the problem, challenge unhelpful beliefs about the problem and enhance the patient's individual motivation and confidence to exercise. These aspects can be enhanced by designing exercise programmes in ways that take into consideration personal preferences (for example for individual or group-based exercise, or for the type of exercise), the potential benefits of peer support and social interaction, the importance of tailoring exercise for individual patients so that they can appreciate its relevance to their individual problem, agreeing specific and meaningful personal goals for the short and long term, and the role of supervision, review and positive reinforcement.

Working within a biopsychosocial model, it is likely that key goals of an exercise programme will include achievement of specific functional tasks. Of course, most functional activities require a combination of strength, endurance, control, range of movement and balance, and in the case of musculoskeletal pain and dysfunction most therapeutic exercise programmes will include several or all of these targets by prescribing functional exercises, facilitating carry-over into activities of daily living. Given the need to engage in the exercise regularly (at least two to three times per week) most exercise programmes will involve a home exercise programme, tailored for individual patients with persistent musculoskeletal pain, adapted for their home environment and to fit with their individual lifestyle. Any new exercise should be started slowly, increased gradually and performed moderately. The following three sections consider the most common sites of persistent musculoskeletal pain and the role exercise plays in patient management.

EXAMPLE 1: EXERCISE FOR PERSISTENT NON-SPECIFIC LOW BACK PAIN

The problem

Low back pain (LBP) is a very common condition, with lifetime prevalence rates as high as 84% (Walker 2000). In the UK, LBP is the fourth most common reason for consulting a GP after depression, hypertension and upper respiratory tract infection, and is the most common musculoskeletal reason for consultation. Estimates suggest that between 6 and 9% of people registered with a GP consult annually with LBP (Croft et al 1998, Dunn & Croft 2005), which equates to approximately five million people each year in the UK (Maniadakis & Gray 2000). In addition, many people seek care from musculoskeletal therapists, including physiotherapists, osteopaths and chiropractors. Even though it is a non-life threatening and largely self-limiting condition, LBP is responsible for large personal, societal and financial burdens as many patients with LBP develop persistent pain with a relapsing and recurrent pattern to their symptoms. The proportion of patients who continue to experience back pain 12 months after onset is reported to be in the region of 42–75% (Hestbaek et al 2003). It is now recognized that only a small proportion of persistent back pain can be attributed to a specific underlying disease or pathology. For patients with LBP presenting in primary care approximately 1% will have serious spinal pathology such as a systemic inflammatory condition or cancer, and around a further 5% will have nerve root pain/radicular pain (Waddell 2004). These patients often require specific diagnoses and management frequently involves onward referral to secondary care clinicians such as rheumatologists and orthopaedic surgeons. The remainder can be categorized as having non-specific LBP and most will be managed within primary care settings. The evidence synthesis presented below focuses on exercise for adults with persistent non-specific low back pain.

Clinical guidelines

Many clinical guidelines for the management of LBP have been developed in a number of different countries. The quality of clinical guidelines for the management of LBP is improving as time goes by (Bouwmeester et al 2009) and a synthesis of recent guidelines found that exercise is recommended in all the guidelines for persistent LBP (Dagenais et al 2010). The most recently published UK guidelines are the National Institute for Health and Clinical Excellence (NICE) guidance for the early management of persistent non-specific low back pain (NICE 2009). The guidelines recommend advising all patients presenting with persistent non-specific LBP to exercise, be physically active and to carry on with normal activities as much as possible. In addition, one of the three core treatments that the guidelines recommend is the provision of a structured exercise programme (a maximum of eight sessions over a period of up to 12 weeks). Exercise programmes may include aerobic activity, movement instruction, muscle strengthening and postural control, and the programme should be delivered in a group setting unless group exercise is considered inappropriate for a particular person.

Exercise for persistent non-specific LBP: the evidence

Exercise therapies are the most widely used type of non-invasive interventions for the management of LBP. The evidence for exercise in persistent non-specific LBP has expanded rapidly in the last decade and as a result there is now a large body of evidence supporting the use of exercise. Systematic reviews of randomized controlled trials (RCTs) of exercise interventions consistently report exercise as achieving equivalent or better outcomes for patients than comparison interventions.

For example, the systematic review by Hayden et al (2005a) included 43 RCTs (3907 individuals) that investigated the effectiveness of exercise in people with persistent non-specific LBP. Strong evidence (consistent findings in multiple high-quality trials) was found that exercise therapy is as effective as other conservative interventions, although there was conflicting evidence (inconsistent findings in multiple trials) that exercise therapy is superior to other interventions. The meta-analyses showed pooled mean improvements in pain of 10.2 points (95% CI: 1.31 to 19.09) compared to no treatment and 5.93 points (95% CI: 2.21 to 9.65) compared to other conservative interventions. Pooled mean improvements in function were 3.00 points (95% CI: 0.53 to 6.48) compared to no treatment and 2.37 points (95% CI: 0.74 to 4.0) compared to other conservative interventions. The exercise interventions that showed better outcomes than comparison interventions were generally based in healthcare rather than general population settings, were designed and delivered with individual patients, and commonly included strengthening and trunk stability exercises.

In a later systematic review, only higher quality studies of exercise therapy were included to overcome some of the difficulties resulting from including studies with methodological limitations (Hettinga et al 2007). The results indicated that inclusion of smaller RCTs in systematic reviews leads to overestimation of effectiveness. The higher quality studies support the use of exercise, particularly strengthening exercises, aerobic exercises, general exercises, hydrotherapy and McKenzie exercises for individuals with persistent pain. Further support that exercise is beneficial for LBP is provided by the systematic review by Macedo et al (2009), who also highlighted that no one type of exercise appears superior. Motor control exercise for LBP was superior to minimal intervention, with mean differences in pain scores at short term, medium term and long term of −14.3 (95% CI: −20.4 to −8.1), −13.6 (95% CI: −22.4 to −4.1) and −14.4 (95% CI: −23.1 to −5.7), respectively. Improvements in function were also seen but at long-term follow-up only, with a difference to the comparison groups of −10.8 (95% CI: −18.7 to −2.8). However, motor control exercise was not more effective than other forms of exercise for LBP.

A further comprehensive review of RCTs for persistent non-specific LBP included 37 RCTs (3957 individuals) (van Middelkoop et al 2010). Compared to usual care, exercise therapy improved post-treatment pain intensity and disability, and long-term function. The review concluded that evidence from RCTs demonstrates that exercise is effective for persistent LBP, that the effects tend to be small, that

there is no evidence that one particular type of exercise is clearly more effective than others and that it is still unclear which patients benefit most from which type of exercise. Of 11 studies that compared different exercise interventions, only two studies found statistically significant differences in pain and disability outcomes. Aerobic exercise was found to be better than a flexion exercise regime in one low-quality study and motor control exercise was shown to be slightly better than general exercises in one high-quality study. Pooling of data was not undertaken due to the heterogeneity of the interventions in these studies.

In addition to specific exercise regimes, graded activity and graded exposure have been shown to be superior to minimal intervention in both the short and medium term on improving pain (pooled mean change at short term −6.2 95% CI: −9.4 to −3.0, medium term −5.5 95% CI: −9.9 to −1.0) and disability (pooled mean change at short term −6.5 95% CI: −10.1 to −3.0, medium term −3.9 95% CI: −7.4 to −0.4) in individuals with persistent non-specific LBP. However, graded activity and exposure were not better when compared to other forms of exercise (Macedo et al 2010).

Effect of exercise on work disability

Intensive exercise interventions that include aerobic capacity, muscle strength, endurance and coordination training, and have some relation to the work environment have been shown, in a systematic review, to reduce the number of sick days in employed individuals with persistent LBP (Schonstein et al 2003). However, the interventions included in this review also incorporated cognitive–behavioural approaches. More recently, a systematic review and meta-analysis of 23 RCTs showed a statistically significant effect of exercise on work disability in the long term (odds ratio 0.66 95%CI: 0.48 to 0.92), but not short or medium term, compared to usual care or other exercise interventions (Oesch et al 2010). Again there was no evidence of the superiority of any particular type of exercise. In addition, a small effect on sickness absence was found in pooled results (mean difference of −0.18 95%CI: −0.37 to 0.0) of five studies of physical conditioning in workers with persistent non-specific LBP, although conflicting results were found when compared to other exercise interventions (Schaafsma et al 2010).

Factors improving outcomes with exercise

Exercise therapy incorporates a wide range of heterogeneous interventions which in addition to the type of exercise can vary in terms of duration, frequency, setting, dosage and supervised or home-based programmes. A Bayesian meta-regression of 43 trials, where the characteristics of exercise interventions providing the best outcomes were examined, concluded that exercise interventions are more effective when individually designed rather than standardized, when exercise programmes were supervised and when programmes were carried out over longer time periods (Hayden et al 2005b). A separate examination of the impact of a variety of study characteristics on the small but significant improvements of pain and disability seen in included trials showed that only exercise dosage was significantly associated with effect sizes (Ferreira et al 2010).

Safety of exercise in persistent non-specific low back pain

Exercise in persistent non-specific LBP is safe. A large number of RCTs have now been completed and no concerns about safety have been raised, although adverse events are rarely reported.

Summary

In summary, therapeutic exercise is the most commonly used conservative intervention for the management of individuals with persistent non-specific LBP. The variable quality of RCTs still presents challenges to interpreting the evidence, with many published studies having moderate to high risk of bias. Exercise therapy is effective for managing individuals with persistent non-specific LBP, but which individuals benefit most from which exercise is still uncertain. In addition, adherence to exercise regimes is poor and strategies to improve adherence should be considered. The issue of adherence to exercise is considered later in this chapter.

Case study 1: **Low back pain**

A patient with persistent low back pain attends an initial appointment with you. His history and clinical examination findings are presented below.

A 48-year-old warehouse operative has a 6-month history of low back pain with some radiation to the left buttock and thigh. He finds difficulty with prolonged flexion activities but also gets increasing discomfort if he walks for longer than 20 minutes. He has some minimal sleep disturbance when the pain is severe. The pain came on after a particularly busy few days at work 'picking and packing' and since onset has varied greatly both in intensity and location of the pain. When the pain is particularly severe he has taken between 1 and 4 days off work at a time and finds that 'taking it easy' helps to settle the pain. His lifestyle outside of work is sedentary and he has no active hobbies other than some occasional gardening. His general health is fair, although he is on medication for hypertension and high cholesterol.

Today he describes his pain as 4 out of 10 in the lumbar spine and 2 out of 10 in the left buttock. On physical

---

examination he has some limitation of movement into flexion, extension and left side bend. He has local tenderness across the lower lumbar spine and left paravertebral soft tissues. Neurological testing is normal.

Based on the evidence presented, think about the following:
1. What type/s of exercise would you prescribe for this patient and why?
2. How would you deliver the exercise programme?
3. What dose of exercise would you advise (intensity, frequency and duration)?

EXAMPLE 2: EXERCISE FOR KNEE PAIN IN OLDER ADULTS

The problem

Knee pain is a common musculoskeletal complaint caused by both acute injuries such as meniscal tears and ligament ruptures, and chronic conditions such as patello-femoral pain syndrome, rheumatoid arthritis and osteoarthritis. Knee problems in older adults are particularly common, with estimates suggesting that approximately 25% of adults aged 55 years and over suffer with knee pain (Peat et al 2001a). This prevalence is likely to continue to rise as the population ages (Wilmoth 2000) and as levels of obesity, a risk factor, continue to grow (James 2008). Most knee pain in older adults is likely to be attributable to osteoarthritis (OA). Traditionally, OA was believed to be a progressive, degenerative disease, but it is now viewed as a dynamic repair process involving all joint tissues, including cartilage, bone, ligament and muscle (NICE 2008; Peat et al 2001b). There is some discordance between the extent of X-ray changes and clinical symptoms of OA, which can make the diagnosis of 'OA' difficult (Peat et al 2006). Recent UK national guidelines (NICE 2008) propose the following working clinical diagnosis of peripheral joint OA: patients aged 45 and over, with persistent joint pain that is worse with use, and morning stiffness lasting no more than half an hour (NICE 2008). Therefore, this evidence synthesis focuses on exercise for 'knee pain', with the assumption that most older adults with this condition will have a clinical problem of OA, and some will have radiographic changes in the relevant joints.

Persistent knee pain can have a considerable impact at an individual level. Pain, joint stiffness, instability, swelling and muscle weakness can contribute to functional limitations, psychological distress and reduced quality of life (Bennell & Hinman 2011; Hurley 2003; Jordan et al 2003; Neame & Doherty 2005). It can also have wider societal implications. For example, within the UK between 1999 and 2000, £43 million was spent on community services for OA, including patients with knee pain (NICE 2008), and each year 2 million adults visit their GP because of OA (Arthritis Research UK 2002).

Clinical guidelines

Many guidelines now exist to try and optimize health care for patients with knee pain, all of which recommend exercise as a frontline treatment (Zhang et al 2007b). The most recent UK guidelines are the NICE Osteoarthritis Guidelines (NICE 2008). They state that three core treatments should be considered first for every patient with OA: advice and education to enhance understanding of the condition, interventions to achieve weight loss if the person is overweight or obese, and activity and exercise, including local muscle strengthening and general aerobic fitness (NICE 2008). A multidisciplinary group have also developed a set of recommendations that address specific questions about the role of exercise in knee and hip OA, summarized in Table 13.1 (Roddy et al 2005a). These incorporate research-based evidence and expert opinion to evaluate ten propositions about the role of exercise, such as the benefit of specific types of exercises and predictors of response.

Exercise for knee pain: the evidence

A large body of evidence supports the usefulness of exercise for older adults with knee pain. Not only has exercise been shown to improve function and reduce pain (Fransen & McConnell 2008, Roddy et al 2005a), it can also improve physical performance, including walking distance and stair climbing (e.g. Ettinger et al 1997), improve muscle strength, increase joint range of motion and walking speed (e.g. Huang et al 2003, 2005), and increase self-efficacy (e.g. Foster et al 2007). In addition, it has wider health benefits, such as reducing the risk of cardiovascular disease (Haskell et al 2007; Nelson et al 2007). The current evidence base surrounding exercise for knee pain is summarized below, focusing on three key elements of exercise prescription: exercise type, delivery and dose. The safety of exercise and physical activity for knee pain is then explored before considering both the long- and short-term effectiveness of exercise for knee pain.

Type of exercise

Many RCTs have explored the effectiveness of different types of land-based exercise for older adults with knee pain, including both general aerobic exercise such as walking, cycling and tai chi, local knee exercises, including range of movement exercises and muscle strengthening

programmes, balance and coordination programmes, and exercise incorporated into wider self-management programmes. A recent Cochrane review of 32 trials (3616 participants) demonstrated the overall beneficial effects of land-based exercise for pain and function (Fransen & McConnell 2008). A meta-analysis found standardized mean differences (SMD) of 0.40 for pain and 0.37 for physical function, effect sizes similar to those found in two other meta-analyses exploring the efficacy of exercise for hip and knee pain (Zhang et al 2007b, 2010). Although these benefits are small to moderate, they are comparable to reported estimates for current simple analgesics and non-steroidal anti-inflammatory drugs (Fransen & McConnell 2008).

Roddy et al (2005b) completed a systematic review including 13 RCTs to compare the efficacy of aerobic walking and home-based quadriceps exercise in patients with knee pain. Meta-analyses for aerobic walking demonstrated a pooled effect size of 0.52 for pain and 0.46 for disability. Effect sizes for pain and disability for home-based quadriceps strengthening exercises were 0.32 and 0.32, respectively. No advantage of one form of exercise over the other was found on indirect comparison of pooled data and they concluded that as both interventions are effective, offering patients the choice over the type of exercise they complete may have the potential to improve exercise adherence. Also supporting the role of muscle strengthening exercise, an additional systematic review of 18 RCTs (2832 participants) investigated the effectiveness of resistance training for knee pain in older adults (Lange et al 2008). Interventions incorporated dynamic and isotonic training, machine-based resistance training, free weights, therabands (elastic resistance bands) and/or other items around the home (e.g. chairs, stairs, etc.). The number of sets of exercises ranged from one to 10 (most studies prescribed three sets), repetitions of each exercise ranged from three to 20 per set and three training sessions per week was most commonly prescribed (range two to seven weekly sessions). Overall 50–75% of the studies included in the review found knee symptoms, physical function and strength to improve by clinically meaningful amounts with resistance training when compared with usual care. The specifics of the resistance training (modality, duration, volume, frequency, intensity) did not appear to be related to patient outcomes (Lange et al 2008).

Delivery of exercise

Within RCTs of exercise for knee pain, interventions have been delivered individually, in groups and in various settings, including patients' own homes, different community settings and healthcare environments. Fransen and McConnell (2008) explored the influence of the delivery of exercise (home versus supervised individual or class-based exercise sessions) on pain and function. Both home and supervised exercise programmes significantly

Table 13.1 Summary of the 10 propositions included in the exercise recommendations for hip and knee OA

Proposition	Category of evidence (1–41)	Strength of recommendation (A–D2)
Both strengthening and aerobic exercise can reduce pain and improve function and health status in patients with hip and knee OA	Knee 1B Hip 4	A C (extrapolated from knee OA)
There are few contraindications to the prescription of strengthening or aerobic exercise in patients with hip or knee OA	4	C (extrapolated from adverse event data)
Prescription of both general (aerobic fitness training) and local (strengthening) exercises is an essential, core aspect of management for every patient with hip or knee OA	4	D
Exercise therapy for OA of the hip or knee should be individualized and patient-centred, taking into account factors such as age, co-morbidity and overall mobility	4	D
To be effective, exercise programmes should include advice and education to promote a positive lifestyle change with an increase in physical activity	4* 1B	D A
Group exercise and home exercise are equally effective and patient preference should be considered	1A** 4	A D
Adherence is the principal predictor of long-term outcome from exercise in patients with hip or knee OA	4	D
Strategies to improve and maintain adherence should be adopted, e.g. long-term monitoring/review and inclusion of spouse/family in exercise	1B	A
The effectiveness of exercise is independent of the presence or severity of radiographic findings	4	Not recommended
Improvements in muscle strength and proprioception (balance) gained from exercise programmes may reduce the progression of hip and knee OA	4	D

Reprinted from Roddy E, Zhang W, Doherty M, et al (2005) Evidence-based recommendations for the role of exercise in the management of osteoarthritis of the hip or knee – the MOVE consensus, *Rheumatology;* 44(1), with permission from Oxford University Press.
*Category 1B evidence that advice and education can promote lifestyle change and increase physical activity. Category 4 evidence that such techniques are required for exercise programmes to be effective.
**Category 1A evidence to support both group and home exercise with no clear evidence of superiority of one over the other, therefore patient preference should be considered (category 4 evidence).
1. Categories of evidence:
1A: Meta-analysis of RCTs
1B: At least one RCT
2A: At least one clinical trial without randomization
2B: At least one type of quasi-experimental study
3: Descriptive studies (comparative, correlation, case-control)
4: Expert committee reports/opinions and/or clinical opinion of respected authorities
2. Strength of recommendation
A: Directly based on category 1 evidence
B: Directly based on category 2 evidence or extrapolated recommendation from category 1 evidence
C: Directly based on category 3 evidence or extrapolated recommendation from category 1 or 2 evidence
D: Directly based on category 4 evidence or extrapolated recommendation from category 1 or 2 or 3 evidence

improved pain and functional status in participants with knee pain. Although the home exercises had consistently lower effect sizes than supervised exercises (either on a one-to-one basis or within a group), the differences were not statistically significant, perhaps explained by some element of supervision in most home exercise programmes. This supports the proposition within the MOVE exercise recommendations (Table 13.1) that 'group exercise and home exercise are equally effective and patient preference should be considered' (Roddy et al 2005a).

Exercise dose

Evidence about the optimal dose of exercise for older adults with knee pain, including its frequency, intensity and duration, is currently lacking (Bennell & Hinman 2011). A Cochrane review of the effectiveness of different exercise intensities for OA identified only one small RCT that tested the efficacy of low-intensity versus high-intensity stationary bicycling for people with knee pain. High- and low-intensity aerobic exercise was equally effective in improving functional status, gait, pain and aerobic capacity (Brosseau et al 2003). An additional review of the literature identified one subsequent RCT that compared high- and low-intensity strengthening programmes for older adults with knee pain. This also concluded that both exercise intensities were beneficial but that neither was clearly superior for pain, function, walking time and muscle strength over 8 weeks (Bennell & Hinman 2011; Jan et al 2008).

To the authors' knowledge, no RCTs have specifically investigated the optimal frequency and duration of exercise for older adults with knee pain. Within their Cochrane review exploring the efficacy of land-based exercise, Fransen & McConnell (2008) conducted sensitivity analyses to explore the effect of the number of supervised exercise sessions, dichotomized as those with less than 12 directly supervised sessions and those with 12 or more, on pain and function for older adults with knee pain. Both categories achieved significant treatment benefits in terms of pain and function, but the effect sizes for programmes with fewer than 12 supervised sessions were considered small, and the effect sizes for exercise programmes with at least 12 directly supervised sessions were moderate. This difference was statistically significant, and consequently the authors concluded that most people with knee pain need some form of ongoing monitoring or supervision to optimize outcomes from exercise.

Short- and long-term effects of exercise for knee pain

In a systematic review, Pisters et al (2007) explored the long-term effectiveness of exercise therapy in patients with hip and knee pain, defined as 6 months or more after the treatment period ended. In total 11 RCTs were included, incorporating a variety of modes of delivery of exercise and different types of exercises delivered at different doses. Overall, the small to moderate effects of exercise declined over time and finally disappeared at long-term follow-up, and there was strong evidence for no long-term effect of exercise on pain or function. However, adding booster sessions in the period after treatment had a positive influence on the maintenance of long-term effects (Pisters et al 2007). One reason for this may be the effect of booster sessions on exercise adherence over time.

Safety of exercise for knee pain in older adults

The safety of exercise therapy for older adults with knee pain was explored within the MOVE exercise recommendations for hip and knee OA (Roddy et al 2005a). No direct evidence was found concerning contraindications to exercise therapy and serious adverse events caused by exercise, such as falls or fractures, were rare. They therefore concluded that exercise is a safe intervention for older adults with knee pain (Roddy et al 2005a).

A recent systematic review of high-quality prospective cohort studies explored whether exercise can cause knee OA and associated knee pain (Bosomworth 2009). The conclusions were that knee problems occur as commonly in those who exercise and those who do not, and that there is no increase in the rate of progression of knee problems in individuals who exercise compared with those who do not.

Summary

In summary, therapeutic exercise is a recommended core treatment for knee pain in older adults. Evidence suggests that many different types of exercise, of both high and low intensities, delivered in groups or to individuals, are effective and safe for older adults with knee pain. Basing the prescription of exercise on the preferences of individual patients may therefore be the optimal approach. It appears that supervision and long-term follow-up in the form of booster sessions may be key ingredients in optimizing outcomes from exercise programmes. The challenge remains to find effective ways to maintain the beneficial effects of exercise over time. A key target is clearly exercise adherence and this is explored in more detail later in this chapter.

 Case study 2: **Knee pain in older adults**

A patient with knee pain attends an initial appointment with you. Her history and clinical examination findings are presented below.

A 65-year-old woman has a 3-year history of left knee pain, which was of insidious onset and has gradually worsened over time. She is a retired shop manageress and usually enjoys swimming, but this has become difficult due to her knee problem. Her general health is good, despite being overweight and suffering from mild hypertension. She also has pain in both hands.

Today she rates the intensity of her knee pain as 6 out of 10. Descending stairs, bending and rising from sitting all aggravate her knee pain. She has some difficulty when walking, and has started to use a stick outdoors. Her knee is stiff first thing in the morning and after staying in one position for too long. She finds some relief from an anti-inflammatory gel, and takes up to three 200 mg ibuprofen tablets per day.

Despite not having an X-ray she feels her problem is due to arthritis as her father suffered from this. It is her first visit to a healthcare professional and she is optimistic about its outcome. On examination the left knee has a mild effusion and a valgus alignment. Flexion is limited and the quadriceps are weak. The joint line is tender on palpation. No other examination findings are remarkable.

Based on the evidence presented, and the basic physiological and psychological principles of exercise training, think about the following:

1. What type/s of exercise would you prescribe for this patient?
2. How would you deliver the exercise programme?
3. What dose of exercise would you advise (intensity, frequency and duration)?

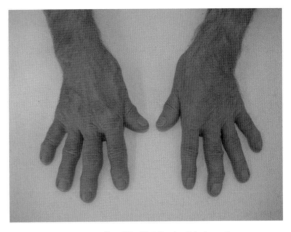

Fig. 13.2 **Photograph of individual with hand osteoarthritis.**

EXAMPLE 3: EXERCISE FOR HAND PAIN IN OLDER ADULTS

The problem

Another common musculoskeletal problem is hand pain. In a large cross-sectional survey of older adults with musculoskeletal hand problems in North Staffordshire, UK, the 1-year period prevalence of hand problems was 47% and the 1-month period prevalence of hand pain was estimated at 30.8% (Dziedzic et al 2007). These figures varied little with age. Severe hand-related disability affected 12.3% and was significantly more common in females than males, and increased in prevalence to the oldest age groups (Dziedzic et al 2007). Sufferers reported significant pain and disability, which affected their everyday lives, and considered the diagnosis of 'hand OA' to represent a serious condition. Hand OA is considered to be the most likely working diagnosis in these older adults.

In the UK it is estimated that at least 4.4 million people have X-ray evidence of moderate to severe OA of their hands (ARMA 2004; Arthritis Research UK 2002). In-depth interviews with patients with hand OA clearly highlighted the personal impact and loss of independence caused by this condition, with disruption of day-to-day activities such as washing, toileting and dressing, together with psychological and emotional distress (Hill et al 2007, 2010). The largest proportion of people treated in primary care for musculoskeletal complaints are older adults with OA (Dziedzic et al 2009) and whilst hand OA (Fig. 13.2) is a common condition (Dahaghin et al 2005a; Mannoni et al 2000; Oliveria et al 1995), many sufferers may never seek medical advice, despite its significant impact and associated disability (Dahaghin et al 2005b; Zhang et al 2002).

Clinical guidelines

Evidence from the NICE OA guidelines (NICE 2008) can be applied to the hand but much of the evidence was developed in studies of knee OA. The European League Against Rheumatism (EULAR) OA Task Force examined the management of hand OA specifically (Zhang et al 2007a). The recommendations were developed using an evidence-based format involving both a systematic review of research evidence and expert consensus. The guidelines recommend that the optimal management of hand OA requires a combination of non-pharmacological and pharmacological treatments, individualized to patients' requirements. Specifically, they state that education concerning joint protection (how to avoid adverse mechanical factors) together with an exercise regimen (involving both range of motion and strengthening exercises) is recommended for all patients with hand OA. This recommendation was based mainly on expert opinion and the research evidence from a trial of 40 patients with hand OA given either active treatment by an occupational therapist – a 45-minute education on joint protection techniques along with 15 minutes' instruction on range of movement exercise – or control, which was an instruction leaflet. The study outcome was at 3 months. It is difficult to ascertain the specific clinical benefit for hand exercises alone. The two elements of treatment were not directly compared and therefore it is not known whether the benefit was derived from the range of motion exercise, the joint protect programme or both. These questions are currently under investigation in a current randomized trial (Arthritis Research UK Self Management in osteoarthritis of the hand, the SMOOTH study ISRCTN33870549).

Local application of heat (paraffin wax and hot pack) is recommended, especially before exercise.

Exercise for hand OA: the evidence

In addition to the EULAR guidelines there are five other systematic reviews of non-surgical treatments for hand OA (Kjeken et al 2011; Mahendira & Towheed 2009; Moe et al 2009; Towheed 2005; Valdes and Marik 2010). Valdes and Marik (2010) examined the quality of the evidence regarding hand therapy interventions between 1986 and 2009. Nine studies (369 participants) examined the role of exercise in the treatment of patients with hand OA (Boustedt et al 2009; Garfinkel et al 1994; Lefler & Armstrong 2004; Moratz et al 1986; Rogers & Wilder 2007, 2009; Stamm et al 2002; Veitiene & Tamulaitiene 2005; Wajon & Ada 2005). Eight of the nine studies found that subjects who performed exercises demonstrated gains in grip strength ranging from 1.94 kg to a 25% improvement over baseline. However, the studies of exercise were of moderate methodological quality and provide limited support for exercise in increasing hand strength and decreasing pain.

The EULAR recommendations highlighted one RCT in particular (Stamm et al 2002) comparing a joint protection programme plus home-based hand exercise (focused on range of motion) versus information alone in 40 patients with hand OA. The number needed to treat (NNT) for improvement in patient global function was 2 (95% CI 1 to 6), suggesting significant clinical benefit from the combined treatment at 3 months (Zhang et al 2007a).

The limitations of existing studies mean that it is difficult to be certain of the clinical benefit of specific doses and intensities of hand exercises for hand OA in the short or long term. Following a recent systematic review by Kjeken et al (2011) to describe the specific doses of hand exercises and a consensus study with occupational therapists to recommend doses and intensities (Kjeken 2011) a new trial is currently underway to test the clinical benefit of such protocols (Kjeken, personal communication).

Whilst the benefit of exercise is demonstrated for lower limb OA (NICE 2008) and recommended for hand OA, there is currently limited evidence for the clinical benefit of hand exercises alone or whether hand exercises are more beneficial in combination with other approaches. New studies (e.g. the SMOOTH study) may shed further light on this evidence.

Even though the available recommendations support the use of simple, easily accessible interventions to manage hand pain, in practice patients are not receiving this care (Porcheret et al 2007). The first approach to improve the primary care of patients with OA is the integration of and continued support for self-management strategies (Dziedzic et al 2009). Encouraging the use of self-management strategies is particularly important for patients with mild hand OA as these patients are generally overlooked. If the goal of intervention is to reduce pain, improve activities of daily living and increase grip strength in hand OA, consider the use of exercise, joint protection education and heat modalities (Valdes & Marik 2010). Specific hand exercises can include

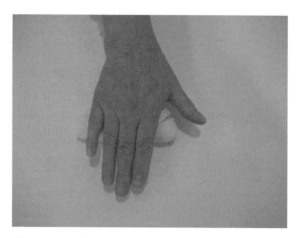

Fig. 13.3 **Specific hand exercises can include dough squeezing and rolling.**

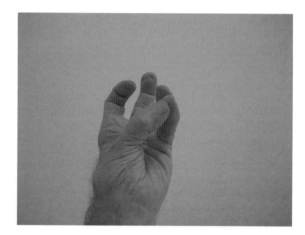

Fig. 13.4 **Specific hand exercises can include active range of movement exercises.**

dough squeezing and rolling (e.g. Fig. 13.3), and active ROM exercises (e.g. Fig. 13.4), all performed at a low pain level (Valdes & Marik 2010).

Summary

In summary, therapeutic exercise is a recommended treatment for hand pain in older adults. There is moderate evidence supporting hand exercises for pain reduction, increased grip strength, improved function and improved range of movement (Valdes & Marik 2010). Prescribing exercise alongside other self-management strategies, joint protection education and heat therapy is likely to provide additional benefits. The specific clinical benefit of hand exercise programmes alone is under-researched to date and new studies in progress will provide further evidence in this area.

Case study 3: **Hand pain in older adults**

A patient with hand pain attends an initial appointment with you. His history and clinical examination findings are presented below.

A 54-year-old farmer presents with pain radiating down his left thumb and is left handed. He has difficulty with everyday tasks, from holding a hammer to grasping a button on his shirt. He finds these difficulties very frustrating and hates asking his wife for help with simple jobs. His GP has given him topical anti-inflammatory gel to rub on his thumb base and has referred him to occupational therapy for advice on joint protection and looking after his hand joints. His GP has mentioned that a steroid joint injection may be indicated but has recommended hand exercises in the first instance. On examination there is evidence of subluxation and adduction of the carpometacarpal (CMC) joint of both hands, prominent nodes and enlargements of all interphalangeal joints, and thenar muscle wasting of the left hand. On palpation of the left CMC joint bony changes are confirmed and there is some evidence of changes in the right CMC joint. Palpation of the left CMC joint provokes pain. There are no signs of Dupuytren's contracture, carpal tunnel syndrome or triggering of tendons on testing, so his signs and symptoms can be attributed to hand OA.

Based on the evidence presented, think about the following:
1. What type/s of exercise would you prescribe for this patient and why?
2. How would you deliver the exercise programme?
3. What dose of exercise would you advise (intensity, frequency and duration)?

EXERCISE ADHERENCE

Given that exercise is clearly a core management option for those with persistent pain, achieving early engagement with, and longer-term adherence to, exercise programmes is crucial. Exercise adherence can be defined as 'the extent to which a person's behaviour corresponds with agreed recommendations from a health care provider' (World Health Organization 2003 from Jordan et al 2010). The importance of adherence in determining clinical outcomes from exercise programmes for chronic musculoskeletal pain is becoming increasingly recognized (NICE 2008, Roddy et al 2005b). A number of studies of patients with low back pain and knee pain have shown significant associations between exercise adherence and the effectiveness of exercise therapy: those with higher adherence levels obtain significantly better improvements in pain and function (Ettinger et al 1997, Hayden et al 2005b, Petrella & Bartha 2000), with some evidence of dose-response

effects (Thomas et al 2002). There is also evidence that continued adherence to exercise programmes and physical activity over the longer term, i.e. after the treatment period has ended, results in better long-term improvements in pain, physical function and self-perceived effect (Pisters et al 2010). When designing a therapeutic exercise programme for patients with chronic musculoskeletal pain, it is therefore crucial not only to ensure that it is based on sound physiological and psychological principles, but that it facilitates early engagement and longer-term adherence over time in ways that work for the individual in pain. In the final section of this chapter, the following questions are addressed:

1. How can exercise adherence be assessed?
2. What factors can influence exercise adherence?
3. How can adherence to exercise be enhanced?

Assessment of exercise adherence

No gold standard for assessing adherence to exercise exists (Treuth 2002) and as adherence can change over time, and patients can have differing levels of adherence to different parts of an exercise programme (for example they may continue with certain exercises and not others or may complete all of the exercises but at a lower intensity or less frequently than prescribed), the accurate assessment of exercise adherence is challenging. Within clinical settings, when time is often limited, physiotherapists frequently report measuring exercise adherence by observing a patient's exercise technique or by simply asking patients about their exercise behaviour (Holden et al 2008). Although these methods are simple and inexpensive, each has disadvantages. Self-reported exercise levels may be overestimated by the patient in an attempt to be viewed positively by the healthcare professional (Marks & Allegrante 2005) and exercises performed under direct observation and in an unfamiliar healthcare environment may not reflect accurately how the exercises are performed at home (Meichenbaum & Turk 1987). Use of a daily exercise diary, an example of which can be found in Box 13.1, may overcome some of these potential problems as patients record their 'real–time' behaviour. In addition, use of a diary might in itself have a positive influence on exercise adherence (Hughes et al 2004). However, an exercise diary still requires patients to be motivated to complete the diary and complete it accurately (Melanson & Freedson 1996). Using an objective assessment of exercise adherence, in the form of a pedometer (to measure step count) or accelerometer (to measure total activity count) can reduce the potential biases associated with self-report data (Paul et al 2007). Yet their relatively high cost, sometimes complex data interpretation requirements and inability to capture information on all domains of exercise behaviour (for example the number of sets and repetitions of a strengthening exercise

Box 13.1 **Example exercise diary**

Instructions

Please:

1. Try to fill your diary in regularly.

2. Every time you complete a set of exercises place a tick in the appropriate box.

3. Record how hard you felt the exercises were (using the scale on the next page).

4. There is a comments box for you to write any thoughts or feelings you have each day. For example, you could record if the exercises are becoming easier, or if you find any exercises particularly difficult.

If you did not manage to complete any exercises that day you can note why, and your physiotherapist can help you to work around any obstacles you uncover.

Below is an example of what part of a week might look like:

	Sets of each exercise completed (please tick)						How the exercises feel	Comments
	Exs. 1	Exs. 2	Exs. 3	Exs. 4	Exs. 5	Exs. 6		
Monday	✓	✓	✓	✓	✓	✓	5	*Exercise 1 was easy, 2 was difficult*
	✓		✓	✓	✓	✓		

'How the exercises feel' scale

1. Very, very easy / no problem

2. Very easy

3. Fairly easy

4. **Moderate/ beginning to feel hard**

5. Fairly hard

6. **Hard**

7. Very hard

8. Very, very hard

9. Extremely hard

10. Maximum

The exercises should feel between level 4 ("moderate/ beginning to feel hard") and level 6 ("Hard"). Below this you are not getting the maximum benefit and above this you are working harder than you need to.

REMEMBER

- It is very important to build up your exercises gradually
- Work at a level/pace that is right for you
- After exercise, it is normal to experience some discomfort around in your muscles, and this may last for a couple of days. BUT, if the discomfort is severe, or lasts for longer than this, reduce your exercises and contact your physiotherapist.

Week commencing:......./......./......./

	Sets of each exercise completed (please tick)						How the exercises feel	Comments
	Exs. 1	Exs. 2	Exs. 3	Exs. 4	Exs. 5	Exs. 6		
Monday								
Tuesday								
Wednesday								
Thursday								
Friday								
Saturday								
Sunday								

Week commencing:......./......./......./

	Sets of each exercise completed (please tick)						How the exercises feel	Comments
	Exs. 1	Exs. 2	Exs. 3	Exs. 4	Exs. 5	Exs. 6		
Monday								
Tuesday								
Wednesday								
Thursday								
Friday								
Saturday								
Sunday								

Developed by the BEEP trial team, Arthritis Research UK Primary Care Centre, Keele University, UK

programme completed) can make these inappropriate or difficult for clinicians and researchers to use (Myers & Midence 1998, Paul et al 2007). In summary, there is no 'right' way to assess exercise adherence, but the simple use of exercise diaries has much merit within clinical practice, offering some advantages over other commonly used approaches. The adherence measure used will depend on the exact content of the exercise programme prescribed, and the time, resources and skill of the clinician or researcher to analyse the data obtained.

Factors that influence exercise adherence

Non-adherence to exercise programmes may be unintentional, for examples in those cases where the individual forgets to do the exercise or is unable to follow the agreed recommendations, or intentional, occurring when a patient decides not to follow treatment as agreed, and is a result of rational decision making (Horne 1997). For example, if a patient decides that following an exercise programme poses more risk than benefit, from the patient's perspective, the rational decision would be to stop following the prescribed regime. Yet adherence behaviour is a complex phenomenon not only influenced by the attitudes and beliefs of patients, but also by many other factors. The WHO (2003) categorize factors that can influence adherence to medical regimes into five interacting dimensions: patient related factors, social and economic factors, healthcare team and system-related factors, condition-related factors, and therapy-related factors (see Box 13.2). It is clear

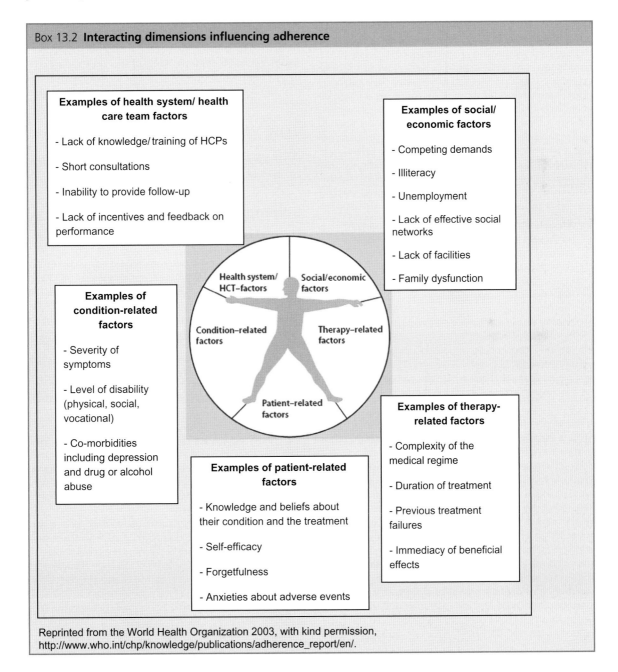

Box 13.2 **Interacting dimensions influencing adherence**

Examples of health system/ health care team factors

- Lack of knowledge/ training of HCPs

- Short consultations

- Inability to provide follow-up

- Lack of incentives and feedback on performance

Examples of social/ economic factors

- Competing demands

- Illiteracy

- Unemployment

- Lack of effective social networks

- Lack of facilities

- Family dysfunction

Examples of condition-related factors

- Severity of symptoms

- Level of disability (physical, social, vocational)

- Co-morbidities including depression and drug or alcohol abuse

Examples of patient-related factors

- Knowledge and beliefs about their condition and the treatment

- Self-efficacy

- Forgetfulness

- Anxieties about adverse events

Examples of therapy-related factors

- Complexity of the medical regime

- Duration of treatment

- Previous treatment failures

- Immediacy of beneficial effects

Health system/ HCT–factors
Social/economic factors
Condition–related factors
Therapy–related factors
Patient–related factors

Reprinted from the World Health Organization 2003, with kind permission, http://www.who.int/chp/knowledge/publications/adherence_report/en/.

therefore that for any individual patient many factors influence their level of exercise adherence, and rather than 'blaming' them for non-adherence to exercise recommendations, healthcare professionals need to assess how they can best support patients in pain to initiate exercise and maintain more active lifestyles over the longer term.

Strategies to enhance adherence to exercise

A recent Cochrane systematic review has summarized interventions that can improve adherence to exercise and physical activity in adults with chronic musculoskeletal pain (Jordan et al 2010). The review included 42 trials (8243 participants) and individual trials were grouped into five categories, based on the characteristics of their interventions, that explored the effect of the following on exercise adherence: type of exercise therapy or physical activity, delivery of exercise, exercise combined with a specific 'adherence' component, self-management programmes and interventions based on cognitive and/or behavioural principles. Overall, only 18 of the 42 trials indicated that the intervention improved adherence to exercise or physical activity. Strategies that positively influenced exercise adherence included:

- adherence-enhancing strategies such as problem solving, goal setting, systematic feedback, skills building, individualization of exercise (e.g. choice of activity and exercise setting), reinforcement messages, exercise diaries and pedometers
- supervision of exercise
- supplementing exercise programmes with refresher or booster sessions or by providing audiotapes or videotapes of exercises
- incorporating exercise into wider self-management programmes
- using behavioural graded activity programmes (increasing physical activity in a time-contingent manner).

Interestingly, the type of exercise (e.g. strengthening versus aerobic exercise) did not appear to be an important factor influencing adherence.

Other systematic reviews of adherence-enhancing interventions for exercise and physical activity have predominantly focused on healthy populations but their findings may be of relevance. Foster et al (2005) used 17 trials (6255 adults) to compare the effectiveness of different strategies to encourage sedentary, community dwelling adults to become more physically active. Results showed that physical activity could be enhanced in the short to mid-term, and that professional guidance and self-direction, plus ongoing professional support, are effective strategies. In a meta-analysis of 8 trials and 18 observational studies, Bravata et al (2007) investigated the effect of pedometer use on physical activity among adults in outpatient settings (Bravata et al 2007). Pedometer users significantly increased their daily step count, increased their overall physical activity by 26.9% over baseline and also significantly decreased their body mass index and blood pressure compared to controls. In addition, goal setting and a step diary were found to be key motivational strategies for increasing physical activity (Bravata et al 2007). Finally, Ogilvie et al (2007) completed a meta-analysis of 19 randomized trials and 29 non-randomized studies to explore how best to promote walking. Although pedometers were effective in the short term (up to 3 months), increases in steps were not sustained in the long term (at 6 or 12 months). Together these reviews provide evidence that adherence to exercise and physical activity can be enhanced, and that some of the strategies are relatively simple and inexpensive (use of diaries and pedometers, additional booster sessions with professional support in the longer term). The reviews also highlight the variable quality of previous trials, the inconsistency in measures of exercise adherence and the need for further research with long-term follow-up that explicitly addresses adherence to exercise and physical activity in adults with chronic musculoskeletal pain.

Summary and key points

Therapeutic exercise is clearly a core treatment for persistent musculoskeletal pain, such as that in non-specific low back pain, knee pain and hand pain related to osteoarthritis. However, the evidence synthesis in this chapter highlights that exercise overall tends to result in small to moderate effects on pain and function, and that a key challenge is that these effects most often decline over time, probably explained by poor adherence to exercise in the long term.

IMPLICATIONS FOR CLINICAL PRACTICE

Healthcare professionals can confidently recommend and prescribe exercise for persistent musculoskeletal pain patients, such as those with non-specific low back pain, or knee or hand pain related to OA. The type of exercise does not appear to be as important as previously thought for adults with persistent pain, at least when investigated in heterogeneous groups of patients with low back pain or knee pain. Therefore, patient preferences for the type of exercise may well be a useful guide upon which to base interventions in the hope of maximizing motivation and the likelihood of exercise behaviour. The characteristics of exercise programmes that appear to differentially influence clinical outcomes appear to be more to do with how the exercise is delivered, for example whether the exercise is individualized, supervised and regular (intensive). In particular, exercise adherence is crucial if the benefits of exercise are to be realized in patients with persistent musculoskeletal pain. Best available evidence challenges some healthcare services which offer brief interventions and simple advice to exercise, with little supervision and no follow-up of patients in the longer term. Simply advising patients to exercise is unlikely to be effective for many patients with persistent musculoskeletal pain.

IMPLICATIONS FOR RESEARCH

There are many questions still to be answered by research in order to assist physiotherapists and other healthcare professionals in designing exercise programmes and in maximizing the potential of exercise for their patients with persistent pain. For example, it is not yet clear how exercise outcomes might be mediated by exercise type, exercise programme length, intensity or duration in musculoskeletal pain problems. We do not yet know enough about how to identify individuals who might do well with exercise versus other treatments, or who might be best to receive one particular exercise approach over another. Studies that test ways to better match exercise treatments to individual patients are needed, following the early

examples from Hicks et al (2005), Brennan et al (2006) and Long et al (2004). In addition, since studies have underlined the highly individual nature of preferences for different types of exercise and physical activities, future research should test how to incorporate these preferences into clinical decision making in ways that might achieve better outcomes for patients. Promising early research in this area includes the development of an exercise preferences questionnaire and a trial comparing preference-based exercise with usual exercise prescription (Slade & Keating 2009). Finally, there are clear challenges to optimizing patients' outcomes from exercise and physical activity in the long term and studies that develop and test ways to support patients with persistent musculoskeletal pain to adhere to long-term exercise and physical activity behaviour are needed.

ACKNOWLEDGEMENTS

The authors would like to thank the BEEP (Best Evidence for Exercise in knee Pain) trial team for providing the example exercise diary.

REFERENCES

ACSM, 2006. American College of Sports Medicine's guidelines for exercise testing and prescription, sixth ed. Williams & Wilkins, Lippincott.

APTA, 2001. American Physical Therapy Association Guide to Physical Therapist Practice, 2nd edn. Phys. Ther. 81 (1), 9–746.

ARMA, 2004. Arthritis and Musculoskeletal Alliance Standards of Care for people with osteoarthritis. Arthritis and Musculoskeletal Alliance, London.

Arthritis Research, U.K, 2002. Arthritis: the big picture. Arthritis Research Campaign, London.www.arc.org.uk.

Bandura, A., 1977. Self-efficacy: Towards a unifying theory of behaviour change. Psychol. Rev. 84, 191–215

Bennell, K.L., Hinman, R.S., 2011. A review of the clinical evidence for exercise in osteoarthritis of the hip and knee. J. Sci. Med. Sport 14 (1), 4–9.

Bosomworth, N.J., 2009. Exercise and knee osteoarthritis: benefit or hazard? Can. Fam. Physician 55, 871–878.

Boustedt, C., Nordenskiold, U., Nilsson, A.L., 2009. Effects of a hand-joint protection programme with an addition of splinting and exercise. Clin. Rheumatol. 28, 793–799.

Bouwmeester, W., van Enst, A., van Tulder, M., 2009. Quality of low back pain guidelines improved. Spine 34, 2562–2567.

Bravata, D.M., Smith-Spangler, C., Sundaram, V., et al., 2007. Using pedometers to increase physical activity and improve health: a systematic review. JAMA. 298, 2296–2304.

Breivik, H., Collett, B., Ventafridda, V., et al., 2006. Survey of chronic pain in Europe: prevalence, impact on daily life, and treatment. Eur. J. Pain 10 (4), 287–333.

Brennan, G.P., Fritz, J.M., Hunter, S.J., et al., 2006. Identifying subgroups of patients with acute/subacute 'nonspecific' low back pain: results of a randomized clinical trial. Spine 31 (6), 623–631.

Brosseau, L., MacLeay, L., Robinson, V., et al., 2003. Intensity of exercise for the treatment of osteoarthritis.

Cochrane Database Syst. Rev. 2, CD004259.

Croft, P.R., Macfarlane, G.J., Papageorgiou, A.C., et al., 1998. Outcome of low back pain in general practice: a prospective study. Br. Med. J. 316, 1356–1359.

Dagenais, S., Tricco, A.C., Haldeman, S., 2010. Synthesis of recommendations for the assessment and management of low back pain from recent clinical practice guidelines. Spine J. 10, 514–529.

Dahaghin, S., Bierma-Zeinstra, S.M.A., Reijman, M., et al., 2005a. Prevalence and determinants of one month hand pain and hand related disability in the elderly (Rotterdam study). Ann. Rheum. Dis. 64, 99–104

Dahaghin, S., Bierma-Zeinstra, S.M.A., Ginai, A.Z., et al., 2005b. Prevalence and pattern of radiographic hand osteoarthritis and association with pain and disability (the Rotterdam study). Ann. Rheum. Dis. 64, 682–687.

Dunn, K.M., Croft, P.R., 2005. Classification of low back pain in primary care: Using 'bothersomeness' to identify the most severe cases. Spine 30, 1887–1892.

Dziedzic, K., Thomas, E., Hill, S., et al., 2007. The impact of musculoskeletal hand problems in older adults: findings from the North Staffordshire Osteoarthritis Project (NorStOP). Rheumatology 46 (6), 963–977.

Dziedzic, K.S., Hill, J.C., Porcheret, M., et al., 2009. New models for primary care are needed for osteoarthritis. Phys. Ther. 89 (12), 1371–1378.

Ettinger Jr., W.H., Burns, R., Messier, S.P., et al., 1997. A randomized trial comparing aerobic exercise and resistance exercise with a health education program in older adults with knee osteoarthritis. The Fitness Arthritis and Seniors Trial (FAST). JAMA. 277 (1), 25–31.

Ferreira, M.L., Smeets, R.J., Kamper, S.J., et al., 2010. Can we explain heterogeneity among randomized clinical trials of exercise for chronic back pain? A meta-regression analysis of randomized controlled trials. Phys. Ther. 90, 1383–1403.

Foster, C., Hillsdon, M., Thorogood, M., 2005. Interventions for promoting physical activity. Cochrane Database Syst. Rev. 1, CD003180.

Foster, N.E., Thomas, E., Barlas, P., et al., 2007. Acupuncture as an adjunct to exercise based physiotherapy for osteoarthritis of the knee: randomised controlled trial. Br. Med. J. 335, 436.

Fransen, M., McConnell, S., 2008. Exercise for osteoarthritis of the knee. Cochrane Database Syst. Rev. 8 (4), CD004376.

Friedrich, M., Gittler, G., Arendasy, M., et al., 2005. Long-term effect of a combined exercise and motivational program on the level of disability of patients with chronic low back pain. Spine 30 (9), 995–1000.

Garfinkel, M.S., Schumacher, H.R., Husain, A., et al., 1994. Evaluation of a yoga based regimen for treatment of osteoarthritis of the hands. J. Rheumatol. 21, 2341–2343.

Glynn, A., Fiddler, H., 2009. The physiotherapist's pocket guide to exercise assessment, prescription and training. Elsevier, London.

Haskell, W.L., Lee, I.M., Pate, R.R., et al., 2007. Physical activity and public health: updated recommendation for adults from the American College of Sports Medicine and the American Heart Association. Med. Sci. Sports Exerc. 39, 1423–1434.

Hayden, J.A., van Tulder, M.W., Malmivaara, A., 2005a. Exercise therapy for treatment of non-specific low back pain. Cochrane Database Syst. Rev. 3, CD000335.

Hayden, J.A., van Tulder, M.W., Tomlinson, G., 2005b. Systematic review: Strategies for using exercise therapy to improve outcomes in chronic low back pain. Ann. Intern. Med. 142, 776–785.

Hestbaek, L., Leboeuf, Y.C., Manniche, C., 2003. Low back pain: what is the long-term course? A review of studies of general patient populations. Eur. Spine J. 2, 149–165.

Hettinga, D.M., Jackson, A., Moffett, J.K., et al., 2007. A systematic review and synthesis of higher quality evidence of the effectiveness of exercise interventions for non-specific low back pain of at least 6 weeks' duration. Phys. Ther. Rev. 12, 221–232.

Hicks, G.E., Fritz, J.M., Delitto, A., et al., 2005. Preliminary development of a clinical prediction rule for determining which patients with low back pain will respond to a stabilization exercise program. Arch. Phys. Med. Rehabil. 86 (9), 1753–1762.

Hill, S., Dziedzic, K., Thomas, E., et al., 2007. The illness perceptions associated with health and behavioural outcomes in people with musculoskeletal hand problems: findings from the North Staffordshire Osteoarthritis Project (NorStOP). Rheumatology 46 (6), 944–951.

Hill, S., Dziedzic, K.S., Ong, B.N., 2010. The functional and psychological impact of hand osteoarthritis. Chronic Illn. 6 (2), 101–110.

Holden, M.A., Nicholls, E.E., Hay, E.M., et al., 2008. Physical therapists' use of therapeutic exercise for patients with clinical knee osteoarthritis in the United kingdom: in line with current recommendations? Phys. Ther. 88 (10), 1109–1121.

Horne, R., 1997. Representation of medication and treatment: advances in theory and measurement. In: Petrie, K.J., Weinman, J.A. (Eds.), Perceptions of health and illness. Hardwood Academic Press, Amsterdam.

Huang, M.H., Lin, Y.S., Yang, R.C., et al., 2003. A comparison of various therapeutic exercises on the functional status of patients with knee osteoarthritis. Semin. Arthritis Rheum. 32, 398–406.

Huang, M.H., Lin, Y.S., Lee, C.L., et al., 2005. Use of ultrasound to increase effectiveness of isokinetic exercise for knee osteoarthritis. Arch. Phys. Med. Rehabil. 86, 1545–1551.

Hughes, S.L., Seymour, R.B., Campbell, R., et al., 2004. Impact of the fit and strong intervention on older adults with osteoarthritis. Gerontologist 44, 217–228.

Hurley, M.V., 2003. Muscle dysfunction and effective rehabilitation of knee osteoarthritis: what we know and what we need to find out. Arthritis Care Res. 49, 444–452.

Hurley, M.V., Bearne, L.M., 2009. The principles of therapeutic exercise and physical activity. In: Dziedzic, K., Hammond, A. (Eds.), Rheumatology. Elsevier, Edinburgh.

James, W.P., 2008. The epidemiology of obesity: the size of the problem. J. Intern. Med. 263, 336–352.

Jan, M., Lin, J., Liau, J., et al., 2008. Investigation of clinical effects of high- and low-resistance training for patients with knee osteoarthritis: a randomised controlled trial. Phys. Ther. 88, 427–435.

Jordan, K.M., Arden, N.K., Doherty, M., et al., 2003. Standing Committee for International Clinical Studies Including Therapeutic Trials ESCISIT. EULAR Recommendations: an evidence based approach to the management of knee osteoarthritis: report of a task force of the standing committee for international clinical studies including therapeutic trials (ESCISIT). Ann. Rheum. Dis. 62, 1145–1155.

Jordan, J.L., Holden, M.A., Mason, E.E., et al., 2010. Interventions to improve adherence to exercise for chronic musculoskeletal pain in adults. Cochrane Database Syst. Rev. Jan 20 (1), CD005956.

Kjeken, I., 2011. Occupational therapy-based and evidence-supported recommendations for assessment and exercises in hand osteoarthritis. Scand. J. Occup. Ther. 18 (4), 265–281.

Kjeken, I., Smedslund, G., Moe, R., et al., 2011. A systematic review of design and effects of splints and exercise programs in hand osteoarthritis. Arthritis Care Res. 59, 1488–1494.

Lange, A.K., Vanwanseele, B., Singh, M.A.F., 2008. Strength training for treatment of osteoarthritis of the knee: a systematic review. Arthritis Care Res. 59, 1488–1494.

Lefler, C., Armstrong, W.J., 2004. Exercise in the treatment of osteoarthritis in the hands of the elderly. Clin. Kinesiol. 58, 13–17.

Long, A., Donelson, R., Fung, T., 2004. Does it matter which exercise? A randomized control trial of exercise for low back pain. Spine 29 (23), 2593–2602.

Macedo, L.G., Maher, C.G., Latimer, J., et al., 2009. Motor control exercise for persistent, nonspecific low back pain: A systematic review. Phys. Ther. 89, 9–25.

Macedo, L.G., Smeets, R.J., Maher, J., et al., 2010. Graded activity and graded exposure for persistent nonspecific low back pain: a systematic review. Phys. Ther. 90, 1538–6724.

Mahendira, D., Towheed, T.E., 2009. Systematic review of non-surgical therapies for osteoarthritis of the hand: an update. Osteoarthritis Cartilage 17, 1263–1268.

Maniadakis, N., Gray, A., 2000. The economic burden of back pain in the UK. Pain 84, 95–103.

Mannoni, A., Briganti, M.P., Di Bari, M., et al., 2000. Prevalence of symptomatic hand osteoarthritis in community-dwelling older persons: the ICARe Dicomano study. Osteoarthritis Cartilage 8, S11–S13.

Marcus, B.H., Rakowski, W., Rossi, J.S., 1992. Assessing motivational readiness and decision-making for exercise. Health Psychol. 22, 3–16.

Marks, R., Allegrante, J.P., 2005. Chronic osteoarthritis and adherence to exercise: a review of the literature. J. Aging Phys. Act. 13, 434–460.

McArdle, W.D., Katch, F.I., Katch, V.L., 1996. Exercise physiology: energy, nutrition and human performance, fourth ed. Williams & Wilkins, Baltimore, Maryland.

McAuley, E., 1992. The role of efficacy cognitions in the prediction of exercise behaviour in middle aged adults. J. Behav. Med. 15, 65–88.

Meichenbaum, D., Turk, D., 1987. Facilitating treatment adherence. Plenum Press, New York.

Melanson, E.L., Freedson, P.S., 1996. Physical activity assessment: a review of methods. Crit. Rev. Food Sci. Nutr. 36, 385–396.

Moe, R.H., Kjeken, I., Uhlig, T., et al., 2009. There is inadequate evidence to determine the effectiveness of nonpharmacological and nonsurgical interventions for hand osteoarthritis: an overview of high-quality systematic reviews. Phys. Ther. 89, 1363–1370.

Moratz, V., Muncie, H.L., Miranda-Walsh, H., 1986. Occupational therapy in the multidisciplinary assessment and management of osteoarthritis. Clin. Ther. 9, S24–S29.

Myers, L.B., Midence, K., 1998. Methodological and conceptual issues in adherence. In: Myers, L.B., Midence, K. (Eds.), Adherence to treatment in medical conditions. Haywood Academic Publishers.

Neame, R.L., Doherty, M., 2005. Osteoarthritis update. Clin. Med. 5, 207–210.

Nelson, M.E., Rejeski, W.J., Blair, S.N., et al., 2007. Physical activity and public health in older adults: recommendations from the American College of Sports Medicine and the American Heart Association. Med. Sci. Sports Exerc. 39, 1435–1445.

NICE, 2008. National Collaborating Centre for Chronic Conditions. Osteoarthritis: National Clinical Guideline for Care and Management in Adults. National Institute for Health and Clinical Excellence, Royal College of Physicians, London.

NICE, 2009. Low back pain: early management of persistent non-specific low back pain. Clinical guideline 88. National Institute for Health and Clinical Excellence, London. www.nice.org.uk/CG88.

Oesch, P., Kool, J., Hagen, K.B., et al., 2010. Effectiveness of exercise on work disability in patients with non-acute non-specific low back pain: Systematic review and meta-analysis of randomised controlled trials. J. Rehabil. Med. 42, 193–205.

Ogilvie, D., Foster, C.E., Rothnie, H., et al., 2007. Scottish Physical Activity Research Collaboration. Interventions to promote walking: systematic review. Br. Med. J. 334, 1204–1207.

Oliveria, S.A., Felson, D.T., Reed, J.I., et al., 1995. Incidence of symptomatic hand, hip and knee osteoarthritis among patients in a health maintenance organization. Arthritis Rheum. 38, 1134–1141.

Paul, D.R., Kramer, M., Moshfegh, A.J., et al., 2007. Comparison of two different physical activity monitors. BMC Med. Res. Methodol. 7, 26.

Peat, G., McCarney, R., Croft, P., 2001a. Knee pain and osteoarthritis in older adults: a review of community burden and current use of primary health care. Ann. Rheum. Dis. 60, 91–97.

Peat, G., Croft, P., Hay, E., 2001b. Clinical assessment of the osteoarthritis patient. Best Practice and Research Clinical Rheumatology. 15, 527–544.

Peat, G., Thomas, E., Wilkie, R., et al., 2006. Multiple joint pain and lower extremity disability in middle and old age. Disabil. Rehabil. 28, 1543–1549.

Petrella, R.J., Bartha, C., 2000. Home based exercise therapy for older patients with knee osteoarthritis: a randomised clinical trial. J. Rheumatol. 27, 2215–2221.

Pisters, M.F., Veenhof, C., van Meeteren, N.L., et al., 2007. Long-term effectiveness of exercise therapy in patients with osteoarthritis of the hip or knee: a systematic review. Arthritis Care Res. 57, 1245–1253.

Pisters, M.F., Veenhof, C., Schellevis, F.G., et al., 2010. Exercise adherence improving long-term patient outcome in patients with osteoarthritis of the hip and/or knee. Arthritis Care Res. 62, 1087–1094.

Porcheret, M., Jordan, K., Jinks, C., with the Primary Care Rheumatology Society, 2007. Primary care treatment of knee pain a survey in older adults. Rheumatology 46, 1694–1700.

Roddy, E., Zhang, W., Doherty, M., et al., 2005a. Evidence-based recommendations for the role of exercise in the management of osteoarthritis of the hip or knee – the MOVE consensus. Rheumatology 44, 67–73.

Roddy, E., Zhang, W., Doherty, M., 2005b. Aerobic walking or strengthening exercise for osteoarthritis of the knee?

A systematic review. Ann. Rheum. Dis. 64, 544–548.

Rogers, M.W., Wilder, F.V., 2007. The effects of strength training among persons with hand osteoarthritis: a two-year follow-up study. J. Hand Ther. 20, 244–250.

Rogers, M.W., Wilder, F.V., 2009. Exercise and hand osteoarthritis symptomatology: a controlled crossover trial. J. Hand Ther. 22, 10–18.

Schaafsma, F., Schonstein, E., Whelan, K.M., et al., 2010. Physical conditioning programs for improving work outcomes in workers with back pain. Cochrane Database Syst. Rev. 1, CD001822.

Schonstein, E., Kenny, D.T., Keating, J.L., et al., 2003. Work conditioning, work hardening and functional restoration for workers with back and neck pain. Cochrane Database Syst. Rev. 1, CD001822.

Slade, S.C., Keating, J.L., 2009. Effects of preferred-exercise prescription compared to usual exercise prescription on outcomes for people with non-specific low back pain: a randomized controlled trial [ACTRN12608000524392]. BMC Musculoskelet. Disord. 10, 14.

Stamm, T.A., Machold, K.P., Smolen, J.S., et al., 2002. Joint protection and home hand exercises improve hand function in patients with hand osteoarthritis: a randomized controlled trial. Arthritis Rheum. 47, 44–49.

Thomas, K.S., Muir, K.R., Doherty, M., et al., 2002. Home based exercise programme for knee pain and knee osteoarthritis: randomised controlled trial. Br. Med. J. 325, 752.

Towheed, T.E., 2005. Systematic review of therapies for osteoarthritis of the hand. Osteoarthritis Cartilage 13, 455–462.

Treuth, M.S., 2002. Applying multiple methods to improve the accuracy of activity assessments. In: Welk, G.J. (Ed.), Physical activity assessments for health related research. Human Kinetics Publishers, Champaign, IL.

Valdes, K., Marik, T., 2010. A systematic review of conservative interventions for osteoarthritis of the hand. J. Hand Ther. 23 (4), 334–335.

Van Middelkoop, M., Rubinstein, S.M., Verhagen, A.P., et al., 2010. Exercise therapy for chronic nonspecific low-back pain. Best Practice Research Clinical Rheumatology 24, 193–204.

Veitiene, D., Tamulaitiene, M., 2005. Comparison of self-management methods for osteoarthritis and rheumatoid arthritis. J. Rehabil. Med. 37, 58–60.

Waddell, G., 2004. The back pain revolution, second ed. Churchill Livingstone, Edinburgh.

Wajon, A., Ada, L., 2005. No difference between two splint and exercise and exercise regiments for people with osteoarthritis of the thumb: a randomised controlled trial. Aust. J. Physiother. 51, 245–249.

Walker, B.F., 2000. The prevalence of low back pain: systematic review of the literature from 1966 to 1998. J. Spinal Disord. 13, 205–217.

White, K.P., Harth, M., 1999. The occurrence and impact of generalized pain. Baillieres Best Pract. Res. Clin. Rheumatol. 13, 379–389.

Wilmoth, J.R., 2000. Demography of longevity: past, present and future trends. Exp. Gerontol. 35, 1111–1129.

World Health Organization, 2003. Adherence to long-term therapies: evidence for action. WHO Library.

Zhang, Y.Q., Niu, I.B., Kelly-Hayes, M., et al., 2002. Prevalence of symptomatic hand osteoarthritis and its impact on functional status among the elderly – the Framingham Study. Am. J. Epidemiol. 156, 1021–1027.

Zhang, W., Doherty, M., Leeb, B.F., et al., 2007a. EULAR evidence based recommendations for the management of hand osteoarthritis: report of a task force of the EULAR Standing Committee for International Clinical Studies Including Therapies (ESCISIT). Ann. Rheum. Dis. 66 (3), 377–388.

Zhang, W., Moskowitz, R.W., Nuki, G., et al., 2007b. OARSI recommendations for the management of hip and knee osteoarthritis: Part I: critical appraisal of existing treatment guidelines and systematic review of current research evidence. Osteoarthritis Cartilage 15, 981–1000.

Zhang, W., Nuki, G., Moskowitz, R.W., et al., 2010. OARSI recommendations for the management of hip and knee osteoarthritis: Part III: changes in evidence following systematic cumulative update of research published through January 2009. Osteoarthritis Cartilage 18, 476–499.

Chapter | 14 |

Transcutaneous electrical nerve stimulation and acupuncture

Mark I. Johnson and Carole A. Paley

LEARNING OUTCOMES

- To overview the use of TENS and acupuncture for pain management, including indications, contraindications and risks.
- To outline the principles underpinning various techniques of TENS and acupuncture.
- To describe the research supporting the analgesic mechanisms of action of TENS and acupuncture.
- To summarize clinical research evidence on clinical effectiveness for TENS and acupuncture.
- To discuss why clinical experience of outcome when using TENS and acupuncture sometimes differs from some of the clinical research findings.

OVERVIEW

Transcutaneous electrical nerve stimulation (TENS) and acupuncture are techniques that stimulate peripheral nerves in order to relieve pain. They are standard therapy in physical therapy and pain clinics, and are becoming more widely used in other healthcare settings. There is strong evidence from electrophysiological studies that both techniques inhibit onward transmission of nociceptive information in the central nervous system. However, their effectiveness has been a matter of much debate.

Part 1: Transcutaneous electrical nerve stimulation

TENS is a non-invasive technique for symptomatic relief of pain (Table 14.1). A portable battery-powered device passes electrical currents transcutaneously across the intact surface of the skin via adhesive electrode pads in order to stimulate non-nociceptive peripheral afferents (Fig. 14.1). TENS is also used for non-painful conditions such as postoperative nausea and vomiting, wound and bone

© 2014 Elsevier Ltd.

Table 14.1 Painful conditions commonly treated using TENS

Acute pain	Chronic pain
Post-operative pain Procedural pains such as colonoscopy Childbirth pain Dysmenorrhoea Angina pectoris Orofacial pain such as dental procedures Physical trauma, including fractured ribs	Musculoskeletal pains such as osteoarthritis, rheumatoid arthritis, low back pain and myofascial pain Neuropathic pains such as amputee stump and phantom pain, post-herpetic and trigeminal neuralgias, post-stroke pain, complex regional pain syndrome Nociceptive pain such as inflammatory pains and chronic wound pain Cancer pain associated with the disease such as cancer bone pain or with its treatment

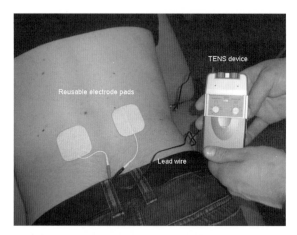

Fig. 14.1 TENS being used to treat chronic low back pain.

healing, incontinence, constipation and dementia. TENS is popular and devices can be purchased without prescription from retail outlets in many countries or over the internet.

When used to relieve pain TENS is given as a stand-alone treatment or in combination with other types of pain relief. Approximately 50% of chronic pain patients who try TENS gain benefit in the short term, although this declines in the long term (Davies et al 1997). Reasons for discontinuing TENS include effects wearing off over time and a discrepancy between effort and pain relief. Hence, patient evaluation and education is critical for successful TENS therapy.

TENS effects are rapid in onset and can occur within minutes for some patients. This may be useful to manage severe breakthrough or incident pain. TENS does not produce many of the side effects associated with drugs, such as sedation, dizziness, nausea and disorientation. There is no potential for toxicity so it can be used for long periods of

time without the fear of overdose. Interactions with drugs are few so TENS is often used in combination with analgesic medication to reduce drug dosage, side effects and costs (Bjordal et al 2003). TENS is most effective when patients administer it as required, following appropriate instruction by a healthcare professional.

DEFINITION

By definition, anything that delivers electricity across the surface of the skin with the purpose of activating underlying nerves is TENS. In health care the term 'TENS' is used to describe stimulation using a standard TENS device.

Standard TENS device

In general, standard TENS devices deliver biphasic pulsed currents at amplitudes between 1 and 60 milliamperes (mA), pulse durations (widths) between 50 and 500 μs and pulse frequencies (rates) between 1 and 250 pulses per second (pps). Pulse patterns include continuous (normal), burst (intermittent trains of pulses) and modulated amplitude, modulated frequency and modulated pulse duration (Table 14.2 and Fig. 14.2). Technical output specifications

Table 14.2 The technical specifications of a standard TENS device

Dimensions	Small device = 6 × 5 × 2 cm Large device = 12 × 9 × 4 cm (50–250 g)
Cost	£15–150
Pulse waveform	Symmetrical or asymmetrical biphasic Monophasic
Pulse amplitude	Most devices deliver constant current output that is adjustable between 1 and 50 mA into a 1-kΩ load
Pulse duration	Adjustable between 50 and 500 μs
Pulse frequency (adjustable)	Adjustable between 1 and 200 pps
Pulse pattern	Adjustable continuous, burst (random frequency, modulated amplitude, modulated frequency, modulated pulse duration)
Channels	One or two
Batteries	PP3 (9 V) or AA
Additional features	Timer Some devices provide a range of pre-programmed settings

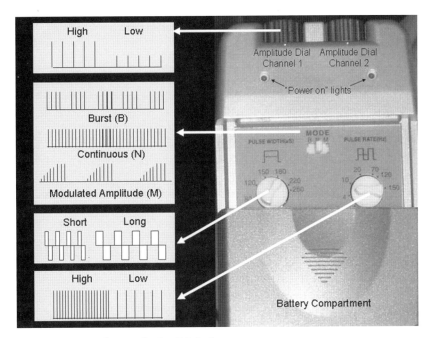

Fig. 14.2 **Electrical characteristics of a standard TENS device.**

of standard TENS devices differ between manufacturers with only limited impact on physiological effects.

TENS-like devices

A variety of TENS-like devices are available (Table 14.3). Some deliver microampere (μA) currents, much lower than a standard TENS device, some use pen-like electrodes, some deliver currents trans-cranially or trans-spinally. Critical reviews conclude that manufacturers' claims about TENS-like devices are over-ambitious and practitioners should use a standard TENS device in the first instance. The remainder of this chapter will focus on a standard TENS device and will use the term 'TENS' to refer to a standard TENS device.

PRINCIPLES UNDERPINNING TENS

Electricity has been used to relieve pain since 2500 BC, when electrogenic fish were used to treat painful conditions. The development of electrostatic generators promoted the use of medical electricity in mainstream medical practice in the 18th century although it fell out of favour by the 20th century because of variable clinical results and the development of pharmacological treatments. In 1965, Melzack and Wall provided a physiological rationale for electro-analgesia and this was followed by clinical observations that chronic pain could be relieved in patients by electrical stimulation of nerve fibres in the skin, dorsal columns in the spinal cord and periaquadctal grey in the midbrain. Initially, TENS was used to predict the success of spinal cord stimulation implants but it was quickly realized that TENS could be used successfully as a treatment in its own right.

The purpose of TENS is to selectively activate different populations of nerve fibres to initiate physiological responses that lead to pain relief. As the current amplitude of TENS is increased, large diameter myelinated non-nociceptive axons (Aβ) are activated first because they have lower thresholds of excitation (Fig. 14.3). The sensation experienced beneath the electrodes is often described as a 'tingling' or 'pins and needles' sensation (electrical paraesthesia) with an intensity that is non-painful. If current amplitude is increased further smaller diameter myelinated (Aδ) and unmyelinated (C-fibre) afferents become active and the user experiences a painful sensation, which is not desirable. Activation of low threshold (Aβ) axons without concurrent activation of higher threshold (Aδ and C-fibre) afferents is achieved using currents with small amplitudes (i.e. low intensity) and pulse durations between 50 and 500 μs. More nerve impulses can be generated in the axon by increasing the pulse frequency of TENS, although at higher frequencies this is limited by the absolute and relative refractory periods for the axon. In theory, TENS frequencies below 200 pps should be optimal.

Most TENS devices use biphasic electrical pulse waveforms, resulting in zero net current flow between the

Table 14.3 Examples of commonly available TENS-like devices (adapted from Johnson 2008)

Device	Characteristics
Action Potential Simulation (APS) (Odendaal & Joubert 1999)	Monophasic square pulse with exponential decay delivered by two electrodes Pulse amplitude low (<25 mA), duration long (800 μs to 6.6 ms), frequency fixed at 150 pps
Codetron (Herman et al 1994)	Pulsed square wave delivered randomly to one of six electrodes Pulse amplitude low, duration long (1 ms), frequency low (2 pps)
H-Wave Stimulation (Blum et al 2008)	'Unique' biphasic wave with exponential decay delivered by two electrodes Pulse amplitude low (<10 mA), duration long (fixed at 16 ms), frequency low (2–60 pps)
Interferential therapy (interference currents) (Palmer & Martin 2008)	Two out-of-phase currents that interfere with each other to generate an amplitude modulated wave Traditionally, delivered by four electrodes; some devices have amplitude modulated waves that are premodulated within the device (two electrodes) Pulse amplitude low, amplitude modulated frequency 1–200 Hz, (carrier wave frequencies approximately 2–4 kHz)
Microcurrent, including transcranial stimulation and 'acupens' (Koopman et al 2009, Tan et al 2006)	Modified square direct current with monophasic or biphasic pulses changing polarity at regular intervals (0.4 s) delivered by two electrodes Pulse amplitude low (1–600 μA with no paraesthesia), frequency depends on manufacturer (1–5000 pps) Many variants exist (e.g. transcranial stimulation for migraine and insomnia, acupens for pain)
Transcutaneous Spinal Electroanalgesia (TSE) (Palmer et al 2009)	Differentiated wave delivered by two electrodes positioned on spinal cord at T1 and T12 or straddling C3–C5 Pulse amplitude high yet no paraesthesic sensation generated, duration very short (1.5–4 μs), frequency high (600–10 000 pps)
Pain®Gone (Asbjorn 2000, Ivanova-Stoilova & Howells 2002)	Hand-held pen device using piezoelectric elements to deliver a low-ampere high-voltage single monophasic spiked pulse (e.g. 6 μA/15 000 V) Delivered by giving 30–40 individual shocks at the site of pain or on acupuncture points to generate non-noxious to mild noxious pin-prick sensation, repeated whenever pain returns
InterX® (Gorodetskyi et al 2007)	High-amplitude, short pulse width, dynamic waveform delivered by closely spaced metal electrodes moved across the surface of the skin Technology claims to identify changes in tissue properties to identify optimal treatment locations
Limoge current (Limoge & Dixmerias-Iskandar 2004, Limoge et al 1999)	High-frequency pulses interrupted with repetitive low-frequency cycle delivered by three electrodes (negative electrode between eyebrows and two positive electrodes in retro-mastoid region) Use to potentiate effects of opiates

Adapted and reprinted by permission from MacMillan publishers Ltd: Nature Reviews Rheumatology. Johnson MI, Walsh DM, Pain: continued uncertainty of TENS's effectiveness for pain relief; 6(6); copyright 2010.

electrodes and thus preventing skin irritation. In devices using monophasic waveforms, the cathode electrode (normally the black lead) is placed proximal to the anode because the cathode activates the axonal membrane and generates the nerve impulse. Also, skin offers high impedance to TENS so currents tend to remain superficial and stimulate cutaneous rather than deep-seated tissue. By reducing pulse duration and placing electrodes over muscles or muscle efferents it is possible to generate muscle contractions without a strong TENS sensation.

CLINICAL TECHNIQUE

TENS outcome depends on stimulation technique, including choice of location, number and type of electrodes, and the electrical characteristics of currents. Protocols provided in manufacturers' materials should be used to guide decisions rather than used as an inflexible regimen. TENS effects are dependent on pulse amplitude, because of its

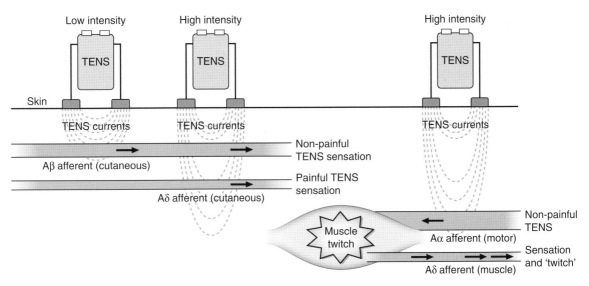

Fig. 14.3 Fibre recruitment by increasing the amplitude of electrical currents administered during conventional TENS.

relationship to axon recruitment, and selective recruitment of different nerve fibres is achieved by the user titrating pulse amplitude whilst monitoring TENS intensity. Two commonly used TENS techniques are conventional TENS and acupuncture-like TENS (AL-TENS) (Table 14.4).

Conventional TENS (low intensity, high frequency)

The International Association for the Study of Pain (IASP) defines conventional TENS as high frequency (50–100 Hz), low intensity (paraesthesia, not painful), small pulse width (50–200 μs). The purpose of conventional TENS is to activate low-threshold non-noxious transmitting afferents (Aβ) as this reduces onward transmission of nociceptive information in the central nervous system (see section on the mechanism of action). TENS amplitude is increased to achieve a strong, comfortable, non-painful electrical paraesthesia beneath the electrodes or in the relevant body part. Frequencies between approximately 10 and 200 pps, pulse durations between 50 and 200 μs and a continuous pulse pattern are initially used.

Acupuncture-like TENS

AL-TENS was first described in the 1970s as a means to harness the mechanisms of action of TENS and acupuncture (Eriksson & Sjölund 1976). IASP defines AL-TENS as 'hyperstimulation' using currents that are low frequency (2–4 Hz), higher intensity (to tolerance threshold) and longer pulse width (100–400 μs). Often, AL-TENS is used to generate non-painful muscle twitching, which subsequently generates impulses in small-diameter peripheral afferents from deeper structures and activates descending

pain inhibitory pathways and the release of endogenous opioids in the central nervous system (Johnson 1998).

AL-TENS is achieved using single pulses at frequencies below 10 pps (usually 1–4 pps) or intermittent trains or bursts (2–4 Hz) of high-frequency pulses (∼100 pps) at the painful site, over muscles, motor points, acupuncture points and trigger points. AL-TENS generates prolonged post-stimulation effects and is useful for patients resistant to conventional TENS (Eriksson & Sjölund 1976) and preferential to conventional TENS for radiating neurogenic pain, pain arising from deep structures and pain associated with altered skin sensitivity (for review see Johnson 1998).

Other TENS techniques

Intense TENS delivers currents at painful intensities for short periods of time and is used as a counterirritant for short painful procedures, such as wound-dressing changes, suture removal and venepuncture. Acu-TENS is the application of TENS to acupuncture points and is offered as a non-invasive alternative to acupuncture. There is inconsistency in Acu-TENS technique and few good-quality studies.

CONTRAINDICATIONS, PRECAUTIONS AND ADVERSE EVENTS

Safety guidelines for TENS are available in Australia, the UK and the USA, and an excellent web-based resource is available at http://www.electrotherapy.org. Active implants such as pacemakers and ventricular assist devices (artificial hearts) are absolute contraindications for TENS, although TENS has been used in these situations following approval

Table 14.4 The characteristics of different TENS techniques

Characteristic	Conventional TENS	AL-TENS
Peripheral action	Generally stimulates cutaneous non-noxious afferents	Generally stimulates cutaneous and muscle nerves, leading to activity in small-diameter muscle and cutaneous afferents
Patient experience	Non-painful TENS paraesthesiae (minimal muscle activity)	Strong pulsating TENS sensation with simultaneous muscle twitching
Electrode location	Straddle site of pain (dermatomal) but if not successful try main nerve bundle, across spinal cord or contralateral positions	Over muscle belly or motor nerves (myotomal) at site of pain but if not successful try contralateral positions, trigger points or acupuncture points
Pulse amplitude (intensity)	Low (non-painful)	High (non-painful twitching)
Pulse frequency	High (10–200 pps) determined by patient preference	Low (<5 pulses per second or <5 bursts per second)
Pulse duration	Usually 50–200 μs determined by patient preference	Usually 100–200 μs Lower pulse width will generate a weaker TENS sensation yet still create muscle twitching
Pulse pattern	Continuous in first instance but determined by patient preference	Burst in first instance; if not successful or uncomfortable try amplitude modulated
Dose	Use as much and as often as needed, but have a break every hour or so	Use for no more than 30 minutes at a time a few times a day as muscle fatigue may develop. Delayed onset muscle soreness may occur the following day
Time course of pain relief	Rapid onset and offset of effects Pain relief tends to be spinal	Rapid onset delayed offset of effects Pain relief tends to be a combination of spinal and supraspinal

from the medical specialist. TENS interferes with internal cardiac defibrillators, producing inadvertent shocks (Holmgren et al 2008), and generates artefacts on fetal monitoring equipment (Bundsen & Ericson 1982). TENS should not be administered over the abdomen during pregnancy, on the neck or head for patients with epilepsy, or close to bleeding tissue, malignancy (except in palliative care) or active epiphysis. TENS can be used over metal implants, although care should be taken as there is one case report of skin burn after interferential therapy (Ford et al 2005). TENS appears to be safe when used with stents, percutaneous central catheters or drainage systems, although consideration must be given to mechanical stresses resulting from TENS-induced muscle contractions. TENS should be used with caution for patients on an anticoagulant treatment and not delivered close to transdermal drug-delivery systems because they may iontophoretically drive the drug through the skin, leading to toxicity. TENS should not be used while operating hazardous equipment, including motor vehicles.

Serious adverse events from TENS are rare and include respiratory compromise when using electrodes positioned on the anterior and posterior chest (Mann 1996) and repetitive epileptic seizures in individuals with coexisting psychomotor disturbances (Rosted 2001). There are reports of skin burns whilst using TENS-like devices due to inappropriate technique (Satter 2008). Contact dermatitis with redness and minor skin irritation may also occur. It is important to monitor the extent of this. TENS worsens pain in some individuals and may produce a vasovagal response, leading to nausea, dizziness and even syncope.

Principles of electrode placement

TENS electrodes are made of knitted stainless-steel fibres with adhesive gel, which enables flexibility across body contours. Sizes vary but 5×5 cm is most common. There is some evidence to suggest that small electrodes (0.8×0.8 cm^2) are more comfortable for thin fat layers (0.25 cm) and stimulating superficial nerves, and larger electrodes (4.1×4.1 cm^2) are more comfortable for thicker fat layers (2 cm) and stimulating deeper nerves (1.1 cm) (Alon et al 1994). Glove, sock and belt electrodes are also available, and more recently array electrodes have been developed in an attempt to target stimulation more precisely.

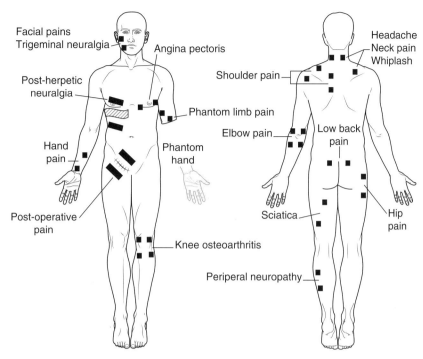

Fig. 14.4 Common electrode placement sites during conventional TENS.

It is necessary to site electrodes on healthy skin with functional nerves and normal sensation, so a sharp-blunt skin test should be conducted before use. Electrodes can be placed up to ~15 cm apart and a dual-channel TENS device with four electrodes used for large areas of pain or for simultaneously treating pains at two body sites. During conventional TENS, electrodes are positioned so that TENS paraesthesiae cover the pain (Fig. 14.4). When this is not possible TENS should be positioned at alternative sites, including:

- over main nerves proximal to the site of pain (this is especially useful to project TENS sensations to distal body parts)
- on skin from an ipsilateral or contralateral dermatome
- paravertebrally at the spinal segment related to the location of the pain.

Electrodes should not be placed over:

- skin with increased sensitivity to touch (i.e. tactile allodynia) or dysaesthesia because it may aggravate the pain, although paradoxically this is not always the case
- an open wound, frail skin due to eczema, radiotherapy or reconstructive surgery
- the abdomen of a pregnant woman
- the anterior neck, because stimulation of baroreceptors at the carotid sinus may cause a hypotensive response and stimulation of laryngeal nerves may cause a laryngeal spasm

- the eyes, because it may increase intraocular pressure
- internally except in specific circumstances and with a specially designed device for dental analgesia or incontinence
- through the chest using electrodes placed on the anterior and posterior thorax as this interferes with intercostal muscle activity, leading to severely compromised breathing.

As neuropathic pain conditions often present with hypersensitivity, electrodes should initially be placed over peripheral nerves proximal to the pain. Likewise, electrodes should be placed along the main nerves proximal to the site of pain if TENS sensation cannot be produced at the site of pain because of diminished skin sensitivity resulting from nerve damage (e.g. numbness following peripheral neuropathy). For postoperative pain, 'strip-like' electrodes can be placed either side of the incision scar providing there is no hypersensitivity. It is also possible to place electrodes along the main nerve trunk in the residual limb to project TENS sensation into the phantom limb pain. Paravertebral electrode positions at spinal segments related to the pain or on the skin of dermatomes related to the pain can also be used. For example, during childbirth, electrodes are positioned on the back at spinal segments over afferents arising from the cervix and lower uterine segment for the first stage of labour, and afferents arising from the pelvis and perineum for the second stage of labour.

Principles of choosing electrical characteristics for TENS

Despite much being written about the optimal TENS settings for different conditions, no relationship has been determined. The critical determinant of outcome is pulse amplitude (intensity) and studies using healthy pain-free human volunteers show that strong non-painful TENS is superior to barely perceptible TENS (Lazarou et al 2009). Electrophysiological research suggests that different frequencies of TENS activate different neurophysiological mechanisms at submotor thresholds (see DeSantana et al 2008a for review). A systematic review of studies using pain-free volunteers exposed to experimentally induced pain concluded that hypoalgesia during strong non-painful TENS was not influenced by pulse frequency, although most studies were underpowered (Chen et al 2008). Subsequently, appropriately powered studies have found that strong non-painful TENS at 80 pps was superior to 3 pps at reducing experimental mechanical pain and ischaemic pain in healthy participants (Chen & Johnson 2010), although 3 pps was superior to 80 pps for cold-pressor pain.

To date, evidence of a relationship between pulse frequency and pattern analgesia or medical diagnosis is limited. Patients appear to have individual preferences for electrical characteristics of TENS based on comfort rather than the amount of pain relief. Encouraging patients to experiment with TENS settings will probably produce the most effective outcome.

Clinical practice and dosage

Pain relief with conventional TENS is rapid in onset and offset, and long-term users report maximal benefit during stimulation so they administer TENS for many hours each day. Sequential TENS delivered by strong non-painful TENS punctuated with more intense TENS using muscle twitching may be clinically useful to mange background pain with incidents of breakthrough pain.

Electrodes are left in situ and the device attached to a trouser belt so that patients can administer TENS intermittently throughout the day on an as-needed basis. The intensity of TENS fades due to habituation, so users increase amplitude to maintain a strong non-painful TENS. Some patients report that TENS effects wear off with repeated use (i.e. tolerance to TENS) and repeated use of TENS generates opioid tolerance in animals, with cholecystokinin and NMDA receptors being involved. Generating a novel stimuli using modulated (Chen & Johnson 2009) and random (Pomeranz & Niznick 1987) delivery of currents has been shown to reduce habituation and tolerance (Hingne & Sluka 2008). Changing electrode placement or temporarily withdrawing TENS may also help.

New TENS patients should be given a supervised trial of TENS to ensure it does not aggravate pain and to educate them on safe technique and expected therapeutic outcome

---

Box 14.1 Safe TENS technique

1. Check contraindications and test skin for normal sensation.
2. Adjust initial TENS settings when device is switched off as follows:
   pulse pattern (mode) = continuous (normal)
   pulse frequency (rate) = mid range (80–100 pps)
   pulse duration (width) = mid range (100–200 µs)
   timer (if available) = continuous
3. Connect electrode lead wires to electrodes.
4. Position electrodes on skin at site of pain or over main nerve bundle.
5. Connect electrode lead wires to TENS device.
6. Switch TENS device on and slowly increase intensity until patient reports first TENS 'tingling' sensation.
7. Ask patient whether the sensation is acceptable.
8. Slowly increase intensity until patient reports a strong but non-painful TENS sensation.
9. Check that the sensation is acceptable and monitor patient for any signs of an autonomic response.
10. Allow patient to experiment with settings by:
    reducing amplitude so TENS barely perceptible, then changing the setting, then increasing the pulse amplitude to a strong non-painful level.
11. Instruct patient to adjust duration of stimulation according to need.

(Box 14.1). Patients should be familiar with operational aspects of the device on leaving the clinic. They should be advised to administer TENS in 30-minute sessions for the first few times and encouraged to use it as much as they like after this. They should be encouraged to experiment with all stimulator settings between and within treatment sessions to achieve the most comfortable stimulation for that moment in time. A point of contact should always be available for patients who encounter problems. Children as young as 4 years of age are able to understand TENS and short-duration treatments have been useful for dental pain, minor procedures such as wound dressing and venepuncture.

MECHANISM OF ACTION

TENS generates impulses in low-threshold afferents that enter the spinal cord and ascend to ipsilateral brainstem nuclei (e.g. nucleus gracilis and nucleus cuneatus) and ultimately to the thalamus and somatosensory cortex. The paraesthesic sensation is generated in the somatosensory cortex by the 'unnatural' (ectopic) patterns of impulses generated by TENS. Pain relief from TENS is due to actions at peripheral, spinal and supraspinal sites.

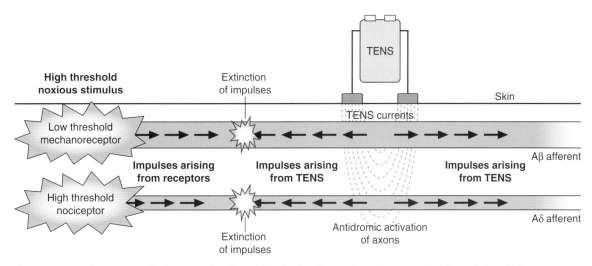

Fig. 14.5 Axonal activation during TENS leading to blockade of nerve impulses travelling in peripheral afferents.

Peripheral mechanisms

TENS generates impulses that travel in both directions along axons (Fig. 14.5). Impulses travelling towards the periphery collide and extinguish impulses arising from sensory receptors activated by natural stimuli (e.g. arising from nociceptors, mechanoreceptors and thermoreceptors) via a 'busy line' effect (Walsh et al 1998).

Spinal mechanisms

Strong non-painful (conventional) TENS activates non-noxious afferents, which branch as they enter the central nervous system and synapse with interneurons, which release inhibitory neurotransmitters (e.g. γ-amino butyric acid (GABA) and met-enkaphalin) and inhibit central transmission of nociceptive information and reduce central sensitization (Sandkühler et al 1997) (Fig. 14.6). This mechanism is rapid in onset and offset, and maximal when TENS is delivered to somatic receptive fields of the central nociceptive transmission cells (i.e. segmental). At higher intensities, longer duration post-stimulation inhibition of central nociceptor cells occurs, which may last up to 2 hours (Sandkühler et al 1997).

Supraspinal mechanisms

AL-TENS activates muscle efferents to generate phasic muscle twitching, which generates impulses in muscle afferents (e.g. proprioceptors). This results in activity in descending pain inhibitory pathways (e.g. periaqueductal grey and ventromedial medulla), which terminate at numerous levels in the spinal cord to inhibit central nociceptive transmission cells (Desantana et al 2009; Fig. 14.7). Stronger and longer lasting inhibition of central nociceptive

transmission occurs when muscle rather than skin afferents are activated. Originally evidence suggested that AL-TENS, but not conventional TENS, was mediated by endorphins, but recent evidence suggests that low-frequency TENS involves μ-opioid receptors, and high-frequency TENS involves δ-opioid receptors (Kalra et al 2001). GABA is a key neurotransmitter for conventional TENS, although cholinergic, adrenergic and serotinergic systems also seem to be involved (for review see DeSantana et al 2008b).

When TENS is delivered at intensities above the pain threshold (i.e. intense TENS) smaller diameter myelinated cutaneous afferents (Aδ) become active, leading to pain relief through counter-irritation via activation of diffuse noxious inhibitory controls (Morton et al 1988). TENS also activates peripheral parasympathetic and sympathetic efferents, leading to the release of acetylcholine and noradrenaline at autonomic effectors, respectively. There has been surprisingly little research into the effects of TENS on the autonomic nervous system and studies are conflicting (Olyaei et al 2004; Reeves et al 2004).

CLINICAL RESEARCH

Most of the existing research consists of case reports or clinical trials lacking control groups, but it is a rich source of documented clinical experience suggesting that TENS is useful. It is not possible to attribute the positive outcomes during TENS to the electrical currents per se. Most randomized controlled trials (RCTs) using placebo TENS delivered using a sham device are underpowered and suffer from methodological limitations. Blinding of active and placebo TENS interventions is a persistent problem because a strong yet non-painful TENS sensation is a pre-requisite of adequate technique (Bjordal et al 2003). Participants may

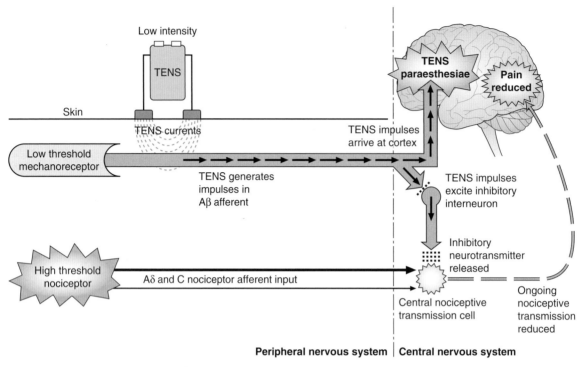

Fig. 14.6 **The mechanism of action of conventional TENS.**

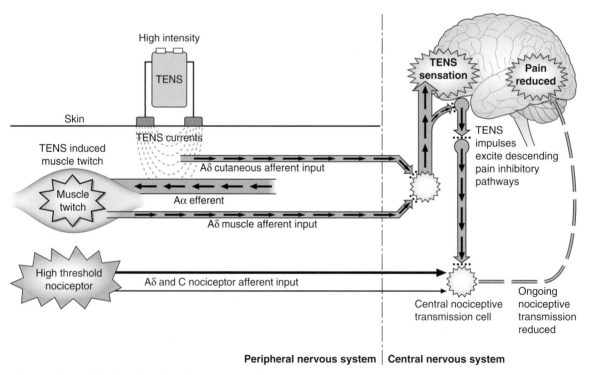

Fig. 14.7 **The mechanism of action of acupuncture-like TENS.**

guess that TENS with no sensation is a placebo, although this can be overcome. A cursory review of the strongest evidence from systematic reviews demonstrates the difficulty in judging the effectiveness of TENS.

TENS and acute pain

The most recent Cochrane review found evidence to be inconclusive for TENS as sole treatment for acute pain (Walsh et al 2009). A systematic review in the mid-1990s reached a similar conclusion (Reeve et al 1996).

TENS and postoperative pain

Systematic reviews in the 1990s concluded that TENS was not effective in postoperative pain (Carroll et al 1996; Reeve et al 1996), but a meta-analysis of 21 RCTs (1350 patients) with a subgroup analysis of 11 trials (964 patients) (Bjordal et al 2003) found larger reductions in analgesic consumption in RCTs using adequate TENS technique (i.e. a strong stimulation at the site of pain). Respected practitioners disagree about its use in perioperative settings.

TENS and labour pain

The most recent Cochrane review concluded there was limited evidence that TENS reduced pain in established labour (Dowswell et al 2009), although the use of TENS at home in early labour was not assessed. Previous systematic reviews concluded that evidence was conflicting (Reeve et al 1996) or suggested lack of effect (Carroll et al 1997). NICE guidelines (NICE 2007) recommend that TENS should not be offered to women in established labour, although it may be beneficial in the early stages of labour.

TENS and other acute pain conditions

A Cochrane review of seven RCTs (213 patients) concluded that high-frequency but not low-frequency TENS was superior to placebo for dysmenorrhoea when delivered at the site of pain (abdomen), on the lower thoracic spine or on acupuncture points (e.g. bladder 21, bladder 29, spleen 6, stomach 36, gallbladder 34, abdomen CV 4) (Proctor et al 2002). TENS may be beneficial for a wide range of acute pain conditions, including orofacial pain, painful dental procedures, fractured ribs, acute lower back pain and angina pectoris. To date there have been no systematic reviews.

TENS and chronic pain

The most recent Cochrane review (25 RCTs, 1281 participants) concluded that it was not possible to determine the effectiveness of TENS for chronic pain (Nnoaham & Kumbang 2008). Pain relief was superior for TENS compared to an inactive control in 13 of 22 studies, although

variations in TENS techniques and methodological quality made meta-analysis impossible. A systematic review of 32 RCTs on TENS and six studies on percutaneous electrical nerve stimulation (PENS) for chronic musculoskeletal pain (1227 patients) concluded that both were effective for chronic musculoskeletal pain (Johnson & Martinson 2007), although the review was criticized for combining multiple diseases states.

TENS and low back pain

The most recent Cochrane review (4 RCTs, 585 patients) (Khadilkar et al 2008) concluded that evidence for pain relief was conflicting, although there was evidence of no effect on functional status.

NICE (2009) concluded that TENS should not be offered for the early management of persistent non-specific low back pain and the Therapeutics and Technology Assessment Subcommittee of the American Academy of Neurology concluded that TENS should not be recommended for the treatment of chronic low back pain (Level A evidence) (Dubinsky & Miyasaki 2010). These reports have been criticized (Johnson & Walsh 2010). In contrast, guidelines generated by the North American Spine Society state that 'Globally, high- and low-frequency TENS appears to have an immediate impact on pain intensity, with results favoring high-frequency TENS' (Poitras & Brosseau 2008).

TENS for arthritic pain

The most recent Cochrane review on osteoarthritic knee pain (18 RCTs, 813 patients) (Rutjes et al 2009) found evidence to be inconclusive, although the meta-analyses revealed a large standard mean difference of -0.85 $(-1.36, -0.34)$, equating to approximately 20 mm on 100 mm VAS. A meta-analysis of seven RCTs administering TENS at optimal doses found that short-term efficacy for TENS was 22.2 mm (95% CI: 18.1 to 26.3) on a 100-mm VAS (Bjordal et al 2007). NICE (2008) recommends TENS as an adjunct to core treatment for osteoarthritic knee pain relief. A Cochrane review of TENS for rheumatoid arthritis of the hand (3 RCTs, 78 people) concluded that evidence was conflicting (Brosseau et al 2003). NICE (2009) and the Ottawa Panel recommended the use of TENS for short-term pain relief (Ottawa 2004).

Chronic neck pain, chronic headache and cancer pain

The most recent Cochrane review on TENS for neck pain concluded that TENS was more effective than placebo (7 RCTs, 88 patients) (Kroeling et al 2009). A Cochrane review of non-invasive physical agents for chronic recurrent headache (i.e. migraine and tension-type headache) was unable to determine whether electrical stimulation in combination with other modalities was effective (3 RCTs)

(Bronfort et al 2004). A Cochrane review of two small RCTs concluded that there was insufficient available evidence to determine the effectiveness of TENS in treating cancer-related pain (Robb et al 2008). More recently a feasibility study on the use of TENS for cancer-induced bone pain provided preliminary evidence that TENS may be of benefit (Bennett et al 2010).

Part 2: Acupuncture

CONTEXT

Acupuncture is a peripheral nerve stimulation technique that uses fine disposable steel needles inserted into the skin at selected points to relieve a wide variety of pains of any origin (Fig. 14.8). It may be used as a standalone treatment or in combination with pain medication and other non-pharmacological techniques. Acupuncture also has a role in the management of other symptoms, such as nausea and vomiting, respiratory conditions, vasomotor symptoms (e.g. hot flushes), allergies, local skin conditions, xerostomia, dyspnoea, radiation rectitis, ulcers which fail to heal, intractable fatigue and insomnia (Harding et al 2009; White et al 2008b).

Acupuncture can be provided by either a qualified acupuncturist or a healthcare professional with supplementary training. Pain relief is often slower in onset and offset compared with TENS, and the main pain-relieving effects are often obtained after acupuncture needles have been removed. Normally patients receive a course of acupuncture treatment that involves one or more sessions each week for at least a month. Acupuncture is relatively safe, with few reports of serious adverse effects.

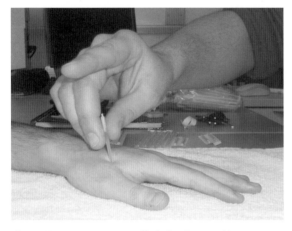

Fig. 14.8 **Acupuncture needle being inserted into LI 4 using a guide tube.**

There is a wealth of evidence to support a neurophysiological basis for acupuncture, for example by inhibiting onward transmission of nociceptive information in the spinal cord. Clinical evidence is often conflicting, however, so despite its widespread use acupuncture continues to be a controversial treatment.

DEFINITION

Acupuncture, derived from the Latin term *acus* ('with a needle') and *pungere* ('to prick'), is the technique of inserting fine disposable steel needles (typically 0.12–0.34 mm in diameter and 7–125 mm long) into the skin at specific points to stimulate skin, nerve, muscle, connective tissue and sometimes periosteum. Stronger stimulation is achieved by manipulating (rotating, flicking or pecking) the needle, heating needles (moxibustion) or passing electrical currents through pairs of needles (electroacupuncture). Alternatively, acupuncture points can be stimulated without needles by using pressure (acupressure), seeds or studs, magnets or low-level laser.

The two main approaches to acupuncture are traditional Chinese medicine (TCM) using oriental clinical reasoning or Western acupuncture using reasoning based on physiology. Most of this chapter will focus on the use of Western medical acupuncture.

Traditional Chinese acupuncture

TCM uses a model of vital energy or qi ('chi') flowing along energy channels (meridians) around the body. Each channel has a series of acupuncture points on or near the surface of the body. Illness is conceptualized as a disturbance in qi. Acupuncture treatment can be seen as normalization of qi and re-balancing of complementary aspects of healthy function referred to as yin and yang. Stimulation of the points achieves de qi (needle sensation), which is often reported as aching, numbness, tingling, heaviness and 'fullness'.

Acupuncture points were named and numbered according to the traditional concept of meridians and this nomenclature is still in use today. Abstract concepts such as qi, yin and yang have fuelled scepticism about acupuncture and the authenticity of traditional diagnosis has been challenged. It is suggested that these concepts might be more understandable for Western clinicians if yin and yang were considered to represent homeostatic mechanisms such as autonomic balance, and qi were taken as a descriptor of bodily functions rather than as a substance.

Western medical acupuncture

Although English medical literature did not reference acupuncture until 150 years ago, it is suspected that acupuncture was practiced as early as the 21st century BC in China. President Nixon's visit to China in 1973 awakened interest in mainstream medicine to the potential use of acupuncture in the West. In 1991 a human body preserved for 5200 years in the Alps revealed widespread arthritis and tattoos corresponding to acupuncture points, suggesting a much longer history of acupuncture use in Europe.

Most western acupuncturists base their diagnosis on an orthodox medical history, examination and reasoning process. They may use a mix of traditional acupuncture points, trigger points and segmental points appropriate to symptoms and pain location. Like TENS, acupuncture is mostly seen as a way of stimulating peripheral nerves, so point selection tends to be based on neuroanatomy. Stimulation is thought to initiate endogenous neuronal and molecular actions, leading to pain relief (see the section on mechanism of action).

Needles are inserted in subcutaneous, intramuscular and periosteal tissues in order to stimulate non-pathological neurones. Needling can activate sensory, motor and autonomic elements of peripheral nerves. The resulting afferent activity is thought to inhibit ongoing nociceptive transmission in the central nervous system via spinal and supraspinal mechanisms (see Chapter 6). To achieve stimulation of the spinal segment which innervates the target tissues, points are selected in dermatomes, myotomes and sclerotomes. Supraspinal points from traditional Chinese acupuncture, trigger points and tender points may be used to increase the effect (Carlsson 2002). Myofascial trigger points (MTPs) may be needled for the relief of local myofascial pain and musculoskeletal problems. Interestingly, the locations of many common trigger points correspond with known acupuncture points. Acupuncture analgesia may be slow in onset but can persist for several days or weeks once the needles have been removed (Sandkühler 2000).

TYPES OF ACUPUNCTURE STIMULATION

Manual stimulation

During manual acupuncture needles are inserted and often manipulated using bi-directional rotation, lifting, thrusting, flicking or 'pecking' to facilitate stimulation. Semipermanent needles are sometimes used to prolong the effects of acupuncture for cancer pain (Filshie & Rubino 2004), dyspnoea and vasomotor symptoms, particularly those associated with cancer treatments (Harding et al 2009). Semi-permanent needles may be applied to the external ear (auricular acupuncture), secured using adhesive tape and left in situ for days. This technique is contraindicated where patients are immunocompromised because of its risk of infection.

Electroacupuncture

Electroacupuncture (EA) uses mild electric currents passed through pairs of needles to generate a strong but nonpainful sensation. EA is used to increase stimulation intensity for intractable pain problems (White 1998). Different brain activation patterns have been found when compared with manual acupuncture and the effects of EA appear to be frequency dependent. Low frequency EA (2–4 Hz) has been found to increase release of enkephalin and cortisol, while high frequency EA (50–200 Hz) increases serotonin (5-HT) and dynorphin (Han 2003). Two common variations of EA are Ryodoraku, a Japanese form of EA which measures skin impedance to aid diagnosis, and percutaneous electrical nerve stimulation (PENS), which may be applied symptomatically over or away from acupuncture points. Finally, EA is different from AL-TENS, which does not involve needles.

Auricular acupuncture

Auricular acupuncture involves needling points on the outer ear, which is thought to have a somatotopic representation of the body. This idea has been challenged, but it may be relevant that the concha of the ear is innervated by the vagus nerve and therefore has a neural link with the viscera. Auricular acupuncture has been used for habitual drug abuse and smoking cessation, although evidence to support effectiveness is not strong (White et al 2006b). Auricular acupuncture may be effective in certain pain conditions, including post-operative pain (Usichenko et al 2008) and cancer pain (Alimi et al 2003). Other microsystems used for acupuncture include the scalp and the hand.

Moxibustion

Moxibustion uses heat to enhance the effect of acupuncture by burning clumps of moxa, made from dried leaves of *Artemisia vulgaris*. No high-quality studies exist for moxibusion as a treatment for pain and there is a risk of burning the skin.

Acupressure

Acupressure is non-invasive, involving applying pressure to acupuncture points, and can be self-administered. Acupressure at PC6 (median nerve) has been shown to be useful for chemotherapy-induced and postoperative nausea and vomiting (Ezzo et al 2006) and for chronic obstructive pulmonary disease (Maa et al 2007). There is limited evidence that acupressure is effective in treating hemiplegic shoulder pain (Shin & Lee 2007), low back pain (Hsieh et al 2006), labour pain (Lee & Ernst 2004) and acute trauma pain (Kober et al 2002).

Laser acupuncture

Laser acupuncture uses a low-level laser (LLL) device to stimulate acupuncture points. LLL therapy is non-invasive and has been shown to modulate biochemical markers of inflammation in a dose-dependent manner when administered at the site of a painful soft tissue injury (Bjordal et al 2006). Studies on laser acupuncture found reductions in peri-articular swelling (Yurtkuran et al 2007), chronic tension-type headache (Ebneshahidi et al 2005) and radicular pain (Kreczi & Klingler 1986).

The remainder of this chapter will discuss manual acupuncture unless otherwise stated.

POINT SELECTION

Western practitioners choose points from innervated regions according to known anatomical structures such as peripheral nerves, dermatomes, myotomes or sclerotomes. Optimal point selection and the depth of needling are achieved through a careful process of trial and error, within safe limits. Distant supraspinal points may be added for their cumulative effect on the response of the central nervous system (Fig. 14.9). Needles may also be placed proximal to the site of nerve damage, above and below affected segments. Contralateral 'mirror' points may be used where acupuncture is locally contraindicated in conditions such as lymphoedema (Filshie & Hester 2006).

The 'surrounding the dragon' technique involves the insertion of needles into areas of normal skin around a local lesion. Its effect relies on the release of neuropeptides via the axon reflex and a consequent increase in blood flow (Carlsson 2002), which may be useful for hyperaesthetic areas or where the skin is broken or infected. MTPs may be needled directly for their local effect.

Patients often report acupuncture needle sensations (de qi) such as heaviness, soreness, dull ache, referred pain, numbness and/or paraesthesia around and radiating from the needle during acupuncture. Deep insertion and rotation of the needle have been shown to generate more intense needle sensations in experimental settings (Benham & Johnson 2009). Claims that acupuncture needle sensations are important indicators of outcome are yet to be confirmed by research.

CLINICAL PRACTICE AND DOSAGE

Needles tend to be left in place from a few seconds to 30 minutes and manipulated intermittently to facilitate stimulation. The onset of pain relief may be delayed by a day or two and occasionally patients experience a temporary exacerbation of pain. Pain relief may outlast needling by several days or weeks and may be cumulative over time, so a typical course could consist of 6–12 treatments once or twice per week. When an acceptable level of pain relief is achieved patients may either require no further treatment or occasional 'top-up' sessions. Acupuncture may be applied in combination with other approaches such as physiotherapy, TENS and medication.

There is a lack of agreement as to what constitutes an adequate dose of acupuncture, and this may depend on what condition is being treated and how the individual responds. A critical review of 47 systematic reviews identified the need for attention to the adequacy of acupuncture technique with respect to the number of needles used, technique, needle sensation, the number of treatment sessions and the experience of the acupuncturist (White et al 2008a). A systematic review which defined an adequate dose of acupuncture and excluded studies that did not meet the dose criteria recommended that acupuncture should be performed at least once per week, using at least four points for at least 20 minutes (Ezzo et al 2000).

CONTRAINDICATIONS AND PRECAUTIONS

Acupuncture is an invasive technique and the use of an informed consent form prior to acupuncture treatment is

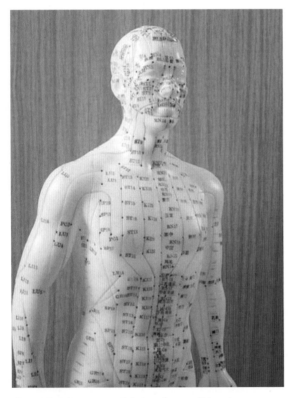

Fig. 14.9 A human model showing traditional acupuncture points.

Box 14.2 **Contraindications to acupuncture**

Contraindications

- patients who are severely immunocompromised
- patients who have a factor 2/prothrombin deficiency
- patients who are on anticoagulants with an unstable INR or who have a clotting disorder such as haemophilia.

Relative contraindications include:

- epilepsy – patients should not be left unattended
- the first trimester of pregnancy – it is advised that strong stimulation is avoided
- extremely thin patients – low body fat can predispose to trauma, particularly over the chest wall, where there is a danger of pneumothorax
- patients with no clear diagnosis – there is a danger of masking symptoms of serious illness and potentially delaying diagnosis.

Absolute contraindications

- Needling over a pregnant uterus must be avoided to prevent damage to the fetus or spontaneous abortion.
- Electroacupuncture is contraindicated for patients with cardiac pacemakers and intracardiac defibrillators.
- Semi-permanent needles are contraindicated for patients with valvular heart disease, neutropenia or after splenectomy because they are a potential source of bacteraemia, which can cause subacute bacterial endocarditis (Filshie & Hester 2006).
- In cancer, acupuncture should not be given where lymphoedema is present because of a hypothetical risk of infection and cellulitis (Filshie & Hester 2006).
- Needling around the spine is contraindicated in patients diagnosed with cancer-related spinal instability because muscle spasm may be acting to protect an unstable spine (Filshie & Hester 2006).

recommended. A medical history and comprehensive assessment is required. Contraindications and precautions must be considered (Box 14.2).

Acupuncture has been shown to be a relatively safe procedure. Serious adverse events such as cardiac tamponade, pneumothorax and fatalities due to needle infection are very rare and likely to be the result of poor standards of practice (MacPherson et al 2001; White et al 2001). Needle pain, tiredness, feeling faint and minor bleeding are more common reactions so acupuncture should be introduced cautiously at first. Frail patients or those who cannot tolerate certain positions (e.g. lying flat) may be accommodated by adopting supported sitting or half-lying positions. When removal of clothes is painful or difficult, peripheral points may be used.

Some patients react strongly to acupuncture, resulting in extremes of emotion, an exacerbation of symptoms, dizziness, fainting and, in rare cases, epileptic fits. People who are hypersensitive to sensory stimulation (e.g. those with neuropathic pain, cancer, or people who are very ticklish!) may react strongly, so gentle stimulation using finer gauge needles and avoidance of tender areas or naturally sensitive points such as LI 4 is recommended in the first instance, along with close supervision. So-called *strong reactors* are often good responders, even with minimal stimulation (White et al 2008b).

Finally, there is a potential risk that some patients with incurable conditions such as cancer or arthritis may be looking at acupuncture as a *cure*, so practitioners must encourage patients to continue with prescribed medication and give them realistic advice.

MECHANISM OF ACTION

Evidence for meridians is not convincing, although physiological correlates of some meridians have been reported, such as electrical conductive properties and intermuscular or intramuscular connective tissue planes. A systematic review of 18 studies examining the electrical properties of acupuncture points and meridians concluded that evidence did not support claims that acupuncture points have lower electrical impedance (Ahn et al 2008). However, there may be an association between acupuncture points and MTPs, tendino-muscular and tendino-fascial structures, and nerve bundles (Langevin et al 2007). Most Western practitioners subscribe to a neurophysiological mechanism for acupuncture with actions at peripheral, spinal and supraspinal sites (Fig. 14.10). Specific patterns of brain activity have been found at different acupuncture points, with different durations of stimulation and with sham needling. There is also evidence of a somatotopic representation of acupuncture points in the primary somatosensory cortex.

Peripheral mechanisms

Studies using mice have demonstrated mechanical transduction with manual needle stimulation (Langevin et al 2006). Acupuncture activates polymodal receptors and/or their afferents, and this inhibits onward transmission of nociceptive information in the central nervous system (White 1998). Acupuncture also affects autonomic nervous system activity and generates an immediate and strong local sympathetic response (Sandberg et al 2003). An axon reflex occurs with the release of neuropeptides, notably calcitonin gene-related peptide (CGRP), nerve growth factor (NGF) and neuropeptide Y, resulting in vasodilatation and increased microcirculation. This effect is greater when the needle is advanced beyond the surface of the skin into the underlying muscle (Sandberg et al 2003). Erythema and local fluid exudation may be the result of a local neurogenic inflammatory

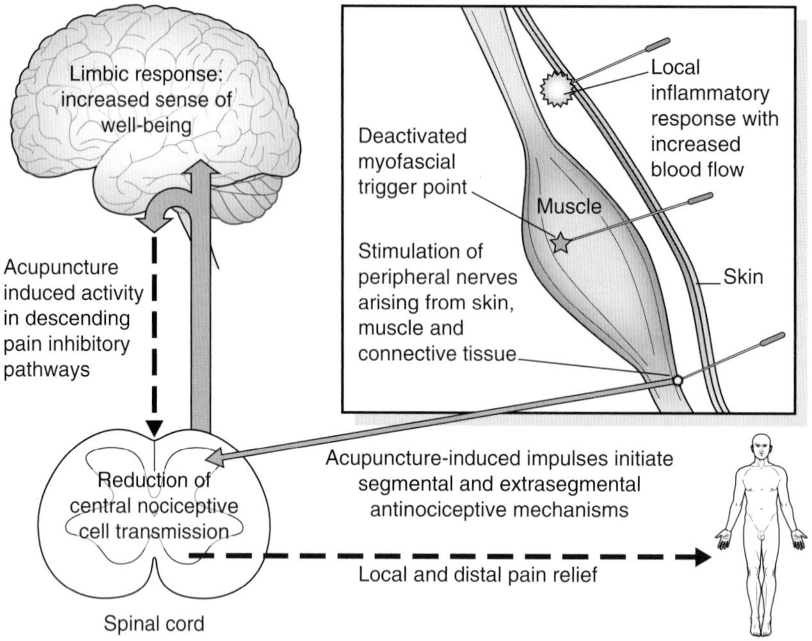

Fig. 14.10 **An overview of the mechanism of action of manual acupuncture.**

reaction caused by the needle (Carlsson 2002). Acupuncture also deactivates MTPs, possibly due to mechanical disruption of the MTP.

Spinal mechanisms

Segmental pain relief is achieved by needling points within the same spinal segment as the origin of the pain. Adjacent segments may also be effective because of overlap of spinal afferents at all levels of the spinal cord. Acupuncture activates small-diameter afferents (Aδ) and activity in these fibres has been shown to inhibit central nociceptive cells for a few hours post-stimulation (Sandkühler et al 1997). Moreover, post-stimulation inhibition of central nociceptive transmission cells occurs during stimulation of connective tissue when compared with skin, and during low-frequency acupuncture and EA (Langevin et al 2007; Sandkühler et al 1997).

Supraspinal mechanisms

Descending pain inhibitory pathways (e.g. ventromedial medulla and periaqueductal grey (PAG)) become active during acupuncture and the subsequent release of neurochemicals inhibits central nociceptive cell transmission (Carlsson 2002). Stimulation of small-diameter myelinated afferents in skin and muscle results in excitation of spinal interneurons and descending pain inhibitory

pathways, and the release of a multitude of endogenous neurochemicals, including opioids, serotonin, noradrenalin, adrenocorticotrophic hormone, cholecystokinin, nerve growth factor and oxytocin in the spinal cord. These neuromodulators reduce activity and sensitization of nociceptive-specific (NS) and wide-dynamic range (WDR) neurones in the central nervous system (see Chapter 6). Prolonged pain relief of many days following acupuncture may be due in part to a positive feedback loop in the mesolimbic system resulting in continuous outflow from descending inhibitory pathways (Han & Xuan 1986). Regular acupuncture enhances gene expression and increased manufacture and storage of opioid peptides (Guo et al 2004). This effect may be frequency dependent as low-frequency EA expresses preproenkephalin mRNA, while high-frequency EA expresses preprodynorphin mRNA. Top-ups of acupuncture may act to maintain gene expression in a 'switched on' mode (Guo et al 1996).

Acupuncture may also be viewed as a counter-irritant which is known to produce widespread reduction in pain via diffuse noxious inhibitory controls (DNIC; see Chapter 6). The required strong stimulus may cause discomfort and may be responsible for painful components of needle sensation (Benham & Johnson 2009). DNIC may explain why strong needle stimulation can be applied anywhere on the body to produce an analgesic effect.

Brain-imaging studies suggest that acupuncture affects brain activity differently in normal and inflammatory states, and in pain patients compared with healthy controls. Acupuncture affects a matrix of brain structures, including systems involved in emotion and reward such as the anterior cingulate, hippocampus, insula, amygdala and nucleus accumbens (Chen et al 2006). This may account for the pleasurable feelings associated with acupuncture and reports from some patients that acupuncture makes pain less unpleasant.

CLINICAL EFFECTIVENESS

Acupuncture for painful conditions

Clinical experience suggests that acupuncture may be beneficial for many types of pain. It can offer options for patients who have not responded to other treatments, are resistant to high-dosage pain medication, experience unacceptable levels of side effects associated with pain medication or require adjunctive treatment alongside conventional analgesia.

There are many RCTs and systematic reviews, consequently making sense of clinical research evidence has become a discipline in itself. Evidence-based guidelines often disagree on whether acupuncture should be offered as a treatment. The Centre for Reviews and Dissemination in the UK has suggested that there is sufficient evidence to justify the use of acupuncture in chronic pain, but only as a second- or third-line treatment. The UK institute NICE recommends the use of acupuncture for non-specific low back pain based on the available evidence but not for osteoarthritis of the knees, despite a similar evidence base (NICE 2009).

A systematic review of systematic reviews concluded that there was no robust evidence for acupuncture for any condition (Derry et al 2006), although a high-quality critique concluded that acupuncture improves symptoms associated with nausea and vomiting (postoperative and chemotherapy-related), insomnia, fibromyalgia, osteoarthritis of the knee, non-specific back pain, dental pain, epicondylitis and idiopathic headache (Ernst 2006). It was acknowledged, however, that inadequate control of placebo effects could have resulted in false-positive data for these conditions. Various other shortcomings of existing studies have been noted (White et al 2008a).

The difficulties in interpreting existing evidence were highlighted in two meta-analyses on osteoarthritis of the knee published 6 months apart. White et al (2007) concluded that 'acupuncture that meets criteria for adequate treatment is significantly superior to sham acupuncture and to no additional intervention in improving pain and function in patients with chronic knee pain', whereas Manheimer et al (2007) concluded that 'sham-controlled trials show clinically irrelevant short-term benefits of acupuncture for treating knee osteoarthritis'.

Systematic reviews evaluating acupuncture are mixed. Reviewers indicate positive findings for pain relief in chronic low back pain (Furlan et al 2005), chronic knee pain, including knee osteoarthritis (Manheimer et al 2007, White et al 2006a), peripheral joint osteoarthritis (Kwon et al 2006) and postoperative pain (Usichenko et al 2008). Evidence is inconclusive for mixed populations of chronic pain (Ezzo 2000), shoulder pain (Green et al 2005) and cancer-related pain (Lee et al 2005). In general, systematic reviews support the use of acupuncture for pain relief over and above no treatment. Evidence that acupuncture is superior to sham is less conclusive, but the concept of sham needling is called into question because of the lack of clarity over the exact nature of acupuncture points and the existence of DNIC. The failure of many studies to address the problem of dose adequacy weakens the research findings (White et al 2008a). Many studies are under-powered and lack methodological rigour, and there is often a high degree of heterogeneity between studies.

CONCLUSION

There is an ongoing debate about the effectiveness of TENS and acupuncture because evidence from RCTs is conflicting or inconclusive. There is little consensus in guidelines for the use of TENS or acupuncture for painful conditions, causing much confusion in policy development and clinical practice. This could impact negatively on patient care TENS and acupuncture are relatively inexpensive, safe and readily accessible, and both modalities are supported by strong evidence from electrophysiological studies and clinical experience. TENS and acupuncture should therefore be considered as treatment options until sufficient gold standard clinical research concludes otherwise.

Q | **Self-test questions**

1. List the contraindications and relative contraindications for TENS and acupuncture.
2. Identify and prioritize the risks that patients face when using TENS and provide simple patient advice to manage these risks.
3. Outline to a patient with non-specific low back pain how to administer TENS at home and what they should expect in terms of pain relief.
4. List three major differences between traditional Chinese and Western style acupuncture.
5. Describe, briefly, the main physiological mechanisms by which TENS and acupuncture relieve pain.
6. List reasons why clinical research on TENS and acupuncture is still not conclusive.

REFERENCES

Ahn, A.C., Colbert, A.P., Anderson, B.J., et al., 2008. Electrical properties of acupuncture points and meridians: a systematic review. Bioelectromagnetics 29, 245–256.

Alimi, D., Rubino, C., Pichard-Leandri, E., et al., 2003. Analgesic effect of auricular acupuncture for cancer pain: a randomized, blinded, controlled trial. J. Clin. Oncol. 21, 4120–4126.

Alon, G., Kantor, G., Ho, H.S., 1994. Effects of electrode size on basic excitatory responses and on selected stimulus parameters. J. Orthop. Sports Phys. Ther. 20, 29–35. Online. Available at: http://www.biomednet.com/db/medline/94362725.

Asbjorn, O., 2000. Treatment of Tennis Elbow with Transcutaneous Nerve Stimulation (TNS). Online. Available at: http://www.paingone.com/.

Benham, A., Johnson, M.I., 2009. Could acupuncture needle sensation be a predictor of analgesic response? Acupunct. Med. 27, 65–67.

Bennett, M.I., Johnson, M.I., Brown, S.R., et al., 2010. Feasibility study of transcutaneous electrical nerve stimulation (TENS) for cancer bone pain. J. Pain 11 (4), 351–359.

Bjordal, J.M., Johnson, M.I., Ljunggreen, A.E., 2003. Transcutaneous electrical nerve stimulation (TENS) can reduce postoperative analgesic consumption. A meta-analysis with assessment of optimal treatment parameters for postoperative pain. Eur. J. Pain 7, 181–188.

Bjordal, J.M., Johnson, M.I., Iversen, V., et al., 2006. Photoradiation in acute pain: a systematic review of possible mechanisms of action and clinical effects in randomized placebo-controlled trials. Photomed. Laser Surg. 24, 158–168.

Bjordal, J.M., Johnson, M.I., Lopes-Martins, R.A., et al., 2007. Short-term efficacy of physical interventions in osteoarthritic knee pain. A systematic review and meta-analysis of randomised placebo-controlled trials. BMC Musculoskelet. Disord. 8, 51.

Blum, K., Chen, A.L., Chen, T.J., et al., 2008. The H-Wave device is an effective and safe non-pharmacological analgesic for chronic pain: a meta-analysis. Adv. Ther. 25, 644–657.

Bronfort, G., Nilsson, N., Haas, M., et al., 2004. Non-invasive physical treatments for chronic/recurrent headache. Cochrane Database Syst. Rev. CD001878.

Brosseau, L., Judd, M.G., Marchand, S., et al., 2003. Transcutaneous electrical nerve stimulation (TENS) for the treatment of rheumatoid arthritis in the hand. Cochrane Database Syst. Rev. CD004377.

Bundsen, P., Ericson, K., 1982. Pain relief in labor by transcutaneous electrical nerve stimulation. Safety aspects. Acta Obstet. Gynecol. Scand. 61, 1–5.

Carlsson, C., 2002. Acupuncture mechanisms for clinically relevant long-term effects – reconsideration and a hypothesis. Acupunct. Med. 20, 82–99.

Carroll, D., Tramer, M., McQuay, H., et al., 1996. Randomization is important in studies with pain outcomes: systematic review of transcutaneous electrical nerve stimulation in acute postoperative pain. Br. J. Anaesth. 77, 798–803.

Carroll, D., Tramer, M., McQuay, H., et al., 1997. Transcutaneous electrical nerve stimulation in labour pain: a systematic review. Br. J. Obstet. Gynaecol. 104, 169–175.

Chen, C.C., Johnson, M.I., 2009. An investigation into the effects of frequency-modulated transcutaneous electrical nerve stimulation (TENS) on experimentally-induced pressure pain in healthy human participants. J. Pain 10, 1029–1037.

Chen, C.C., Johnson, M.I., 2010. An investigation into the hypoalgesic effects of high- and low-frequency transcutaneous electrical nerve stimulation (TENS) on experimentally-induced blunt pressure pain in healthy human participants. J. Pain 11, 53–61.

Chen, A.C., Liu, F.J., Wang, L., et al., 2006. Mode and site of acupuncture modulation in the human brain: 3D (124-ch) EEG power spectrum mapping and source imaging. Neuroimage 29, 1080–1091.

Chen, C., Tabasam, G., Johnson, M., 2008. Does the pulse frequency of Transcutaneous Electrical Nerve Stimulation (TENS) influence hypoalgesia? A systematic review of studies using experimental pain and healthy human participants. Physiotherapy 94, 11–20.

Davies, H.T., Crombie, I.K., Brown, J.H., et al., 1997. Diminishing returns or appropriate treatment strategy? An analysis of short-term outcomes after pain clinic treatment. Pain 70, 203–208. Online. Available at: http://www.biomednet.com/db/medline/97294538.

Derry, C.J., Derry, S., McQuay, H.J., et al., 2006. Systematic review of systematic reviews of acupuncture published 1996–2005. Clin. Med. 6, 381–386.

Desantana, J.M., Santana-Filho, V.J., Guerra, D.R., et al., 2008a. Hypoalgesic effect of the transcutaneous electrical nerve stimulation following inguinal herniorrhaphy: a randomized, controlled trial. J. Pain 9, 623–629.

Desantana, J.M., Walsh, D.M., Vance, C., et al., 2008b. Effectiveness of transcutaneous electrical nerve stimulation for treatment of hyperalgesia and pain. Curr. Rheumatol. Rep. 10, 492–499.

Desantana, J.M., Da Silva, L.F., De Resende, M.A., et al., 2009. Transcutaneous electrical nerve stimulation at both high and low frequencies activates ventrolateral periaqueductal grey to decrease mechanical hyperalgesia in arthritic rats. Neuroscience 163 (4), 1233–1241.

Dowswell, T., Bedwell, C., Lavender, T., et al., 2009. Transcutaneous electrical nerve stimulation (TENS) for pain relief in labour. Cochrane Database Syst. Rev. CD007214.

Dubinsky, R.M., Miyasaki, J., 2010. Assessment: efficacy of transcutaneous electric nerve stimulation in the treatment of pain in neurologic disorders (an evidence-based review): report of the Therapeutics and Technology Assessment Subcommittee of the American Academy of Neurology. Neurology 74, 173–176.

Ebneshahidi, N.S., Heshmatipour, M., Moghaddami, A., et al., 2005. The effects of laser acupuncture on chronic tension headache – a randomised controlled trial. Acupunct. Med. 23, 13–18.

Eriksson, M., Sjölund, B., 1976. Acupuncture-like electroanalgesia in TNS resistant chronic pain. In: Zotterman, Y. (Ed.), Sensory functions of the skin. Pergamon Press, Oxford/New York.

Ernst, E., 2006. Acupuncture – a critical analysis. J. Intern. Med. 259, 125–137.

Ezzo, J., 2000. Is acupuncture effective for the treatment of chronic pain: a systematic review. Pain 86, 217–225.

Ezzo, J., Berman, B., Hadhazy, V.A., et al., 2000. Is acupuncture effective for the treatment of chronic pain? A systematic review. Pain 86, 217–225.

Ezzo, J.M., Richardson, M.A., Vickers, A., et al., 2006. Acupuncture-point stimulation for chemotherapy-induced nausea or vomiting. Cochrane Database Syst. Rev. CD002285.

Filshie, J., Hester, J., 2006. Guidelines for providing acupuncture treatment for cancer patients – a peer-reviewed sample policy document. Acupunct. Med. 24, 172–182.

Filshie, J., Rubino, C., 2004. Promising results of auriculoacupuncture in the treatment of cancer pain. Focus on Alternative & Complementary Therapies 9, 132–133.

Ford, K.S., Shrader, M.W., Smith, J., et al., 2005. Full-thickness burn formation after the use of electrical stimulation for rehabilitation of unicompartmental knee arthroplasty. J. Arthroplasty 20, 950–953.

Furlan, A.D., van Tulder, M., Cherkin, D., et al., 2005. Acupuncture and dry-needling for low back pain: an updated systematic review within the framework of the cochrane collaboration. Spine 30, 944–963.

Gorodetskyi, I.G., Gorodnichenko, A.I., Tursin, P.S., et al., 2007. Non-invasive interactive neurostimulation in the post-operative recovery of patients with a trochanteric fracture of the femur. A randomised, controlled trial. J. Bone Joint Surg. Br. 89, 1488–1494.

Green, S., Buchbinder, R., Hetrick, S., 2005. Acupuncture for shoulder pain. Cochrane Database Syst. Rev. CD005319.

Guo, H.F., Tian, J., Wang, X., et al., 1996. Brain substrates activated by electroacupuncture of different frequencies (I): Comparative study on the expression of oncogene, c-fos and genes coding for three opioid peptides. Brain Res. Mol. Brain Res. 43, 157–166.

Guo, Z.L., Moazzami, A.R., Longhurst, J.C., 2004. Electroacupuncture induces c-Fos expression in the rostral ventrolateral medulla and periaqueductal gray in cats: relation to opioid containing neurons. Brain Res. 1030, 103–115.

Han, J.S., 2003. Acupuncture: neuropeptide release produced by electrical stimulation of different frequencies. Trends Neurosci. 26, 17–22.

Han, J.S., Xuan, Y.T., 1986. A mesolimbic neuronal loop of analgesia: I. Activation by morphine of a serotonergic pathway from periaqueductal gray to nucleus accumbens. Int. J. Neurosci. 29, 109–117.

Harding, C., Harris, A., Chadwick, D., 2009. Auricular acupuncture: a novel treatment for vasomotor symptoms associated with luteinizing-hormone releasing hormone agonist treatment for prostate cancer. BJU Int. 103, 186–190.

Herman, E., Williams, R., Stratford, P., et al., 1994. A randomized controlled trial of transcutaneous electrical nerve stimulation (CODETRON) to determine its benefits in a rehabilitation program for acute occupational low back pain. Spine 19, 561–568.

Hingne, P.M., Sluka, K.A., 2008. Blockade of NMDA receptors prevents analgesic tolerance to repeated transcutaneous electrical nerve stimulation (TENS) in rats. J. Pain 9, 217–225.

Holmgren, C., Carlsson, T., Mannheimer, C., et al., 2008. Risk of interference from transcutaneous electrical nerve stimulation on the sensing function of implantable defibrillators. Pacing Clin. Electrophysiol. 31, 151–158.

Hsieh, L.L.C., Kuo, C.H., Lee, L.H., et al., 2006. Treatment of low back pain by acupressure and physical therapy: randomised controlled trial. Br. Med. J. 332, 696–700.

Ivanova-Stoilova, T., Howells, D., 2002. The usefulness of PainGone pain killing pen for self-treatment of chronic musculoskeletal pain - a pilot study. The Pain Society. Annual Scientific Meeting, Bournemouth UK.

Johnson, M., 1998. The analgesic effects and clinical use of Acupuncture-like TENS (AL-TENS). Phys. Ther. Rev. 3, 73–93.

Johnson, M., 2008. Transcutaneous electrical nerve stimulation. In: Watson, T. (Ed.), Electrotherapy: Evidence Based Practice. Churchill Livingstone, Edinburgh, pp. 253–296.

Johnson, M., Martinson, M., 2007. Efficacy of electrical nerve stimulation for chronic musculoskeletal pain: a meta-analysis of randomized controlled trials. Pain 130, 157–165.

Johnson, M., Walsh, D., 2010. Pain: continued uncertainty of TENS effectiveness for pain relief. Nature Reviews Rheumatology 6, 314–316.

Kalra, A., Urban, M.O., Sluka, K.A., 2001. Blockade of opioid receptors in rostral ventral medulla prevents antihyperalgesia produced by transcutaneous electrical nerve stimulation (TENS). J. Pharmacol. Exp. Ther. 298, 257–263.

Khadilkar, A., Odebiyi, D.O., Brosseau, L., et al., 2008. Transcutaneous electrical nerve stimulation (TENS) versus placebo for chronic low-back pain. Cochrane Database Syst. Rev. CD003008.

Kober, A., Scheck, T., Greher, M., et al., 2002. Prehospital analgesia with acupressure in victims of minor trauma: a prospective, randomized, double-blinded trial. Anesth. Analg. 95, 723–727table of contents.

Koopman, J.S., Vrinten, D.H., Van Wijck, A.J., 2009. Efficacy of microcurrent therapy in the treatment of chronic nonspecific back pain: a pilot study. Clin. J. Pain 25, 495–499.

Kreczi, T., Klingler, D., 1986. A comparison of laser acupuncture versus placebo in radicular and pseudoradicular pain syndromes as recorded by subjective responses of patients. Acupuncture and Electrotherapy Research 11, 207–216.

Kroeling, P., Gross, A., Goldsmith, C.H., et al., 2009. Electrotherapy for neck pain. Cochrane Database Syst. Rev. CD004251.

Kwon, Y.D., Pittler, M.H., Ernst, E., 2006. Acupuncture for peripheral joint osteoarthritis: A systematic review and meta-analysis. Rheumatology (Oxford) 45, 1331–1337.

Langevin, H.M., Storch, K.N., Cipolla, M.J., et al., 2006. Fibroblast spreading induced by connective tissue stretch involves intracellular redistribution of alpha- and beta-actin. Histochem. Cell Biol. 125, 487–495.

Langevin, H.M., Bouffard, N.A., Churchill, D.L., et al., 2007. Connective tissue fibroblast response to acupuncture: dose-dependent effect of bidirectional needle rotation. J. Altern. Complement. Med. 13, 355–360.

Lazarou, L., Kitsios, A., Lazarou, I., et al., 2009. Effects of intensity of transcutaneous electrical nerve stimulation (TENS) on pressure pain threshold and blood pressure in healthy humans: a randomized, double-blind, placebo-controlled trial. Clin. J. Pain 25, 773–780.

Lee, H., Ernst, E., 2004. Acupuncture for labor pain management: A systematic review. Am. J. Obstet. Gynaecol. 191, 1573–1579.

Lee, H., Schmidt, K., Ernst, E., 2005. Acupuncture for the relief of cancer-related pain – a systematic review. Eur. J. Pain 9, 437–444.

Limoge, A., Dixmerias-Iskandar, F., 2004. A personal experience using Limoge's current during a major surgery. Anesth. Analg. 99, 309.

Limoge, A., Robert, C., Stanley, T.H., 1999. Transcutaneous cranial electrical stimulation (TCES): a review 1998. Neurosci. Biobehav. Rev. 23, 529–538.

Maa, S.H., Tsou, T.S., Wang, K.Y., et al., 2007. Self-administered acupressure reduces the symptoms that limit daily activities in bronchiectasis patients: pilot study findings. J. Clin. Nurs. 16, 794–804.

MacPherson, H., Thomas, K., Walters, S., et al., 2001. The York acupuncture safety study: prospective survey of 34 000 treatments by traditional acupuncturists. Br. Med. J. 323, 486–487.

Manheimer, E., Linde, K., Lao, L., et al., 2007. Meta-analysis: acupuncture for osteoarthritis of the knee. Ann. Intern. Med. 146, 868–877.

Mann, C., 1996. Respiratory compromise: a rare complication of transcutaneous electrical nerve stimulation for angina pectoris. J. Accid. Emerg. Med. 13, 68.

Morton, C., Du, H., Xiao, H., et al., 1988. Inhibition of nociceptive responses of lumbar dorsal horn neurones by remote noxious afferent stimulation in the cat. Pain 34, 75–83.

NICE, 2007. Intrapartum care: care of healthy women and their babies during childbirth. NICE clinical guideline 55. National Institute for Health and Clinical Excellence, London.

NICE, 2009. Early management of persistent non-specific low back pain. NICE clinical guideline 88. National Institute for Health and Clinical Excellence, London.

Nnoaham, K.E., Kumbang, J., 2008. Transcutaneous electrical nerve stimulation (TENS) for chronic pain. Cochrane Database Syst. Rev. CD003222.

Odendaal, C., Joubert, G., 1999. APS therapy - a new way of treating chronic headache - a pilot study. S. Afr. J. Anaesthesiol. Analg. 5, 1–3.

Olyaei, G.R., Talebian, S., Hadian, M.R., et al., 2004. The effect of transcutaneous electrical nerve stimulation on sympathetic skin response. Electromyogr. Clin. Neurophysiol. 44, 23–28.

Ottawa, P., 2004. Ottawa Panel evidence-based clinical practice guidelines for electrotherapy and thermotherapy interventions in the management of rheumatoid arthritis in adults. Phys. Ther. 84, 1016–1043.

Palmer, S., Cramp, F., Propert, K., et al., 2009. Transcutaneous electrical nerve stimulation and transcutaneous spinal electroanalgesia: a preliminary efficacy and mechanisms-based investigation. Physiotherapy 95, 185–191.

Palmer, S., Martin, D., 2008. Interferential current. In: Watson, T. (Ed.), Electrotherapy. Evidence-Based Practice, 12th ed. Churchill Livingstone Elsevier, Edinburgh.

Poitras, S., Brosseau, L., 2008. Evidence-informed management of chronic low back pain with transcutaneous electrical nerve stimulation, interferential current, electrical muscle stimulation, ultrasound,

and thermotherapy. Spine J. 8, 226–233.

Pomeranz, B., Niznick, G., 1987. Codetron, a new electrotherapy device overcomes the habituation problems of conventional TENS devices. American Journal of Electromedicine. 1, 22–26.

Proctor, M.L., Smith, C.A., Farquhar, C.M., et al., 2002. Transcutaneous electrical nerve stimulation and acupuncture for primary dysmenorrhoea. Cochrane Database Syst. Rev. CD002123.

Reeve, J., Menon, D., Corabian, P., 1996. Transcutaneous electrical nerve stimulation (TENS): a technology assessment. Int. J. Technol. Assess. Health Care 12, 299–324. Online. Available at: http://research.bmn.com/medline/search/results?uid=MDLN.96293007.

Reeves 2nd, J.L., Graff-Radford, S.B., Shipman, D., 2004. The effects of transcutaneous electrical nerve stimulation on experimental pain and sympathetic nervous system response. Pain Med. 5, 150–161.

Robb, K.A., Bennett, M.I., Johnson, M.I., et al., 2008. Transcutaneous electric nerve stimulation (TENS) for cancer pain in adults. Cochrane Database Syst. Rev. CD006276.

Rosted, P., 2001. Recurring epileptic seizures – a possible side effect of transcutaneous electric nerve stimulation. Ugeskr. Laeger 163, 2492–2493. Online. Available at: http://research.bmn.com/medline/search/results?uid=MDLN.21271413.

Rutjes, A.W., Nuesch, E., Sterchi, R., et al., 2009. Transcutaneous electrostimulation for osteoarthritis of the knee. Cochrane Database Syst. Rev. CD002823.

Sandberg, M., Lundeberg, T., Lindberg, L.G., et al., 2003. Effects of acupuncture on skin and muscle blood flow in healthy subjects. Eur. J. Appl. Physiol. Occup. Physiol. 90, 114–119.

Sandkühler, J., 2000. Long-lasting analgesia following TENS and acupuncture: Spinal mechanisms beyond gate control. In: Devor, M., Rowbotham, M.C., Wiesenfeld-Hallin, Z. (Eds.), Progress In Pain Research And Management. IASP Press, Seattle.

Sandkühler, J., Chen, J.G., Cheng, G., 1997. Low-frequency stimulation of afferent A-delta fibers induces long-term depression at primary afferent synapses with substantia gelatinosa neurons in the rat. J. Neurosci. 17, 6483–6491.

Satter, E.K., 2008. Third-degree burns incurred as a result of interferential current therapy. Am. J. Dermatopathol. 30, 281–283.

Shin, B.C., Lee, M.S., 2007. Effects of aromatherapy acupressure on hemiplegic shoulder pain and motor power in stroke patients: a pilot study. J. Altern. Complementary Med. 13, 247–251.

Tan, G., Rintala, D.H., Thornby, J.I., et al., 2006. Using cranial electrotherapy stimulation to treat pain associated with spinal cord injury. J. Rehabil. Res. Dev. 43, 461–474.

Usichenko, T.I., Ch, L., Ernst, E., 2008. Auricular acupuncture for postoperative pain control: a systematic review of randomised clinical trials. Anaesthesia 63, 1343–1348.

Walsh, D.M., Lowe, A.S., McCormack, K., et al., 1998. Transcutaneous electrical nerve stimulation: effect on peripheral nerve conduction, mechanical pain threshold, and tactile threshold in humans. Arch. Phys. Med. Rehabil. 79, 1051–1058.

Walsh, D., Howe, T., Johnson, M., et al., 2009. Transcutaneous electrical nerve stimulation for acute pain. Cochrane Database Syst. Rev. 138, 1–72.

White, A., 1998. Electroacupuncture and acupuncture analgesia. In: Filshie, J., White, A. (Eds.), Medical Acupuncture. A Western Scientific Approach. Churchill Livingstone, Edinburgh.

White, A., Hayhoe, S., Hart, A., et al., 2001. Survey of adverse events following acupuncture (SAFA): a prospective study of 32,000 consultations. Acupunct. Med. 19, 84–92.

White, A., Foster, N., Cummings, M., et al., 2006a. The effectiveness of acupuncture for osteoarthritis of the knee – a systematic review. Acupunct. Med. 24 (Suppl), S40–S48.

White, A.R., Rampes, H., Campbell, J.L., 2006. Acupuncture and related interventions for smoking cessation. Cochrane Database Syst. Rev. CD000009.

White, A., Foster, N.E., Cummings, M., et al., 2007. Acupuncture treatment for chronic knee pain: a systematic review. Rheumatology 46, 384–390.

White, A., Cummings, M., Barlas, P., et al., 2008a. Defining an adequate dose of acupuncture using a neurophysiological approach – a narrative review of the literature. Acupunct. Med. 26, 111–120.

White, A., Cummings, M., Filshie, J., 2008b. An Introduction to Western Medical Acupuncture. Churchill Livingstone Elsevier, Edinburgh.

Yurtkuran, M., Alp, A., Konur, S., et al., 2007. Laser acupuncture in knee osteoarthritis: a double-blind, randomized controlled study. Photomed. Laser Surg. 25, 14–20.

Chapter | 15 |

Complementary therapy approaches to pain

Peter A. Mackereth, Ann Carter and Jacqui Stringer

LEARNING OBJECTIVES

The objectives of this chapter are:

1. To develop the reader's understanding of the role and limitations of complementary therapies in pain management.
2. To consider the evidence base for specific complementary therapies interventions for patients living with pain.
3. To explore key practical and professional issues in the integration of complementary therapies within clinical practice.
4. To identify possible sources of information and guidance to help increase the reader's knowledge and awareness of this area of work.

OVERVIEW

The aim of this chapter is to give the reader a clear understanding of how complementary therapies can be a useful addition to the supportive care of a patient in pain. Health professionals, like the general population, may turn to complementary and alternative medicine (CAM) therapies as a means of alleviating pain where conventional medical approaches appear to have failed. Equally, patients and their carers often ask for advice and information regarding the appropriateness of CAM therapies for pain relief. Additionally, clinical staff are taking the initiative, ranging from training in 'simple to use' techniques through coordinating CAM services for patients, to taking a lead in clinical research work. This chapter is not intended as a definitive guide to pain management using CAM; rather the aim is to review the evidence base and theoretical perspectives, and to provide some examples and case studies illustrating good clinical practice. The context for the work reflects the authors' clinical practice, namely cancer care and long-term health conditions. Additionally, emphasis is on how pain is perceived and influenced by broader considerations, for

© 2014 Elsevier Ltd.

example patient anxiety, the therapeutic relationship and expectations of patients and carers.

POPULARITY OF COMPLEMENTARY AND ALTERNATIVE MEDICINE

CAM is used globally, with different practices reflecting local cultural health beliefs and values. Internationally, training varies enormously from skills passed on amongst communities to formalized accredited programmes within colleges and university settings. The attitudes of the medical establishment are changing from dismissal of CAM to demands for greater regulation and evidence of safety and efficacy to support further integration. Surveys conducted in the UK and Australia indicate that 25–50% of the general population use CAM on a regular basis, often at their own expense (Ernst & White 2000; Thomas et al 2001). Complementary therapies popular with patients in the UK include aromatherapy, massage, medical acupuncture (discussed in Chapter 14), reflexology, creative imagery and relaxation; these lend themselves to greater integration within mainstream health care. Alternative disciplines, such as herbal medicines, homeopathy, traditional Chinese medicine, reiki and spiritual healing, are more common in private practice settings, with some limited access in publically funded healthcare services. This chapter focuses on the use of complementary therapies (CTs).

The term 'complementary' encompasses a wide range of treatments and products. National guidelines for the use of CTs in supportive and palliative care uses the term to broadly describe therapies used alongside conventional health care (Tavares 2003). Stone (2001) suggests that in both the UK and the USA there has been a significant shift towards 'integrated or integrative health care' (p. 55) and greater tolerance towards the inclusion of CTs within private and public healthcare services. The Foundation of Integrated Medicine's discussion document on integrated healthcare (Foundation for Integrated Medicine 1997), established by HRH the Prince of Wales, examined practical ways in which conventional and complementary therapists could develop a working partnership. Over a decade later, challenges with funding and the building of an evidence base still continue to be issues for this integrative movement that prevent widespread provision of CTs to patients within the NHS. Pockets of good practice do exist, although these are often highly dependent on committed practitioners, support from clinical champions and access to charitable funds.

Resistance to greater integration of CTs comes from conventional practitioners who question their efficacy and validity, particularly where there is a cost to the service provider and/or the patient. Because of the term 'CAM', CTs are often linked to the use of 'alternative' therapies by patients and concerns that they will abandon

recommended (and evidence-based) conventional medicine, with potential consequences for disease progression and/or other harmful consequences. Cassileth et al (2001) suggest that 'alternative therapies' may be defined as unproven treatments promoted to treat the disease itself, whereas 'complementary therapies' represent adjunctive therapies aimed at symptom management and enhancement of quality of life. Swisher et al (2002) claim that most patients who use alternative therapies do so in conjunction with standard medical therapy, with only a small minority choosing alternative therapy to the exclusion of standard medical treatment. The recommendations and therapeutic practices discussed in this chapter focus on the best of CTs working in conjunction with high-quality conventional medicine, equally *alternative therapies are NOT recommended as curative modalities by the authors.* Importantly, it is advised that within practice settings the CTs used with patients and carers are:

1. delivered by appropriately trained, supervised and insured practitioners
2. adapted skilfully for the individual, who is informed and has consented for the intervention offered
3. provided by practitioners who work in collaboration with conventional health professionals to deliver high-quality, accountable and evaluated care
4. most importantly: when there any concerns about safety or risks of harm to the patient, the interventions are not offered.

REASONS FOR USING CTs

When reviewing the literature, multiple reasons are given for the tremendous use of CTs amongst patients who have cancer and long-term conditions. Cassileth (1998) suggests that CAM is used for a variety of reasons ranging from supporting patients' psychological needs to dissatisfaction with the medical system and/or the nature of the relationship with the physician. Coss et al (1998) undertook a telephone survey of cancer patients (n = 503) in California. They suggest that people turn to CAM for the following reasons: a desire to be treated as a whole person, to be able to participate in his or her own care and through a sense that traditional medicine has failed to meet their spiritual or psychological needs.

WORKING WITH THE WHOLE PERSON IN PAIN

Bollentino (2001, p. 101) reminds us 'each person is an organic whole, with inseparable physical, intellectual, psychological, social, creative, and spiritual aspects.' Working holistically acknowledges the uniqueness of the individual and his or her response to pain. Meeting the whole person requires the development of the therapeutic relationship, well recognized within the field of health care and CAM. Erskine et al (1999) recommend that this relationship should be nurtured and entered into fully for its potential for psychological well-being. Clarkson (1992) takes this further by referring to working at the transpersonal relationship level with people facing challenging symptoms and life-threatening illness.

Relationships develop between people and within a certain environment – a 'therapeutic space' can be created anywhere, even in a busy ward or clinic. Creating and maintaining this 'special space' allows us to go beyond the physical. Bion (1962) uses the term 'containment' to encompass 'being there' and 'attuning' with another in their pain and suffering. Importantly, this includes an ability to both witness and 'hold' any emotional material that might arise. A patient will only feel safe if he or she knows that the practitioner will not be overwhelmed by it. Viewing pain in the physical domain alone ignores the potential of engaging the patient and with his or her own resources and capacities, be they spiritual, psychological and/or social.

PSYCHONEUROIMMUNOLOGY, IMAGERY AND PAIN

The use of imagery has developed in the field of cancer care and is part of the growing field of psychoneuroimmunology (PNI). The connection between the immune system and imagery has been studied in some depth. There is now enough evidence on the mind (psychology), the brain (neurology) and the body's natural defences (immunology) to suggest that the mind and body communicate with each other (Ader 1996; Evans et al 2000). This has been made possible through a rapid advance in scientific understanding of the immune system over the past 30 years. Watkins (1997) asserts that PNI research has generated hard scientific data that provide irrefutable evidence that virtually all the body's defence systems are under the control of the central nervous system. This research was the beginning of more extensive research on the mind–body connection.

The concept that every thought, idea and belief is part of the mind–body pathways raises interesting questions into the role of these in maintaining health and fighting disease. Although much of this work is in its infancy, the potential for its use is proving to be an exciting area. Simonton et al (1980) pioneered the use of imagery to treat cancer patients with advanced disease. Their study involved 225 participants where imagery was used in combination with traditional medical treatment. The imagery involved encouraging patients to imagine and draw their cancer, immune defences and medical treatments. The aim of this approach was for the patients to see the disease as weak and the host resistance and treatment as strong and therefore more likely to overcome the disease. The findings demonstrated that the median survival time of the clients in the experimental group was 18–19 months longer than the national average for persons with breast, bowel and lung cancer. However, there has been much debate over the findings of this particular study and other similar ones. Cunningham (2000) questions whether it is the technique which can heal, or whether the positive outcome is due to the patient gaining a sense of control. Further research is required to test these hypotheses.

A study described by Giedt (1997) suggests how the use of guided imagery as a nursing intervention using psychoneuroimmunology (PNI) principles can assist in the management of distressing symptoms such as pain, which is a common problem associated with cancer. Giedt (1997) states that pain causes both a physical sensation and a mental image, so paying attention to the metaphors used by the patient to describe the pain sensation may have an effect on the pain.

Imagery is potentially important in healing because it may in some circumstances act as a blueprint or set of instructions to the body, as an intermediary between thoughts and physiological changes. For example, fearful images can stimulate the stress response (Cunningham 2000). Davis-Brigham et al (1996) suggest that imagery goes on at all times in all individuals, both at a conscious and unconscious (and maybe even cellular) level. They suggest that when assessing a patient's suitability for imagery, an important starting point would be to explore the imagery already in place in relation to disease, health, values, fears and what the person sees as occurring in the body. They recommend that any guided imagery must be syntonic with the individual's core beliefs. It needs to fit in with their deepest values and not be contradictory with their view of the world. An example would be to avoid aggressive imagery, such as attacking the cancer, when a more gentle approach would better suit the individual.

PLACEBO, NOCEBO AND PAIN

Hope can have powerful effects on the experience of a symptom such as pain and can be linked to the concept of placebo: an inert substance or supposedly ineffective treatment may result in a perceived or physiological improvement in symptoms. This is called the *placebo effect* (Benedetti 2009). The phenomenon is related to the patient's expectation; if the substance is viewed as helpful, it can help, but if it is viewed as harmful, it can cause negative effects. This is known as the *nocebo effect*.

Because of the potential impact of these psychological processes which link expectation to a treatment's potency, the information given to a patient and, most importantly, *how* it is conveyed in both written and verbal form, must be

Box 15.1 **Four components of placebo (and potentially nocebo)**

1. Treatment characteristics, e.g. colour, size and shape of drug.
2. Practitioner characteristics, e.g. empathy, status, treatment and illness belief.
3. Patient characteristics, e.g. treatment and illness beliefs, anxiety state and trait, coping strategies.
4. Patient–practitioner interactions, e.g. therapeutic alliance, length of consultation, costs including time, disclosures and information provided/requested.
(Mackereth & Maycock 2010; Peters 2001)

carefully considered for its psychological interpretation. This is particularly relevant with respect to informed consent, which is required for all medical and CT interventions.

Originally, the term 'placebo' was attributed to benefits from 'pleasing the patient' rather than as a result of the intervention itself (Beecher 1955). Expectation of outcome is argued to be a key component of placebo, with signals such as the colour, shape and name of a pill being significant. Importantly, confidence in who prescribes and what is said about the intervention can also influence perception of the potency of the treatment (Kienle & Kiene 1997). Other important interactive components between a therapist and a client which may be influenced by the placebo/nocebo effect include the patient's ability to manage or contain anxiety, the therapeutic relationship itself and the characteristics of the practitioner. Important here is the language, non-verbal cues and paralinguistic components of the practitioner–patient interaction. For example, if the practitioner is hesitant, does not maintain good eye contact and infers by speech that the intervention 'might help' (i.e. 'may not'), the patient may be less than confident about the therapeutic benefits. There is a delicate balance to be struck between inspiring confidence and being realistic. Highly anxious patients may worry about side effects or have high expectations of not responding well to the treatment (Box 15.1).

TOUCH: A TOOL FOR ACKNOWLEDGING AND RELIEVING DISTRESS AND PAIN

The therapeutic use of touch by nurses and other health professionals has been well discussed in the literature, with acknowledgment that we touch patients for a variety of reasons, such as washing, applying dressings and holding during medical procedures. *Intention* is a key issue in relation to touch and in the past healthcare practice has been criticized for being largely task orientated in touching behaviours. Supportive empathic touch works on a physical and intuitive level and provides comfort that is a physical expression of 'being there and with the patient'. Provided with openness and sensitivity, another person's touch can be profound in its humanizing effects and is often moving for both the patient and the practitioner. If overburdened and time deprived, health professionals may avoid this intimate act, unsure of their capacity to be in the moment and open to being really present with another person, particularly if their distress is palpable. They may additionally feel unsure of their ability to manage any emotional responses from the patient which occur as a result of the encounter. Equally, a patient may not always welcome the therapeutic use of touch, however well intentioned. Closing down to physical touch can occur when an individual feels their body has become a painful battleground invaded by investigations, medical devices and treatments. Touch history is important, and sometimes painful and/or abusive touch experiences may have shaped how receptive a person is to physical contact. Receptivity and appropriateness can only be assessed by viewing touch as a negotiated activity, with the patient able and fully aware that they can say 'no' at any point. This golden rule, which respects autonomy, Mackereth (2000) argues should apply to any therapeutic or clinical activity involving touch.

SPECIFIC PATIENT-FOCUSED THERAPIES

The manipulation of soft tissue, in the form of massage, aromatherapy or reflexology, carries with it many possible benefits, some as yet not fully understood or evaluated within clinical care. In relation to pain, some of the improvements following touch can be linked to the gate theory of pain perception (see Chapter 6). The work of the Touch Research Institutes (see resources section) and others have helped to clarify the benefits of massage for people with cancer and to diminish safety concerns. Using a number of validated physiological and psychological measures, massage has been demonstrated to reduce cortisol levels, levels of anxiety and the perception of pain (Stringer et al 2008). The following section will examine the evidence for specific therapies, with examples of research illustrating the growing evidence base and identifying the outcomes and limitations of the studies (see Table 15.1). They represent only a sample of the work available and readers are recommended to conduct a more in-depth search to supplement these observations.

Table 15.1 Therapy-specific research

Authors	Condition	Design	Interventions	Measures	Findings	Limitations
Aromatherapy						
Gedney et al (2004)	Sensory and affective pain discrimination after inhalation of essentials oils	Randomized crossover design (n = 26)	A thermal pain stimulus was delivered to the right masseter and right upper trapezius, and the ischemic pain procedure involved cuff inflation on the right arm Each subject was exposed to three experimental conditions before and during pain stimulation: 1. lavender inhalation 2. rosemary inhalation 3. distilled water (control)	Quantitative sensory measures of contact heat, pressure and ischaemic pain BP, HR and pre- and post-treatment salivary cortisol Post-treatment questionnaires, including VAS: 1. properties of odour 2. pain intensity 3. pain unpleasantness	No difference for 'sex' No statistical difference in quantitative measures for each intervention Significant difference in the qualitative data: 1. pain intensity 2. pain unpleasantness with the lavender intervention and marginally reduced with rosemary when compared with the control intervention	Selection bias as the subjects were already familiar with the testing measures Small sample size Essential oil exposure was for a short time with no choice as to the selection
Hypnotherapy						
Lang et al (2008)	To determine the effect of hypnosis and empathic attention on pain, anxiety, drug use and adverse events during percutaneous tumour treatment	Randomized control trial (n = 201)	1. Hypnosis group 2. Attention group 3. Standard care Group 1 also received empathic attention	Pain VAS, anxiety VAS, measured every 15 minutes Medication usage Incidence of adverse events	Hypnosis group reported significantly less pain and anxiety compared to other groups and used less analgesia Attention-only group experienced 48% adverse event rate	High adverse events in attention-only group led to trial being discontinued Researchers provided interventions Clinicians aware of allocation

Continued

Table 15.1 Therapy-specific research—cont'd

Authors	Condition	Design	Interventions	Measures	Findings	Limitations
Hypnotherapy						
Saadat et al (2006)	To examine the effects of hypnosis on preoperative anxiety	Randomized control trial (n = 76)	1. Hypnosis group 2. Attentive listening 3. Standard care	STAI, anxiety VAS, BP, HR pre- and post-treatment on entry to operating room	Hypnosis group were significantly less anxious (STAI) post-treatment On entry to operating room hypnosis group reported a reduction in baseline anxiety – other groups reported an increase (VAS) No significant difference with BP or HR	Assessor blinded to intervention Limited detail of surgical procedure No longer-term follow-up
Massage						
Cassileth & Vickers (2004)	Change in cancer-related symptom scores from pre- to post-massage therapy	Survey (n = 1290)	Analysis of data from symptom cards (which use rating scales)	Rating scales relating to several symptoms, including pain, fatigue, nausea and depression	Symptom scores were reduced in approximately 50% of patients Benefits persisted, especially in outpatients	Large variation in patients, for example some were inpatients and some were outpatients
Post-White et al (2003)	To evaluate the effectiveness of MT and HT at reducing the side effects of cancer treatment	Randomized, prospective, cross-over intervention study (n = 230)	Four weekly 45-minute sessions of assigned intervention plus four weekly sessions of standard care (control) Order of sessions was randomized After four sessions in one condition they received four sessions in the other condition	HR, RR, BP, one item score (0–10) of current pain and current nausea, BPI, BNI, POMS, assessment of analgesic and antiemetic use, satisfaction with care through self-devised questionnaires	MT and HT are more effective than P alone or standard care at reducing pain, fatigue and mood disturbance in patients with cancer receiving chemotherapy	29% attrition rate (n = 164) completed all 8 sessions Question-mark over appropriateness of study design in such poorly patients

Progressive muscle relaxation training and guided imagery

Study	Design	Intervention	Measures	Results	Limitations
Chen & Francis (2010)	Randomized trial (n = 19)	1. 30-minute abbreviated progressive muscle relaxation followed by home practice using personalized audiotapes 2. Usual care (GP)	McGill Pain Questionnaire VAS, Mental Health DASS 21, Quality of Life (Rand-36) pain diary (VAS) GAS and record of home practice	Trends for improvements in pain (McGill and VAS), mental health, all domains of quality of life and sleep	Eight participants withdrew Small sample, inadequate power Need for an improvement in the protocols
Kwekkeboom et al (2008)	Randomized trial (n = 40)	Crossover: 1. relaxation day 1, imagery day 2 2. imagery day 1, relaxation day 2	Imaging ability questionnaire, relaxation ability questionnaire, outcome expectancy scale, primary pain outcome, secondary pain outcome, perceived control over pain	Both PMR and analgesic imagery produced greater improvements in pain intensity, pain-related distress and perceived control over pain than the control conditions There were ability responder differences with guided imagery but not PMR	Interventions provided only short-term effects Subjective measures only – may have been useful to include a physiological measure
Baird & Sands (2004)	Randomized trial (n = 28)	1. Listening twice a day to 10–15 minute audiotaped script with guided imagery and PMR 2. Usual care	Pain Scale (AIMS2) Assessment of mobility (seven items)	Treatment group reported a significant reduction in pain and mobility difficulties	Small sample Compliance with protocol issues – participants reported falling asleep before completing GI with PMR

Reflexology

Study	Design	Intervention	Measures	Results	Limitations
Brown & Lido (2008)	Case series (n = 10)	All participants received six sessions of reflexology followed by six sessions of training and then six sessions of self-treatment	Pain diaries, HADS, lifestyle changes	Self-reported improvements in phantom limb pain and lifestyle Changes maintained at 12 months follow-up	No control groups limit conclusions Researcher provided treatments
Tsay et al (2008)	Randomized controlled trial (n = 63)	1. Three 20-minute reflex therapy sessions plus usual care 2. Usual care only	McGill Pain Questionnaire, usage of medication, HADS	Significantly less pain and anxiety in the reflexology group	Comparison only with usual care Only three sessions

Continued

Table 15.1 Therapy-specific research—cont'd

Authors	Condition	Design	Interventions	Measures	Findings	Limitations
Reflexology						
Poole et al (2007)	Investigation of the effectiveness of reflexology on chronic low back pain	Randomized controlled trial (n = 63)	1. Reflexology (six sessions) 2. Relaxation (six sessions) 3. Usual care (via GP)	SF-36 Pain, Oswestry Disability Questionnaire	No significant differences between groups	Reflexologist provided the treatment Trends in the data showed pain reduction greater in reflexology group
Stephenson & Weinrich (2000)	To assess the effects of reflexology on pain and anxiety in patients with lung and breast cancer	Quasi-experimental crossover trial (n = 23)	1. Reflexology 2. No intervention period	Pain (SF– MPQ), anxiety (VAS)	Significant decrease in anxiety following reflexology for both groups Significant decrease in pain for breast cancer group	Only 2 out of the 10 lung cancer patients reported pain compared to 11 out of 13 in the breast cancer group Gender difference in the group and effects of pain relief makes it difficult to interpret results
Grealish et al (2000)	To assess the effects of foot massage on nausea, pain and relaxation in hospitalized patients with cancer	Crossover randomized controlled trial (n = 87)	1. Two sessions of foot massage 2. Quiet resting	HR, pain (VAS), nausea (VAS), self- report of relaxation (VAS)	Significant difference in all measures, improving relaxation and reducing nausea and pain	No control for medication No exploration of lasting effects Numbers in each group not given 10-minute sessions only Therapists were trained as reflexologists

Terms: AIMS2, arthritis impact measures; BNI, Brief Nausea Index; BP, blood pressure; BPI, Brief Pain Inventory; DASS, depression anxiety and stress scale; GAS, individual global achievement Scales; GI, HADS, Hospital Anxiety and Depression Score; HR, heart rate; HT, healing touch therapy; MT, massage therapy; P, caring presence; POMS, Profile of Mood States; PMR, progressive muscle relaxation; RR, respiratory rate; SF-36, social functioning 36; SF–MPQ, Short-form McGill Pain Questionnaire; STAI, State Trait Anxiety Inventory; VAS, Visual Analogue Scale;

Aromatherapy and the clinical use of essential oils

Aromatherapy is the systematic use of essential oils in treatments to improve physical and emotional well-being (National Occupational Standards for Aromatherapy 2002). Within the UK, essential oils are usually applied as part of a massage in low concentrations using carrier oils, creams or lotions as vehicles for application. When used in this way, they are unlikely to have a direct physiological effect on a person's perception of pain. However, essential oils are potent reinforcers of positive sensation as the olfactory system is the most primitive of the senses and closely linked to the limbic system or 'emotional centre' of the brain stimulating memory and emotion. An example would be giving an aromatherapy massage to someone where muscular tension is contributing to their pain. The feeling of relaxation and release of muscular tension will reduce the sensation of pain and the continuing aroma will reinforce such sensations – this may be all that is required in certain patient populations (Stringer 2000). Recently the use of aromatic inhaler 'aromasticks' has become widespread, and this allows the practitioner to provide the client with a way of triggering the positive sensations felt at the time of the massage. Physical effects can be caused either by arousing smell memory or by the odour molecules infiltrating the patient's vascular system (Kutlu et al 2008). Stringer & Donald (2010) reported on a group of patients with cancer (n = 123) using aromasticks and noted that they appeared to assist in reducing anxiety and stress, plus some patients reported the aromasticks were helpful during painful and distressing medical procedures. Numerous aromatherapy studies have reported improvements in mood and well-being through the use of a combination of massage and essential oils (Steflitsch & Steflitsch 2008). Attempts have been made to compare massage with and without essential oils, with some studies indicating a statistical difference (Corner et al 1995; Evans 1995; Wilkinson 1995). These studies, however, did have limitations in terms of control related to therapist–patient interactions and the use of premade essential mixes, which would not reflect the practice of individualizing essential oil prescriptions. In another palliative study (Wilcock et al 2004) participants (n = 46) received a series of aromatherapy massages (weekly for four sessions) and were compared with conventional day care (attention only). While there were no significant differences in mood, physical symptoms and quality of life, the aromatherapy group's qualitative feedback was extremely positive, with requests to continue with the intervention.

Gedney et al (2004) reported on a randomized controlled trial (n = 26) comparing effects on sensory and affective pain discrimination using essential oils. Quantitative analysis did not show any difference when comparing the treatment groups (lavender and rosemary) to a control (distilled water). However, qualitative data indicated reduction in perception of the intensity and unpleasantness of pain with the use of lavender, but less so with rosemary oil (see Table 15.1).

Essential oils can also be used topically in concentrated form to have direct physiological effects. When used in this way it is the chemical constituents of the oils that are important in the therapist's choice of oils, as opposed to merely the pleasantness of the aroma. When used topically (often in creams and ointments for slow release of the oils) oils are used for their pharmacological properties. Eugenol (e.g. in clove oil or *Syzygium aromaticum*) and menthol (e.g. in peppermint oil or *Mentha piperita*) are examples of components of certain essential oils well known for their local anaesthetic properties. Many others have components such as methyl salicylate (e.g. wintergreen or *Gaultheria procumbens*), which is a potent anti-inflammatory agent. Due to the high doses of oils often required and the associated safety risks, therapists working at this level of practice require much more advanced training. This mode of working (using oils as medicinal products) is commonplace in Europe, where oils may be prescribed by physicians, but still relatively unusual within the UK. Developments in the clinical use of essential oils have been reported to assist with mucositis, neuropathic pain, itch and skin lesions (Stringer 2006; Tavares 2011). Box 15.2 describes a case study illustrating a clinical approach to managing distressing odour and pain associated with metastatic breast cancer.

A number of individual oils have been subjected to in vitro analysis of efficacy for certain clinical issues and the drug industry makes regular use of (often synthetic versions) of many essential oil components. However, the clinical application of blended essential oils for specific conditions is an area with a paucity of scientific data requiring formal evaluation.

Box 15.2 **Case study**

Louise, age 63, was admitted to the ward with a right breast fungating lesion. Apart from the pain, soreness and inflammation around the site the odour was distressing to family members and other patients. A base cream, which contained lavender (*Lavandula angustifolia*), Roman chamomile (*Chamaemelum nobile*) and tea tree (*Melaleuca alternifolia)* was applied. A secondary dressing containing citrus oils was applied to help reduce the odour. The goal of the treatment was to reduce pain, soreness and distress.

Over a period of a week, the odour almost disappeared, and the skin around the wound was much improved. Louise reported less pain, and her mobility increased; she appeared more and more relaxed and able to socialize with her family and other patients.

Hypnotherapy

Hypnotherapy may be described as the deliberate use of the trance state to effect change in both the conscious and unconscious states of the mind (Rankin-Box 2010). It is important to note that the purpose of using hypnotherapy should be to assist in managing rather than eradicating pain. Suggestions can be made to affect the perception of pain rather than to numb it totally. The therapist's role is to assist the patient in identifying useful strategies to cope with, be distracted from or avoid being overwhelmed by pain. Importantly, pain is a warning mechanism and the patient should be able to detect a change in their pain experience so that they can take necessary actions and/or seek further medical advice. In chronic pain states hypnotherapy can be used to affect mood, promote healthy lifestyles (e.g. stopping smoking, which can affect pain) and improve sleep so as to improve resilience. Hypnotherapy is ideal for situations where patients require a temporary hypnotic state to facilitate the successful completion of distressing and painful medical procedures (see Box 15.3).

Donald (2010) reviewed the use of hypnotherapy for pain relief and identified a number of pilot studies and literature reviews. A key paper by Patterson & Jensen (2003) found numerous laboratory studies reporting temporary analgesia achieved through hypnotherapy. A common observation was that the more suggestible a patient

was the more benefit he or she gained from the intervention. In reviewing the trials that focused on acute pain, hypnotherapy was shown to be effective, but in some of the studies hypnotherapy did not produce any greater difference when compared to outcomes for the control groups. Additionally, hypnotherapy was only superior half of the time when compared to relaxation training or distraction. A number of reasons have been identified for such discrepancies, including standardization of induction techniques, the skill of the practitioner and number and the length of sessions offered.

Chronic pain studies have shown hypnosis to be equivalent to acute pain management when compared to controls. However, hypnosis has not routinely outperformed other therapies such as autogenic and relaxation training. Studies on chronic headaches have demonstrated positive outcomes, but have also concluded that further studies with other causes of chronic pain are needed. It was acknowledged, in the studies reviewed, that for people living with chronic pain, the activities of daily living, mood and well-being were often compromised and these issues needed addressing. The authors concluded that hypnotherapy was a useful supportive intervention in the management of both acute and chronic pain. Recent studies using positron emission tomography (Faymonville et al 2006) and functional magnetic resonance imaging (Derbyshire et al 2009; Mohr et al 2005,) support these findings, showing hypnotically modified neural activity. These researchers concur that areas of the limbic system, such as the anterior cingulate cortex, seem to be involved in the temporary analgesic effect and perception of suffering (see Chapter 6. There is generally a growing body of scientific evidence indicating that hypnotherapy has a clinical benefit in relation to pain perception as well as clear physiological effects.

Box 15.3 **Case study**

Dawn, aged 45, was attending for three weekly sessions of chemotherapy and by her fourth session she reported needle anxiety. Dawn described being fearful about the pain of needling but was also concerned that cannulation attempts would all fail. On arrival Dawn was hyperventilating and her hands were cold.

Progressive muscle relaxation (PMR) training was offered and used as an induction method, a means of interrupting the hyperventilation response and a useful way of reducing 'flight or fight' hormones. During hypnosis Dawn was guided to envisage her veins as flowing rivers and the procedure was completed successfully in her own time. A squeezable stress ball was used to pace and anchor the PMR instructions. Guided to indicate when she was ready to begin the procedure, the nurse was encouraged to join in with the PMR so everyone involved was calm and focused. After 5 minutes Dawn indicated her readiness and a distended and ideal vein was successfully cannulated with minimal discomfort.

By anchoring (positive link or trigger to deepen and reinforce a calm state) a squeezable stress ball to the successful cannulation, Dawn became confident to self-hypnotize with minimal support at subsequent chemotherapy sessions; all cannulations were successful and undertaken with minimal discomfort.

Massage

'Massage' is a general term for a variety of manipulative soft tissue techniques, which may involve a mixture of stroking, kneading and applied pressure. Practitioners may draw on a variety of massage styles and philosophies (Tavares 2003). For example, Shiatsu is normally provided through cloth with the client lying on a mat (note that this is not always suitable for patients with mobility issues). Bailey (2006), a physiotherapist and Shiatsu practitioner, recommends taking account of fatigue and limited mobility by adapting timing, position and techniques, for example sitting a patient in a chair for treatment. Box 15.4 describes the use of the ergonomic massage chair, which not only facilitates a good position but is also portable for use by the bedside or in the day room (Campbell et al 2006).

A team of researchers who stand out in their contribution to understanding the power of touch through massage is led by Dr Tiffany Field. They are based at the Touch

Box 15.4 **Case study**

Ron, aged 47, with a history of chronic back pain, was in attendance with his partner, who was dying from ovarian cancer. He had not slept or been able to sit for long at the bedside. His two sons were also present but were sitting away from the bed. The nursing staff ask for Ron to be offered a back massage as he was agitated and pacing the room constantly. On arrival the therapist invited Ron to sit on an ergonomic massage chair. He took off his shirt and positioned himself. The therapist oiled his back and gently massaged for 20 minutes. Towards the end Ron was snoring loudly. Wrapping him in a blanket he was gently awoken and guided to the bedside. Ron snuggled into his partner and tears started to flow. His sons stood behind him resting their hands on his shoulders.

Research Institutes (TRI), which is part of the University of Miami, Florida, USA. For two decades they have been producing research that has consistently shown massage to reduce levels of pain and distress in a variety of settings. They are perhaps best known for their pioneering work looking at the effects of massage on preterm infants. They have documented that regular massage for adults and children suffering from chronic conditions such as juvenile rheumatoid arthritis and fibromyalgia reduces symptoms of stress and the perception of pain (Field et al 1997, 2002). One of the methodological concerns regarding the otherwise meticulous studies from TRI investigating the effects of massage is their limited sample sizes. Two studies from other workers have gone some way to address this concern and validate TRI's findings, showing the positive effects of massage on the perception of pain. Cassileth & Vickers (2004) reported the effects of massage on over 1000 cancer patients from the Sloan–Kettering Cancer Centre over a period of 3 years. They concluded that massage had an immediate and substantiative beneficial effect by reducing symptoms of anxiety, depression, pain and nausea. In a second study, again with cancer patients, Post-White and colleagues (2003) showed massage to reduce ratings in several measures, including anxiety and perception of pain in 230 patients.

Reflexology

Reflexology is an ancient practice in which areas of the feet and sometimes the hands are worked with pressure-based techniques. Integral to the theoretical basis of reflexology are maps showing how body regions and organs are represented on the feet and hands, which therapists use to guide their practice. Explanations for reported effects have been attributed to overlaps with acupressure points and endorphin release from the manipulation of the soft tissue,

which is highly innervated in hands and feet. As with massage, such theories are linked with the gate theory (Tiran 2011). Additionally, critics argue that the time, attention and interactions between patient and therapist may add significant therapeutic benefits (Ernst et al 2011; Mackereth 2010). Typically, reflexology treatments last 45–60 minutes and patients are advised to attend for a course of 6–10 weekly sessions to obtain cumulative effects. Requiring access only to feet and/or hands this therapy is popular with some patients as they do not need to undress or move to a treatment couch/chair. Areas are worked either dry or with a very small amount of oil, avoiding excessive slippage. Relaxation movements are included between pressure to specific areas to promote a pleasurable and calm experience. Some example studies evaluating the effect reflexology can have on pain are briefly summarized in Table 15.1. The case study in Box 15.5 identifies gradual improvement for a patient living with peripheral neuropathy after cancer treatment. It could be argued that the condition may have improved over time without treatment, but the patient also noticed other benefits, which may have speeded his recovery. Further research is needed to formally evaluate this intervention.

Relaxation

Evidence from a number of research studies suggests that muscle relaxation techniques can make a difference to pain perception and coping ability. Several therapies have been classified as physical relaxation techniques, including various forms of progressive muscle relaxation, deep breathing and paced respiration. The overall aim of these techniques is to achieve relaxation and ultimately to reduce stress, which may be linked to pain, e.g. in tension headache. According to Lutgendorf et al (2000), relaxation is achieved once a set of physiological changes have occurred. The aim is to slow respiration, lower pulse and blood pressure, increase alpha wave brain activity and possibly reduce the body's inflammatory response mechanisms. This physiological process, related with activation of the parasympathetic nervous system, can have a positive impact on

Box 15.5 **Case study**

Ian, aged 57, had completed chemotherapy and radiotherapy treatment for lymphoma. Unfortunately he had been left with peripheral neuropathy, affecting sensation of his lower limbs and feet. He described a mixture of numbness and pain. Ian attended weekly for reflexology for 10 weeks and then reduced to fortnightly for 3 months. Ian noticed a gradual improvement in sensation and a reduction in pain. Additionally, he felt less anxious and noticed improvements in sleep and a lessening of fatigue.

health and improve symptoms in many acute and chronic conditions, including pain. Stress and anxiety can exacerbate pain through, for example, extreme muscular tension/spasm. This can become a vicious cycle as pain tends to cause more stress and anxiety, and therefore muscle tension. This downward spiral may be counteracted if the patient can be helped to relax. Although using relaxation techniques may not always eradicate pain, they can provide patients with an element of control. A particularly useful physical approach is progressive muscle relaxation (PMR), which can be easily learned by patients and then adapted to suit the individual patient (Mackereth & Tomlinson 2010). Patients are guided to work through different groups of muscles, tensing with inspiration and releasing muscles during expiration. Battino (2007) suggests that to deepen the effects of physical relaxation techniques some guided imagery can be beneficial to pain management. He suggests that the session could start with 10–20 minutes of physical relaxation followed by 10 minutes of guided imagery.

Devine & Westlake (1995) conducted a meta-analysis of 116 studies involving patients who have cancer receiving relaxation training, with statistically significant reductions reported for levels of anxiety, depression, mood, nausea, vomiting and pain. Carroll & Seers (1998) completed a systematic review of relaxation studies involving patients with acute pain. Only seven (362 patients) out of a possible 40 studies were eligible for inclusion. When considering pain outcomes, three out of the seven reported significantly less pain in the relaxation groups. Brief summaries of specific studies related to pain management are provided in Table 15.1.

Complementary therapists often have training in a number of different therapies and in practice may combine these, for example using essential oils with reflexology and/or providing a short visualization at the end of treatment. Carter (2006) combined selected approaches from several therapies, which involve touch with very simple 'imagery' methods designed to involve the patient in the relaxation process. She called the therapeutic approach HEARTS, which is an acronym for **h**ands on, **e**mpathy, **a**romatherapy, **r**elaxation, **t**extures and **s**ound. The aim is to help patients and carers to easily achieve a state of relaxation and feeling of well-being. HEARTS always involves physical touch and empathy, and relies largely on the involvement of the patient and the skills of the therapist rather than a predetermined set of techniques (see Box 15.6).

THE PAIN OF LOSS: CARING FOR CARERS

Burnout and work-related stresses are well acknowledged in the nursing literature. Providing on-site services for staff has been the subject of evaluation and research studies.

> **Box 15.6 Case study**
>
> Bill, aged 70, with lung cancer, was attending a day-care hospice. He complained of pain in the right upper arm and shoulder. Bill was taking medication but this did not help with a 'gnawing' sensation, particularly when trying to sleep. Bill appeared fatigued, breathless on exertion and anxious on arrival. He was made comfortable on the couch in a supported upright position.
>
> The therapist began the session by fully supporting the right arm. The therapist talked to the arm, inviting it to become 'relaxed and heavy', slowly repeating this statement at short intervals. After a few minutes Bill's breathing eased and he began to drift into what he later described as a 'zonked out' state. Bill was asked to describe the painful area's colour, shape, sensation and any sound. He said it was 'purple, jagged, rough and it hums'. The therapist suggested he convert these to their opposites – these became gold, smooth, round and silent. During a gentle clothed massage the process of changing the sensory perception of the pain was repeated. He practiced this process at home whilst lying in a comfortable position morning and evening. His wife rang a few days later thanking the therapist and said he was really hooked on his 'zonking' treatment; his sleep and pain had improved.

Researchers have reported that 15-minute sessions of chair massage can reduce stress and enhance the electroencephalogram pattern of alertness in subjects. Field et al (1996) identified that a group of 26 subjects receiving chair massage twice a week for 5 weeks had more reduced anxiety levels, lowered cortisol readings, improved alertness and higher scores in computational tasks after treatment than the control group of 24 subjects. A key finding in a study by Cady & Jones (1997) was the significant lowering of both systolic and diastolic blood pressure in employees following a 15-minute on-site massage, although there was no control group for this study. Importantly for healthcare workers, Field et al (1997) conducted a study in which hospital workers were given a 10-minute chair massage, after which decreases in anxiety, depression and fatigue were reported as well as increases in vigour. Katz et al (1999) conducted a small pilot study evaluating eight sessions of on-site chair massage also given to hospital staff. Relaxation and profile of mood states were scored better after the treatment, along with reduced tension and pain intensity.

In another larger study by Hodge et al (2002) involving 100 healthcare workers, subjects were randomized into two groups. One group (n = 50) received 20 minutes of chair massage and the control group (n = 50) rested for an equal time period. Subjects who received chair massage exhibited decreases in blood pressure recordings, anxiety and sleep disturbances, and improvements in well-being and emotional control. Carers may have limited time to receive massage, often because they are reluctant to spend time away from their loved ones (see Box 15.4). A service providing massage to carers has been the subject of a published evaluation in the USA (Oregon Hospice Association and East–West College of Healing Arts 1998). Thirteen caregivers were given an average of six massages, after which 85% reported emotional and physical stress level reduction, 77% reported physical pain reduction and 54% reported better patterns of sleep. In the UK a massage service for family members of patients receiving palliative care has been well evaluated by subjects participating in focus groups (Penson 1998).

Legal, professional and managerial issues

Although not usually perceived as core activities within healthcare services, CTs are nonetheless interventions that require managing and delivery by skilled and accountable therapists. Those making referrals to therapists are delegating treatment to patients and require to be satisfied that it is both beneficial and not harmful. Stone (2002) asserts that the ethical duty to provide benefit to patients is enshrined in the legal concept of duty of care, which behoves therapists to treat their patients with all due skill and care. As many CTs involve touch, the civil action of battery (or trespass to the person), which upholds respect for the patient's bodily autonomy, is of importance. Battery is said to occur when touch is given to a patient, e.g. in the course of the treatment, without first having obtained consent (Stone 2002).

RECOMMENDATION FOR BEST PRACTICE IN DELIVERING COMPLEMENTARY THERAPIES

Currently, provision of CTs within the healthcare service is largely on an ad hoc basis, delivered by existing healthcare staff or as part of research projects. In areas where funding has been obtained therapies may thrive and provide useful evaluative information. The authors of this chapter manage an established team of therapists within a large cancer care trust, providing a range of therapies and conducting audits, services evaluations and innovative research work. Some centres and hospices may have to rely on sessional therapists or even volunteer therapists who visit wards and departments, are supervised by clinical staff and provide only short treatments without any remuneration to selected patients. Some patients request that their own practitioners be allowed to provide private treatment whilst in hospital. In view of this situation, it is difficult to make recommendations for best practice which would

fit all environments. It is very important, however, that whatever arrangements, protocols and policies are put in place each therapist is suitably trained for the therapies they are providing. Therapists need to have adequate insurance cover for their practice and all treatments must be carried out with the permission (through informed consent) of the patient and their specialist. In most cases this will be required in writing, with a record of treatment sessions kept in the patient's hospital notes.

CONCLUSION

CTs should not be seen as the last resort or only for the end of life when all other measures have failed. Education is required to ensure the role of CTs is understood in terms of both benefits and limitations. Where a patient is requesting *alternative* therapies it presents dilemmas for both complementary and conventional practitioners. Patients with their own resources will inevitably make their own decisions, but it is essential to provide information that enables them to consider the possible consequences and risks. Public access to information through the world wide web and other forms of media has opened the door to numerous hoped-for possibilities for someone living with pain; knowing what can be helpful or harmful requires skilled judgment and critical appraisal.

This chapter has endeavoured to share insights into the role of CTs in pain management. There are continuing challenges in providing equitable access to these types of therapies. What we know is that it is the patients who are driving their greater inclusion in healthcare settings. It is essential for health professionals to inform themselves about the evidence base for CTs. In addition, we believe, exposure to the integration of therapies can enable health professionals to fully appreciate their contribution to patient care.

Q | Questions for consideration

1. What is the potential of specific complementary therapies to assist with pain management in your speciality?
2. How does the content of this chapter affected your professional view of complementary therapies, specifically the interventions you would need to investigate?
3. What essential steps might you need to take if you propose to introduce one or more complementary therapies within your specialty?
4. How can you access further information to critically evaluate the potential of specific complementary therapies in your work context?

REFERENCES

Ader, R., 1996. Historical perspectives on psychoneuroimmunology. In: Friedman, H., Klein, T.W., Friedman, A.L. (Eds.), Psychoneuroimmunology, stress and infection. CRC Press, Boca Raton, FL.

Bailey, J., 2006. Shiatsu for symptom management. In: Mackereth, P., Carter, A. (Eds.), Massage & Bodywork: adapting therapies for cancer care. Churchill Livingstone, London.

Baird, C.L., Sands, L., 2004. A pilot study of the effectiveness of guided imagery with progressive muscle relaxation to reduce chronic pain and mobility difficulties of osteoarthritis. Pain Manag. Nurs. 5 (3), 97–104.

Battino, R., 2007. Guided Imagery and other approaches to healing. Wales Crown House Publishing, Cardiff.

Beecher, H.K., 1955. The powerful placebo. J. Am. Med. Assoc. 159, 1602–1606.

Benedetti, F., 2009. Placebo effects. Understanding the mechanisms in health and disease. Oxford University Press, Oxford.

Bion, W.R., 1962. A Theory of Thinking. Int. J. Psychoanal. 43 (Parts 4–5), 306–310.

Bollentino, R.C., 2001. A model of spirituality for psychotherapy and other fields of mind–body medicine. Adv. Mind Body Med. 17, 90–107.

Brown, C.A., Lido, C., 2008. Reflexology treatment for patients with lower limb amputations and phantom limb pain – An exploratory pilot study. Compl. Ther. Clin. Pract. 14, 124–131.

Cady, S.H., Jones, G.E., 1997. Massage therapy as a workplace intervention for reduction of stress. Percept. Mot. Skills. 84 (1), 157–158.

Campbell, G., Mackereth, P., Sylt, P., 2006. Adapting chair massage for carers, staff and patients. In: Mackereth, P., Carter, A. (Eds.), Massage & Bodywork: adapting therapies for cancer care. Elsevier Science, London.

Carroll, D., Seers, K., 1998. Relaxation for the relief of chronic pain: a systematic review. J. Adv. Nurs. 27, 476–487.

Carter, A., 2006. The HEARTS Process. In: Mackereth, P., Carter, A. (Eds.), Massage and Bodywork: adapting

therapies for cancer care. Elsevier Science, London.

Cassileth, B.R., 1998. The alternative medicine handbook: the complete guide to alternative medicine. Norton, New York.

Cassileth, B.R., Vickers, A.J., 2004. Massage therapy for symptom control: outcome study at a major cancer centre. J. Pain Symptom Manage. 28 (3), 244–249.

Cassileth, B.R., Schraub, S., Robinson, E., et al., 2001. Alternative medicine use worldwide: The International Union against cancer survey. Cancer. 91 (7), 1390–1393.

Chen, Y.L., Francis, A.J., 2010. Relaxation and imagery for chronic, nonmalignant pain: effects on pain symptoms, quality of life, and mental health. Pain Manag. Nurs. 11 (3), 159–168.

Clarkson, P., 1992. Transactional Analysis Psychotherapy, an Integrated Approach. Routledge, London.

Corner, J., Cawley, N., Hildebrand, S., 1995. An evaluation of the use of massage and essential oils on the well-being of cancer patients. Int. J. Palliat. Nurs. 1, 67–73.

Coss, R.A., McGrath, P., Caggiano, V., 1998. Alternative care: patient choices fro adjunct therapies within a cancer centre. Cancer Pract. 3, 176–181.

Cunningham, A.J., 2000. The Healing Journey. Overcoming The Crisis Of Cancer. Key Porter Books, Toronto.

Davis-Brigham, D., Davis, A., Cameron-Sampey, D., 1996. Imagery for Getting Well: Clinical Applications of Behavioural Medicine. Norton, New York.

Derbyshire, S.W., Whalley, M.G., Oakley, D.A., 2009. Fibromyalgia pain and its modulation by hypnotic and non-hypnotic suggestion: An fMRI analysis. Eur. J. Pain. 13 (5), 542–550.

Devine, E.C., Westlake, S., 1995. The effects of psych-educational care provided to adults with cancer: meta-analysis of 116 studies. Oncol. Nurs. Forum. 22, 1369–1381.

Donald, G., 2010. Research and hypnotherapy. In: Integrative Hypnotherapy – Complementary approaches in clinical care. Elsevier, London.

Ernst, E., White, A., 2000. The BBC survey of complementary therapy medicine used in the UK. Complement. Ther. Med. 8, 32–36.

Ernst, E., Posadzki, P., Lee, M.S., 2011. An update of a systematic review of randomised clinical trials. Maturitas. 68, 116–120.

Erskine, R.G., Moursund, P., Trautmann, R.J., 1999. Beyond empathy: A therapy of contact-in-relationship. Edwards Brothers, Michigan.

Evans, B., 1995. An audit into the effects of aromatherapy massage and the cancer patient in palliative and terminal cancer. Complement. Ther. Med. 3 (4), 239–241.

Evans, P., Hucklebridge, F., Clow, A., 2000. Mind Immunity and Health: The Science of Psychoneuroimmunology. Free Association Books, London.

Faymonville, M., Boly, M., Laureys, S., 2006. Functional neuroanatomy of the hypnotic state. J. Physiol. (Paris) 99 (4–6), 463–469.

Field, T., Ironson, G., Scafidid, F., et al., 1996. Massage therapy reduces anxiety and enhances EEG pattern of alertness and maths computations. Int. J. Neurosci. 86 (3–4), 197–205.

Field, T., Quintino, O., Henteleff, T., et al., 1997. Job stress reduction therapies. Alternative Therapies. 3 (4), 54–56.

Field, T., Diego, M., Cullen, C., et al., 2002. Fibromyalgia pain and substance P decreases and sleep improves after massage therapy. J. Clin. Rheumatol. 8, 72–76.

Foundation for Integrated Medicine, 1997. Integrated Healthcare: A Way Forward for the Next Five Years. FIM, London.

Gedney, J.J., Glover, T.L., Fillingim, R.B., 2004. Sensory and affective pain discrimination after inhalation of essential oils. Psychosom. Med. 66, 599–606.

Giedt, M.S., 1997. Guided imagery. A psychoneuroimmunological intervention in holistic nursing practice. Journal of Holistic Nursing Association. 15, 112–127.

Grealish, L., Lomasney, A., Whiteman, B., 2000. Foot Massage: a nursing intervention to modify the distressing symptoms of pain and nausea in patients hospitalised with cancer. Cancer Nurs. 23 (3), 237–243.

Hodge, M., Robinson, C., Boechemer, J., 2002. Employee outcomes following work-site acupressure and massage. Massage Ther. J. 39 (3), 48–64.

Katz, J., Wowk, A., Culp, D., et al., 1999. Pain and tension are reduced among hospital nurses after on-site massage treatments: a pilot study. J. Perianesth. Nurs. 14 (3), 128–133.

Kienle, G.S., Kiene, H., 1997. The powerful placebo effect: fact or fiction? J. Clin. Epidemiol. 50 (12), 1311–1318.

Kutlu, A.K., Yilmaz, E., Cecen, D., 2008. Effects of aroma inhalation on examination anxiety. Teach. Learn. Nurs. 3 (4), 125–130.

Kwekkeboom, K.L., Hau, H., Wanta, B., et al., 2008. Patients' perceptions of the effectiveness of guided imagery and progressive muscle relaxation interventions used for cancer pain. Compl. Ther. Clin Pract. 14, 185–194.

Lang, E.V., Berbaum, K.S., Pauker, S.G., et al., 2008. Beneficial effects of hypnosis and adverse effects of empathic attention during percutaneous tumour treatment when being nice does not suffice. J. Vasc. Interv. Radiol. 19 (6), 897–905.

Lutgendorf, S.K., Logan, H., Kirchner, H.L., et al., 2000. Effects of relaxation and stress on the capsaicin-induced local inflammatory response. Psychosom. Med. 62, 524–534.

Mackereth, P., 2000. Tough places to be tender: contracting for happy or 'good enough' endings in therapeutic massage/bodywork. Complement. Ther. Nurs. Midwifery. 6 (3), 111–115.

Mackereth, P., 2010. Psychological basis for therapeutic outcomes of reflexology. In: Tiran, D., Mackereth, P. (Eds.), Clinical Reflexology, second ed. Elsevier Science, London.

Mackereth, P., Maycock, M., 2010. In: Cawthorne, A., Mackereth, P. (Eds.), Integrative Hypnotherapy – Complementary approaches in clinical care. London, Elsevier.

Mackereth, P., Tomlinson, L., 2010. Progressive muscle relaxation: a remarkable tool for therapists and patients. In: Cawthorne, A., Mackereth, P. (Eds.), Integrative Hypnotherapy – Complementary approaches in clinical care. Elsevier, London.

Mohr, C., Binkofski, S., Erdmann, C., et al., 2005. The anterior cingulate cortex contains distinct areas dissociating external from self-administered painful stimulation: a parametric fMRI study. Pain. 114 (3), 347–357.

National Occupational Standards for Aromatherapy. 2002. Healthwork UK (now Skills for Health), London.

Oregon Hospice Association and East–West College of Healing Arts, 1998. Massage as a respite intervention for primary caregivers. Am. J. Hosp. Palliat. Care. Jan/Feb: 43–47 (in text but abbreviated).

Patterson, D.R., Jensen, M.P., 2003. Hypnosis and clinical pain. Psychol. Bull. 129 (4), 495–521.

Penson, J., 1998. Complementary therapies: making a difference in palliative care. Complement. Ther. Nurs. Midwifery. 4 (3), 77–81.

Peters, D. (Ed.), 2001. Understanding the placebo effect in complementary medicine: theory, practice and research. Churchill Livingstone, London.

Poole, H., Glenn, S., Murphy, P., 2007. A randomised controlled study of reflexology for the management of chronic low back pain. Eur. J. Pain. 11, 878–887.

Post-White, J., Kinney, M.E., Savik, M.S., et al., 2003. Therapeutic massage and healing touch improve symptoms in cancer. Integr. Cancer Ther. 2 (4), 332–344.

Rankin-Box, D., 2010. The Development of Hypnotherapy in Healthcare. In: Cawthorn, A., Mackereth, P. (Eds.), Integrative Hypnotherapy – complementary approaches in clinical care. Elsevier, London.

Saadat, H., Drummond-Lewis, J., Maranets, I., et al., 2006. Hypnosis reduces preoperative anxiety in adult patients. Anaesthesia & Analgesia. 102 (5), 1394–1396.

Simonton, O.C., Matthews-Simonton, S., Sparks, T.F., 1980. Psychological interventions in the treatment of cancer. Psychosomatics. 21, 226–233.

Steflitsch, W., Steflitsch, M., 2008. Clinical aromatherapy. Journal of Men's Health. 5 (1), 74–85.

Stephenson, N.L.N., Weinrich, S.P., 2000. The effects of foot reflexology on anxiety and pain in patients with breast and lung cancer. Oncol. Nurs. Forum. 27 (1), 67–72.

Stone, J., 2001. How might traditional remedies be incorporated into discussions of integrated medicine? Complement. Ther. Nurs. Midwifery. 7 (2), 55–58.

Stone, J., 2002. Identifying ethicolegal and professional principles. In: Mackereth, P., Tiran, D. (Eds.), Clinical Reflexology: a guide for health professionals. Churchill Livingstone, Edinburgh.

Stringer, J., 2000. Massage and aromatherapy on a leukaemia unit. Complement. Ther. Nurs. Midwifery. 6, 72–76.

Stringer, J., 2006. Massage and essential oils in haemato-oncology. In: Mackereth, P., Carter, A. (Eds.), Massage and Bodywork: adapting therapies for cancer care. Elsevier Science, London.

Stringer, J., Donald, G., 2010. Aromasticks in cancer care: an innovation not to be sniffed at. Compl. Ther. Clin. Pract. 17 (2), 116–121.

Stringer, J., Swindell, R., Dennis, M., 2008. Massage in patients undergoing intensive chemotherapy reduces serum cortisol and prolactin. Psychooncology. 17, 1024–1031.

Swisher, E.M., Cohn, D.E., Goff, B.A., et al., 2002. Use of complementary and alternative medicine among women with gynecological cancers. Gynecol. Oncol. 84, 363–367.

Tavares, M., 2003. National Guidelines for the Use of Complementary therapies in Supportive and Palliative Care. Foundation for Integrated Health, London.

Tavares, M., 2011. Integrating Clinical Aromatherapy in Specialist Palliative Care – the use of essential oils for symptom management. Self-published, Toronto.

Thomas, K.J., Nicholl, J.P., Fall, M., 2001. Access to complementary medicine via general practice. Br. J. Gen. Pract. 51 (462), 25–30.

Tiran, D., 2011. The physiological basis for therapeutic outcomes of reflexology. In: Tiran, D., Mackereth, P. (Eds.), Clinical Reflexology, second ed. Elsevier Science, London.

Tsay, S.L., Chen, H.L., Chen, S.C., et al., 2008. Effects of reflextherapy on acute postoperative pain and anxiety amongst patients with digestive cancer. Cancer Nurs. 31 (2), 109–115.

Watkins, A., 1997. Mind–body medicine: a clinician's guide to psycho-immunology. Churchill Livingstone, New York.

Wilcock, A., Manderson, C., Weller, R., et al., 2004. Does aromatherapy massage benefit patients with cancer attending a specialist palliative care day centre? Palliat. Med. 18 (4), 287–290.

Wilkinson, S., 1995. Aromatherapy and massage in palliative care. Int. J. Palliat. Nurs. 1 (1), 21–30.

RESOURCES/CONTACTS

Acupuncture Association of Chartered Physiotherapists www.aacp.uk.com

The Association of Chartered Physiotherapists in Reflex Therapy christenherbert@christen.f9.co.uk

Association of Reflexologists www.reflexology.org

American Massage Therapy Association www.amtamassage.org

British Massage Therapy Council www.bmtc.co.uk

British Holistic Medical Association www.bhma.org

British Medical Acupuncture Society www.medical-acupuncture.org.uk

Federation of Holistic Therapists www.FHT.org

International Federation of Professional Aromatherapists www.ifparoma.org

Research Council for Complementary Medicine www.rccm.org.uk

Medical School Hypnosis Association www.mhsa.org.uk

National Council for Hypnotherapy www.hypnotherapist.org.uk

National Center for Complementary and Alternative Medicine (USA) www.http:nccam.nih.gov

Shiatsu Society www.shiatsu.org

Touch Research Institutes, Miami, USA www.miami.edu/touch-research

College of Medicine (UK) www.collegeofmedicine.org.uk

Chapter | 16 |

Workplace rehabilitation

Libby Gibson and Jenny Strong

LEARNING OBJECTIVES

At the end of this chapter readers will have an understanding of:
1. The role of the workplace rehabilitation consultant in helping the injured worker to return to work.
2. Ways in which the injured worker, co-workers, employers and other relevant parties can all contribute to the overall success of a return-to-work programme.
3. The steps involved in a return-to-work programme for the injured worker.
4. Different models and assessments that can be applied to assist a worker in need of rehabilitation.
5. Ways in which workloads and/or workplaces can be adapted to suit the needs of the returning worker.

HIGH COST OF PAIN AND WORK DISABILITY

The high incidence of musculoskeletal disorders around the world tells us that many workers are either off work or working with pain. When a worker incurs an injury, work-related or not, that causes pain, there can be high costs, both to him or her personally and to the wider society. It is well established that pain has a high price in terms of its economic impact on a workforce and society (Access Economics 2007, Dagenais et al 2008) and that a small proportion of cases can contribute to a high proportion of the costs (Chou et al 2007, Maetzel & Li 2002). Therefore, there is increasing consensus that countries around the world need to implement strategies to reduce the costs of post-injury return to work (RTW), primarily by early intervention (Waddell & Burton 2005).

There is international recognition of the effectiveness of early intervention to keep workers with pain at work. However, how or whether such intervention is implemented is largely affected by the prevailing legislation and systems in place in that country, or even state, province or regional jurisdiction. This, in turn, impacts on the role that a health professional has assisting the worker with pain to stay at, or return to, work.

© 2014 Elsevier Ltd.

ALLIED HEALTH PROFESSIONAL ROLE

Around the world, the role of the health professional can be greatly influenced by the systems in place for intervention for workers with pain. They may only have a role in medical treatment and intervention, and little involvement with the workplace. They may be involved only if the worker claims workers' compensation, and collaborate with the claimant and the insurer to develop a suitable or modified duties programme to get the worker back to functional employment. The allied health professional (AHP) may work with people with persistent pain who cannot return to their usual occupation and are considering returning to the workforce in a new occupation. At the other end of the spectrum, they may be heavily involved at the place of employment, liaising with workers and managers to provide workplace-based early intervention and injury prevention interventions (see Fig. 16.1).

The roles can be condensed into two broad categories of prevention and rehabilitation. Rehabilitation can be further categorized into the areas of occupational rehabilitation and vocational rehabilitation. These two types of workplace rehabilitation can have varying definitions around the world. Workplace rehabilitation is 'a managed process involving timely intervention with appropriate and adequate services based on assessed need, and which is aimed at maintaining injured or ill employees in, or returning them to, suitable employment' (Heads of Workers' Compensation Authorities 2009, p. 5).

However, no matter what the definitions, the role of the AHP tends to depend on whether the person has a job to which he or she is aiming to return (usually called occupational rehabilitation) or the person is returning to the workforce in a different job or occupation (often called vocational rehabilitation). In the latter instance, the person may be unable to return to their prior occupation due to a work-related disability and, therefore, may still be covered by workers' compensation or other insurance schemes, or the person may have developed a pain-related disability from non-work causes and is receiving welfare payments and rehabilitation to get back into the workforce after a period of disability. In many parts of the world, the spectrum of practice outlined earlier is referred to as disability management (Williams & Westmorland 2002). This spectrum is being extended further in some countries to encompass absenteeism management, where early intervention is provided no matter what the reason for days off work and whether the cause is work-related or not. It is even being extended to management of presenteeism, for workers who do not take time off work but are not at full productivity due to injury, illness or disability (Calkins et al 2000).

This chapter will primarily cover the roles of AHPs working as workplace rehabilitation consultants (WRCs) with people with pain where either (a) the person with pain, acute or persistent, has a job to which they are aiming to return, so is still within the worker role (worker), and/or (b) the person with pain, typically persistent, is looking at returning to the workforce usually in a new or different occupation and is therefore usually in a job-seeker role, receiving either welfare or workers' compensation payments (job-seeker).

The role of the WRC is to coordinate services to '... achieve a cost effective, safe, early and durable return to work' for the injured worker or job-seeker (Heads of Workers' Compensation Authorities 2009, p. 6). This chapter will cover broad principles and services used in workplace rehabilitation to get the worker or job-seeker back to work and follow the common pathways for these clients

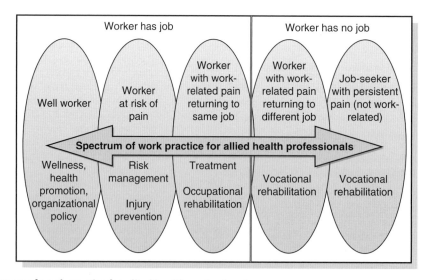

Fig. 16.1 **Spectrum of work practice for allied health professionals.**

in the workplace rehabilitation process. Two cases will be used to illustrate the typical presentation of the injured worker and job-seeker with persistent pain. An overview of some of the common strategies used in the WRC's toolbox will be presented and current evidence-based principles presented for the reader to consider for practice.

KNOWLEDGE AND SKILLS REQUIRED FOR WORKPLACE REHABILITATION

The AHP needs a range of knowledge and skills for their role in workplace rehabilitation. When working as a WRC, knowledge of the prevailing legislation, such as workers' compensation, occupational health and safety, disability discrimination and welfare legislation, is essential, at least in terms of the implications of this legislation and related policies for the worker or job-seeker with whom they are working. There is also a need for a strong grounding in the nature, prognosis and functional impact of the pain-related injury, including the implications of current treatments for RTW issues, e.g. the effect of pain medications on driving (see Box 16.1). WRCs also need an understanding of measurement principles and programme evaluation to be able to demonstrate the evidence for their practice (Gibson et al 2002).

Given this varied role and the significant number of systems around the world, this chapter will focus on broad principles for RTW and explore some of the current services being used by WRCs to assist workers to return to, or stay at, work. It will look at some of the models that can be used for RTW interventions and some of the emerging trends for the field of workplace rehabilitation.

Prior to this, however, it is important to address a key issue that can be a major barrier for people returning to work. The role described above assumes health professionals accept that workers who have pain usually can indeed work. Some experts in the field have raised concerns that treating health professionals can at times compound the issues for workers returning to work, for example by certifying workers as unfit for all duties or by providing

---

Box 16.1 **RTW coordination role: evidence-based competencies**

- Ergonomic and workplace assessment
- Clinical interviewing
- Social problem-solving
- Workplace mediation
- Knowledge of business and legal aspects
- Knowledge of medical conditions

(Shaw et al 2008)

---

inaccurate education about resuming activity (Waddell & Burton 2006). Health professionals can also achieve this by concentrating, contrary to prevailing international evidence-based practice guidelines, on symptom management in the early and not-so-early stages after onset of work-related pain (Hush 2008), rather than explaining the benefits of staying at work (McGuirk & Bogduk 2007) and being actively engaged with the worker's workplace to facilitate a safe and efficient RTW. In defence of health professionals, this can occur merely because they themselves need better education about work and workplaces (Royal Australasian College of Physicians 2009) or need systems that reimburse their time for such engagement with the workplace. However, no matter what role the health professional may have in their contact with the worker who has pain, he or she needs to be cognisant of the messages they give to the worker and how influential such messages can be for safe, early and effective RTW.

THE WORKER'S PERSPECTIVE

What about the worker with pain? The societal value of work cannot be underestimated. This is recognized by the World Health Organization's (WHO) International Classification of Functioning, Disability and Health (ICF) (World Health Organization 2001), which includes participation in work as a major valued role. Workers with disabilities can face many barriers in returning to work, and some of the most influential can be attitudinal.

Qualitative research on the perspectives of workers with injuries in the workers' compensation system and job-seekers with persistent pain gives insight to some of the major barriers people can face (Friesen et al 2001; Lippel 2007; Patel et al 2007). For example, a qualitative study of the effect of the workers' compensation process on workers in Quebec found the stigma attached to being an injured worker a major barrier, with participants reporting that they need to deal with prejudice against injured workers and stereotypes about them playing the system (Lippel 2007). They also described the difficulty they experience in dealing with the imbalance of power in the workers' compensation system, feeling 'like David against Goliath' (Lippel 2007, p. 435). These participants reported a high incidence of mental health issues during the workers' compensation process, sadly with often greater disabling consequences than the initial injury itself. Despite these negative health effects, participants also identified the positive health effects of being in the process, such as more expedient access to health care and a valuable, supportive relationship with someone in power, such as a health professional or caseworker, who knew the system and the process.

Similarly, job-seekers with persistent pain reported appreciating the benefits they received through the welfare support system (Patel et al 2007). However, they reported feeling frustrated at the limited understanding of case-workers and employers about persistent pain and its consequences for work ability, and at healthcare providers not taking their problem seriously (Patel et al 2007).

EVIDENCE-BASED PRINCIPLES FOR RETURN TO WORK FOR ALL STAKEHOLDERS

Before exploring the roles of AHPs in assisting workers or job-seekers with pain to RTW, this chapter will first explore seven principles that are needed for workplaces to achieve successful RTW after work disability (Institute for Work & Health 2007) (Box 16.2). These principles are particularly important for workplaces and employers, but can also inform the role of the AHP in supporting such RTW. These principles confirm the value of early and safe modified work, also called work accommodation or suitable duties programmes (SDPs), as the cornerstone of successful RTW (principle 2). The principles probably have the most implications for employers and workplaces in terms of their advocacy of a strong health and safety culture (1), with support of supervisors for work disability prevention and RTW planning in their duties (4), including early communication with injured or ill workers (5).

Box 16.2 **Seven 'principles' for successful return to work**

1. The workplace has a strong commitment to health and safety which is demonstrated by the behaviours of the workplace parties.
2. The employer makes an offer of modified work (also known as work accommodation) to injured/ill workers so they can return early and safely to work activities suitable to their abilities.
3. RTW planners ensure that the plan supports the returning worker without disadvantaging co-workers and supervisors.
4. Supervisors are trained in work disability prevention and included in RTW planning.
5. The employer makes an early and considerate contact with injured/ill workers.
6. Someone has the responsibility to coordinate RTW.
7. Employers and healthcare providers communicate with each other about the workplace demands as needed, and with the worker's consent.

Institute for Work & Health, Toronto, Canada, March 2007.
© Copyright 2007 Institute for Work & Health http://www.iwh.on.ca/files/seven_principles_rtw_2007.pdf.

However, the principles also provide implications for AHPs in their roles with workers who have work-related pain. These implications include the need for healthcare providers to communicate with employers, with the worker's consent, about workplace demands and the potential impact on the worker's condition (7). These may include AHPs who are not traditionally involved in the RTW process, such as treating medical specialists or treating physiotherapists. AHPs who are directly involved in the RTW planning process need to ensure the modified duties are safe, suitable to the worker's abilities and enacted as soon as is safely possible (2) without disadvantaging co-workers and supervisors (3).

Beyond the implications these principles have for AHPs assisting workers once they have incurred injury, they also have implications for a potential role working with employers to help them improve their commitment to health and safety (1), to educate management and line supervisors about work disability prevention and RTW planning (3 and 4), and to assist them to develop processes for early communication (5) and effective in-house RTW coordination processes (6).

The challenges are many when working with employers to implement organizational change (Amick et al 2000; Whysall et al 2006). Consultants to employers may need to apply attitude and behaviour change theories, such as a transtheoretical approach to change, for individuals and organizations, and provide practical tools and techniques to enable managers to measure and tackle behavioural change. Employers also need to provide more budgetary control and time to managers to deal with health and safety issues, and flatten the hierarchy of decision-making systems about health and safety (Whysall et al 2006).

THE WORKPLACE REHABILITATION PROCESS

The basic common steps of the workplace rehabilitation process are outlined in Figure 16.2. The names and numbers of steps can vary around the world and with different systems; these are based on a national framework currently in place in Australia and cover the basic steps in most processes of getting workers or job-seekers back to work.

The following section explains each of the steps in the process. It goes into more depth in some sections, such as planning (3), where an introduction to some models to assist planning and an overview of common services are provided. The steps are also illustrated by a companion case study (see Box 16.4) that provides further details of the individual processes followed within the overall process, such as conducting an initial needs assessment and developing a rehabilitation plan and SDP.

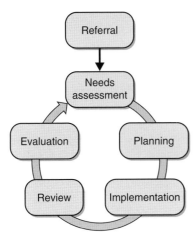

Fig. 16.2 Workplace rehabilitation process continuum.
Adapted from Heads of Workers' Compensation Authorities (2009).

1. Referral

Referral may come from several sources depending on the prevailing system in any one country, state or province. These sources include the insurer or workers' compensation authority, the person's treating medical practitioner, the employer, other health or welfare professionals, solicitors/ attorneys, the injured worker or job-seeker with a disability, and their family. Regardless of the referral source, the programme needs to be funded. It is in the interests of all stakeholders to resolve the issue of payment early and to have the client return to productive work as quickly and safely as possible.

2. Rehabilitation needs assessment

Box 16.3 provides a summary of the sort of information that may be gathered in the initial needs assessment with the worker or job-seeker. How much depth is needed in each area will depend on the case and the type of workplace rehabilitation being undertaken. When the person is a job-seeker and cannot return to work, detailed information about aspects such as their work and education history will be needed. When the person is a worker who has a job available for a RTW programme less of such history is needed, if any, and more information about the current work duties and environment would be taken. Information about performance in daily living and leisure activities is sought, not necessarily to consider what interventions can be provided to improve these, as workplace rehabilitation may not cover such interventions, but to establish a sense of the functional effects of the pain-related injury or disability, especially when the person is not currently working.

Box 16.3 **Initial needs assessment**

1. Demographic information:
   - Age
   - Current working status
   - Income support, e.g. workers' compensation/ centrelink benefit/other
   - Litigation
2. History of injury/disability
   - Onset/cause
   - Medical history and treatment to date
   - Current treatment
   - Medication
3. Effect of injury/disability
   - Perceived abilities and limitations, especially for work
   - ADL and IADL*
   - Leisure*
   - Fitness
   - Use of time
   - Psychosocial issues, e.g. yellow/blue/black flags (formally screen if indicated)
4. Current working situation and goals for RTW
   - Reported work duties and tasks, hours and environment (specialist workplace assessment may be indicated)
   - Work tasks
   - Perceived demands of the job
   - Perceived potential for RTW
   - Current expectations of RTW
5. Education/employment history
   - Highest education
   - Prior jobs
   - Work interests
6. Social situation
   - Relationships
   - Engagement in social situations/activities
   - Responsibilities
7. Observations
   - Presentation
   - Communication skills
   - Affect
   - Behavioural factors
8. Recommendations
   - RTW hierarchy of goals
   - Eligibility for services
   - Further assessment required
   - Recommended action plan

---

*Information is obtained about activities of daily living (ADL), instrumental activities of daily living (IADL) and leisure only in terms of assessing the impact of the injury on current function, not necessarily for intervention purposes.

Leanne is an administrative officer in the office of a large vocational education college. She is currently off work on workers' compensation benefits and has been referred by an insurer's case manager (CM) to a rehabilitation provider for a rehabilitation programme to get her back to her normal job and duties.

Note: The following steps are the ones that could be followed by the workplace rehabilitation consultant (WRC) managing the rehabilitation process. As such, it is described as the role that a generic case WRC could manage, i.e. one with any appropriate qualification. Specialist roles will be described for specialist services provided as part of the rehabilitation programme.

Step 1: Referral

The first steps for the WRC would be to obtain any available background information from the referrer and arrange to meet Leanne and her supervisor as soon as possible, preferably at her workplace. In this case, an occupational therapist was assigned as her WRC/CM and approval sought for a workplace assessment as part of the initial needs assessment.

Step 2: Needs assessment

The following is the sort of information that would be gathered at the initial workplace meeting with Leanne and her supervisor, and from the referral information:

1. Demographic information
   - Leanne is 47 years old.
   - Leanne was initially off work for 1 month, and then attempted a full-time return to work on full duties, which lasted 2 weeks. She then had another month off, then came back part-time for 1 month, still on full duties, and is now off again with persistent pain in her low back.
   - Leanne is receiving workers' compensation and not pursuing litigation.

2. Social situation
   - Leanne is married with two children, a 12-year-old son and a 16-year-old daughter. Her husband works in his own business and travels interstate regularly for his work.
   - She has friends that she plays weekly tennis with, attends a monthly book club with work friends and is friends with parents from her children's school.
   - Leanne says she really needs to return to work to help with paying their mortgage as they recently purchased a small holiday house at the beach.

3. History of injury/disability
   - Leanne has been experiencing episodes of back pain in her lumbar and left sacro-iliac regions on and off for over 3 months, since she had to manually handle a student in her capacity as first-aid officer for the school.
   - She says she was in considerable pain while working, having to take regular breaks and lie down on the staff room floor at lunch times.
   - Her GP has referred her to an orthopaedic surgeon. She has been attending a chiropractor on and off for treatment and having massages for pain relief.

- Commencement of anti-inflammatory medication in the last week has reportedly resulted in markedly reduced pain levels; she also takes paracetamol as required.

4. Reported effect of injury/ disability
   - Since her injury, Lenne has been hiring a cleaner to clean her house fortnightly, and relying on her husband and children as much as possible for other household tasks, such as doing the laundry, grocery shopping and meal preparation. She has had trouble driving, as she owns a manual car and has difficulty operating the clutch with her left leg. While working, she was able to get lifts from a co-worker when her husband was away, or catch the bus, which aggravated her back pain.
   - Leanne usually enjoys weekly tennis with friends and walking in her local area. She likes to read and do scrap-booking, but has found even reading difficult as the pain interrupts her concentration. She has mostly been resting at home and watching television since her last attempt to return to work, fearful that activity might re-aggravate her injury.
   - She reports that she is afraid to carry out too much movement or exercise for fear of re-injuring her back.

5. Current working situation and goals for return to work
   - Work duties: Leanne is one of three general administration officers in the college office, responsible for the parent and student enquiries counter, telephone enquiries, general word-processing for the principal (e.g. college newsletter, data entry of student details), photocopying, book-keeping and management of accounts, and management of petty cash, including handling of student payments for fees/excursions. Leanne is also one of two first-aid officers for the college.
   - Work hours: Her normal work hours are 8:15 am to 4:00 pm, with 45 minutes for lunch. during which she is often interrupted to attend to first-aid duties, and 15 minutes for morning tea. Leanne works 5 days per week with most of the school holidays off.
   - Leanne is starting to get anxious that she will be unable to return to her job. She says she is losing confidence about her capacity for even daily tasks, let alone working, but is very motivated and determined to return to work.
   - The college principal highly values her skills and dedication to her work, and is very supportive about getting Leanne back to work. Leanne's direct supervisor works with her, managing the school office. Leanne feels that her direct supervisor is supportive of her, but that she has concerns about her ability to return to full-time work. This supervisor and the other administration officer have needed to cope with the extra duties in Leanne's absence.

6. Education/employment history
   - Leanne has worked in her role at the college for 12 years, since her younger child started school. She had paid time off when her children were young, and before that

worked as a secretary in a law firm. She completed high school then obtained a certificate in office studies.

7. Observations
- At the work visit, Leanne presents as a little anxious but speaks passionately about her job. She says she loves working with the students and her colleagues at the college, and enjoys the sense of belonging to the college community.
- She describes her work duties and expresses some concerns about her ability to handle some of the duties, like first aid, where she incurred her injury. She also expresses concerns about dealing with the busy times of her day, such as morning tea and lunch times, when the student queries increase, and the busy times of year, such as the end of the college year, which is approaching, when the principal's need for her administrative support peaks.

After gathering essential background information, the next step would be to view and assess Leanne's workstations in the office and observe her briefly at these workstations. This may be conducted at the first meeting, if given prior approval by the funder of the programme, or may require a separate visit after funder approval is obtained via the approved rehabilitation plan.

Summary of workstation assessment

Note: This could be assessed in more detail in an ergonomic workplace assessment.

The college office is located on the ground floor of the administration block, accessed by two stairs. Leanne's workstations include the enquiries counter, a computer workstation and a clerical workstation. There is little adjustability in these workstations, apart from the computer workstation, which has a manually adjustable desk and an adjustable chair for use at both computer and clerical workstations, which Leanne moves from one desk to the other. The enquiries counter has cupboards below, with no clearance for a stool. Leanne's first-aid duties also involve working in the first-aid/sick-bay room, which contains reclined lounges, a bed and a supply cupboard. The lounges and bed are low and not adjustable, so require low bending or squatting to access.

8. Recommendations

On the basis of the visit, the information gathered and the basic assessment of Leanne's duties and work environment, recommendations would be made to the insurer for a rehabilitation plan.

Step 3: Rehabilitation programme planning

The first step is to discuss and agree on a RTW goal from the hierarchy of RTW (see Fig. 16.3) As Leanne has a job available for her, the goal would be 'same job, same employer'.

If not already provided, the WRC would need to obtain Leanne's consent to acquire further information from other key stakeholders in the RTW rehabilitation process, such as the treating medical practitioners, chiropractor and family members.

The next step is to develop a rehabilitation plan to be approved by the payer and then, given approval, to implement and monitor the plan.

In developing the plan, the WRC would consider the facilitators or positive factors and barriers or negative factors in Leanne's situation for RTW.

Facilitators/strengths	Barriers
Job available	Persistent pain (>12 weeks)
Supportive employer and supervisor	Direct supervisor concerned about ability for RTW
Claim accepted and referred for rehabilitation	Worker fearful about activity and currently not active
Sound work history	Carer responsibilities as mother to school-aged children
Motivated for RTW	Difficulty with travel to work
Strong sense of belonging at workplace	Potential aggravators at work of physical demands and unsuitable physical environment, e.g. prolonged sitting and standing, non-adjustable multiuser workstations, manual handling of people and awkward postures

Another consideration in the development of the plan is what the current evidence is recommended for effective RTW. The seven principles of RTW, developed by the IWH, are helpful for the WRC in the development of a rehabilitation plan. For a case like Leanne's, where pain has persisted and she has had some failed attempts at RTW but no rehabilitation support to date so is becoming fearful and anxious about her chances of returning to full-time duties, the evidence supports the need for a safe and supported modified duties programme as soon as possible, wherein she can return to her duties gradually.

Step 4: Implementation and coordination of programme

See Rehabilitation plan. In addition to a suitable duties programme, the Plan is likely to include ergonomic equipment and training, communication with key stakeholders, education of Leanne about self-management of her condition, education of co-workers about the SDP, evaluation, travel and monitoring. It may also include a monitored exercise program, psychological counselling and workplace modifications if indicated.

Steps 5 and 6: Review and evaluation

The final steps in Leanne's case might be reported as follows:

Regular reviews were set up to monitor Leanne's SDP until she achieved a return to full-time hours and duties within 6 weeks, with restricted first-aid duties. On follow-up 13 weeks after the end of her programme, Leanne was maintaining her job and another staff member was trained for the first-aid role. Recommendations were made to the workplace for risk management training of staff for their duties, particularly in the manual handling of people, and this was conducted for the staff.

There are standardized tools available for gathering such information. One is the Worker Role Interview (WRI) (Velozo et al 1998). This tool, a semi-structured interview based on the Model of Human Occupation, is designed to evaluate the psychosocial and environmental aspects of work in the initial rehabilitation assessment process for the injured worker (Velozo et al 1998).

At this stage a formal screening of psychosocial factors may be indicated, particularly if there has been delayed RTW or unsuccessful prior attempts at RTW. Psychosocial factors are covered in-depth elsewhere in this book. The sorts of factors that may need screening or further formal measurement include those found to be risk factors for the development of chronicity from pain-related disability. These include perceived functional disability, pain-related fears, catastrophizing, depression, poor problem-solving, low expectancies of RTW and low self-efficacy for work-related activities (Sullivan et al 2005). A plethora of tools is now available for measurement of such factors (Foster et al 2010). Some composite tools are often advocated for early screening, for example the Örebro Musculoskeletal Pain Questionnaire (Linton & Boersma 2003), and show some good predictive properties, but are limited in helping identify the relative contribution of the variables they cover (Nicholas 2010). Recent evidence has challenged which of the psychosocial factors are most predictive of outcome, at least for people with back pain at the primary care stage (Foster et al 2010). This research challenged common assumptions about measuring only the 'usual suspects' (Nicholas 2010) of catastrophizing, fear-avoidance beliefs, anxiety and depression in showing that other factors, such as illness perceptions and self-efficacy, were most predictive of outcome.

It is important for WRCs to keep in mind these so-called 'yellow flags', as well as any possible 'blue' (worker's perception of the workplace) or 'black' (organizational or policy) flags, early in and throughout the workplace rehabilitation process (Main 2002; Shaw et al 2009). A useful step-by-step guide and recommendations for this screening were provided by a panel of experts in Shaw et al (2009).

For the job-seeker with pain, there are also some tools that may be useful to the WRC in this early stage of rehabilitation needs assessment. One is the Job-seeking Self-efficacy scale (Strauser & Berven 2006), which asks the job-seeker about their confidence in a range of areas, including self-presentation, handling disability and barriers in the job-seeking process and in executing the job search.

It is at this stage that, if not already provided by the referrer, consent is obtained from the worker to contact other important stakeholders in the rehabilitation process, such as the treating medical practitioner and other treatment providers (physiotherapists, chiropractors, etc.), the employer, the union representative if applicable, family members and so forth. In many cases, especially where the person has a job available, approval may be given for a workplace assessment to be conducted in conjunction with the initial needs assessment so that a modified RTW programme can begin as soon as possible.

3. Planning

Developing the RTW goal

An important part of managing the overall RTW process is developing the RTW goal and plan in conjunction with the worker, employer, treating medical practitioner and other key parties. The WRC needs to be able to select and consult appropriate members of a multidisciplinary team, including the person's medical practitioners, in order to propose and then monitor and review the RTW programme (Gibson et al 2002).

In developing the RTW goal, the WRC needs to consider the preferred hierarchy of RTW goals (see Fig. 16.3) 'but not at the expense of the worker's needs or the employer's capacity' (Heads of Workers' Compensation Authorities 2009, p. 7).

The formats for rehabilitation plans vary in different schemes. However, plans commonly include the items contained in Table 16.1, that is, the agreed goal, the objectives for achieving the goal, the services or actions proposed to achieve those objectives, the timeframe and cost for the services, and who is responsible for providing the service (CRS Australia 2006). Different schemes may have particular approved services for workplace rehabilitation and, when this is the case, the WRC needs to be careful not to fall into the trap of choosing services from the approved list, like ingredients for a recipe. Instead, the WRC needs to consider the facts for each individual case and develop the most cost-effective means of addressing the agreed goal from the RTW hierarchy. The

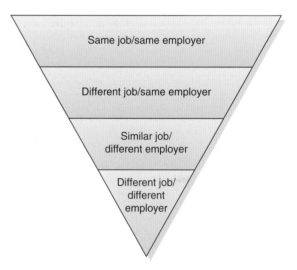

Fig. 16.3 Hierarchy of RTW goals.
Adapted from Heads of Workers' Compensation Authorities (2009).

Table 16.1 Rehabilitation plan format

Worker's name:			
Goal (from RTW hierarchy):			
Objective	Service/ action	Timeframe	Cost
(Will do what/why?)	(How?) Who		
Worker's signature:		Date:	
Rehabilitation consultant's signature:		Date:	

main concern for the approver of the plan is that they need to know who is doing what for how long, for how much and why, that is, how it is going to achieve the necessary outcome of RTW for the least amount of money. Plans need to be clear, concise and easy to read, especially for lay readers, such as the worker, employer or funder.

In developing the plan, the WRC can consider the strengths, facilitators or positive factors for the person's RTW, as well as the associated barriers, risks or negative factors (CRS Australia 2006). The WRC can also consider the current evidence for achieving effective RTW programmes. The seven principles of RTW, developed by the IWH, are helpful for the WRC in the development of a rehabilitation plan.

In the past there has been a strong focus on assessing the compatibility between the demands of the job and the capacities of the worker. Although this can be a helpful approach in guiding the development of a rehabilitation plan for getting a worker back to work, it may be that, just as unnecessary sickness certification can delay RTW at a critical window for early and safe RTW, so can an over-emphasis on assessment. The complexity of the nature of work, including the impact of psychosocial factors, can make accurate matching of functional capacities to job demands difficult (Pransky et al 2004). This is not to say that workers should return to duties that are not deemed safe and suitable for their capacities. Safety of the injured worker and co-workers is still paramount in designing a RTW programme. However, a new emphasis may be needed to ensure effective and durable RTW outcomes.

A NEW PARADIGM: AN EMPHASIS ON COMMUNICATION

Pransky et al (2004) provided a useful outline of four models of work disability prevention and management that have prevailed in recent years: (1) the medical model,

where the RTW plan is determined by the treating medical practitioner, who decides when and how the injured worker or job-seeker with a disability returns to work, (2) the physical rehabilitation model, where the worker or job-seeker improves their fitness for work through work simulation and physical conditioning activities, (3) the job-match model, as described above, where the worker's or job-seeker's functional abilities are assessed and matched against the physical demands of the job, and (4) the managed care model, where population norms of RTW for different injuries or disabilities are used as guidelines for RTW strategies.

In the absence or limited availability of evidence supporting these models and in light of emerging evidence about the value of early and effective communication in getting workers back to work, Pransky et al (2004) proposed a greater emphasis on communication at both individual and organizational levels for both injured workers in the occupational rehabilitation systems and job-seekers in the vocational rehabilitation system.

With a greater emphasis on communication, occupational rehabilitation requires SDPs developed as soon as possible and facilitation of workplace communication by key stakeholders, very similar to that supported by the IWH's seven principles of RTW. For the job-seeker with an injury, the evidence for programmes for job-seekers with severe mental health problems may apply as a useful model for other job-seekers, such as those with persistent pain. These programmes provide early, intensive job-seeking support, including peer-directed worksite visits and the training of job-seekers in effective communication skills such as prioritizing and assertiveness.

Subsequent evidence has confirmed the importance of early communication by the healthcare provider with the injured worker and the workplace, including the provision of RTW recommendation including a specific date for the expected RTW and proactive communication about preventing a recurrence of the injury (Kosny et al 2006).

OTHER MODELS

Another alternative model that may challenge current practice and enhance outcomes is the Readiness for Return-To-Work (RRTW) scale (Franche et al 2007), based on Prochaska and DiClemente's Readiness for Change Model (Prochaska & DiClemente 1983). Franche et al developed the RRTW scale to help gauge the worker or job-seeker's degree of acceptance of their situation, as well as their readiness for change and action for RTW.

The ICF also provides a framework that can be considered in planning RTW (Heerkens et al 2004). The ICF framework is used later in this chapter to illustrate the vocational rehabilitation process for a job-seeker with persistent pain needing to retrain for a new occupation.

RETURN-TO-WORK PROGRAMME HIERARCHY

Another approach to contemplating the worker or job-seeker's needs in getting back to the workforce is to consider a RTW hierarchy of strategies (Fig. 16.4). Based on the risk-control hierarchy that proposes the most effective means for reducing injury from hazards in the workplace, this hierarchy can be used as a guide in considering how to tackle and address any barriers to RTW for the worker with pain.

In the first instance, the WRC considers whether any potentially aggravating tasks can be eliminated or avoided, at least in the short term. Next, he or she thinks about how the workstation and/or wider workplace environment and/or tasks can be redesigned so that the worker can do the tasks with minimal aggravation. This will have a longer-term benefit as it will minimize the likelihood of re-injury and may have carry-over effects to preventing injury to other workers who use the same workstations. Failing this, the WRC considers whether adaptive strategies can be used to minimize the aggravation of discomfort, such as the worker gradually returning to work rather than all at once, using assistive technology or adaptive or personal protective equipment, or, if all else fails, educating the worker in how to perform the tasks for maximal comfort.

The RTW hierarchy is best used on the basis of the findings of a sound assessment of the workplace and the job duties, tasks, hours and environment. Such a workplace assessment, also referred to as an ergonomic assessment or job analysis, often provides the foundation for a workplace rehabilitation programme, especially where there is a job available and the potential exists for the worker to return to that job. The next section will outline this and other key services commonly provided in workplace rehabilitation programme plans.

Different jurisdictions can have different standards about which professionals can provide particular services (Heads of Workers' Compensation Authorities 2009). For example, in some jurisdictions, only particular professionals can provide workplace ergonomic assessments, functional capacity evaluations (FCEs) or vocational assessments, or set up SDPs. Specific systems can also set the costs for these different services and the approved time allowed for their provision.

WORKPLACE ASSESSMENT AND MODIFIED WORK/SUITABLE DUTIES PROGRAMMES

Although this chapter has raised concerns about the perils of over-assessment, there seems to be little argument in practice about, or evidence against, the value of a sound workplace assessment of the person's job, especially as a basis for the development of a modified work or suitable duties programme. Anema et al (2003) described a promising approach to workplace assessment for the development of modified work programmes based on the participatory ergonomics approach successfully used in injury prevention.

In this approach, the worker and supervisor are interviewed separately about the job and then the worker is observed in the workplace performing work tasks. A joint meeting to develop solutions for RTW then follows. In the separate interviews, the tasks and their resultant problems for the injured worker are noted, and the frequency

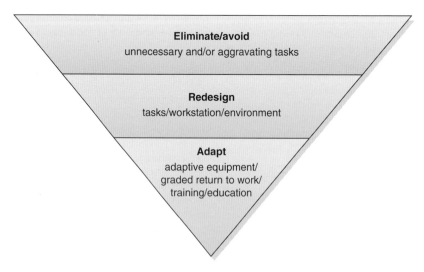

Eliminate/avoid
unnecessary and/or aggravating tasks

Redesign
tasks/workstation/environment

Adapt
adaptive equipment/
graded return to work/
training/education

Fig. 16.4 **RTW programme hierarchy of strategies.**

and severity of each problem is rated then prioritized. In the observations, checklists are used to note the physical demands of the job, the anthropometrical dimensions of equipment and tasks, collaboration with others, skills required on the job, and the materials and equipment used. In the joint meeting, the possible solutions are brainstormed separately then prioritized jointly based on their existence, feasibility and problem-solving capability. The value of such an approach may be in no small part due to the collaborative nature of the process and the fact that the worker and supervisor 'own' the solution, with the expert's input used to facilitate the solutions, rather than this input being imposed externally.

A cornerstone of this approach is the analysis of the physical demands of the job. Although recent evidence has identified the strength of psychosocial factors in influencing RTW, for workers with persistent pain the physical demands of the job can contribute to the cause and ongoing aggravation of discomfort at work and work-related disability (Hoogendoorn et al 2002; Shaw et al 2009). For workers with persistent pain who report significant concerns about their workplace for RTW, a worksite visit and more detailed assessment are indicated (Shaw et al 2009).

A number of standardized and non-standardized tools can be used by specialist professionals to assess the workplace (Innes 2008). The reader is directed to consult specialist resources or texts for further guidance on assessment of the workplace (e.g. Holmes 2007; Innes 2008).

SUITABLE DUTIES PROGRAMMES: THE CORNERSTONE OF RETURN-TO-WORK PROGRAMMES

This chapter has already argued a strong case for the provision of modified duties programmes to workers and job-seekers with pain, but the challenge for the WRC is how to develop them and where to start. The answer to this is both a science and an art, that is, it is based on a skilled sound assessment and some common principles, but getting them right is often simply a matter of trial and error. These principles include the following (Innes 1997):

1. Based on the right goal from the hierarchy of goals: Sometimes the worker at least needs to attempt a return to their job to determine whether he or she can indeed perform that job and sustain that performance. The best of assessments cannot replace the gold standard test of doing the actual job.
2. Compatible with the person's functional abilities, or the person at least has the potential to perform them in a modified way.
3. Safe: Safety is of utmost importance not just for the worker but also for co-workers.

4. Meaningful and productive: The duties have a purpose and contributes to the role, process or business of the workplace.
5. Compatible with the worker's age, education, skills and experience: When workers are from high-level physically demanding jobs in physically demanding industries, such as labouring jobs in construction, and may have little education, it is inappropriate for workers on SDPs to be placed in what are considered 'lighter' office jobs that require higher level literacy. It can be challenging for such companies to find alternative duties, but 'lighter' does not necessarily mean 'different duties.
6. Developed with the input of all key stakeholders: The importance of involving the worker and the supervisor has already been noted. It is also important that the worker's treating medical practitioner be consulted about the suitability of duties in terms of potential medical contraindications or precautions. Some jurisdictions require the signed approval of the treating medical practitioner on the SDP plan. The person's co-workers and/or the union or labour representative may also need to be consulted if the duties impact on other workers.
7. Well-graded: The challenge for the developer of the SDP can be choosing starting duties and hours, as it is important to start the worker at a level appropriate to their capacities without the likelihood for aggravation of the injury, but also productive enough to contribute to the work process without being disruptive. When deciding on the starting point and subsequent grading of the worker's duties, the WRC can consider choosing and grading specific duties, specific tasks within the duties, and hours and days of work. Duties and tasks can be graded from light to heavy and/or occasional to frequent. The WRC can be creative with days, hours and shifts. For example, it can be worthwhile considering a mid-week start for an SDP so that the person can work 3 days then have a weekend off for recovery in the critical commencement stage of the programme. In increasing hours, duties or days, it is important to try to change as little at a time as possible so that, if aggravations of the pain occur, the WRC and worker can more easily pinpoint the likely cause of the aggravation.
8. Monitored regularly: Monitoring can be conducted formally (e.g. using checklists or diaries) and informally through phone calls to the worker or supervisor or both.

The power of self-efficacy was mentioned previously in this chapter in terms of outcome. It may be that well-graded SDPs work well because they are an instrument of improving self-efficacy for RTW. SDPs may fit within Bandura's model of self-efficacy, which advocated four means of improving self-efficacy: (1) performance accomplishments, (2) vicarious learning, (3) emotional arousal and

(4) social persuasion (Bandura 1977, 1982, Betz 2004). Through the WRC supporting the worker to RTW gradually in a well-graded and safe way, is it that the SDP is a form of performance accomplishment with some social persuasion added? Through the supported performance of suitable duties, the person approaches their concerns rather than avoids them, and is required to persist in their performance, which feeds on itself to further improve confidence for RTW.

IMPROVING THE WORK ENVIRONMENT

After SDPs, workplace modification and provision of workplace aids and equipment or assistive devices are some of the most commonly provided services in work rehabilitation practice (Deen et al 2002). All of these strategies are aimed at improving the physical environment for the worker or job-seeker with pain-related disability. It must be noted that recent evidence for such interventions is not strong, but that the quality and quantity of the evidence is low. For example, a recent review challenged the benefit of devices such as lifting equipment for prevention of back pain disability (Martimo et al 2008); another recent systematic review of the effectiveness of physical and organizational ergonomic interventions on low back pain and neck pain found low to moderate quality evidence for such interventions being no more effective than no intervention (Driessen et al 2010). There is evidence that provides some support for devices such as standing aids (mats, foot-rests and sit-stand chairs) (Cham & Redfern 2001; Konz & Rys 2003; Krumwiede et al 1998) and ergonomic seating for some populations (Driessen et al 2010).

More high-quality research is needed to determine whether ergonomic modifications to the work environment are an effective strategy for durable RTW outcomes. WRCs need to keep up to date with emerging evidence about different technologies, devices and approaches. One of the key implications for practice, emerging from the limited evidence available to date, is that training and education are critical for successful and sustained use of workplace equipment. de Jonge and Gibson (2009) provide an overview of a user-centred process to develop solutions for improving the work and work environment fit using assistive technology. Further detail can be found in de Jonge et al (2007).

EDUCATION

Education of the worker with pain formerly had a focus on using so-called correct technique, for example for lifting objects and minimizing aggravation of pain. However, recent advances in neuroscience have demonstrated the complexity of the persistent pain experience and indicate the need for new approaches to education of the worker with pain (see Chapter 17). The AHP and WRC collaborating with a worker or job-seeker with pain need to know about these advances and be aware of the influence that his or her language and content of education can have on the worker or job-seeker. Current guidelines require simple messages of encouragement for the worker to stay active and at work (McGuirk & Bogduk 2007) and reassurance that he or she cannot expect to be pain-free before or during RTW (Royal Australasian College of Physicians 2009). It is critical that workers and job-seekers with pain obtain accurate information about their condition that allays unfounded fears of pain, re-injury, movement and work activities (McGuirk & Bogduk 2007).

Recent evidence also challenges the 'current widespread practice of advising workers on correct lifting technique' (Martimo et al 2008, p. 1). Indeed, there is conflicting evidence about which technique is indeed 'correct' (Straker 2003). The key role for the WRC in education may be in the role he or she provides in the rehabilitation process: to support and reassure the worker or job-seeker that they can indeed work or RTW, and to educate the other key stakeholders about how to make it happen.

OTHER SERVICES

Other services commonly provided in workplace rehabilitation programmes include FCEs, vocational assessment and work training or host employment. These services can be of particular value for the job-seeker needing to get into alternative employment.

The case of Stan (see Box 16.5) provides an example of how these services can be used to assist a job-seeker with a disability to return to employment in a new job with a new employer. It summarizes a programme using the ICF framework to illustrate how a programme can operate at different levels to achieve a durable RTW outcome.

Functional capacity evaluation

FCEs are assessments of a person's ability to perform a range of activities or tasks, such as lifting, standing, reaching, walking and carrying, from which recommendations are made about the person's capacity to perform these activities in the workplace (for the worker) or a potential job (for the job-seeker) (Innes & Straker 2002; James & Mackenzie 2009).

There has been a burgeoning of literature and evidence about FCE in the last decade and in a number of approaches. Innes (2006) provided a review of the psychometric properties of the many commercially available approaches. Step-by-step guides to the FCE process can be found in Chappell et al (2006) and Gibson (2009). Although the establishment of

---

Box 16.5 Case study: Stan – Example of vocational rehabilitation process (job-seeker) using ICF framework

Goal: New job/new employer

Background information:

- 32-year-old man with persistent back pain and sciatica since work incident lifting steel on job as dogger (rigger) 6 months earlier (interstate).
  - Medically certified as unable to return to heavy occupation as a dogger.
  - Received conservative treatment after accident; had a recent consultation with local neurosurgeon that showed no spinal pathology.

- Social situation:
  - Immigrated from eastern Europe 10 years before.
  - Married to Australian-born woman who works as teacher; 18-month-old son.
  - Limited social contacts outside immediate family and wife's local family.
- Employment history:
  - Education to grade 10 equivalent.
  - Fitter and turner apprenticeship overseas.
  - Manual labouring jobs since move to Australia.

	Impairment	Activity	Participation	Personal	Environmental
	Pain Reduced fitness	Unable to perform heavy physical demands of previous occupation	Unable to return to previous job; needing new job with different employer	Non-English-speaking background Highly motivated to return to work	Socially isolated since move interstate with young family
Assessments	Medical report Physiotherapy assessment	Functional capacity evaluation Workplace assessment of job activities	Vocational assessment of work history, interests and transferable skills	Interview about motivation for RTW Job-specific literacy assessment	Workplace assessment of workplace environment
Interventions	Physiotherapy Home fitness programme	Graded RTW activities Functional education in workplace	Work training with host employers in engine reconditioning Supported job search	Case management and support for RTW Literacy training for administrative duties of job	Workplace equipment (trolley) to reduce manual handling on job

---

the predictive validity of FCEs remains elusive, with some evidence questioning their predictive value (e.g. Gross & Battie 2005; Streibelt et al 2009), there is also some support for their utility in making RTW recommendations (Oesch et al 2006, Wind et al 2006, 2009).

FCEs are often used in conjunction with a vocational assessment (explained later in this chapter) to help the multidisciplinary process of determining alternative vocational options for workers with no job to which they can return (Innes & Straker 2002). An example of their utility in practice is illustrated in the job-seeker case (Stan), where knowing Stan's specific capacities for manual handling gave the WRCs the confidence to support him in job-seeking and on-the-job training in the area of engine reconditioning.

On-the-job training

On-the-job training (CRS Australia) – also called work training schemes or host employment placements (WorkCover Qld, 2005) can be a powerful tool for getting job-seekers with a disability into new jobs. These schemes vary in different systems and countries, but the principles are much the same. The schemes allow employers the opportunity to give the job-seeker with a disability a trial on the job without having to pay them (the job-seeker remains on welfare, workers' compensation or insurance payments) and without risk of exposure to workers' compensation claims for any aggravation of the injury, as the schemes cover the job-seeker for workers' compensation, sometimes for all claims, but at least for aggravation of pre-existing injuries. This can be an excellent way for a job-seeker with a disability to trial employment and to demonstrate to employers that they can perform the duties of the job.

The principles for developing and monitoring SDPs outlined earlier in this chapter could also be applied to the development and monitoring of work training.

Vocational assessment

Sometimes, job-seekers with persistent pain who cannot return to their previous occupation have no existing or suitable transferable skills that they can draw on to gain employment. In these cases, a vocational assessment may be required to help ascertain potential new occupations for the job-seeker and the need for training. Such assessment can include exploration of work interests, values and transferable skills. It may be carried out as a formal assessment of intelligence and aptitudes (Power 2000) through use of standardized tests, such as questionnaires and profiles, or it may take a naturalistic form, using interviews and on-the-job assessments (Hagner 2010).

IMPLEMENTATION, REVIEW AND EVALUATION

The final steps of the workplace rehabilitation process are by no means the least. They are where effective and timely communication can be critical to ensure a durable RTW. Different schemes have different provisions for the time and costs attached to such services, but these stages can be the most critical to the programme's success. The WRC needs to maintain regular reviews to ensure that services are mobilized in a timely and cost-effective manner, streamlining with any concurrent treatment services and avoiding duplication of services (Heads of Workers' Compensation Authorities 2009). This phase is where dialogue between key parties can be critical to prevent possible breakdowns in communication and ensure prevention of re-injury.

The last step in the process is evaluation or outcome measurement or management. This is where objective measures are used to determine the efficiency and/or effectiveness of interventions (Clifton 2005). Efficiency usually relates to administrative aspects (Clifton 2005) such as cost and length of programme. Effectiveness can include outcomes such as durable RTW and satisfaction with the service. Different schemes may have different outcome evaluation requirements, for example that a person sustains a return to employment for 13 weeks before the case can be closed or payment forwarded by the funder to the rehabilitation provider. On case closure, the WRC needs to consider and advise on any ongoing or potential future needs of the worker for maintenance of employment (Heads of Workers' Compensation Authorities 2009), such as health services or equipment maintenance or replacement.

Q Study questions/questions for revision

1. What are some physical/emotional/social/financial problems an injured worker might face when returning to work, and how can the WRC help to combat these?
2. What are some problems employers and/or co-workers might face in relation to an injured worker returning to work, and how can the WRC help to address these?
3. Which assessments might the WRC perform to establish the needs and preferences of the injured worker or job-seeker?
4. Which assessments might the WRC perform to establish the suitability of a workplace/workload for the injured worker or job-seeker?
5. What steps are involved in achieving a successful RTW programme?

REFERENCES

Access Economics, 2007. The high price of pain: The economic impact of persistent pain in Australia. Available: http://www.accesseconomics.com.au/publicationsreports/search.php?searchfor=chronic+pain&from=0 (11.09.08).

Amick, B.C., Habeck, R.V., Hunt, A., et al., 2000. Measuring the impact of organizational behaviors on work disability prevention and management. J. Occup. Rehabil. 10 (1), 21–38.

Anema, J.R., Steenstra, I.A., Urlings, I.J.M., et al., 2003. Participatory ergonomics as a return-to-work intervention: A future challenge? Am. J. Ind. Med. 44 (3), 273–281.

Bandura, A., 1977. Self-efficacy: Toward a unifying theory of behavioural change. Psychol. Rev. 84 (2), 191–215.

Bandura, A., 1982. Self-efficacy mechanism in human agency. Am. Psychol. 37 (2), 122–147.

Betz, N.E., 2004. Contributions of self-efficacy theory to career counselling: A personal perspective. Career Development Quarterly. 52 (4), 340–353.

Calkins, J., Lui, J.W., Wood, C., 2000. Recent developments in integrated disability management: Implications for professional and organisational development. J. Vocat. Rehabil. 15 (1), 31–37.

Cham, R., Redfern, M.S., 2001. Effect of flooring on standing comfort and fatigue. Hum. Factors. 43 (3), 381–391.

Chappell, I., Henry, A., McLean, A., et al., 2006. In:Strong, S. (Ed.), The Functional Capacity Evaluation: A Clinician's Guide. Canadian Association of Occupational Therapists, Ottawa.

Chou, R., Qaseem, A., Snow, V., et al., for the Clinical Efficacy Assessment Subcommittee of the American College of Physicians and the American College of Physicians/American Pain Society Low Back Pain Guidelines Panel, 2007. Diagnosis and treatment of low back pain: A joint clinical practice guideline from the American College of Physicians and the American Pain Society. Ann. Intern. Med. 147 (7), 478–491.

Clifton, D.W., 2005. Outcomes management. In: Clifton, D.W. (Ed.), Physical Rehabilitation's Role in Disability Management: Unique Perspectives for Success. Elsevier Saunders, St Louis, MO.

CRS Australia (compiled), 2006. Case Management: A Framework for Success. CRS Australia, Braddon, ACT.

CRS Australia, List of our services. Available: http://www.crsaustralia. gov.au/list_of_our_services.htm#voc_axmt.

Dagenais, S., Caro, J., Haldeman, S., 2008. A systematic review of low back pain cost of illness studies in the United States and internationally. Spine J. 8 (1), 8–20.

Deen, M., Gibson, L., Strong, J., 2002. A survey of occupational therapy in Australian work practice. Work 19 (2), 219–230.

de Jonge, D., Gibson, L., 2009. Effective utilization of assistive devices in the workplace. In: Kumar, S. (Ed.), Ergonomics for Rehabilitation Professionals. First, ed. Taylor & Francis, Boca Raton FL.

de Jonge, D., Schere, M.J., Rodger, S., 2007. Assistive Technology in the Workplace. Mosby Elsevier, St Louis, MO.

Driessen, M.T., Proper, K.I., van Tulder, M.W., et al., 2010. The effectiveness of physical and organisational ergonomic interventions on low back pain and neck pain: A systematic review. Occup. Environ. Med. 67 (4), 277–285.

Foster, N.E., Thomas, E., Bishop, A., et al., 2010. Distinctiveness of psychological obstacles to recovery in low back pain patients in primary care. Pain 148 (3), 398–406.

Franche, R.L., Corbière, M., Lee, H., et al., 2007. The Readiness for Return-To-Work (RRTW) scale: Development and validation of a self-report staging scale in lost-time claimants with musculoskeletal disorders. J. Occup. Rehabil. 17 (3), 450–472.

Friesen, M.N., Yassi, A., Cooper, J., 2001. Return-to-work: The importance of human interactions and organizational structures. Work 17 (1), 11–22.

Gibson, L., Allen, M., Strong, J., 2002. Reintegration into work. In: Strong, J., Unruh, A., Wright, A., Baxter, G.D. (Eds.), Pain: A textbook for therapists. Harcourt, Edinburgh, pp. 67–287.

Gibson, L., 2009. Functional capacity evaluation: An integrated approach to assessing work activity limitations. In: Söderback, I. (Ed.), International Handbook of Occupational Therapy Interventions. Springer Science + Business Media, Inc, Dordrecht, pp. 497–505.

Gross, D.P., Battie, M.C., 2005. Functional capacity evaluation performance does not predict sustained return to work in claimants with chronic back pain. J. Occup. Rehabil. 15 (3), 285–294.

Hagner, D., 2010. The role of naturalistic assessment in vocational rehabilitation. J. Rehabil. 76 (1), 28–34.

Heads of Workers' Compensation Authorities, 2009. Nationally Consistent Approval Framework for Workplace Rehabilitation Providers. Available: http://www.hwca.org.au/projects.php.

Heerkens, Y., Engels, J., Kuipers, C., et al., 2004. The use of the ICF to describe work related factors influencing the health of employees. Disabil. Rehabil. 26 (17), 1060–1066.

Holmes, J., 2007. Vocational Rehabiltation. Blackwell Publishing, Oxford, Malden, MA.

Hoogendoorn, W.E., Bongers, P.M., de Vet, H.C.W., et al., 2002. High physical work load and low job satisfaction increase the risk of sickness absence due to low back pain: Results of a prospective cohort study. Occup. Environ. Med. 59 (5), 323–328.

Hush, J.M., 2008. Clinical management of occupational low back pain in Australia: What is the real picture? J. Occup. Rehabil. 18 (4), 375–380.

Innes, E., 1997. Work assessment options and the selection of suitable duties: An Australian perspective. N. Z. J. Occup. Ther. 48 (1), 14–20.

Innes, E., 2006. Reliability and validity of functional capacity evaluations: An update. Int. J. Disabil. Manag. Res. 1 (1), 135–148

Innes, E., 2008. Ergonomics and work assessments. In: Jacobs, K. (Ed.), Ergonomics for Therapists, third ed.

Elsevier Mosby, St Louis, MO, London, pp. 48–72.

Innes, E., Straker, L., 2002. Workplace assessments and functional capacity evaluations: Current practices of therapists in Australia. Work 18 (1), 51–56.

Institute for Work & Health, 2007. Seven 'principles' for successful return to work. Institute for Work & Health. Online. Available: http://www.iwh.on.ca/files/seven_principles_rtw_2007.pdf (2.05.07).

James, C., Mackenzie, L., 2009. Health professional's perceptions and practices in relation to functional capacity evaluations: Results of a quantitative survey. J. Occup. Rehabil. 19 (2), 203–211.

Konz, S.A., Rys, M.J., 2003. An ergonomics approach to standing aids. Occupational Ergonomics 3 (3), 165–172.

Kosny, A., Franche, R.L., Pole, J., et al., 2006. Early healthcare provider communication with patients and their workplace following a lost-time claim for an occupational musculoskeletal injury. J. Occup. Rehabil. 16 (1), 25–37.

Krumwiede, D., Konz, S., Hinnen, P., 1998. Standing comfort on floor mats. Occupational Ergonomics 1 (2), 135–143.

Linton, S.J., Boersma, K., 2003. Early identification of patients at risk of developing a persistent back problem: the predictive validity of the Örebro Musculoskeletal Pain Questionnaire. Clin. J. Pain 19 (2), 80–86.

Lippel, K., 2007. Workers describe the effect of the workers' compensation process on their health: A Quebec study. Int. J. Law Psychiatry 30 (4–5), 427–443.

Maetzel, A., Li, L., 2002. The economic burden of low back pain: A review of studies published between 1996 and 2001. Best Pract. Res. Clin. Rheumatol. 16 (1), 23–30.

Main, C., 2002. Concepts of treatment and prevention in musculoskeletal disorders. In: Linton, S.J. (Ed.), New Avenues for the Prevention of Chronic Musculoskeletal Pain and Disability., Pain Research and Clinical Management, vol. 12. pp. 47–63.

Martimo, K.P., Verbeek, J., Karppinen, J., et al., 2008. Effect of training and lifting equipment for preventing back pain in lifting and handling:

Systematic review. Br. Med. J. 336 (7641), 429–431.

McGuirk, B., Bogduk, N., 2007. Evidence-based care for low back pain in workers eligible for compensation. Occup. Med. 57 (1), 36–42.

Nicholas, M.K., 2010. Obstacles to recovery after an episode of low back pain; the 'usual suspects' are not always guilty. Pain 148 (3), 363–364.

Oesch, P.R., Kool, J.P., Bachmann, S., et al., 2006. The influence of a Functional Capacity Evaluation on fitness for work certificates in patients with non-specific chronic low back pain. Work. 26 (3), 259–271.

Patel, S., Greasley, K., Watson, P.J., 2007. Barriers to rehabilitation and return to work for unemployed chronic pain patients: A qualitative study. Eur. J. Pain 11 (8), 831–840.

Power, P.W., 2000. A Guide to Vocational Assessment, third ed. Pro-Ed, Austin, TX.

Pransky, G.S., Shaw, W.S., Franche, R.L., et al., 2004. Disability prevention and communication among workers, physicians, employers, and insurers – current models and opportunities for improvement. Disabil. Rehabil. 26 (11), 625–634.

Prochaska, J.O., Di Clemente, C.C., 1983. Towards a comprehensive model of change. In: Prochaska, J.O., DiClemente, C.C. (Eds.), A Transtheoretical Approach: Crossing the Traditional Boundaries of Therapy. Dow Jones, Homewood, IL.

Royal Australasian College of Physicians, Australasian Faculty of Occupational and Environmental Medicine, 2009. Realising the Health Benefits of Work – Draft AFOEM Position Statement for Comment. Available: http://afom.racp.edu.au/page/media-and-news/news-and-announcements/realising-the-health-benefits-of-work-draft-afoem-position-statement-for-comment.

Shaw, W., Hong, Q., Pransky, G., et al., 2008. A literature review describing the role of return-to-work coordinators in trial programs and interventions designed to prevent workplace disability. J. Occup. Rehabil. 18 (1), 2–15

Shaw, W.S., van der Windt, D.A., Main, C.J., et al., Decade of the Flags Working Group, 2009. Early patient screening and intervention to address individual-level occupational factors ('blue flags') in back disability. J. Occup. Rehabil. 19 (1), 64–80.

Straker, L.M., 2003. A review of research on lifting techniques for lifting low-lying objects: 2. Evidence for a correct technique. Work 20 (2), 83–96.

Strauser, D., Berven, N.L., 2006. Construction and field testing of the Job Seeking Self-Efficacy Scale. Rehabil. Counsel. Bull. 49 (4), 207–218

Streibelt, M., Blume, C., Thren, K., et al., 2009. Value of functional capacity evaluation information in a clinical setting for predicting return to work. Arch. Phys. Med. Rehabil. 90 (3), 429–434.

Sullivan, M.J., Feuerstein, M., Gatchel, R., et al., 2005. Integrating psychosocial and behavioral interventions to achieve optimal rehabilitation outcomes. J. Occup. Rehabil. 15 (4), 475–489.

Velozo, C., Kielhofner, G., Fisher, G., 1998. A user's guide to Worker Role Interview (WRI) (Version 9.0) Model of Human Occupational Clearinghouse. Department of Occupational Therapy, College of Health and Human Development Sciences, University of Illinois at Chicago, Chicago, IL.

Waddell, G., Burton, A.K., 2005. Concepts of rehabilitation for the management of low back pain. Best Pract. Res. Clin. Rheumatol. 19 (4), 655–670.

Waddell, G., Burton, A., 2006. Is work good for your health and well-being? The Stationery Office, London.

Whysall, Z., Haslam, C., Haslam, R., 2006. Implementing health and safety interventions in the workplace: An exploratory study. International J. Indust. Ergonom. 36 (9), 809–818

Williams, R.M., Westmorland, M., 2002. Perspectives on workplace disability management: A review of the literature. Work 19 (1), 87–93.

Wind, H., Gouttebarge, V., Kuijer, P.P.F.M., et al., 2006. The utility of functional capacity evaluation: The opinion of physicians and other experts in the field of return to work and disability claims. Int. Arch. Occup. Environ. Health 79 (6), 528–534.

Wind, H., Gouttebarge, V., Kuijer, P.P.F.M., et al., 2009. Complementary value of functional capacity evaluation for physicians in assessing the physical work ability of workers with musculoskeletal disorders. Int. Arch. Occup. Environ. Health 82 (4), 435–443.

WorkCover Qld, 2005. Host suitable duties – six-month exemption. Available: https://www.workcoverqld.com.au/Formsa362sheets/Hostsu559tsheet.pdf.

World Health Organization, 2001. International classification of functioning, disability and health. ICF, Geneva.

Section | 3 |

Special issues

Chapter | 17 |

Pain education for professionals

Emma Briggs and Sarah E. Henderson

LEARNING OBJECTIVES

By the end of this chapter readers will be able to:
- Assess their current learning needs around pain management and identify effective learning strategies.
- Discuss the skills needed and opportunities for interprofessional learning and working in pain management.
- Outline the issues and opportunities in undergraduate, postgraduate and in-service pain education.
- Describe the need for continuing professional development and opportunities for further study.

OVERVIEW

In 2010, the International Association for the Study of Pain (IASP; International Association for the Study of Pain 2010) launched the Declaration of Montreal, an important statement highlighting the fundamental human right to an appropriate assessment by healthcare professionals, access to pain relief and specialist referral where relevant. A major knowledge deficit in healthcare professionals was one of the reasons IASP gave for inadequate pain management worldwide. Education can be a powerful solution to addressing gaps in knowledge, but having an understanding of pain is only part of the picture. Providing patients with effective pain management also requires a range of skills, understanding our own attitudes, limitations and insight into our own learning needs. This chapter focuses on the education of healthcare professionals, helping readers to refine their skills for supporting patients in pain, discusses collaborative learning and working, highlights important issues for undergraduates and postgraduates, and signposts readers to further educational resources. The chapter is aimed at both learners and those delivering pain education to professionals.

BUILDING A KNOWLEDGE BASE AND IDENTIFYING KEY SKILLS

Managing patients in pain is a complex process; an interaction between two (or more) people with different

© 2014 Elsevier Ltd.

experiences of pain in their lifetime, different family and cultural backgrounds, different communication styles, knowledge base, attitudes and skills around pain. It is easy to assume that patients and healthcare professionals are working towards the same target, but they may not have negotiated specific goals and may have different expectations. An assessment is required; identification of the likely mechanisms and contributing factors, decisions and negotiations on appropriate treatments and referrals, there is patient education needed and later an evaluation of treatments provided. Healthcare professionals require several core skills to help patients manage pain and so understanding our educational needs starts with identifying current skills, knowledge and attitudes.

Identifying specific learning needs involves assessing your current strengths in managing pain and identifying priority areas for development. An interesting starting point is to evaluate attitudes and feelings around pain which can have a significant impact on the way we interact and support others. Spend a few minutes considering the points in Box 17.1, which should lead you to think about your own attitudes and may challenge existing thinking.

Learning pain management skills and knowledge is more effective if the starting point is acknowledged and people identify their current learning needs. Table 17.1 presents a skills profile with some key pain management areas to start thinking about strengths and areas for development. Writing goals can help to identify the next steps, taking into account the educational resources you have access to.

Once you have identified your learning needs and have a specific plan, you may want to access independent learning resources on pain management. Table 17.2 highlights a few of the available resources.

Learning experiences and strategies

We all have experienced successful learning moments where we were inspired, motivated to learn and there is a positive outcome. A number of factors may have contributed to this situation (an interesting topic, an inspirational teacher) but one tool that can accelerate learning in pain management is metacognition. Metacognition is often referred to as 'learning about learning' or 'knowing about knowing' (Postholm 2011) and it describes the knowledge of your preferred approach to learning and skills in choosing a learning technique in a given situation. For example, Philippe is a year 3 undergraduate who has met a patient on placement with complex regional pain syndrome, a condition he wants to learn more about. Philippe is aware that his learning is most effective when there are visual and auditory stimuli so plans his learning accordingly, choosing to access an online video first. He later supplements this with written material and presents the patient as case study to his peers as a way of evaluating his own understanding and sharing his learning. Study skills textbooks can provide valuable resources and information to refine your metacognitive skills, provide useful tools to assess learning styles and preferences as well as advice on maximizing learning from different experiences such as lectures, group work etc. (e.g. Burns & Sinfield 2008; Cottrell 2008).

Formal pain education may come in different forms and employs a range of learning strategies; including lectures, seminars, e-learning or blended learning (a purposeful mix of face-to-face and e-learning). People may prefer one strategy over another but they all have a contribution to make in enhancing particular knowledge and skills. Here, a few recommendations are given to maximize your learning using face-to-face and online experiences.

Making the most of lectures

Whether you are attending a study day, seminar or a formal programme of study, lectures will form a key part of pain management education. Preparation and using key techniques during and after the lecture can make the learning much deeper. Beforehand, read through any previous lecture notes and key texts to get a sense of the topic and the key terms. Write down any terms that are unclear and questions you would like to ask, leaving space for the

---

> **Box 17.1 Reflection point: What is your attitude towards pain?**
>
> Spend 5–10 minutes considering the following points on attitudes and expression of pain:
>
> - Think of a recent pain experience. How do you express pain and how do the people around you react?
> - How do you react to pain expressed by your friends and family?
> - How do you react to pain expressed by patients and is it different from the way you react to friends and family?
> - Suja is in severe pain, crying loudly and pleading for someone to help her. The therapist assessing her is a quiet person who is stoical when he experiences pain. How might the therapist react to this pain expression that is different from his own?
> - Consider your opinion around the following topics:
>   - Pain arising for surgery compared to persistent pelvic pain with no history of trauma or surgery.
>   - Administering opioids to a cancer patient compared to giving opioids to someone with a history of substance misuse.
>   - Think about why you hold these beliefs. Is it because of experience with a particular patient, media stories, knowledge of the topic? Do you have any research evidence or national guidelines to support or challenge your belief or assumption?

Table 17.1 Pain management knowledge and skills profile

Knowledge/skill	Confidence rating			
	None/limited confidence	**Some confidence**	**Fairly confident**	**Confident**
Core skills				
Effective communication skills with people in pain				
Perform a comprehensive pain assessment				
Problem solving and decision making in pain management				
Assess the patient's educational level (health literacy) and needs				
Negotiate goals and provide appropriate patient education				
Liaise with the interprofessional team and make appropriate referrals				
Ensure effective documentation				
Locate and evaluate published research on pain management				
Reflect critically on practice, identifying potential barriers				
Other:				

	No/limited knowledge	**Some knowledge**	**Good knowledge**	**Very good knowledge**
Core knowledge and understanding				
Pain neuroanatomy and physiology				
Impact of pain and influencing factors				
Psychology and sociology of pain				
Pain assessment tools and frameworks				
Specific pain types Nocicpetive/inflammatory pain Neuropathic pain Generalized/dysfunctional pain				
Pharmacology				
Cognitive-based interventions				
Physical/manual therapies				
Role of specialist pain teams				
Other:				
Actions Identify the areas for development, describing how these can be achieved (e.g. further reading, electronic resources, rehearsals in practice) and a target date. Try to ensure that goals are SMART (specific, measurable, achievable, realistic, time management; Egan 1986)				

Table 17.2 Resources for independent learning about pain

Resource	Examples
Books	An enormous range of books is available, including general introductory texts, condition-specific and patient education books. These can be accessed through public, NHS and university libraries
Journals	British Journal of Pain European Journal of Pain Journal of Pain and Symptom Management Pain
Websites of professional organizations	British Pain Society, International Association for the Study of Pain
Pain-related charities	
general	Pain UK
condition specific	Pelvic Pain Support Network, Pain Community Centre website
Online videos or lectures publically available	SlideShare, Henry Stewart Lectures Series
Lectures series that require an institutional subscription	British Pain Society publications
National guidelines	National Institute for Heath & Clinical Excellence, Scottish Intercollegiate Guidelines Network

answers (Cottrell 2008). Suggestions for making notes more meaningful include:

- Use key headings and list the points – avoid writing everything down. Details can be obtained later from a textbook and this will help you listen.
- Try to actively make connections with existing knowledge and ask questions (Is this always the case? Do I agree?).
- Consider using the pattern note-making system (similar to mind maps; see Burns & Sinfield 2008 for details) where you identify keywords and link them together to create a visual representation of the topic. This is an active learning strategy that promotes the connections of ideas and concepts.
- As soon as possible after the lecture, read through lecture notes and add any additional detail from other sources and discuss the ideas explored with other people (Burns & Sinfield 2008; Cottrell 2008).

Group work

Group works offers an opportunity for collaborative learning, shared workload and responsibility and social support (Burns & Sinfield 2008; Cottrell 2008). Interpersonal skills and techniques such as negotiation, giving and receiving feedback, problem solving and summarizing arguments are skills that can be rehearsed and refined. Any aspect of interprofessional learning (two or more professions learning and working together) will involve group work, reflecting the skills needed for pain management practice.

Effective group work relies on motivated members who are willing to share ideas to clarifying their own thinking but also willing to listen to others and arrive at a consensus. It is essential that that group members work together to:

- understand the task required
- brainstorm, make notes and plan how the end goal will be reached
- follow the agreed action plan
- offer positive and constructive feedback
- review findings and leave time to proof-read and practice presentations (Burns & Sinfield 2008).

Early on in group work, it is useful to establish the ground rules, decide how you will communicate outside of meetings (e.g. email, web discussion board, social networking site) and identify key roles to assist the team to engage and successfully complete the activity or assignment. These may include group chair, note-taker and coordinator for completed tasks. Ensure that the workload is evenly spread and everyone has a chance to contribute. Regularly review the group's progress: How supportive are the group? Do one or two people dominate the discussion? Could the discussion have been organized differently? How well did you contribute? Always aim to be a supportive, critical friend who is 'a trusted person who asks provocative questions, provides data to be examined through another lens, and offers critiques of a person's work as a friend. A critical friend takes the time to fully understand the context of the work presented and the outcomes that the person or group is working towards. The friend is an advocate for the success of that work. (Costa & Kallick 1993, p. 49)

E-learning

Technology-enhanced learning is a feature of most university courses and study days. E-learning can take place individually or as a group, will use a range of online resources and have specific learning outcomes. Be aware of the resources you have available to you at university and the personal equipment that would aid your learning. Check the technological system requirements before staring courses, including adequate connectivity (for downloading videos and online lectures) and access to an appropriate mobile or computing device. E-learning may include:

- using a virtual learning environment (a web-based programme for resources, discussions and assessments)

- downloadable lecture notes, podcasts and presentations
- e-communications – email, live chat (synchronous discussion in real time), discussion boards (asynchronous discussion)
- use of web cams and video links
- simulation and interactive materials
- activities such as wikis (a website that allows collaborative working, contributions and editing) and blogs (an online discussion thread by an individual or group) or creating an e-portfolio
- computer assisted assessment (based on Cottrell 2008).

E-learning is an active learning process that may be challenging, especially if unfamiliar systems and new activities are used. Approach these new experiences with an open mind and willingness to learn about how to learn in this new way as well as taking away new pain-management knowledge and skills. One of the great benefits of e-learning is an ability to personalize your learning around pain based on identified needs or your skills profile. For example, in the classroom, an introductory session on pain physiology can be revisited for revision but then further resources may help people apply this to new knowledge to areas such the neurophysiology of pain in children. Try to treat e-learning on pain in the same was as other learning methods: create a physical or electronic file, gathering resources and making notes. If e-learning is new to you, Cottrell (2008) provides a good chapter on making learning more effective.

UNDERGRADUATE EDUCATION

Undergraduates can have very different experiences of how, when and what they learn about pain management as part of the pre-registration programmes. This section describes what we know about pain education in the UK and explores strategies for learners and academics to maximize learning and enhance pain management in the curricula.

The amount of pain education in undergraduate programmes for healthcare professions varies enormously. A UK survey of 19 universities (108 undergraduate programmes) revealed that students had between 2 and 158 hours on pain management although the average was just 12 hours (Briggs et al 2011). Some programmes offered separate pain modules (n = 11, 14.8%), although most of these were optional rather than core to all students. The predominant learning strategies used were lectures (n = 65, 87.8%) and case studies (n =, 78.4%) with around a third using e-learning resources. How learning is encouraged can make a difference. All learning strategies have their strengths and weaknesses, but lectures in particular have been criticized as promoting a passive rather than active learning experience, encouraging surface learning (knowledge recall) rather than deep learning (engaging, problem solving, making connections between ideas)

and does not help people apply or analyse new knowledge (Light et al 2009; Ramsden 2003). As we have seen earlier, healthcare professionals involved in pain management need a range of skills, knowledge and education needs to encourage this development. Learners, clinicians and academics can all do something to improve the learning experience around pain.

Learners on undergraduate programmes

As well as understanding your own learning needs and refining the metacognitive skills, there are other things that learners can do individually or as a group to maximize their learning around pain. First, use your skills profile and take a proactive approach to learning opportunities as they arise on your programme. This could involve reading around the topic, seeking out case studies before lectures to provide you with a 'scaffold' upon which to apply new knowledge and make new connections in the classroom.

The curriculum will involve a broad range of topics and conditions, and pain will feature in many cases. Try to consider the pain-related issues in every situation, reflecting on the impact it has on people and the management of their condition. Think about the professionals that may be involved in their care and their role in that situation. For example, the topic of human immunodeficiency virus (HIV) could be studied in terms of the virology, diagnosis, impact and recommended treatment and care. However, up to 69.4% will experience painful HIV-related neuropathy (Ghosh et al 2012) and this will need to be explored and understood along with an insight into the role of the interprofessional team.

Take opportunities to feed back on the pain teaching and learning provided and highlight areas for development. This can be done individually or in a group or cohort. Seeking opportunities in practice to refine pain management and collaborative skills will also help your professional development. Short placement experiences with specialist teams that provide inpatient, outpatient or community pain services can offer a rich opportunity to accelerate your learning of pain management. Finally, continue to develop your skills and knowledge after graduation by attending in-service education and postgraduate programmes (see the section on postgraduate education for a detailed discussion).

Academics and clinicians promoting pain education

Introducing changes to the curriculum can present a number of challenges and it is important to identify and try to predict the issues so that they can hopefully be addressed. Gibbins et al (2009) interviewed curriculum coordinators in 50% of UK medical schools to explore the factors that help or hinder the introduction of palliative care into their

Box 17.2 Developing pain in the curriculum (based on the themes from Gibbins et al 2009)

- Identify a champion to speak for speciality and influence curriculum leaders.
- Gather evidence – map out where pain is in the curricula.
- Use key documents to provide evidence, including:
  - research data (e.g. Briggs et al 2011; Watt-Watson et al 2009)
  - national policy documents to drive change (e.g. Chief Medical Officer's Report, Donaldson 2009; National Pain Summit documents (www.painsummit.org.uk)
  - patient/charity group reports that recommend improvements in education (e.g. Help the Aged & British Pain Society 2008; Patient's Association 2010)
  - guidance from professional regulators around pain management competencies where available (e.g. General Medical Council 2009)
- Assess current student knowledge and attitudes using questionnaires.
- Gather student feedback on pain management teaching in their programme.
- Aim to make major changes when the curriculum is under review and being redeveloped.
- Foster partnerships between clinical and academic settings.
- Develop placement opportunities where students can experience specialist pain services.
- Try to incorporate pain management in all parts of the learning journey, including academic and clinical assessments.
- Review the paper and electronic resources available, including internet resources.

programmes. The themes that emerged are familiar issues and transferable to the topic of pain. These have been used as a basis for the recommendations in Box 17.2, which contains suggestions for supporting change.

The perceived importance of pain management by the wider academic community may have an important role to play in the lack of emphasis in undergraduate courses. One author (EB) was asked at a conference how to respond to the dean of a health school who had been asked by his faculty staff to introduce pain teaching sessions. The dean replied to the request by saying; 'I have a huge number of penguins on the iceberg, which one do you want me to push off to fit pain in?' Changing perceptions and attitudes can take time, relationship building, interpersonal skills and a specific strategy.

The strategy should involve identifying the key stakeholders, including students, academics, curriculum leads and clinical partners. Reviewing existing teaching and learning strategies and content, and building a case (one that keeps the patient experience and the importance of pain management at the centre of the argument) can be helpful. Box 17.2 also contains some useful documents with statistics that can assist in building this case. Patient/user groups can also be strong advocates for change and can advise on curriculum content as well as contributing to the actual delivery of sessions, thus having a powerful impact on learners (see Terry 2012 for example).

Building discipline-specific and interprofessional networks locally and with national groups can provide support for champions of pain education as well as continuous professional development opportunities. Special interest groups (SIGs) may be generic (e.g. the Higher Education Academy Interprofessional SIG) or specific to pain (e.g. British Pain Society or IASP Pain education SIGs). Discipline-specific networks exist, such as the Pain Physiotherapy Association and the Royal College of Nursing Pain and Palliative Care Forum (see web links at the end of this chapter).

INTERPROFESSIONAL LEARNING AND WORKING

The World Health Organization (2010) highlighted the need for a collaborative, practice-ready work force, professionals who have learned to work together in order to provide better services for patients and improve health outcomes. Pain management is an interprofessional activity and requires understanding of each other's roles and close collaboration to provide effective management. Interprofessional education (IPE) has key role to play in this and the Centre for Advancement of Interprofessional Education (Centre for the Advancement of Interprofessional Education 2002) considers IPE as occurring in work-based or academic settings 'when two or more professions learn with, from and about each other to improve collaboration and the quality of care'.

National and international initiatives have encouraged the development of IPE in the curriculum of health undergraduates, education that should:

- focus on the needs of individuals, families and communities to improve their quality of care, health outcomes and well-being
- apply equal opportunities within and between the professions and all with whom they learn and work
- respect individuality, difference and diversity within and between the professions and all with whom they learn and work
- sustain the identity and expertise of each profession
- promote parity between professions in the learning environment
- instil interprofessional values and perspectives throughout uniprofessional and multiprofessional learning (Barr & Low 2011).

Box 17.3 Case study: Interprofessional Pain Management Learning Unit at King's College London

The King's College London (KCL) Interprofessional Pain Management Learning Unit was launched in 2011 for second-year undergraduates from dentistry, medicine, midwifery, nursing, pharmacy and physiotherapy. The unit was designed to enhance the pain management knowledge and skills, challenge existing attitudes and assumptions, improve interprofessional collaboration and understanding of roles as well as contributing to the suite of interprofessional learning available. Around 1000 students complete the unit annually, which consists of an e-learning module and interprofessional workshops. Students work collaboratively online and in the classroom to devise a pain management plan for a particular case study. Specific learning outcomes are:

- Discuss the physiology of pain and the impact on the individual, their family and society.
- Plan a holistic assessment for people experiencing pain.
- Identify the main pharmacological strategies and the mechanism of action, cautions and contraindications.
- Discuss the role of non-pharmacological approaches to pain management.

- Plan pain management strategies that promote independence.
- Discuss the role of interprofessional and specialist teams in providing effective pain relief.

Eight virtual, animated patients are available online and the students are allocated to a patient with one of the following pain conditions: post-operative pain, post-herpetic neuralgia, trigeminal neuralgia, persistent headaches, tooth abscess, osteoarthritis, postnatal pain and back pain from metastatic cancer. The patients are a range of ages, ethnic backgrounds, vary in their response to pain and present in a range of healthcare settings. Online, the students design a pain assessment strategy and they work in their interprofessional teams (six to eight in each team) in the workshop to explore the nature and impact of pain, and agree the assessment strategy, pharmacological interventions and non-pharmacological approaches. An informal presentation to remaining students in the workshop (around 25–30) ensures that the students gain an insight into the management of a range of painful conditions.

The topic of pain management lends itself to interprofessional education, and developments have been pioneered in Canada where students from six disciplines experience a 20-hour interprofessional pain week (Watt-Watson et al 2004). The week includes multiprofessional introductory sessions, uniprofessional seminars to explore discipline specific issues and students working together to form an interprofessional pain management plan for case studies. This successful model has demonstrated significant increases in student knowledge and satisfaction (Hunter et al 2008). Box 17.3 presents an example of interprofessional pain education from the UK.

Despite these successful initiatives, survey results revealed that IPE in pain management has not been widely developed in the UK or Canada (Briggs et al 2011; Watt-Watson et al 2009). In the UK survey of 108 undergraduate programmes, only 18.9% (n = 14) of disciplines shared content with another health programme (Briggs et al 2011). This was predominantly medicine, occupational therapy and physiotherapy sharing an average of 5.5 hours of lectures, suggesting that students learned alongside one another (multiprofessional learning) rather than interprofessional learning where people are learning with, from and about each other. There are a number of barriers that may be hindering developments in this area, including difficulties with the logistics of timetabling, availability of rooms and administrative support as well as variations in local expertise and champions for change in the curriculum. We need to address these challenges in order to promote a practice-ready workforce that can work collaboratively and skillfully to manage pain.

Examples of interprofessional postgraduate education have also emerged over the last decade, offering one-off workshops with community practitioners on opioids (Allen et al 2011) or a longer programme of workshops (4.5 days) for hospital staff (Carr et al 2003). Initial results from these small-scale studies suggest favourable results; staff reported greater confidence, self-efficacy (belief in their own competence) and communication with interprofessional colleagues. Similar to undergraduate IPE, further research is needed to explore the role of interprofessional education on pain and the impact on pain management and patient care.

One opportunity for interprofessional working and learning is seeking mentorship from a member of a different discipline. The role of a mentor in this context is to promote interprofessional learning opportunities by negotiating goals and expectations (linked to competencies for all professions) and facilitate opportunities for collaborative practice. Interprofessional mentors can support undergraduates and qualified staff helping a discipline-specific mentor and foster a culture of collaborative mentorship (Deutschlander & Suter 2011). A guide for students and mentors on interprofessional mentoring is available online (see http://www.caipe.org.uk/silo/files/interprofessional-mentoring-guide.pdf).

Evaluating the impact on IPE represents an interesting challenge. Current research focuses on the effect education can have on knowledge and attitudes, typically measuring these before and after an educational session or programmes. Carr and Watt-Watson (2012) offer a detailed critique of interprofessional pain education, reviewing the current evidence and future directions.

Resources for promoting interprofessional learning and working in pain management continue to be developed. IASP (International Association for the Study of Pain 2012) have published an interprofessional core curriculum outlining a list of recommendations for key areas and skills that all healthcare professionals should achieve as an undergraduate. The British Pain Society Education SIG will also publish a guide to accompany this and help integrate IPE around pain into the curriculum. Further resources on general IPE are available at the end of this chapter.

POSTGRADUATE EDUCATION

In the UK, higher education courses and qualifications are delivered through a wide variety of institutions, mostly universities and colleges, and despite no clear or single definition of 'postgraduate' or 'higher education', the terms are often used interchangeably to describe advanced academic study undertaken by people with a first or undergraduate degree-level qualification. Students will typically study either full or part time for up to 6 years, and programmes of study may be based in research, taught by coursework or use a combination of both. The terms are frequently used to refer to qualifications such as master's and doctoral studies, but also include qualifications such as Postgraduate Certificate and Postgraduate Diploma, which are taught to a more academically demanding standard than undergraduate certificates and diplomas (Higher Education Policy Institute 2010). It is important to note, however, that postgraduate level education may not necessarily be in the same subject area as one's first or undergraduate degree. Professionals who work in pain management will have entered the field from a diverse range of undergraduate subject areas, including social work, education, medicine, nursing, health economics, biology and pharmacy. As the field of pain covers a broad spectrum of subspecialities, master-level study is an opportunity for study at an equally broad level of complexity and depth, from Postgraduate Certificates through to PhDs and beyond, into post-doctoral study.

Across the UK there are increasing numbers of students actively engaged in postgraduate education and continued growth in the areas of medicine, dentistry and subjects allied to medicine, with currently over 78,000 postgraduate students studying at UK higher education institutions (Higher Education Statistics Agency 2013). These statistics suggest that there is an increased demand for postgraduate level study driven by a number of factors, including educational, clinical, increased competition for employment opportunities and increased marketing by higher educational institutions.

Improved education is generally seen as a positive exercise and something that is of value, whether clinical, personal, societal, monetary or even political value. On a larger scale, increased levels of education can transform lives by improving economic conditions and health outcomes for populations, including patients in pain, and personal employment prospects.

Personal benefits of higher level study

The motivations for undertaking postgraduate education are varied and complex, but findings from the Higher Education Academy (2011, 2012) provide some key insights:

- to progress in one's chosen career path and to fulfil their employment and/or research potential
- to progress towards higher academic qualifications
- to fulfill personal interest and enjoyment in a subject.

These motivations are echoed in the benefits that are often described as coming from postgraduate study (see Box 17.4).

Development of transferable skills for enhanced employability

Postgraduate programmes of study are exceptionally well placed to provide the development of transferable skills that are valued within a range of career paths. These include subject and discipline-specific skills as well as:

- the ability to locate and use information effectively
- time- and project-management skills
- communication and presentation skills
- critical thinking and problem-solving skills
- organization and planning ability
- the development of strong negotiation ability

Box 17.4 Key benefits of higher level/ postgraduate study

- Development of transferable skills for enhanced employability.
- Improved career prospects, career change and identification of development needs.
- Greater confidence and strong independent learning skills.
- Improved research skills.
- The development of a strong academic and vocational profile.
- The development and refinement of practical skills.
- Potential financial reward and increased career options.

Summarized from Higher Education Academy (2011, 2012; Jamieson et al 2009).

- research and data-analysis skills
- demonstration of capability and tenacity to undertake investigative work.

In postgraduate pain management study the acquisition of both generic and specific transferable skills may include a deep and critical understanding of the principles and practice underpinning the biopsychosocial approach, expertise in evidence-based clinical practice, a demonstration of highly specialized pain management skills that are informed by up-to-date research developments and the ability to manage complex issues in the absence of consistent information.

Career progression and the development of a strong academic and vocational profile

Continuing professional development (CPD) is the norm in many employment sectors, including most aspects of healthcare, and in many areas is essential, including law, education, social work and some areas of health care. A number of employers may give preference to those with postgraduate qualifications, particularly if specialist knowledge and skills are coupled with periods of practical work experience either within or outwith the academic programme itself.

The career benefits of advanced study in pain management can be seen in an increasing number of specialist roles for which a postgraduate qualification would be advantageous. Nurses, occupational therapists and physiotherapists may have extended roles as advanced practitioners or gain consultant level status within their profession. Equally, general practitioners and pharmacists may, through postgraduate study, gain additional competencies to become 'practitioners with special interests' (GPwSIs and PhwSIs, respectively).

Potential rewards and career options

A postgraduate qualification will provide an opportunity to explore your strengths and personal and professional interests, and to develop career aspirations and ideas. Postgraduate study also makes extensive demands on personal relationships, time, hobbies and interests yet provides the satisfaction of achievement, sustained motivation and personal challenge.

The skills and qualities that are developed during postgraduate study may enhance employability in an increasingly competitive employment market. A number of reports have suggested that there are strong economic advantages to postgraduate degrees, including increased earnings of up to 23% compared to those with an undergraduate degree only (Higher Education Policy Institute 2010; Sutton Trust 2010).

Equally, a postgraduate qualification may be of benefit if current and future career prospects are no longer in line with aspirations, opportunities or personal circumstances. Transferable skills mean that a postgraduate qualification may be useful in developing new areas of interest within pain management (e.g. a research role) or new career avenues.

Characteristics of postgraduate education

Despite the lack of clear definition of higher or postgraduate education, there is a clear understanding of what education at this level should consist of and the educational aims this level should exemplify. Examples of this can be found in the development from undergraduate programmes to postgraduate level programmes, and can be identified in framework guidelines from the Quality Assurance Agency for Higher Education (Quality Assurance Agency for Higher Education 2008, 2010; Scottish Credit and Qualifications Framework Partnership 2009). These guidelines clearly show the progressive acquisition of desirable attributes, both generic and specialized, such as critical analysis, evaluation and synthesis, the demonstration of originality and creativity in the application of knowledge understanding and practice, and the use of a broad range of advanced and specialized skills appropriate to practice.

One of the key themes from the postgraduate education level is the strong and informed use of the word 'critical' to examine knowledge, understanding and how this can translate into practice. Equally, the emphasis on advanced and specialized skills is highlighted, as is the development of autonomy and initiative – skills that are valued within evolving environments such as health care and pain management.

In practice, studying at postgraduate level translates into healthcare professionals who have gained enhanced career progression, developed specialized clinical practice skills, and increased confidence, a positive attitude towards change and the opening up of new career options and opportunities previously not identified (Stathopoulos & Harrison 2003; Whyte et al 2000). In addition, the perceived enhancement of clinical practice, strong sense of personal achievement and growth along with the increased application of critically analysed theory to practice may provide benefit, directly or indirectly, to patients (Cotterill-Walker 2012). The advanced skills that postgraduate study can bring will be essential in meeting the increasingly diverse roles required of contemporary health care and pain management.

Opportunities for advanced study

Increasingly, higher education institutions are offering postgraduate programmes in either profession specific fields (i.e. physiotherapy, nursing) or subject-specific areas such as pain management and clinical education (see Box 17.5). The diverse range of programmes, offered full

Box 17.5 **UK universities offering Master of Science degrees in pain-management-related subjects***

Birmingham City University
Cardiff University
Keele University
King's College London
Queen's University Belfast
The University of Edinburgh
University of Leicester

*At time of publication

time and part time, provides a wide range of choice to develop both personal and professional interests whilst reaping the broader benefits of a postgraduate qualification.

Further developments in the provision of postgraduate education have capitalized on technology as there is a rapidly developing number of programmes offered by online distance learning so students are able to study and interact with others from across both the country and the world at times that fit with personal and professional commitments. Postgraduate education is no longer limited in its scope and the opportunities for postgraduate education are increasingly limitless.

IN-SERVICE EDUCATION

In addition to undergraduate and postgraduate level education, in-service, community or hospital-based education plays an equally important role in the development of pain management skills, practice and healthcare provision, and, importantly, promotes clinical governance.

In recent years, the National Health Service (NHS) in the UK has placed increasing emphasis on the importance of CPD for all healthcare staff. This drive has stemmed from the development and introduction of national standards of healthcare delivery and clinical governance, the 'system through which NHS organizations are accountable for continuously improving the quality of their services and safeguarding high standards of care by creating an environment in which excellence in clinical care will flourish' (Department of Health 1998; Scally & Donaldson 1998). The remit of clinical governance is broad, but central to the success of its concepts is the understanding and coverage of a number of component working practices, including resource effectiveness, strategic effectiveness, risk-management effectiveness, patient experience, communication effectiveness, clinical effectiveness and learning effectiveness (Nicholls et al 2000).

CPD in pain management and other areas provides a key link to this learning effectiveness as it can provide the mechanisms whereby all staff can be competent in their roles and the development of the skills that are required to maintain up-to-date practice, high-quality care and service delivery (General Medical Council 2012; Health & Care Professions Council 2013; Nursing and Midwifery Council 2006).

The scope of CPD activities that can be undertaken is necessarily broad as it covers a spectrum of healthcare providers, including NHS employees, independent sector healthcare providers, the education sector and social care employers. These activities can include formal and informal learning activities appropriate to the needs of both the individual and the service (Health & Care Professions Council 2013). In practice, the range of activities that can be used as examples of CPD is lengthy and covers areas such as work-based learning, professional activity, formal education, self-directed learning and other activities such as public service and voluntary work. Examples of in-service or work-based activities are listed in Table 17.3.

CPD activities are at the core of professional practice. Just as recipients of health care have the right to safe and effective practices, healthcare professionals are also bound to possess up-to-date knowledge, skills and abilities. The skills developed through CPD activities will enable healthcare practitioners to meet the demands of not only patients, their families and carers, and themselves, but also to provide this care within a rapidly changing healthcare environment.

PROFESSIONAL ORGANIZATIONS

One of the most important, yet underused, resources that healthcare professionals have is access to professional organizations and associations, be they local, regional or international. Have a look at the activity in Box 17.6, which considers the benefits of membership.

Benefits of membership of a professional organization

Belonging to professional organization has long been promoted as an important aspect of career development (Cottrell et al 2009). This membership of a professional organization can be on a variety of levels, from local to international, and from subject-specific (for example the British Pain Society or IASP) to discipline-specific (for example the Royal College of Nursing). However, regardless of the organization, membership of professional organizations brings a number of benefits and educational opportunities (for example Chartered Society of Physiotherapists 2012; College of Occupational Therapists 2011; Royal College of Nursing 2012), many of which are not articulated to new graduates or early career professionals (Mata et al 2010).

Table 17.3 Examples of in-service or work based continuous professional development activities

Work-based learning	Professional activity	Formal/ educational	Self-directed learning
Reflective practice	Involvement in a professional body	Research	Reading journals/articles
Coaching from others	Membership of a specialist interest group	Attending conferences (for example British Pain Society meetings)	Reviewing books or articles
Work shadowing	Mentoring	Writing articles or papers	Updating knowledge through the internet, television or radio (for example Airing Pain)
Journal club	Being an expert witness	Going to seminars (for example British Pain Society Education Special Interest Group meetings)	
Secondments	Organizing accredited courses	Planning or running a course	
Supervising staff or students	Giving presentations at conferences		
Job rotation			
Visiting other departments and reporting back			

Adapted from Health Professions Council (2005).

Box 17.6 Reflection point

Take a moment to think about the educational benefits that membership to your own professional organization brings. Do you feel you are benefiting from membership to your professional organization and if not, what can you do to improve the situation?

If you are uncertain, how can you find out more about these benefits?

Networking opportunities

By joining a professional organization there is an increased opportunity for attending meetings and becoming active within the organization in a number of ways, including the joining of pain-related special interest groups, becoming politically active within the organization and taking on leadership roles to direct the growth and policy of the organization as a whole. By being part of a larger organization there is the opportunity for ongoing development of personal, education and professional goals which has the potential to inspire and open up new opportunities.

These networks are also useful as they form a support system for members, who may be able to take advantage of mentoring systems that are in place. They can also be a useful source of answers and practical solutions as and when needs arise.

Conferences, education and access to online resources

Members of professional organizations such as BPS and IASP often receive advance information about forthcoming conferences and seminars, and often receive 'members only' registration discounts and preferable rates on conference and seminar-related costs such as hotels and airfares.

Many professional organizations offer their members the opportunity to update and develop their academic and clinical skills through study days, clinical education sessions, break-out sessions at conferences and, increasingly, online courses or workshops. In some instances, professional organizations offer scholarships for professional development and continuing educational activities. In addition, the websites of many professional organizations have members-only areas that provide access to message boards, career opportunities, international exchanges, various databases that provide information on numerous healthcare related topics, topic-specific discussion areas as well as areas for new graduates.

Discounted publications

Professional membership usually will include a free subscription to the organization's main and subsidiary publications (e.g. IASP PAIN, Pain: Clinical Updates, IASP Insight, BPS British Journal of Pain, Pain News) and, in many cases, publications of related organizations. This ensures that members are aware of the latest research and best practice as well as opportunities to receive discounts on CDs, educational DVDs, journals and other materials.

Special interest groups

SIGs are an important part of many larger organizations as they provide a mechanism by which members of the organization who have a specific interest are given a forum to discuss their interest in more depth. SIGS are, in many cases, driven by proactive members of the larger organization who feel strongly about developing their particular field. The British Pain Society, for example, has, amongst others, a SIG in pain education for those members who have a particular interest in raising the awareness of the importance of pain education for patients, the public and healthcare professionals. Information about SIGs can be found on the organization's website.

Political and educational interests

Many professional organizations have an interest in the political sphere, particularly where it affects their specific area of interest or business, and are often asked to provide advice, comment and guidance on legislation, government policy and educational development strategies. In many instances, professional organizations can provide significant political pressure that exceeds the voice of any individual member and joining such a professional organization facilitates access to the group's resources and influence.

Protection

Membership of many professional organizations, particularly those that are discipline specific, often includes professional indemnity insurance against claims of clinical negligence. This entitles members of the organization to advice and representation on matters of law that occur in the course of employment. Additionally, there is often union support to provide representation, and support of workplace rights and working conditions.

Benefits of conference attendance

Conference and seminar attendance has a specific place in professional and educational development, and although there has been criticism of the value of such activities (Ioannidis 2012), such activities present opportunities for inter- and intradisciplinary collaboration, experiencing the diversity of the profession, networking, preparing and giving presentations, attending seminars and SIG meetings, and developing relationships with both lay and professional attendees (Mata et al 2010). A variety of pain-related conferences is held every year.

Although initially from the field of health promotion, a useful understanding of the connection between professional development, conference attendance and professional organization membership comes from Mata et al (2010), who see this as an evolutionary process. In the early stages of professional development one may join a professional organization and perhaps later attend local seminars or regional conferences, and later still present at seminars and conferences. Through this process, professionals may develop increased opportunities for collaboration, develop broad networks of fellow professionals and colleagues across professions, and may develop advocacy or educational roles. This development may then have potential for improved knowledge, educational initiatives and strategy planning, and programme development (Mata et al 2010).

Summary

Much of the value in membership of professional organizations can be found in personal professional development and in the aspirations for the growth of one's career, profession and educational development. The connections that are made, whether formal or informal, serve as valuable stepping stones to future activities and development, and the benefits that come with engaging with professional organizations may turn out to be one of the most positive steps in one's career and educational journey.

USING THE INTERNET FOR PAIN EDUCATION AND FURTHER RESOURCES

With the growth of electronic communications and increased access to information, the world wide web and associated websites can be an ever-expanding source of pain education. Access to educational material about pain and other healthcare conditions is no longer restricted to the realm of healthcare professionals, and the public are becoming increasing informed about healthcare conditions, management options and potential treatments (Dutton et al 2009). The growth in internet-based information is important for both professionals and for the public and patients, but the information sought by each group may be different. Healthcare professionals may seek information that is consistent with clinical practice, legislation and guidelines, peer-reviewed current research and professional educational opportunities, whilst patients and the public may seek more generalized healthcare treatment or management. Box 17.7 considers these points further.

Regardless of the purpose for which internet-based educational materials are sought, there is the need to balance quantity of information with quality of information. The quality, accuracy and trustworthiness of information on the internet is a longstanding issue, with key items of concern being trustworthiness, navigation and availability of information (Pletneva et al 2011). A number of organizations (e.g. the American Medical Association, Health on the Net Foundation, Hi-Ethics) have provided general guidelines, although not universally acceptable for both professionals and patients, for assessing the quality and reliability of websites (Clark 2002, Hanif et al 2009). Such guidelines should include clear disclosure of authorship, full disclosure of funding and financial associations and sponsorship, comment on the adherence to ethical standards, identification of online advertising, clear attribution of sources of content and description of methodology, timeliness of information updates, and the appropriateness for audience and overall generalizability (Eysenbach et al 2002). Equally important are the clear use of precautions to keep personal information, including health-related information, secure (Clark 2002).

Given the known difficulties of the quality and accuracy of information on the internet, professionals searching for initial sources of clinical information might be directed towards organizations such as the National Institute for Health and Clinical Excellence (NICE) and Scottish Intercollegiate Guidelines (SIGN) for information on clinical guidelines, treatment and management. Equally, professional organizations, such as the British Pain Society, and the websites of research-driven universities are excellent starting points for up-to-date clinical and research information. Many patients will also seek relevant information and starting points for patients could include websites developed and maintained by the NHS and its associated organizations.

Although the internet is a valuable source of information, provided appropriate care is taken, patient groups and patient organizations provide a valuable source of education information and support for both healthcare professionals and patients. These patient groups can range from local charity groups to large, long-established national groups with many thousands of members and they may or may not have direct links with healthcare professionals. Within the UK some useful resources for pain education for patients are The PainToolkit, Pain Concern, Airing Pain and Pain Association Scotland. An internet search will often highlight patient groups and organizations in regional areas.

The internet is an ever-expanding source of information for patients, patient groups and healthcare professionals and, when used with common sense, appropriate caution and, if necessary, in conjunction with healthcare providers, can be a catalyst for education, patient awareness, communication and sharing of research, and best practice.

CONCLUSION

- Effective learning about pain management begins with assessing our current knowledge, skills and attitude towards pain and making specific plans for enhancing these areas.
- Undergraduate education varies throughout the UK but there are strategies that learners, clinicians and academics can use to improve their own learning and promote curriculum development.
- Postgraduate education in pain management offers a chance for personal growth and challenge, and can provide a range of professional and patient-related benefits.
- Generic and pain-specific organizations can provide continuous professional development and vital networking opportunities, conferences, special interest groups and publications.
- The internet and electronic sources of information can provide a useful source of education for patients and professionals, although the quality varies and trusted sources should be used.

Box 17.7 **Reflection point**

Take some time to think about the sources of information that you use on the internet and consider whether these are directed towards professional or patient use. How do you know?

Think about a particular healthcare condition, for example migraine headache. As a healthcare professional, where would you search for information about the different types of migraine headache and their associated management options if you were not already familiar with them? Is this be the same source of information that you would direct your patients to?

Q Self-test questions

1. Metacognition is:
   a. strategic learning and insight about topic in a particular situation
   b. knowledge of preferred learning approaches and choosing a learning technique in a particular situation
   c. lecturers understanding people's preferred learning approach in particular situations
2. Thinking about your role, describe three ways you can influence the pain education provided (whether you are an undergraduate, qualified clinician, postgraduate or academic staff).
3. The internet can be a valuable source of pain-management information for both patients and healthcare professionals, but which of the following are the most important when seeking out this information? Tick all that apply.
   a. Authorship and source of content.
   b. Design of the website.
   c. Disclosure of funding and advertising.
   d. Publication date of information.
   e. Suitability of content to the audience.
4. Continuing professional development (CPD) activities are the responsibility of all healthcare professionals in order to maintain up-to-date practice, high-quality care and service delivery. Which of the following could be considered CDP?
   a. Journal club.
   b. Mentoring.
   c. Research.
   d. Reviewing books or journals.
   e. Writing articles for publication.
   f. Membership of a special interest group.
   g. All of the above (correct).
5. List five of the transferable skills that you would hope to gain as a result of postgraduate or higher level study. Check your answers again those in the section on development of transferable skills for enhanced employability).

REFERENCES

Allen, M., Macleod, T., Zwicker, B., et al., 2011. Interprofessional education in chronic non-cancer pain. J. Interprof. Care 25, 221–222.

Barr, H., Low, H., 2011. Principles of Interprofessional Education. Centre for Advancement of Interprofessional Education. Online. Available: http://www.caipe.org.uk/resources/principles-of-interprofessional-education/.

Briggs, E., Carr, E., Whittaker, M., 2011. Survey of undergraduate pain curricula for healthcare professionals in the United Kingdom. Eur. J. Pain 15 (8), 789–795.

Burns, T., Sinfield, S., 2008. Essential Study Skills: The Complete Guide to Success @ University, second ed. Sage, London.

Carr, E.J.C., Watt-Watson, J., 2012. Interprofessional pain education: definitions, exemplars and future directions. British Journal of Pain 6 (2), 59–65.

Carr, E.C.J., Brockbank, K., Barrett, R.F., 2003. Improving pain management through interprofessional education: evaluation of a pilot project. Learning in Health and Social Care 2 (1), 6–17.

Centre for the Advancement of Interprofessional Education, 2002.

Defining IPE. Online. Available: www.caipe.org.uk/about-us/defining-ipe (accessed 25.06.12.).

Chartered Society of Physiotherapists, 2012. Benefits. Online. Available: http://www.csp.org.uk/membership/join-csp/full-members/benefits (accessed 25.06.12.).

Clark, E.J., 2002. Health care web sites: Are they reliable? J. Med. Syst. 26 (6), 519–528.

College of Occupational Therapists, 2011. Membership Benefits. Online. Available: http://www.cot.co.uk/join-baot/membership-benefits (accessed 25.06.12.).

Costa, A., Kallick, B., 1993. Through the Lens of a Critical Friend. Educational Leadership 51 (2), 49–51.

Cotterill-Walker, S.M., 2012. Where is the evidence that master's level nursing education makes a difference to patient care? A literature review. Nurse Educ. Today. 32 (1), 57–64.

Cottrell, S., 2008. The Study Skills Handbook, third ed. Palgrave, Basingstoke.

Cottrell, R.R., Girvan, J.T., McKenzie, J.F., 2009. Principles and Foundations of Health Promotion and Education, fourth ed. Pearson Benjamin Cummings, San Francisco.

Department of Health, 1998. A first class service: Quality in the new NHS. Department of Health, London.

Deutschlander, S., Suter, E., 2011. Interprofessional Mentoring Guide for Supervisors, Staff and Students. Online. Available: http://www.caipe.org.uk/silo/files/interprofessional-mentoring-guide.pdf (accessed 25.06.12.).

Donaldson, L., 2009. 150 years of the Annual Report of the Chief Medical Officer: On the State of the Public Health 2008. Department of Health, London.

Dutton, W.H., Helsper, E.J., Gerber, M.M., 2009. Oxford Internet Survey 2009 Report: The Internet in Britain. Oxford Internet Institute, University of Oxford, Oxford.

Egan, G., 1986. The Skilled Helper: Systematic Approach to Effective Helping, third ed. Brooks/Cole, Belmont, CA.

Eysenbach, G., Powell, J., Kuss, O., et al., 2002. Assessing the Quality of Health Information for Consumers on the World Wide Web A Systematic Review. JAMA 287 (20), 2691–2700.

General Medical Council, 2009. Tomorrow's doctors, second ed. General Medical Council, London.

General Medical Council, 2012. Continuing Professional Development. Guidance for all Doctors 2012. General Medical Council, Manchester.

Ghosh, S., Chandran, A., Jansen, J.P., 2012. Epidemiology of HIV-related neuropathy: a systematic literature review. AIDS Res. Hum. Retroviruses 28 (1), 36–48.

Gibbins, J., McCourbrie, R., Maher, J., et al., 2009. Incorporating palliative care into undergraduate curricula: lessons for curriculum development. Med. Educ. 43, 776–783.

Hanif, F., Read, J.C., Goodacre, J.A., et al., 2009. The role of quality tools in assessing reliability of the internet for health information. Information for Health and Social Care 34 (4), 231–243.

Health & Care Professions Council, 2013. Our standards for continuing professional development. Online. Available: http://www.hpc-uk.org/registrants/cpd/standards/(accessed 24.02.13.).

Health Professions Council, 2005. Standards for continuing professional development. Health Professions Council, London.

Help the Aged & British Pain Society, 2008. Pain in Older People: Reflections and experiences from an older person's perspective. Help the Aged & British Pain Society, London. Online. Available: www.britishpainsociety.org/pub_professional.htm#helptheaged (accessed 25.06.12.).

Higher Education Academy, 2011. Postgraduate Research Experience Survey (PRES). The Higher Education Academy, York.

Higher Education Academy, 2012. National findings from the Postgraduate Taught Experience Survey (PTES). The Higher Education Academy, York.

Higher Education Policy Institute, 2010. Postgraduate Education in the United Kingdom. Online. Available: http://www.hepi.ac.uk/466/Reports.html (accessed 25.06.12).

Higher Education Statistics Agency, 2013. Student enrolments on HE courses by level of study, subject area and mode of study 2007/08 to 2011/12. Online. Available: http://www.hesa.ac.uk/ (accessed 23.02.13.).

Hunter, J., Watt-Watson, J., McGillion, M., et al., 2008. An interfaculty pain curriculum: lessons learned from six years experience. Pain 140, 74–86.

International Association for the Study of Pain, 2010. Declaration of Montreal. Online. Available: http://www.iasp-pain.org/Content/NavigationMenu/Advocacy/DeclarationofMontr233al/default.htm (accessed 25.06.12.).

International Association for the Study of Pain, 2012. IASP Interprofessional Pain Curriculum Outline. Online. Available: http://www.iasp-pain.org/Content/NavigationMenu/GeneralResourceLinks/Curricula/Interprofessional/default.htm (accessed 04.02.13.).

Ioannidis, J.P.A., 2012. Are Medical Conferences Useful? And for Whom? J. Am. Med. Assoc. 307 (12), 1257–1258.

Jamieson, A., Sabates, R., Woodley, A., et al., 2009. The benefits of higher education study for part-time students. Studies in Higher Education. 34 (3).

Light, G., Calkins, Cox, R., 2009. Learning and Teaching In Higher Education: The Reflective Professional, second ed. Sage, London.

Mata, H., Latham, T.P., Ransome, Y., 2010. Benefits of professional organization membership and participation in national conferences: Considerations for students and new professionals. Health Promot. Pract. 11 (4), 450–453.

Nicholls, S., Cullen, R., O'Neil, S., et al., 2000. Clinical governance: its origins and its foundations. British Journal of Clinical Governance 5 (3), 172–178.

Nursing and Midwifery Council, 2006. PREP handbook. Nursing & Midwifery Council, London.

Patient's Association, 2010. Public Attitudes to Pain. Patient's Association, London. Online. Available: www.patients-association.com/News/410 (accessed 25.06.12.).

Pletneva, N., Cruchet, S., Simonet, M.A., et al., 2011. Results of the 10th HON survey on health and medical Internet use. Online. Available: http://www.hon.ch/Project/publications.html (accessed 25.06.12.).

Postholm, M.B., 2011. Self-regulated learning in teaching – student's experiences. Teachers and Teaching: Theory and Practice 17 (3), 365–382.

Quality Assurance Agency for Higher Education, 2008. The Framework for Higher Education Qualifications in England. Wales and Northern Ireland. Quality Assurance Agency for Higher Education, Gloucester.

Quality Assurance Agency for Higher Education, 2010. Master's Degree Characteristics. Quality Assurance Agency for Higher, Gloucester.

Ramsden, P., 2003. Learning to Teach in Higher Education. Routledge Falmer, London.

Royal College of Nursing, 2012. Why should nurses and midwives join the RCN? Online. Available: http://www.rcn.org.uk/membership/categories/category01/full_member_benefits (accessed 25.06.12.).

Scally, G., Donaldson, L.J., 1998. Clinical Governance and the drive for quality improvement in the new NHS in England. Br. Med. J. 317, 61–65.

Scottish Credit and Qualifications Framework Partnership, 2009. SCQF Handbook: User Guide. Scottish Credit and Qualifications Framework Partnership. Online. Available: http://www.scqf.org.uk/content/files/resources/SCQF_handbook_FULL_-_amended_Dec_09.pdf (accessed 02.07.12.).

Stathopoulos, I., Harrison, K., 2003. Study at Masters level by practicing physiotherapists. Physiotherapy 89 (3), 158–169.

Sutton Trust, 2010. The Social Composition and Future Earnings of Postgraduates. Interim results from the Centre for Economic Performance at the London School of Economics. Online. Available: http://www.suttontrust.com/research/the-social-composition-and-future-earnings-of-postgraduates/ (accessed 25.06.12.).

Terry, L.M., 2012. Service user involvement in nurse education: A report on using online discussions with a service user to augment his digital story. Nurse Educ. Today 32 (2), 161–166.

Watt-Watson, J., Hunter, J., Pennefather, P., et al., 2004. An integrated undergraduate pain curriculum for six Health Science Faculties. Pain 110, 140–148.

Watt-Watson, J., McGillion, M., Hunter, J., et al., 2009. A survey of pre-licensure pain curricula in health science faculties in Canadian Universities. Pain Res. Manag. 14 (6), 439–444.

Whyte, D.A., Lugton, J., Fawcett, T.N., 2000. Fit for purpose: the relevance of masters preparation for the professional practice of nursing. A 10-year follow-up study of postgraduate nursing courses in the University of Edinburgh. J. Adv. Nurs. 31 (5), 1072–1080.

World Health Organization, 2010. Framework for action on interprofessional education and collaborative practice. Online. Available: www.who.int/hrh/resources/framework_action/en/ (accessed 25.06.12.).

INTERNET RESOURCES – INTERPROFESSIONAL EDUCATION

Centre for the Advancement of Interprofessional Education   www.caipe.org.uk
Centre for Interprofessional E-Learning   www.cipel.ac.uk
European Interprofessional Education Network   www.eipen.org
Higher Education Academy Interprofessional SIG   www.health.heacademy.ac.uk/

PROFESSIONAL ORGANIZATIONS THAT HAVE AN INTEREST IN PAIN EDUCATION

Pain-specific organizations

British Pain Society   http://www.britishpainsociety.org/
British Pain Society Pain Education SIG   www.britishpainsociety.org/members_sigs.htm

International Association for the Study of Pain   http://www.iasp-pain.org
IASP Education SIG   www.iasp-pain.org/sigs
European Federation of IASP Chapters   http://www.efic.org/
Faculty of Pain Medicine   http://www.rcoa.ac.uk/faculty-of-pain-medicine/
Physiotherapy Pain Association   http://ppa.csp.org.uk/
Royal College of Nursing Pain and Palliative Care Forum   www.rcn.org.uk/development/communities/rcn_forum_communities

Generic organizations

British Dental Association   http://www.bda.org/
British Psychological Society   http://www.bps.org.uk/
College of Occupational Therapists   http://www.cot.co.uk/
Chartered Society of Physiotherapists   http://www.csp.org.uk/
Royal College of Anaesthetists   http://www.rcoa.ac.uk/
Royal College of Nursing   http://www.rcn.org.uk/
Royal Pharmaceutical Society   http://www.rpharms.com

Chapter | **18** |

Pain in childhood

Anita M. Unruh and Patrick J. McGrath

LEARNING OBJECTIVES

On completing this chapter readers will have an understanding of:

1. The prevalence of pain in infants, children and adolescents.
2. Measurement tools to assess pain in infants and children.
3. Management of paediatric pain.
4. The family as a vector for learning about pain.
5. Managing school anxiety and school avoidance due to pain.
6. The influence of sex and gender on children's experience and learning about pain.

OVERVIEW

Pain in the paediatric age range (0–16 years of age) is common. It can have serious effects on the child, the family and on healthcare professionals. We have made much progress in the past 30 years in our understanding of pain in children. These advances have changed our view of the physiology of pain in children and the influence of early episodes of pain on the risk for future pain. The development of reliable and valid child-focused measurement tools have greatly improved our capacity to determine when children are in pain. The development and evaluations of interventions enable us to do something about it. We also have elaborated the important social influences on learning about pain through family and school.

In this chapter we will examine some specific problem areas in children's pain, discuss the challenges and give specific suggestions for health professionals.

WHAT IS THE PROBLEM?

Children are not strangers to pain. Virtually all infants will have a heel-prick within the first few days of life to collect the few drops of blood needed for PKU and adrenal screening. Many male infants will be circumcised in the first week of life. For infants (neonates) who have health issues in their first period of life, and spend time in an intensive care unit, the risk for pain sharply increases. A recent Swiss study of ventilated newborns in the first 2 weeks of life (Cignacco et al 2009) logged 38,626 procedures in 120 preterm infants or about 23 procedures per day, per child. Three-quarters of these procedures were considered to be painful (e.g. 17–18 procedures per day per infant). In these very pain sophisticated units, almost all infants were given some form of pain comfort or analgesia. A common approach was pre-emptive oral sucrose, which has been shown to be an effective analgesic in infants (Stevens et al 2004). Oral sucrose is an example of a pain-relieving strategy that has an active physiological benefit to relieve pain in infants but no such effect in adults.

© 2014 Elsevier Ltd.

Even healthy young children are subject to a large number of needle procedures. For example, children in Canada receive about 20 needles for immunization before they turn 5 years of age. Parents may avoid or delay immunizations because of their concern about the child's distress over the needle (Luthy et al 2009). Young children may experience other pain associated with common childhood illnesses and infections such as earache and sore throats.

As children develop their gross motor skills through play and exploration, they experience the many bumps and falls of childhood. Observational studies of such pain among preschoolers and young school-age children on a daycare playground yielded mean rates of between 0.34 and 0.41 incidents per hour per child (Fearon et al 1996; von Baeyer et al 1998). Some children experience pain from less frequent but more serious unintentional injury at home, in cars, on farms, on playgrounds, at daycare centres and at school. Injury prevention programmes are an important step in alerting adults about potential dangers to children but changing behaviours to protect children is challenging. Legislation is often needed to insure that children are sufficiently protected.

Unfortunately, many children still suffer pain and distress because their parents hit them as a form of discipline. A national study in the USA (Straus & Stewart 1999) found that 35% of parents hit infants and 94% hit children ages 3 and 4 years. Just over 50% of American parents hit children at age 12; the rate then decreased. Parents who hit their teenagers averaged doing so about six times during the year. The children most likely to be hit with an object (28%) were 5–12-year-olds. Children who are physically or sexually abused experience pain and suffering in their immediate environment. They are also at risk for chronic pain as adults (Davis et al 2005; Walsh et al 2007).

As children enter the school-age years they become more vulnerable to the commonplace and troublesome pains that also affect adults. Headache and migraine are reported by about 3–7% of school age children but increase in prevalence after puberty, particularly for girls (Unruh & Campbell 1999). 10–15% of children have recurrent abdominal pain. Recurrent abdominal pain in children is common and may be associated with irritable bowel syndrome and chronic abdominal pain in adulthood (Nurko 2009). In a recent prospective study of school-age children, 18% of children had weekly abdominal pain that persisted for more than 12 weeks (Saps et al 2009).

Four percent of school children have limb pains and 15% report growing pains (Goodenough 1998; Naish & Apley 1950). Growing pains are characterized by deep aching sensations in the muscles of the lower limbs late in the day or night. A review (Evans 2008) noted that much of the literature about growing pains is of poor quality and that no one theory has explained its aetiology. Back pain is the most common chronic pain in adults. Although typically considered to be an adult pain, back pain starts early in childhood and has a sharp incline following puberty. In a large Danish community study, 35% of 17-year-old girls and 27% of boys reported back pain in the last month (Bo Andersen et al 2006). The growing problem of childhood obesity in the Western world results in children with a greater risk of physical inactivity, deconditioning, reduced bone mineral content, poor flexibility and coordination, which increases the risk for back pain (Bo Andersen et al 2006). On the other hand, children who are competitive athletes may be at greater risk for injury-related pain that is exacerbated by denial and under-treatment of pain (Nemeth et al 2005).

The incidence and prevalence of pain in children is common throughout the Western world. For example, Huguet & Miro (2008) studied 511 9–17-year-olds in the Catalan region of Spain; 88% of children reported at least one pain episode during the previous 3 months, 38.3% visited the doctor due to the pain and 37.3% suffered chronic pain. Just over 5% had moderate or high functional disability because of pain. Perquin and colleagues (2000) reported that more than 50% of 5424 children in The Netherlands had experienced pain within the previous 3 months. Approximately one-quarter had chronic pain (recurrent or continuous pain for more than 3 months). Chronic pain increased with age and was significantly higher for girls, especially those between 12 and 14 years of age. About 9% of these children experienced frequent and intense pain. In the developing world, children's risk for pain is increased by disease, conflict and war, poverty, malnutrition, and reduced access and availability of health care to treat pain and underlying issues (Finley & Forgeron 2006). King et al (2011) is recent meta-analysis of recurrent pain prevalence in children.

Fortunately, children are less likely than adults to develop serious acute or chronic health conditions that are also associated with pain. Nevertheless, some children do have cancer, HIV/AIDS, neurodegenerative disorders or rapidly progressive forms of cystic fibrosis (Berde & Collins 1999). Children with cancer experience pain due to the growth of tumours and from the procedures used to diagnose and treat their disease. Long-term survivors of childhood cancer may have causalagia, phantom limb pain, postherpatic neuralgia and central pain even though the cancer appears to be cured (Berde & Collins 1999). Neurological degeneration associated with HIV/AIDS may be painful and, as with cancer, the procedures to diagnose and treat this disease may be painful (Hirshfield et al 1996). Headache and chest pain are common in children with cystic fibrosis, especially in the last 6 months of life or if the disease has a rapid progress (Berde & Collins 1999). Sickle cell disease is an inherited blood disorder diagnosed by newborn screening. It is a chronically painful disease with both pain crises and chronic pain (Brousseau et al 2009).

The most common childhood disease that is accompanied by pain is juvenile chronic arthritis (JCA). The prevalence of juvenile rheumatoid arthritis in the community when diagnosed by clinical examination may be as high as 4 in 1000 (Manners & Diepeveen 1996). In the USA, approximately 294,000 children are diagnosed annually with significant paediatric arthritis and other rheumatologic conditions (Sacks et al 2007). Approximately 25% of children with JCA have moderate to severe pain due to the disease (Schanberg et al 1997).

Fibromyalgia is a common chronic pain syndrome in adults marked by widespread non-joint musculoskeletal pain and generalized tender points. This syndrome also affects children, especially teenage girls. Some clinicians and researchers prefer to refer to fibromyalgia as widespread pain. Buskila (2009a,b) has reviewed the research on fibromyalgia and found that in addition to pain, fatigue, non-restorative sleep, difficulties in thinking, irritable bowel syndrome, chronic fatigue, chronic headache and depression often accompany fibromyalgia. Central nervous system sensitization is a major pathophysiologic aspect of fibromyalgia. Trauma and stress often trigger its development. Treatments for fibromyalgia in children include mild to moderate exercise, antidepressants, and antiepileptics and cognitive–behavioural interventions. The outcome for children with fibromyalgia appears more positive than the outcome for adults.

Atypically developing children are probably at higher risk for pain due to underlying issues affecting their development. Clancy et al (2005) surveyed 68 children with spina bifida (30 males, 38 females) between the ages of 8 and 19 years of normal intelligence. Figure 18.1 presents the frequency of pain they reported. She found that 56% of children with spina bifida had pain once a week or more. About one in eight had pain every day.

Similarly, pain is more common in children with developmental delays. McGrath et al (1998) showed that parents and caregivers used behaviours to identify pain in children with cognitive impairments and delays. Using a validated behavioural report by parents (Breau et al 2000), Breau and her colleagues (Breau et al 2003), in a cohort study of 94 children with severe to profound cognitive delay aged 3 to 18 years, found that 73 children (78%) experienced pain at least once in a 4-week period. Accidental, gastrointestinal, infection and musculoskeletal pain were the most common. Children had an average of 9 hours per week of pain. In a subsequent study, Breau et al (2007) reported that in a year when children had more pain, they also had much poorer cognitive and social development, suggesting that pain interferes with development in these children. Such pain has significant impact on quality of life for these children (Oddson et al 2006).

Often the disease or underlying injury is itself painful for the child, but the procedures to treat the problem may also inflict pain. Debridement of dead tissue, hydrotherapy and dressing changes are painful procedures for children recovering from burn injuries. Splinting and range of motion exercises and activities can be painful for children who are recovering the use of a limb from a position of immobility. Lumbar punctures, bone marrow aspirations, injections, heel lances and so on can be painful if not adequately managed. Circumcision, a common procedure for male infants, usually performed for non-medical reasons, is painful if performed without analgesia (Geyer et al 2002).

WHAT ARE THE CHALLENGES?

Access to appropriate pain care is a serious problem. Specialist pain services are available only in some children's

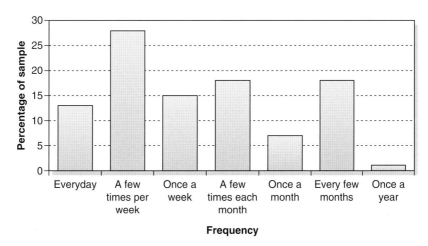

Fig. 18.1 Frequency of pain in children with spina bifida.
Reprinted from Clancy C A, McGrath P J, Oddson B E 2007 Pain in children and adolescents with spina bifida. Developmental Medicine & Child Neurology 47:27–34, with permission from John Wiley & Sons.

hospitals and even in these centres most children with chronic disabling pain are not referred to specialist care. For example, if the child population of the catchment area of the local children's hospital is one million children, then one would expect that at least 5% of these children (e.g. 50,000) would have chronic and disabling pain. Clearly, even in the best funded and staffed centres, specialist pain care will never meet this need. For this reason, every health professional who treats children and young people has an obligation to become competent in assessing and treating paediatric pain to insure that all children, even those not seen through a specialist pain clinic, have access to pain management.

Developmental considerations

Developmental changes are important in paediatric pain. Development affects the biology of pain, the way children learn to think about pain, the types of pain they may experience, the assessment and measurement of pain, and the use of different interventions.

The central and peripheral system is immature in early life but the basic connections in nociceptive and pain pathways are formed before birth (Fitzgerald 2005). There are also important postnatal changes that affect pain sensitivity and perception. The infant does not appear to have the segmental control mechanisms within the spinal cord or the descending controls from the cortex that are present in an adult (Fitzgerald 2005). Because of this neurological immaturity, an infant will have very little, if any, ability to dampen down a pain stimulus using cortical mechanisms. The implication is that infants may be extremely sensitive to all stimuli and may have heightened pain sensitivity and arousal.

Early pain events in infancy and childhood can have an impact on later pain experiences in at least two ways. The first is through memory and learning. Although it is obvious that at some point in our life we remember and learn from negative painful experiences, it is not clear when such learning begins to occur. It is part of neonatal intensive care unit folklore that infants who are subjected to numerous invasive procedures soon develop the tendency to 'go off' when their incubator is approached by anyone (McGrath & Unruh 1993). These babies demonstrate anticipatory anxiety behaviour.

Infants are also capable of developing a physiological memory of pain. In a series of studies, Taddio and colleagues found that male infants who were circumcised had higher pain scores at their routine 4- and 6-month immunizations than male infants who were not circumcised (Taddio et al 1995, 1997). Further, infants who were given EMLA, a local anaesthetic, had lower pain scores at immunizations than infants who were circumcised with a placebo. Taddio (1999) argued that circumcision may produce long-lasting changes in infant pain behaviour because of changes to the infant's central nervous system processing of painful stimuli.

Unfortunately, the belief that infants and children do not remember pain, or if they do remember it, then the memory is not long-lasting, has contributed to the inadequate management of children's pain (Cunningham 1993). Aversive childhood pain experiences can have long-term negative consequences even in adulthood, leading to fears of procedures, health professionals and healthcare settings. Such fear and anxiety can have devastating consequences for children who have chronic health conditions and recurrent or chronic pain.

Children and young people are often vulnerable to beliefs that they are exaggerating their pain or that their pain is psychological in origin, but there is no evidence to support these attitudes. Psychological attributions for pain are more convincing when they are time-locked with the onset and cessation of pain. For example, if a child complains of abdominal pain before going to school, does not complain of pain when allowed to stay home and complains of pain next morning before going to school, then it may be important to enquire about events at school. The abdominal pain may be very real for the child but the causation of the pain may be due to school difficulties.

Children learn about pain through their own pain experiences and the response of others to the pain. They also learn by observing the pain of other people, especially family and friends. Such learning enables children to develop a language to communicate about pain, to understand whether their pain needs attention and the skills to manage the pain.

Sex and gender have an impact on the pain experience of adults and the roots of this influence probably begin in childhood. There is little evidence that the sex of a child affects the prevalence of pain until puberty. After puberty, the prevalence of headache, migraine and abdominal pain increases for girls (Unruh & Campbell 1999). On the other hand, gender may have an important impact on pain through socialization and cultural expectations about pain and gender roles. There is some evidence that boys in particular are socialized to be more stoic in response to pain as part of social expectations about masculinity. Evans et al (2008) found that there was an association between girls' (not boys') complaints of pain and responses to experimental pain with the pain reports of their mothers. Moon et al (2008) reported that fathers were better judges of pain in their children than mothers.

Attitudes of health professionals and others

Blaming patients for their illnesses has a long history (Gunderman 2000). Patient blaming may take many forms, including:

- The child' pain is psychological, it's all in the child's head.

- The child's disability is because the mother or father is not firm enough with him.
- The child's pain is continuing because the child is not doing her therapy.
- The child's pain is because of the family's stress.

Stigmatizing people in pain is widespread by health professionals and others. including teachers, families and friends. Stigmatization appears to be particularly prominent when pain is a bit unusual. It is more likely to occur when there is no known underlying disease or when the underlying disease cannot seem to explain the pain.

Many children and young people who live with chronic pain report that one of the most difficult things to deal with is the attitudes of some health professionals. They report that if their pain cannot be understood, health professionals either directly or indirectly suggest that the pain is 'all in your head'. The tendency to ascribe psychological causes to pain of unknown origin or pain that shows unusual characteristics was described by Wall as a 'leap to the head' (Wall 1989). Leaping to the head for an explanation may take the form of blaming parents for the child's pain (usually the mother). Children with difficult problems, families with complex social issues, families from backgrounds that are dissimilar to those of health professionals and children or families who are seen as difficult because they are anxious or agitated in some way may be more likely to be blamed for the pain. The outcome is a desensitization of empathy between health professionals and the patient that impairs the assessment and management of pain.

Families

Children are usually accompanied by families, usually parents and most often the mother, when they are seen by a health professional about pain. Although health professionals may sometimes prefer to see the child alone, most children prefer to be seen with their parents and parents generally prefer to be with their children (von Baeyer 1997). Advice about how to support children using distraction during a procedure is helpful. Parents are often uncertain about how to best manage and support a child with pain, especially a chronic or recurrent pain. It is not uncommon for parents to be at times overly solicitous and at other times too harsh or demanding. Parents may disagree between themselves about how the child's pain should be managed. In addition, they may be anxious or uncomfortable in the healthcare environment and may be more aggressive or demanding than they intend. Parents often have multiple responsibilities (e.g. employment, other care-giving responsibilities) or other issues (e.g. single parenthood, poverty, language barriers, cultural differences) that may necessitate more care and attention. Managing pain in children is enhanced by a strong, positive relationship between parents and health professionals.

School system

School is an important part of children's lives, and many children and adolescents living with recurrent or chronic pain will have problems managing at school. These problems will be most commonly manifested by school absences. Along with school absences, children experience decreased self-confidence in their academic abilities, decreased academic achievement reduced ability to cope with the many expectations of being at school (Logan & Simons 2010) as well as loss in friendships and social support. Large studies in several countries have shown that approximately 50–75% of children who have chronic pain will have missed at least 1 or 2 days of school in the previous month due to pain and 15–20% miss more than 10 days in a month (Konijnenberg et al 2005; Logan et al 2008; Roth-Isigkeit et al 2005). In addition, some aspects of the school environment, such as carrying heavy school backpacks, poor ergonomic design of desks and computer workstations, and inadequate student lavatories, may put the child at risk for pain or exacerbate pain such as back pain and abdominal pain (Chan et al 2005). Consultation with schools is typically necessary to help children and adolescents, and their parents, overcome school-related problems associated with recurrent or chronic pain. There have been few studies of interventions to improve such children's school functioning. A recent promising study utilized a group-based cognitive–behavioural intervention with 40 adolescents and their parents, and demonstrated improvement in pain, some aspects of depression and improved school attendance (Logan & Simons 2010) but participation was low. Further research with this intervention may enhance its potential effectiveness.

Assessment and measurement of children's pain

Measurement of pain can be a challenge but there have been major advances in pain measurement across the paediatric age range. The January 2009 issue of the Journal of Pain Research and Management (www.pulsus.com/Pain/home.htm) was devoted to paediatric pain measurement and assessment. In addition, there are several meta-analytic reviews examining paediatric pain measurement (e.g. Stinson et al 2006; von Baeyer & Spagrud 2007).

There are three major strategies in measuring pain (see Chapter 7). The first is self-report: what the person says they are feeling. The second is behaviour: how the person reacts to pain. The third is physiological measures: how the person's body reacts to pain.

Self-report is not possible with infants and very young children. There are many different self-report measures that have been validated with older children and adolescents, and these are widely used. The most important issue for each health centre is to choose a standard way of measuring pain

Table 18.1 Recommended pain measures

Age group	Measure	Description	References
Babies	Premature Infant Pain Profile (PIPP)	Behavioural and physiological	Ballantyne et al 1999
	Neonatal Infant Pain Scale (NIPS)	Behavioural	Lawrence et al 1993
Toddlers and children	Children's Hospital of Eastern Ontario Pain Scale (CHEOPS)	Behavioural	McGrath et al 1985
Children 5–7 years	Pieces of Hurt	Five poker chips	Hester 1979
Children 7 years and older	Pain Faces Scale – Revised	Six line-drawn faces Instructions are available in 35 languages	Hicks et al 2001
	Numeric Rating Scale 0–10 (NRS11)	Rate your pain from 0 to 10	Huguet et al 2010 von Baeyer et al 2009

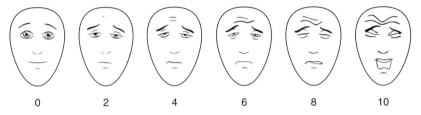

0   2   4   6   8   10

The scale is scored with the first face scored 0 and each one increasing by 2 points to yield a possible range from 0 to 10.

Fig. 18.2 The Pain Faces Scale Revised (Hicks et al 2001).

Hicks, C.L., von Baeyer, C.L., Spafford, P., et al, Faces Pain Scale - Revised: toward a common metric in pediatric pain measurement. PAIN, 2001, 93:173–183. This Faces Pain Scale - Revised has been reproduced with permission of the International Association for the Study of Pain® (IASP). The figure may not be reproduced for any other purpose without permission.

and recording it to facilitate communication. Table 18.1 provides our suggestions for pain measurement for clinicians.

We suggest two self-report scales in Table 18.1. The Pain Faces Scale Revised (Hicks et al 2001) (Fig. 18.2) is available with instructions in 35 different languages, has excellent psychometric properties and can be downloaded from the web (http://painsourcebook.ca/docs/pps92.html). Children like the scale and most children over 7 years of age can use it without difficulty.

The second self-report scale that we would recommend is the Numeric Rating Scale using 0–10 or NRS10. The child is asked, 'On a scale of zero to ten with zero being no pain and ten being the most severe pain, how much pain do you have?'

WHAT CAN HEALTH PROFESSIONALS DO?

Management of pain in infants, children and adolescents works best in a multidisciplinary team that is able to develop an integrated plan to decrease pain, improve function (especially at school) and support the child's physical, emotional and cognitive development. Even when a multidisciplinary team is not available, a sole health professional will achieve better outcomes by using multimodal methods to manage a child's pain and its sequelae. Any intervention is likely to be enhanced and have better outcomes if the parent (s) are involved and supportive. Involving the child and parents in developing a plan they perceive as beneficial is optimal.

Pain in infants and young children

Fortunately most infants and young children do not experience recurrent pain. The exceptions are infants who require intensive care at birth or early infancy. There are now well-established guidelines for management of neonatal pain. For example, Anand et al (2001) developed a consensus statement on neonatal pain and its management. The consensus statement maintains that newborns feel pain and may be more sensitive to pain than older infants and more likely to have long-term effects from exposure to painful events. Further, it notes that sedation does not treat pain and that appropriate pain management, which may include environmental, behavioural and pharmacological approaches, may decrease complications and mortality.

Table 18.2 Type of pain and evidence-based intervention (non-pharmacological)

Type of pain	Evidence-based interventions	Key references
Headaches	Cognitive–behavioural therapy Relaxation training Biofeedback	Trautmann et al 2006 Palermo et al 2010 Larrson et al 1987
Recurrent abdominal pain	Cognitive–behavioural therapy	Palermo et al 2010
	Increased fibre	Feldman et al 1988
Irritable bowel syndrome	Yoga	Kuttner et al 2006
Fibromyalgia	Cognitive–behavioural therapy	Palermo et al 2010
Growing pains	Stretching exercises	Baxter & Dulberg 1988
Needle pain and other procedure pain	Distraction, cognitive–behavioural therapy Hypnosis	Uman et al 2006 MacLaren & Cohen 2007
Post operative pain		Chorney et al 2009 Chorney & Kain 2009 Fortier et al 2010 Fortier et al 2009

In addition, it argues that if a procedure is likely to be painful in an adult, then it should be assumed to be painful in a newborn and treated accordingly.

In addition to general principles, individual pain problems in neonates and infants may have specific approaches that are indicated (Anand 2001). Anand et al (2007) have published a text on this topic.

Pain in children and adolescents

Treatment of pain in children and adolescents depends to a great extent on the type of pain, its severity and its interference with function. Pharmacological pain management is discussed in Chapter 11. Parents benefit from discussion about their concerns regarding the use of pain medication for their children with information about safety, appropriate monitoring and administration.

Table 18.2 outlines types of pain and some of the treatments that have been validated for pain management in children and youth.

Many of these interventions are also used for pain management in adults and are discussed in Chapters 8 and 9. The literature is too extensive to cover all of the possible interventions for paediatric pain or even all of the key references. Here we will focus on the interventions most commonly used in paediatrics: distraction, cognitive–behavioural therapy (CBT) and physiotherapy.

Distraction is an important part of acute pain management, especially management of procedures that may be painful. Many activities can be used for distraction but they should be age appropriate and be of sufficient interest to the child to engage the child's mind. Remembering an event that the child enjoyed, paying special attention to detailed sensory elements, makes the memory more alive. Music and short videos may be helpful. Blowing bubbles may engage a child if the child is able to move part of the body. Parents who are present during a procedure can be trained to use distraction during the procedure to help the child manage the painful situation.

CBT is an important element of most psychological interventions for pain, especially recurrent or chronic pain. It is usually administered by psychologists, but most health professionals, with some additional training, can master the skills to assist most children and adolescents. Very complex problems will need specialist assistance. The essential elements of CBT are given in Table 18.3.

Table 18.3 Elements of CBT for chronic pain in children and adolescents

Session	Topic
Introduction	Discussion of role of stress, fear, avoidance, deconditioning in chronic pain
Learning relaxation	Relaxation using suggestion, tension-release exercises, breathing
Increasing activity	Slow increase in activity Importance of pacing
Cognitive changes	Reducing catastrophizing, using cognitive restructuring
Avoidance reduction	Decreasing avoidance of feared activity
Problem solving	How to manage difficult situations

Box 18.1 **Brenda's story**

Brenda was a shy, 9-year-old girl when she was referred for pain in her right wrist that radiated up her right arm. She had previously fractured her wrist twice in falls from playground equipment and a bike. Brenda described her pain as feeling like pins and needles, aching and burning. Her mother reported that the right hand sometimes changed colour (mottled red), sometimes with activities and at rest, and the pain would then be worse. The pain was most intense with writing for long periods and with colouring activities. Brenda was falling behind in her work at school and found it upsetting. She did not want others to know she received special treatment and was shy about speaking to her teacher.

Brenda was prescribed gabapentin for pain and given neuromobilization exercises by the physiotherapist. A letter was sent to the school principal and her teacher describing Brenda's pain condition and the difficulties it caused her in trying to keep up. The pain team offered to contact the teacher but Brenda's mother preferred to advocate for her daughter with the help of the letter. The strategies suggested in the school letter included more time to complete school work such as tests or assignments during class, extensions for assignments requiring colouring and smaller-sized art projects.

Brenda's teacher followed through on these strategies and also decreased the number of questions on the girl's tests. This approach lessened the pressure on Brenda to complete a long test even if her right wrist and forearm were painful. Additionally the teacher integrated stretching and movement into the class as a whole. She encouraged students to change positions, and provided breaks from writing by standing up to stretch and move their hands. This activity gave Brenda an opportunity to do some of her neuromobilization exercises without attracting the attention of her classmates. Altogether these efforts helped to provide pain relief and kept Brenda interested in her school activities. After 8 months of intervention, which included the 2-month summer holiday, Brenda returned to school pain free and no longer on medication or in need of academic accommodations.

Children and adolescents with chronic pain often have challenges with respect to attendance and performance at school. As a result, they may develop school anxiety and social anxiety that impairs relationships with friends. A goal of intervention should be to reduce school absences due to pain and build a graded return to school where absence has occurred. Developing a programme using pacing of school activity with brief rest, reinforcement of participation and encouragement will be helpful. Education about pain and support for parents and the school through a pain team is often needed. CBT incorporating distraction, breathing, relaxation and positive self-talk has been used successfully to reduce school absenteeism (Robins et al 2005). CBT is commonly used in a self-management programme that encourages the child to identify achievable goals from one week to the next with incremental increases in expectations as goals are met.

Distraction and CBT are available to children from nurses, psychologists and occupational therapists. Each profession may have a somewhat different focus in their use of these strategies but the goal is to help the child manage pain and improve their function and ability to participate in activities.

Along with CBT most children with chronic pain will need help to maintain or increase their physical activity and physical fitness. Activities that use slow gentle movement, such as walking and swimming, will be helpful for children who are fearful that activity will increase pain. There is some preliminary evidence from a randomized controlled trial that activities like yoga may be helpful for some types of pain. Kuttner et al (2006) found that children aged 11–18 years with irritable bowel syndrome who were involved in a yoga programme had lower levels of functional impairment, less emotion-focused avoidance and lower anxiety. Physiotherapy is also often advised for children and will be more beneficial if parents are involved. In a randomized controlled trial for the treatment of growing pains, parents were instructed in muscle-stretching exercises for their children. The children in the stretching group showed rapid and significant reduction in pain whereas the control group reported a slow and less marked decline in pain (Baxter & Dulberg 1988).

Applying these strategies to individual children must be customized to the circumstances of the child and family. The cases studies in Boxes 18.1 and 18.2 illustrate the complexity of managing pain in children and adolescents.

Brenda's and Hannah's stories are fictional but put together from real cases. Both girls have serious pain that interferes with attendance and achievement at school. They required direct treatment of their pain to decrease it sufficiently to develop a plan for reintegration to school. In both cases, the plan was effective because the child, parent and school were involved in developing a plan that began with small achievable steps to ensure success. Brenda and Hannah were active participants in identifying goals. The school was given more information about the nature of the child's pain and agreed to make needed accommodations. Such intervention plans need the participation of all concerned.

RESOURCES FOR HEALTH PROFESSIONALS

Interdisciplinary paediatric pain units are the best solution for the assessment and management of children's pain but there are only a small number of clinics. All health

Box 18.2 **Hannah's story**

Hannah was 15 years old and in grade 10 when she was referred with severe back pain due to juvenile fibromyalgia. She had difficulty sleeping, found it too painful to bend over to tie her shoes and experienced sitting in a chair as extremely painful. She was absent from school for the previous year due to pain but was taking two online courses with a tutor. Hannah wanted to return to school, graduate with her friends and attend university. At the time of referral, she was socially isolated and in touch with only a few friends.

Hannah was prescribed gabapentin, amitriptyline and a non-steriodal drug for pain, taught to use cognitive–behavioural strategies along with the pharmacological regime and began a physiotherapy programme of exercises.

Once Hannah started to have some mild pain relief, a school plan was developed by the team with Hannah and her parents. This plan increased expectations on Hannah to attend school in small incremental steps. The programme started with getting up and getting dressed to go to school but working at home with her tutor and walking short distances. The next step involved talking with Hannah about which course she was most interested in at school and would enjoy attending. A meeting was then held with the school, Hannah, her parents and a team representative to develop a plan for a graduated reintegration to school. The meeting included discussion about the pathology of chronic pain, and the associated psychosocial and academic impact. The agreed reintegration plan began with one course at school in addition to the distance courses. The school board continued to pay for the tutor. The number and size of assignments were decreased and time to complete assignments was increased. Exams were home based and supervised by the tutor to enable Hannah to move about and adjust her position without disturbing other students. Hannah was given a pass to use the school elevator and permitted two sets of textbooks, one for home use. Her school schedule was organized to have free periods for rest at school or at home. She was able to sit at the back of the class to move about without disturbing others. Some school regulations concerning grades and attendance were waived to allow Hannah to join clubs and school social functions to protect against loneliness and depression. In each subsequent semester an additional course was added and the accommodations maintained. Hannah also continued with online courses during the summer months to make up for missed courses. Hannah graduated with her peers and received an entrance scholarship for university, which she currently attends part-time.

professionals who work with infants, children or adolescents need to be attentive to problems associated with children's pain. An invaluable resource for health professionals is the Pediatric Pain Listserv (pediatric-pain@lists.dal.ca or http://listserv.dal.ca/index.cgi?AO=PEDIATRC-PAIN). For many years it has been the go-to resource for healthcare professionals to seek advice from other professionals about their pain patients. The listserv has over 800 members on six continents There is no fee to join. Another resource is the Pediatric Pain Letter (http://childpain.org/ppl). There is a variety of books available specific to pain in infants (e.g. Anand et al 2007), children (e.g. Twycross et al 2009) and adolescents (e.g. Rogers 2008). Lastly, there are two conferences venues for continuing education. The International Pediatric Pain Symposium is organized by the Special Interest Group on Pain in Children of the International Association for the Study of Pain (http://childpain.org/). The International Forum on Pediatric Pain is a theme-based conference on children's pain (http://pediatric-pain.ca).

REFERENCES

Anand, K.J.S., International Evidence-Based Group for Neonatal Pain, 2001. Consensus statement for the prevention and management of pain in the newborn. Arch. Pediatr. Adolesc. Med. 155, 173–180.

Anand, K.J.S., Stevens, B.J., McGrath, P.J. (Eds.), 2007. Pain in neonates and infants, third ed. Elsevier, London.

Ballantyne, M., Stevens, B., McAllister, M., et al., 1999. Validation of the premature infant pain profile in the clinical setting. Clin. J. Pain 15, 297–303.

Baxter, M.P., Dulberg, C., 1988. 'Growing pains' in childhood – a proposal for treatment. J. Pediatr. Orthop. 8, 402–406.

Berde, C.B., Collins, J.J., 1999. Cancer pain and palliative care in children. In: Wall, P.D., Melzack, R. (Eds.), Textbook of Pain, fourth ed. Churchill Livingstone, New York, pp. 967–989.

Bo Andersen, L., Wedderkopp, N., Leboeuf-Yde, C., 2006. Association between back pain and physical fitness in adolescents. Spine 31, 1740–1744.

Breau, L.M., McGrath, P.J., Camfield, C., et al., 2000. Preliminary validation of an observational pain checklist for cognitively impaired, non-verbal persons. Dev. Med. Child Neurol. 42, 609–616.

Breau, L.M., Camfield, C.S., McGrath, P.J., et al., 2003. The incidence of pain in children with severe cognitive impairments. Arch. Pediatr. Adolesc. Med. 157, 1219–1226.

Breau, L.M., Camfield, C.S., McGrath, P.J., et al., 2007. Pain's impact on adaptive functioning. J. Intellect. Disabil. Res. 51, 125–134.

Brousseau, D.C., Panepinto, J.A., Nimmer, M., et al., 2009. The number of people with sickle cell disease in the United States: national and state estimates. Am. J. Hematol. 85, 77–78.

Buskila, D., 2009a. Developments in the scientific and clinical understanding of fibromyalgia. Arthritis Res. Ther. 11, 242–252.

Buskila, D., 2009b. Pediatric fibromyalgia. Rheum. Dis. Clin. North Am. 35, 253–261.

Chan, E.C.C., Piira, T., Betts, G., 2005. The school functioning of children with chronic and recurrent pain. Pediatric Pain Letter 7, 11–16.

Chorney, J.M., Kain, Z.N., 2009. Behavioral analysis of children's response to induction of anesthesia. Anesthesia & Analgesia 109, 1434–1440.

Chorney, J.M., Hammell, C., Blount, R., et al., 2009. Healthcare provider and parent behavior and children's distress and coping at anesthesia induction. Anesthesiology 111, 1290–1296.

Cignacco, E., Hamers, J., van Lingen, R.A., et al., 2009. Procedural pain exposure and pain management in ventilated preterm infants during the first 14 days of life. Swiss Med. Wkly. 139, 226–232.

Clancy, C.A., McGrath, P.J., Oddson, B.E., 2005. Pain in children and adolescents with spina bifida. Dev. Med. Child Neurol. 47, 27–34.

Cunningham, N., 1993. Moral and ethical issues in clinical practice. In: Anand, K.J.S., McGrath, P.J. (Eds.), Pain in Neonates. Elsevier, Amsterdam, pp. 255–273.

Davis, D.A., Luecken, L.J., Zautra, A.J., 2005. Are reports of childhood abuse related to the experience of chronic pain in adulthood: a meta-analytical view of the literature. Clin. J. Pain 21, 398–405.

Evans, A.M., 2008. Growing pains: contemporary knowledge and recommended practice. J. Foot Ankle Res. 1, 4. http://dx.doi.org/10.1186/1757-1146-1-4.

Evans, S., Tsao, T.C.I., Zeltzer, L.K., 2008. Relationship of child perceptions of maternal pain to children's laboratory and nonlaboratory pain. Pain Res. Manag. 1393, 211–218.

Fearon, I., McGrath, P.J., Achat, H., 1996. 'Booboos': the study of everyday pain among young children. Pain 68, 55–62.

Feldman, W., Rosser, W., McGrath, P., 1988. Recurrent abdominal pain in children. Can. Fam. Physician 34, 629–630.

Finley, G.A., Forgeron, P., 2006. Developing pain services around the world. In: Finley, G.A., McGrath, P.J., Chambers, C.T. (Eds.), Bringing pain relief to children: treatment approaches. Humana Press, Totowa, New Jersey, pp. 177–198.

Fitzgerald, M., 2005. The development of nociceptive circuits. Nat. Rev. Neurosci. 6, 507–520.

Fortier, M.A., Chorney, J.M., Rony, R.Y.Z., et al., 2009. Children's desire for perioperative information. Anesthesia & Analgesia 109, 1085–1090.

Fortier, M.A., Weinberg, M., Vitalano, L.M., et al., 2010. Effects of therapeutic suggestion in children undergoing general anesthesia: a randomized controlled trial. Pediatric Anesthesia 20, 90–99.

Geyer, J., Ellsbury, D., Kleiber, C., et al., 2002. An evidence-based multidisciplinary protocol for neonatal circumcision pain management. J. Obstet. Gynecol. Neonatal Nurs. 31, 403–410.

Goodenough, B., 1998. Growing pains. Pediatric Pain Letter 2, 38–41.

Gunderman, R., 2000. Illness as failure. Blaming patients. Hastings Centre Report 30, 7–11.

Hester, N.K.O., 1979. The preoperational child's reaction to immunization. Nurs. Res. 28, 250–254.

Hicks, C.L., von Baeyer, C.L., Spafford, P.A., et al., 2001. The Faces Pain Scale – Revised: toward a common metric in pediatric pain measurement. Pain 93, 173–183.

Hirshfield, S., Moss, H., Dragistic, K., et al., 1996. Pain in pediatric human immunodeficiency virus infection: incidence and characteristics in a single institution pilot study. Pediatrics. 98, 449–452.

Huguet, A., Miró, J., 2008. The severity of chronic pediatric pain: an epidemiological study. J. Pain 9, 226–236.

Huguet, A., Stinson, J.N., McGrath, P.J., 2010. Measurement of self-reported pain intensity in children and adolescents. J. Psychosom. Res. 68, 329–336.

King, S., Chambers, C., Huguet, A., et al. 2011. The epidemiology of chronic pain in children and adolescents revisited: a systematic review. Pain 152, 2729–2738.

Konijnenberg, A.Y., Uiterwaal, C., Kimpen, J., et al., 2005. Children with unexplained chronic pain: substantial impairment in everyday life. Arch. Dis. Child 90, 680–686.

Kuttner, L., Chambers, C.T., Hardial, J., et al., 2006. A randomized trial of yoga for adolescents with irritable bowel syndrome. Pain Res. Manag. 11, 217–223.

Larrson, B.S., Daleflod, B., Hakansson, L., et al., 1987. Therapist-assisted versus self-help relaxation treatment of chronic headaches in adolescents: a school-based intervention. J. Child Psychol. Psychiatry 28, 127–136.

Lawrence, J., Alcock, D., McGrath, P., et al., 1993. The development of a tool to assess neonatal pain. Neonatal Netw. 12, 59–66.

Logan, D.E., Simons, L.E., 2010. Development of a group intervention to improve school functioning in adolescents with chronic pain and depressive symptoms: a study of feasibility and preliminary efficacy. J. Pediatr. Psychol. 35, 823–836.

Logan, D.E., Simons, L.E., Stein, M.J., et al., 2008. School impairment in adolescents with chronic pain. J. Pain 9, 407–416.

Luthy, K.E., Beckstrand, R.L., Peterson, N.E., 2009. Parental hesitation as a factor in delayed childhood immunization. J. Pediatr. Health Care. 23, 388–393.

MacLaren, J., Cohen, L.L., 2007. Interventions for pediatric procedure-related pain in primary care. Paediatrics & Child Health 12, 111–116.

Manners, P.J., Diepeveen, D.A., 1996. Prevalence of juvenile chronic arthritis in a population of 12-year-old children in urban Australia. Pediatrics 98, 84–90.

McGrath, P.J., Unruh, A.M., 1993. Social and legal issues. In: Anand, K.J.S., McGrath, P.J. (Eds.), Pain in

Neonates. Elsevier, Amsterdam, pp. 295–320.

McGrath, P.J., Johnson, G., Goodman, J., et al., 1985. The CHEOPS: a behavioral scale to measure post operative pain in children. In: Fields, H.L., Dubner, R., Cervero, F. (Eds.), Advances in Pain Research and Clinical Management. Raven Press, New York, pp. 395–402.

McGrath, P.J., Rosmus, C., Camfield, C., et al., 1998. Behaviours caregivers use to determine pain in non-verbal, cognitively impaired individuals. Dev. Med. Child Neurol. 40, 340–343.

Moon, E., Chambers, C.T., Larochette, A.C., et al., 2008. Sex differences in parent and child pain ratings during an experimental child pain task. Pain Res. Manag. 13, 225–230.

Naish, J.M., Apley, J., 1950. Growing pains: a clinical study of non-arthritic limb pains inchildren. Arch. Dis. Child 26, 134–140.

Nemeth, R.L., von Baeyer, C.L., Rocha, E.M., 2005. Young gymnasts' understanding of sport-related pain: a contribution to prevention of injury. Child Care Health Dev. 31, 615–625.

Nurko, S., 2009. The tip of the iceberg: the prevalence of functional gastrointestinal diseases in children. J. Pediatr. 154, 313–315.

Oddson, B.E., Clancy, C.A., McGrath, P.J., 2006. The role of pain in reduced quality of life and depressive symptomology in children with spina bifida. Clin. J. Pain 22, 784–789.

Palermo, T.M., Eccleston, C., Lewandowski, A.S., et al., 2010. Randomized controlled trials of psychological therapies for management of chronic pain in children and adolescents: an updated meta-analytic review. Pain 148, 387–397.

Perquin, C.W., Hazebroek-Kampschreur, A.A., Hunfeld, J.A., et al., 2000. Pain in children and adolescents: a common experience. Pain 87, 51–58.

Robins, M., Smith, S., Glutting, J.J., et al., 2005. A randomized controlled trial of a cognitive–behavioral family intervention for pediatric recurrent

abdominal pain. J. Pediatr. Psychol. 30, 397–408.

Rogers, R., 2008. Managing persistent pain in adolescents: a handbook for therapists. Radcliffe, Oxford and New York.

Roth-Isigkeit, A., Thyen, U., Stoven, H., et al., 2005. Pain among children and adolescents: restrictions in daily living and triggering factors. Pediatrics 115, e152–e162.

Sacks, J.J., Helmick, C.G., Luo, Y.H., et al., 2007. Prevalence of and ambulatory health care visits for pediatric arthritis and other rheumatological conditions in the United States 2001–2004. Arthritis Care Res. 57, 1439–1445.

Saps, M., Seshadri, R., Sztainberg, M., et al., 2009. A prospective school-based study of abdominal pain and other common somatic complaints in children. J. Pediatr. 154, 322–326.

Schanberg, L.E., Lefebvre, J.C., Keefe, F.J., et al., 1997. Pain coping and the pain experience in children with juvenile chronic arthritis. Pain 73, 181–189.

Stevens, B., Yamada, J., Ohlsson, A., 2004. Sucrose for analgesia in newborn infants undergoing painful procedures. Cochrane Database Syst. Rev. 3, CD001069.

Stinson, J.N., Kavanagh, T., Yamada, J., et al., 2006. Systematic review of the psychometric properties, interpretability and feasibility of self-report pain intensity measures for use in clinical trials in children and adolescents. Pain 125, 143–157.

Straus, M.A., Stewart, J.H., 1999. Corporal punishment by American parents: national data prevalence, chronicity, severity, and duration, in relation to child and family characteristics. Clin. Child Fam. Psychol. Rev. 2, 55–70.

Taddio, A., 1999. Effects of early pain experience: the human literature. In: McGrath, P.J., Hinley, G.A. (Eds.), Chronic and Recurrent Pain in Children and Adolescents, Progress in Pain Research and Management, vol. 13. pp. 57–74.

Taddio, A., Goldbach, M., Ipp, M., et al., 1995. Effects of neonatal circumcision on pain response during vaccination in boys. Lancet 345, 291–292.

Taddio, A., Stevens, B., Craig, K., et al., 1997. Efficacy and safety of lidocaine-prilocaine cream for pain during circumcision. N. Engl. J. Med. 336, 1197–1201.

Trautmann, E., Lackschewitz, H., Kröner-Herwig, B., 2006. Psychological treatment of recurrent headache in children and adolescents – a meta-analysis. Cephalalgia 26, 1411–1426.

Twycross, A., Dowden, S., Bruce, E. (Eds.), 2009. Managing pain in children: A clinical guide. Wiley- Blackwell, Oxford.

Unruh, A.M., Campbell, M.A., 1999. Gender variation in children's pain experiences. In: McGrath, P.J., Finley, G.A. (Eds.), Chronic and recurrent pain in children and adolescents, Progress in Pain Research and Management, vol. 13. pp. 199–241.

Uman, L.S., Chambers, C.T., McGrath, P.J., et al., 2006. Psychological interventions for needle-related procedural pain and distress in children and adolescents. Cochrane Database Syst. Rev. 18 (4), CD005179.

von Baeyer, C.L., 1997. Presence of parents during painful procedures. Pediatric Pain Letter 1, 56–59.

von Baeyer, C., Spagrud, L.J., 2007. Systematic review of observational (behavioral) measures of pain for children and adolescents aged 3 to 18 years. Pain 127, 140–150.

von Baeyer, C.L., Baskerville, S., McGrath, P.J., 1998. Everyday pain in three- to five-year-old children in day care. Pain Res. Manag. 3, 111–116.

von Baeyer, C.L., Spagrud, L.J., McCormick, J.C., et al., 2009. Three new datasets supporting use of the Numerical Rating Scale (NRS-11) for children's self-reports of pain intensity. Pain 143, 223–227.

Wall, P.D., 1989. Introduction. In: Wall, P.D., Melzack, R. (Eds.), Textbook of pain, second ed. Churchill Livingstone, Edinburgh, pp. 1–18.

Walsh, C.A., Jamieson, E., MacMillan, H., et al., 2007. Child abuse and chronic pain in a community survey of women. J. Interpers. Violence 22, 1536–1554.

Chapter | 19 |

Pain in the elderly

Stephen J. Gibson

LEARNING OBJECTIVES

At the end of this chapter readers will have an understanding of:

1. How the pain experience differs with age.
2. Particular conditions that commonly cause pain among middle-aged and older people.
3. Differences in pain report and coping strategies among people of different age groups.
4. How age-related changes in neurophysiology may alter the pain experience.
5. How the pain experience is unique for older people in special populations, such as those with dementia.
6. How to approach the assessment of pain in elderly persons.
7. Some key points about pain management in elderly people.

OVERVIEW

Throughout the world there has been an increase in the number of people living into old age. Throughout the world the number of people aged over 60 years is anticipated to triple by 2050, and the number over 80 years of age is expected to increase by more than five-fold (Australian Bureau of Statistics 2004). This is relevant for many nations, including Australia, Japan, Korea and the USA. For example, in Korea an escalation of the number of older persons is expected, with older adults expected to increase from 7.2% to 14.3% of the total Korean population by 2018 (Park et al 2009). In the USA it is expected that the population aged 65 and above will double by 2050 (US Census Bureau DIS 2012).

With an ageing population, it is important for healthcare professionals to be cognizant of the prevalence of pain in the elderly, special issues related to pain perception and expression among the elderly, and assessment, treatment and management approaches for elderly people with pain.

© 2014 Elsevier Ltd.

THE EPIDEMIOLOGY OF PAIN ACROSS THE LIFESPAN

Recent reviews of the epidemiologic literature reveal a marked age-related increase in the prevalence of persistent pain (often defined as pain on most days persisting beyond 3 months) up until the seventh decade of life and then either a plateau or slight decline into very advanced age (Helme & Gibson 2001; McBeth & Jones 2007). In contrast, the prevalence of acute pain in the community appears to remain relatively constant at approximately 5% regardless of age (Crook et al 1984; Kendig et al 1996). Absolute prevalence rates of persistent pain vary widely between different studies (7–80%) and depend upon the time interval sampled (days, weeks, months, lifetime), the time in pain during this interval (pain everyday, most days, at least weekly, any pain during the period), the severity of pain needed for inclusion as a case (mild, moderate, bothersome, activity limiting, etc.) and the sampling technique (telephone, interview, questionnaire). Nonetheless, with one exception (Crook et al 1984), all studies show a progressive increase in pain prevalence throughout early adulthood (7–20%), with a peak prevalence during late middle age (50–65; 20–80%) followed by a plateau or decline in the 'old' old (75–85) and 'oldest' old (85+) adults (25–60%) (Andersson et al 1993; Bassols et al 1999; Blyth et al 2001; Brattberg et al 1989, 1997; Herr et al 1991; Kendig et al 1996; Kind et al 1998; Magni et al 1993; Tsang et al 2008).

When considering pain at specific anatomical sites, a slightly different picture emerges. Foot and leg pain have been reported to increase with advancing age well into the ninth decade of life (Benvenuti et al 1995; Herr et al 1991; Leveille et al 1998). The prevalence of articular joint pain (particularly of weight-bearing joints) also doubles in adults over 65 years of age (Barberger-Gateau et al 1992; Bergman et al 2001; Harkins et al 1994; Sternbach 1986; Von Korff et al 1990). Conversely, the prevalence of headache (Andersson et al 1993; D'Alessandro et al 1988; Kay et al 1992; Sternbach 1986), abdominal pain (Kay et al 1992; Lavsky-Shulan et al 1985) and chest pain (Andersson et al 1993; Sternbach 1986; Tibblin et al 1990; Von Korff et al 1988) all peak during later middle age (45–55) and decline thereafter. Oral pain may not change in prevalence over the lifespan (Leung et al 2008). Studies of age-specific rates of back pain are mixed, with some reports of a progressive increase over the lifespan (Dionne et al 2006; Harkins et al 1994; Von Korff et al 1988) and others of a reverse trend after a peak prevalence at 40–50 years (Andersson et al 1993; Borenstein 2001; Sternbach 1986; Tibblin et al 1990). While the site of pain does seem to influence the age-related pattern of pain prevalence, with the exception of joint pain, a consensus view from these studies would still support the notion of peak pain prevalence in late middle age and then a decline in persistent pain into very advanced age.

The very high prevalence of pain noted in older segments of the community has clear resource implications for the provision of pain management, but it is important to understand that not all persistent pain will be bothersome or of high impact. Indeed, many older persons will not seek treatment for pain and will manage pain symptoms without help. For this reason, several recent studies have started to focus on pain termed as 'clinically relevant' or 'clinically significant'. Large epidemiologic surveys show that approximately 14% of adults over 60 years suffer from moderate-severe or significant pain, defined as continuous, needing professional treatment and occurring on most days in the past 3 months (Breivik et al 2006; Smith et al 2001). Adults aged 75+ have been found to be four times more likely to suffer from a significant pain problem than young adults. Similarly, 15% of residents in nursing homes have moderate-severe pain and almost half of these have been judged to have inadequate pain management (Teno et al 2003). It appears, therefore, that 'clinically relevant' pain also shows a major age-related increase in prevalence, and that older segments of the community are in most need of state-of-the-art treatment services for the management of bothersome pain.

AGE DIFFERENCES IN PAIN AS A PRESENTING SYMPTOM OF CLINICAL DISEASE

Another source of information on age-related changes in the pain experience can be derived from the patterns of symptom presentation in those clinical disease states that are known to have pain as a usual component (Gibson & Helme 2001; Pickering 2005). The majority of studies in this area have focused on somatic or visceral pain complaints and particularly myocardial pain, abdominal pain associated with acute infection and different forms of malignancy. Variations in the classic presentations of 'crushing' myocardial pain in the chest, left arm and jaw are known to be much more common in older adults. Indeed, approximately 35–42% of adults over the age of 65 years experience apparently silent or painless heart attack (Konu 1977; MacDonald et al 1983). For many patients with coronary artery disease, strenuous physical exercise will induce myocardial ischaemia as indexed by a 1 mm drop in the ST segment of the electrocardiogram. By comparing the onset and degree of exertion-induced ischaemia with subjective pain report, it is possible to provide an experimentally controlled evaluation of myocardial pain across the adult lifespan. Several studies have documented a significant age-related delay between the onset of ischaemia and the report of chest pain

(Ambepitiya et al 1993, 1994; Miller et al 1990; Rittger et al 2010). Adults over 70 years take almost three times as long as young adults to first report the presence of pain (Ambepitiya et al 1993, 1994; Rittger et al 2010). Moreover, the severity of pain report is reduced even after controlling for variations in the extent of ischaemia. Collectively, these findings provide strong support for the view that myocardial pain may be somewhat muted in adults of advanced age.

With regard to pain associated with various types of malignancy, a retrospective review of more than 1500 cases revealed a marked difference in the incidence of pain between younger adults (55% with pain), middle-aged adults (35% with pain) and older adults (26% with pain) (Cherng et al 1991). With one exception (Vigano et al 1998), most studies also note a significant decline in the intensity of cancer pain symptoms in adults of advanced age (70+ years) (Brescia et al 1992; Caraceni & Portenoy 1999; McMillan 1989). The presentation of clinical pain associated with abdominal complaints such as peritonitis, peptic ulcer and intestinal obstruction shows a similar pattern of age-related change. Pain symptoms become more occult after the age of 80 years and, in marked contrast to young adults, the collection of clinical symptoms (nausea, fever, tachycardia) with the highest diagnostic accuracy does not even include abdominal pain. (Albano et al 1975; Wroblewski & Mikulowski 1991). From these uncontrolled studies, it is difficult to ascertain whether the apparent decline in pain reflects some age difference in disease severity and/or the willingness to report pain as a symptom, or whether it reflects an actual age-related change in the pain experience itself.

Other reports of atypical pain presentation have been documented for pneumonia, pneumothorax and postoperative pain. For instance, several studies suggest that older adults report a lower intensity of pain in the postoperative recovery period even after matching for the type of surgical procedure and the extent of tissue damage (Morrison et al 1998; Oberle et al 1990; Thomas et al 1998). This change is thought to be clinically significant and is in the order of a 10–20% reduction per decade after the age of 60 years (Morrison et al 1998; Thomas et al 1998). Older men undergoing prostatectomy reported less pain on a present pain intensity scale and McGill Pain Questionnaire (but not on a visual analogue scale) in the immediate post-operative period and used less patient-controlled opioid analgesia than younger men undergoing the same procedure (Gagliese & Katz 2003). Recent studies of chronic musculoskeletal pain have also started to address the issue of age differences. This is of considerable importance given that more than three-quarters of persistent pain states are of musculoskeletal origin. Unfortunately, the findings are quite equivocal, with reports of increased severity of arthritic pain in older adults (Chiou et al 2009; Harkins et al 1994), decreased pain severity (Lichtenberg et al 1984; Parker et al 1988) and no change

(Gagliese & Melzack 1997; Yunus et al 1988). Some caution is needed when interpreting these findings, as the studies cited do not indicate that pain is reduced in older persons when it is actually reported. On the contrary, a report of pain is probably greater evidence of discomfort in older persons who do choose to report it and, even though pain symptoms may be more occult, the demonstrated age-related increase in disease prevalence (including in those cases mentioned above) suggests a corresponding increase in the prevalence of pain in older adults, at least until very advanced age.

SUMMARY OF EPIDEMIOLOGIC STUDIES ON AGE DIFFERENCES IN PAIN

The findings from numerous large-sample epidemiologic studies as well as retrospective case reviews of clinical pain presentation in various somatic and visceral disease states suggest that pain is most common during the late middle-aged phase of life, and that this is true regardless of the anatomical site or the pathogenic cause of pain. The one exception appears to be degenerative joint disease (e.g. osteoarthritis), which shows an exponential increase up until at least 90 years of age. Studies of clinical disease and injury would suggest a relative absence of pain, often with an atypical presentation and a reduction in the intensity of pain symptoms, with very advanced age.

EPIDEMIOLOGY OF PAIN IN SPECIAL OLDER POPULATIONS

Persistent pain is typically more common in institutional settings such as residential care facilities and nursing homes. Almost 5% of the older adult population will reside in nursing homes or long-term care settings in developed countries, and over half of these will suffer from cognitive impairment or dementia (Gibson 2007). As a result, it is important to characterize the epidemiology of pain in these special older populations. A number of studies demonstrate an exceptionally high prevalence of pain in residential aged care facilities, with as many as 58–83% of residents suffering from some persistent pain complaint (Ferrell 1995; Parmelee et al 1993; Weiner et al 1998). Using the minimum data set from all nursing homes in the USA (representing almost 2.2 million residents), approximately 15% of residents had 'clinically significant' pain of moderate or severe intensity and 3.7% had excruciating pain on at least one day in the previous week (Teno et al 2001, 2004).

There is some evidence to suggest a lower prevalence of pain in persons with cognitive impairment or dementia

(Parmelee et al 1993; Proctor & Hirdes 2001; Walid & Zaytseva 2009). A significant inverse relationship between pain report and cognitive impairment has been shown in nursing home residents (Cohen-Mansfield & Marx 1993; Parmelee et al 1993). Both the prevalence and severity of pain were reduced in those with more severe cognitive impairment, and the magnitude of difference was quite large. For instance, pain was detected in just 31.5% of cognitively impaired residents, compared to 61% of cognitively intact residents, despite both groups being equally afflicted with potentially painful disease (Proctor & Hirdes 2001). Subsequent work has confirmed that the observed decrease in pain occurs when using either self-report pain assessment (Leong & Nuo 2007; Mäntyselkä et al 2004) or, with one exception (Feldt et al 1998), observational pain scales or proxy nurse ratings of a resident's pain (Leong & Nuo 2007; Sawyer et al 2007; Wu et al 2005). Given the similar findings with both self-report and observational assessments, it might be deduced that the reduced levels of pain prevalence and intensity are not simply due to deterioration in verbal communication skills with advancing dementia. There is also reduced pain report in those with dementia following acute medical procedures, including venipuncture (Porter et al 1996) and injection (Defrin et al 2006), as well as a possible reduction in the prevalence of post-lumbar puncture headache (Blennow et al 1993). There have been relatively few studies to examine pain report in different subtypes of dementia, although patients with Alzheimer's disease indicate a significant decrease in self-rated pain intensity and affect when compared to age-matched controls (Scherder et al 1999, 2001), and the reduction in self-reported or observational pain scores has not been found to differ according to dementia diagnosis (vascular, Alzheimer's disease, mixed) (Husebo et al 2008; Mäntyselkä et al 2004).

EXPLAINING AGE DIFFERENCES IN PAIN PREVALENCE AND REPORT

The age-related increase in pain prevalence until late middle age is easy to explain given that the highest rates of surgery, injury and painful degenerative disease are found in the older segments of the population. However, the unexpected drop in pain prevalence during very advanced age is perhaps more difficult to understand, as the rates of injury and disease continue to climb over the entire adult lifespan. Indeed, several recent systematic reviews of the epidemiology of radiographic osteoarthritis demonstrate a continual and escalating rise in incident disease with advancing age (Arden & Nevitt 2006). Osteoarthritis of weight-bearing joints (hips, knees, feet) is present in the majority of individuals by age 65 years and affects more than 80% of persons over 75 years of age. This single entity could be expected to lead to a massive age-related increase in the

presence of persistent pain. However, it is widely acknowledged that joints affected by osteoarthritis often remain asymptomatic (pain-free) despite the presence of radiographic change, and this apparent discordance between symptoms and disease (Hannan et al 2000) mirrors the situation of more occult pain symptoms in many other clinical conditions (see above). In explaining differences in pain perception and report one needs to consider age differences in the neurophysiological aspects underlying the experience of pain, and the role of psychological and social mediators of pain in older persons.

AGE DIFFERENCES IN PSYCHOSOCIAL ASPECTS OF PAIN

Modern conceptualizations of pain emphasize a biopsychosocial perspective in which biological, psychological and social factors all play a relevant role in shaping the experience and reporting of pain. As a result, changes to any one of these systems are likely to help account for the observed age-related changes in pain.

It has been suggested that older adults perceive pain as something to be expected and just a normal part of old age (Hofland 1992). With some exceptions (Gagliese & Melzack 1997; McCracken 1998), empirical studies of pain appraisals and ageing provide clear support for this view (Liddell & Locker 1997; Fahey et al 2008; Ruzicka 1998; Stoller 1993; Weiner & Rudy 2002) and the idea that older adults are often more accepting of mild pain symptoms (Appelt et al 2007; Gignac et al 2006). For instance, when compared to arthritis patients aged 50–59 years, adults aged greater than 70 years were 2.3 times more likely to agree with the statement that 'arthritis is just a natural part of growing old' and 5.2 times more likely to endorse the statement that 'people should expect to have to live with pain as they grow old' (Appelt et al 2007). This style of misattribution has important implications, as older people appear less threatened by mild pain symptoms and are less likely to seek treatment (Stoller 1993). However, this mistaken accreditation of pain symptoms to normal ageing only occurs for mild-moderate aches and pains. If pain is severe, older persons are more likely to interpret the experience as a sign of serious illness and are more likely to seek rapid medical care than their younger counterparts (Leventhal & Prohaska 1986; Stoller 1993).

Attention has also started to focus on age differences in other types of pain beliefs, such as stoicism, control over pain and beliefs in finding a cure. The conviction that organic issues are important in determining the pain experience have been reported as similar between younger and older chronic pain patients (Gagliese & Melzack 1997), although older patients may be less inclined to acknowledge that pain leads to emotional disturbance (Cook et al 1999). In addition, older adults appear to endorse a greater conviction in finding a medical cure for pain and have a lesser belief that persistent pain is disabling (Gibson 2003). The locus of control scale has been used to examine age differences in cognitive factors related to control over pain. Older chronic pain patients have a greater belief in pain severity being controlled by factors of chance or fate (Gibson & Helme 2000) when compared to younger pain patients, who seem more likely to endorse their own behaviours and actions as the strongest determinant of pain severity. Older patients with chronic pain also express more stoicism toward pain (Yong 2006; Yong et al 2001, 2003), with higher reported stoic-fortitude and a greater cautious self-doubt for pain report. This finding is consistent with other studies of stoic attitudes in older pain patients (Machin & Williams 1998) and provides strong empirical support for the widely held view that older cohorts are generally more stoic in response to pain.

In order to deal with the negative impacts of persistent pain on quality of life, patients often develop a variety of coping strategies. The self-perceived efficacy in being able to use coping methods to successfully manage pain does not appear to change with advancing age (Corran et al 1994; Gagliese et al 2000; Keefe & Williams 1990; Keefe et al 1991; Watkins et al 1999). The findings on age differences in coping strategies have somewhat mixed results. Studies by Keefe and colleagues have shown no age differences in the frequency of coping strategy use, although there was a strong trend for older adults to engage more with praying and hoping than young people (Keefe & Williams 1990; Keefe et al 1991). Conversely, older people with chronic pain have been found to report fewer cognitive coping strategies and an increased use of physical methods of pain control when compared to young adults (Sorkin et al 1990). Corran et al (1994) examined a large sample of outpatients attending a multidisciplinary pain treatment centre and found a significantly higher prevalence of praying and hoping as well as fewer incidences of ignoring pain in adults aged greater than 60 years. Watkins et al (1999) also reported clear age differences for patients in mild pain, with middle-aged and older adults reporting more catastrophizing, praying and hoping, but less frequent use of self-coping statements, than younger adults. Further research is needed to help document the extent and type of age differences in coping efforts and the exact circumstances under which this might occur.

Overall, there does appear to be some age differences in pain beliefs, coping, attributional style and attitudes towards pain. If a pain symptom is mild or transient in older adults, it is likely to be attributed to the normal ageing process, be more readily accepted and be accompanied by a different choice of strategy to cope with pain. These factors are likely to diminish the importance of mild aches and pains, and actually alter the meaning of pain symptoms. More stoic attitudes to mild pain and a stronger belief in chance factors as the major determinant of pain severity are likely to lead to the under-reporting of pain symptoms

by older segments of the adult population. However, many of the age differences in coping, misattribution and beliefs disappear if pain is persistent or severe.

AGE-RELATED CHANGES IN NEUROPHYSIOLOGY

Any age-related change in the function of nociceptive pathways would also be expected to alter pain sensitivity and therefore alter the perception of noxious events and the prevalence of pain complaints over the adult lifespan. Recent reviews by Gibson (2003), Gibson & Farrell (2004) and Gagliese & Farrell (2005) summarize the age-related changes that occur in pain perception and the underlying neurophysiology of nociception. In general, the nervous system of older persons shows extensive alterations in structure, neurochemistry and function of both peripheral and central nervous systems, including a neurochemical deterioration of the opioid and serotonergic systems. Therefore, there may be changes in nociceptive processing, including impairment of the pain inhibitory system.

Peripheral nerves show a decrease in density (both myelinated and, particularly, unmyelinated peripheral nerve fibres), and there is an increase in the number of fibres with signs of damage or degeneration. A slowing of conduction velocity and reductions in substance P, calcitonin gene-related peptide (CGRP) and somatostatin levels have been reported (Helme & McKernan 1985; Li & Duckles 1993; Ochoa & Mair 1969). Studies of the perceptual experience associated with activation of nociceptive fibres indicate a selective age-related impairment in Aδ-fibre function and a greater reliance on C-fibre information for the report of pain in older adults (Chakour et al 1996). Given that Aδ fibres subserve the epicritic, first warning aspects of pain, while the C-fibre sensation is more prolonged, dull and diffuse, one might reasonably expect some changes in pain quality and intensity in older adults.

Consistent with these changes in peripheral nociceptive function, a number of studies using experimental pain stimuli have shown that pain threshold, or the minimum intensity of noxious stimulation required to elicit a report of just noticeable pain, is increased in older persons (i.e. they are less sensitive to faint pain). The magnitude of age-related change depends on a number of factors, including the modality of stimulation used, and, regardless of stimulus modality, the age-related change appears to be modest and somewhat inconsistent. Nonetheless, a meta-analysis of all 50+ studies of pain threshold does demonstrate a significant overall increase in pain threshold in older adults (Gibson 2003). Older people tend to have higher thresholds for thermal stimuli and a minor increase with electrical stimuli (Gibson 2003), while pressure pain thresholds may actually decrease (Lautenbacher et al 2005).

The significance of these observations in the clinical setting, where pain is a pathophysiological process, remains uncertain, although it could indicate some deficit in the early warning function of pain and contribute to a greater risk of delayed diagnosis of injury or disease (Gibson & Farrell 2004).

Similar structural and neurochemical changes have been noted in the central nervous system of older humans. There are sensory neuron degenerative changes and loss of myelin in the dorsal horn of the spinal cord, as well as reductions in substance P, CGRP and somatostatin levels. Decreases in noradrenergic and serotonergic neurons may contribute to the impairment of descending inhibitory mechanisms and may underlie the decrease in pain tolerance observed in the elderly (see below). Age-related loss of neurons and dendritic connections is seen in the human brain, particularly in the cerebral cortex, including those areas involved in nociceptive processing, synthesis, axonal transport and receptor binding of neurotransmitters also change. Opioid receptor density is decreased in the brain but not in the spinal cord, and there may be decreases in endogenous opioids. An investigation of the cortical response to painful stimulation has documented some changes in adults over 60 years. Using the pain-related encephalographic response in order to index the central nervous system processing of noxious input, older adults were found to display a significant reduction in peak amplitude and an increased latency of response (Gibson et al 1990). These findings might suggest an age-related slowing in the cognitive processing of noxious information and a reduced cortical activation. More recently, Cole and colleagues (2009) used neuroimaging techniques (fMRI) to examine the brain regions activated during noxious mechanical stimulation. Both younger and older adults showed significant pain-related activity in a common network of areas, including the insula, cingulate, posterior parietal and somatosensory cortices. However, compared with older adults, young subjects showed significantly greater activity in the contralateral putamen and caudate, which could not be accounted for by increased age-associated atrophy in these regions. The age-related difference in pain-evoked activity was suggested to reflect a reduced functioning of striatal pain modulatory mechanisms with advancing age and a possible impairment in endogenous pain inhibitory networks (see below).

Variations in pain sensitivity depend not only on activity in the afferent nociceptive pathways but also endogenous pain inhibitory control mechanisms that descend from the cortex and midbrain onto spinal cord neurons. Two studies have reported that the analgesic efficacy of this endogenous inhibitory system may decline with advancing age (Edwards et al 2003; Washington et al 2000). Following activation of the endogenous analgesic system, young adults showed an increase in pain threshold of up to 150%, whereas the apparently healthy older adult group increased pain threshold by approximately 40%. Such age differences in the efficiency of endogenous

analgesic modulation are consistent with many earlier animal studies (see Bodnar et al 1988 for review) and would be expected to reduce the ability of older adults to cope with severe or strong pain. It is not surprising, therefore, that there is also convincing evidence that all 13 studies of experimental pain tolerance (or the intensity of stimulation tolerated before withdrawing from further stimulation), across several different modalities of stimulation, show a reduced pain tolerance in older adults (Gibson 2003).

AGE DIFFERENCES IN PAIN PROCESSING UNDER PATHOPHYSIOLOGIC CONDITIONS

Recently there has also been research directed at developing a better understanding of age differences in pain neurophysiology under pathophysiological conditions. Such studies are needed as all clinical pain states associated with injury or disease involve some pathophysiological changes in the nociceptive system. Three studies have shown that the temporal summation of noxious input may be altered in older persons (Edwards & Fillingim 2001; Farrell & Gibson 2007; Harkins et al 1996). Temporal summation refers to the enhancement of pain sensation associated with repeated stimulation. Using experimental pain stimuli, it can be shown that the threshold for temporal summation is lower in older persons (Edwards & Fillingim 2001; Gibson & Farrell 2004; Harkins et al 1996). In subjects given trains of five brief electrical stimuli of varying frequency (ranging from two pulses every second through to one pulse every 5 seconds), older subjects showed temporal summation at all frequencies of stimulation, whereas summation was not seen at the slower stimulation frequencies in younger subjects (Farrell & Gibson 2007). Temporal summation of thermal stimuli was increased in older adults compared with younger subjects (Edwards & Fillingim 2001; Lautenbacher et al 2005) and was considerably prolonged in duration (Edwards & Fillingim 2001), but temporal summation of pressure pain showed no age-related effects (Lautenbacher et al 2005). Temporal summation is known to result from a transient sensitization of dorsal horn neurons in the spinal cord and is thought to play a role in the development and expression of post-injury tenderness and hyperalgesia. The increased responses and prolonged duration of central sensitization in older adults, even when stimuli are delivered further apart, may indicate that it is more difficult to reverse the pathophysiological changes in the nociceptive system once they have occurred (Farrell & Gibson 2007). Zheng et al (2000) offer complementary findings using a different experimental model by comparing the intensity and time course of post-injury hyperalgesia in younger (20–40) and older (73–88) adults. While the intensity and area of hyperalgesia was similar in both groups, the state of mechanical tenderness persisted for a much longer duration in the older group. The mechanical tenderness was not altered by the application of local anaesthetic (Zheng et al 2009), confirming previous research which shows that mechanical tenderness is mediated by sensitized spinal neurons. These findings may indicate a reduced capacity of the aged central nervous system to reverse the sensitization process once it has been initiated. The clinical implication is that post-injury pain and tenderness will resolve more slowly in older persons. However, in combination with the studies of temporal summation, these findings provide strong evidence for an age-related reduction in the functional plasticity of spinal nociceptive neurons following an acute noxious event.

In summary, the evidence from numerous neurophysiologic and psychophysical studies suggests a small, but demonstrable, age-related impairment in the early warning functions of pain. The increase in pain perception threshold and the widespread change in the structure and function of peripheral and central nervous system nociceptive pathways may place the older person at greater risk of undiagnosed injury or disease. Moreover, the reduced efficacy of endogenous analgesic systems, a decreased tolerance of pain, a greater propensity to central sensitization of the nociceptive system and the slower resolution of post-injury hyperalgesia with a heightened sensitivity to pain may make it more difficult for the older adult to cope once injury has occurred.

PAIN PROCESSING IN PERSONS WITH DEMENTIA

Dementia may exacerbate age-related impairments in pain processing, and there is growing international debate as to whether persons with a dementing illness actually feel less pain than age-matched peers (Scherder et al 2009). As discussed previously, the prevalence and severity of clinical pain appear to be reduced in persons with cognitive impairment when using self-report, observational pain scales or proxy ratings. There are blunted autonomic reactions to acute medical procedures, such as injection and venipuncture, but increased facial expression of pain and enhanced withdrawal reflexes in those with Alzheimer's disease (Defrin et al 2006; Porter et al 1996). Pain threshold appears to remain unchanged in persons with Alzheimer's disease, but pain tolerance may be increased (Benedetti et al 1999; Gibson et al 2001), suggesting a selective deterioration in the affective-motivational aspects of pain (Scherder et al 2009). However, a recent neuroimaging study of central nervous system processing revealed significantly greater pain-related activations in various regions for patients with Alzheimer's disease, including regions known to be involved in the cognitive and affective components of pain processing (i.e. dorsolateral prefrontal cortex, mid cingulate cortex and insula) (Cole et al 2006).

It is somewhat difficult to reconcile these divergent findings of increase, decrease and no change in pain perception and associated physiological responses. It seems likely that the severity of dementia may help to explain this disparate evidence base, as most experimental studies have been conducted in those with mild disease, whereas clinical measures of pain are also taken from those with more advanced disease. At present, it appears dementia may impair pain perception at least in more severe cases, but the extent of change in pain perception with the progression of dementia remains unclear. Further research is needed in order to answer this important question.

Key points from the case study:

- Older people may have multiple health conditions which make good assessment and management more difficult.
- Older people with cognitive impairments may not be able to articulate that they are in pain, and where so.
- Good observation skills are critical in understanding pain in cognitively impaired persons.
- Gathering data from family members assists in better understanding the client.

Assessment of pain in older people

The key points regarding assessment of pain have been covered earlier in Chapter 7. As noted, chronic pain requires a multifaceted, comprehensive assessment, including due attention to pain intensity, quality and variations over time and situation, the extent of psychological disturbance, the degree of functional impairment in activities of daily life and the social impacts of chronic pain. In older persons, it is also argued that taking a prior medical history, a full physical examination and an assessment of all co-morbid disease is of particular importance (Herr 2005). Considerable work has been undertaken in this area, and documents such as the Interdisciplinary Expert Consensus Statement on Assessment of Pain in Older Persons (Hadjistavropoulos et al 2007) provide important information, including recommendations for physical evaluation, recommendations for assessing pain using self-report procedures, recommendations for functional assessment and recommendations for the assessment of emotional functioning. Other consensus statements on the most suitable types of pain assessment for older adults have been published and highlight simple word descriptor scales (i.e. weak, mild, moderate, strong) and numeric rating scales (1–10) as the tools of first choice for pain assessment in older adults (American Geriatrics Society Panel on Pharmacological Management of Persistent Pain in Older Persons 2009; APS 2005; Royal College of Physicians et al 2007; Herr 2005). A number of other scales also have demonstrated merit (i.e. box scales, pain thermometer, faces pain scales, McGill Pain Questionnaire), but may be less preferred by some older people (Herr 2005).

Visual analogue scales are generally not recommended for use in older adults as they typically have a higher failure rate (Hadjistavropoulos et al 2007; Herr 2005). More comprehensive pain assessment tools that monitor pain intensity and the biopsychosocial impacts of pain (on mood, function, sleep, quality of life, etc.) have also been developed (APS 2005; Hadjistavropoulos et al 2007). The Brief Pain Inventory, Pain Disability Index, Multidimensional Pain Inventory and Geriatric Pain Measure have been effectively used with older adults, although there has been relatively limited testing of reliability and validity, and further studies within the clinical setting are required (Royal College of Physicians et al 2007; Herr 2005).

Pain assessment strategies for those with cognitive impairment, sensory loss or lacking in verbal skills must seek to capitalize on the available communication repertoire of the individual. While self-report has become the de facto gold standard for pain assessment, other non-verbal methods (i.e. behavioural measures, observational tools) can provide important and clinically relevant information, and may be the preferred assessment choice in cases of moderate-severe impairment. Cognitive impairment can potentially interfere with self-report, although several recent studies have shown that such scales can remain valid and reliable in those with mild to moderate impairment (Hadjistavropoulos 2005; Herr 2005; Pautex et al 2005). There has been a rapid proliferation of new observer-rated scales for pain assessment in those with dementia over the last 5–10 years (Hadjistavropoulos 2005). Most scales grade the presence or absence of various behaviours that are thought to be indicative of pain. For instance, combinations of facial expressions, negative vocalizations, altered body language (e.g. rubbing, limping) and physiologic signs (e.g. blood pressure) can be scored to provide an index of likely pain intensity. More recently, there have even been some direct comparisons of the relative strengths and weaknesses of different observer-rated measures (Aubin et al 2007; Zwakhalen et al 2006). These measures represent an important advance in pain assessment of demented older adults, although further work is required to validate the new measures across different settings and older populations.

MANAGING PAIN IN OLDER PERSONS

Persistent pain is known to be most common in the older segments of the population, yet the vast majority of pain treatment studies and intervention trials have been conducted in young adult populations. The degree to which standard pain treatment approaches might need to be modified in order to meet the special needs of the older person has not been systematically examined and possible age differences in treatment efficacy have rarely been considered. Nonetheless, in recent years several useful guidelines have been developed by key organizations such as the American Geriatric Society (American Geriatrics Society Panel on Persistent Pain in Older Persons 2002; American Geriatrics Society Panel on Pharmacological Management of Persistent Pain in Older Persons 2009), the Australian Pain Society (2005) and the American Medical Directors Association (2003) to guide practitioners working with older persons who may experience pain. See, for example, the American Geriatrics Society's 2009 document on Pharmacological Management of Persistent Pain in Older Persons (American Geriatrics Society Panel on Pharmacological Management of Persistent Pain in Older Persons 2009). These guidelines document a wide range of treatments and include the following broad recommendations. The selection of appropriate analgesics for the older person requires an understanding of age-related pharmacokinetic and pharmacodynamic changes and must account for the impact of co-morbid disease and concurrent medication use. For this reason, simple analgesics (i.e. paracetamol) are the pharmacologic treatment of choice for the management of mild-moderate persistent pain and particularly musculoskeletal conditions. Non-steroidal compounds (NSAIDs and COX2) should be used with caution and all medications, including opioids and adjuvant analgesics (i.e. anticonvulsants, antidepressants), carry a balance of benefits and risks that must be weighed up for each older individual. Most guidelines emphasize that pharmacological therapy for persistent pain is always more effective when combined with non-pharmacological approaches. For certain selected patients interventional treatments (including joint injection techniques, orthopaedic surgery, indwelling pumps for intrathecal administration of analgesic compounds or use of spinal cord stimulation techniques for the management of refractory pain) might also be considered and have been shown to play a useful role in the management of chronic pain in older persons.

Non-pharmacological approaches with evidence of efficacy in older populations include physical therapies (i.e. graded exercise programme, heat/cold, TENS), psychological methods (i.e. relaxation, cognitive–behavioural therapy), education programmes, social support interventions and certain types of complementary therapies (i.e. glucosamine, acupuncture). However, the lack of an appropriate evidence base and the urgent need for further research on most treatment modalities is universally acknowledged in all of these guidelines. Multidisciplinary pain programmes that combine several modes of pharmacological and non-pharmacological treatment have demonstrated efficacy for the management of persistent pain in older adults (Ersek et al 2003; Katz et al 2005), including for those in residential aged care (Cook 1998). This treatment approach is considered to be state of the art for chronic pain management but appears to be under-utilized at present. Older patients are under-represented in pain management clinics, are less likely to be offered treatment and receive fewer treatment options when attending such clinics (Kee et al 1998). There have been some attempts to move the essential features of a multidisciplinary pain management programme so that it can be delivered as a home-based service (Kung et al 2000). Initiatives such as this should help to improve access to multidisciplinary treatment and ultimately improve pain-management options for those frail, incapacitated or institutionalized older persons who suffer from persistent and bothersome pain.

CONCLUSIONS

With the rapid ageing of the world's population, there is a clear need to be fully informed about any age-related change in pain perception and report as this is likely to affect options for the best available assessment and treatment approaches. The literature shows that pain, particularly of the joints, is very common in older adults. However, there is also clear evidence for a greater proportion of atypical presentations of usually painful disease states, including a relative absence of pain symptoms and a reduced intensity of pain when it is actually reported. Older persons with dementia represent a special population of older adults and generally show an even greater magnitude of change in pain perception and report.

Evidence suggests that older persons are more accepting of mild aches and pains, have altered pain beliefs and attitudes, including increased stoicism, and are less likely to seek medical attention. There are also a demonstrable age-related decline in pain sensitivity to mild noxious stimuli and some impairment in the structure and function of nociceptive pathways (both peripheral and central nervous system). These changes may partly compromise the early warning functions of pain, leading to the underreporting of mild pain, and may place the older person at greater risk of undiagnosed disease or injury. Conversely, experimental studies show that the endogenous analgesic system (e.g. endorphins) may be less efficient in persons of advanced age, and that tolerance of strong pain is reduced. Prolonged pain and tenderness after injury and poorer repair mechanisms also indicate that the older person may be more vulnerable to the negative impacts of strong, persistent pain. Thus, there are many reasons for age-related changes in pain, including physiological and psychological influences, but the current pool of knowledge in this area remains incomplete. A better understanding of age-related differences and similarities in the pain experience will ultimately contribute to a more rational and effective management of pain and suffering in older persons.

> **Q Study questions/questions for revision**
>
> 1. Which conditions are common in middle-aged and older people?
> 2. What are some of the psychosocial factors that might affect older people's beliefs about and/or strategies for dealing with pain?
> 3. What are some of the physiological factors that might affect older people's experience of pain?
> 4. How might the experience of pain differ for an older person suffering from dementia?
> 5. What are the ways you can use to determine if an older person has pain?
> 6. What are some key principles about managing pain in elderly people?

ACKNOWLEDGEMENTS

This work was supported by grants from the National Health and Medical Research Council of Australia.

REFERENCES

Albano, W., Zielinski, C.M., Organ, C.H., 1975. Is appendicitis in the aged really different? Geriatrics 30, 81–88.

Ambepitiya, G.B., Iyengar, E.N., Roberts, M.E., 1993. Silent exertional myocardial ischaemia and perception of angina in elderly people. Age Ageing 22 (4), 302–307.

Ambepitiya, G.B., Roberts, M., Ranjadayalan, K., 1994. Silent exertional myocardial ischemia in the elderly: a quantitative analysis of anginal perceptual threshold and the influence of autonomic function. J. Am. Geriatr. Soc. 42, 732–737.

American Geriatrics Society Panel on Persistent Pain in Older Persons, 2002. Clinical practice guidelines: The management of persistent pain in older persons. J. Am. Geriatr. Soc. 50, S205–S224.

American Geriatrics Society Panel on Pharmacological Management of Persistent Pain in Older Persons, 2009. Pharmacological management of persistent pain in older persons. J. Am. Geriatr. Soc. 57 (8), 1331–1346.

American Medical Directors Association, 2003. Chronic pain management in the long-term care setting. AMDA, San Diego, CA.

Andersson, H., Ejlertsson, G., Leden, I., et al., 1993. Chronic pain in a geographically defined general population: Studies of differences in age, gender, social class, and pain localization. Clin. J. Pain 9 (3), 174–182.

Appelt, C.J., Burant, C.J., Siminoff, L.A., et al., 2007. Arthritis-specific health beliefs related to aging among older male patients with knee and/or hip osteoarthritis. J. Gerontol. A Biol. Sci. Med. Sci. 62A (2), 184–190.

Arden, N., Nevitt, M.C., 2006. Osteoarthritis: Epidemiology. Clin. Rheumatol. 20 (1), 3–25.

Aubin, M., Giguère, A., Hadjistavropoulos, T., et al., 2007. The systematic evaluation of instruments designed to assess pain in persons with limited ability to communicate. Pain Res. Manag. 12 (3), 195–203.

Australian Bureau of Statistics, 2004. 4102.0 – Australian Social Trends. Online. Available at: http://www.abs.gov.au/ausstats/abs@.nsf/0/95560b5d7449b135ca256e9e001fd879? Online. (accessed 27.07.10.).

Australian Pain Society, 2005. Pain in residential aged care facilities: management strategies. Australian Pain Society, Sydney.

Barberger-Gateau, P., Chaslerie, A., Dartigues, J., et al., 1992. Health measures correlates in a French elderly community population: The PAQUID study. J. Gerontol. 47 (2), S88–S95.

Bassols, A., Bosch, F., Campillo, M., et al., 1999. An epidemiologic comparison of pain complaints in the general population of Catalonia (Spain). Pain 83 (1), 9–16.

Benedetti, F., Vighetti, S., Ricco, C., et al., 1999. Pain threshold and tolerance in Alzheimer's disease. Pain 80 (1,2), 377–382.

Benvenuti, F., Ferrucci, L., Guralnik, J.M., et al., 1995. Foot pain and disability in older persons: An epidemiologic survey. J. Am. Geriatr. Soc. 43 (5), 479–484.

Bergman, S., Herrström, P., Högström, K., et al., 2001. Chronic musculoskeletal pain, prevalence rates, and sociodemographic associations in a Swedish population study. J. Rheumatol. 28 (6), 1369–1377.

Blennow, K., Wallin, A., Häger, O., 1993. Low frequency of post-lumbar puncture headache in demented patients. Acta Neurol. Scand. 88 (3), 221–223.

Blyth, F.M., March, L.M., Brnabic, A.J.M., et al., 2001. Chronic pain in Australia: A prevalence study. Pain. 89 (2,3), 127–134.

Bodnar, R.J., Romero, M.T., Kramer, E., 1988. Organismic variables and pain inhibition: Roles of gender and aging. Brain Res. Bull. 21 (6), 947–953.

Borenstein, D.G., 2001. Epidemiology, etiology, diagnostic evaluation, and treatment of low back pain. Curr. Opin. Rheumatol. 13 (2), 128–134.

Brattberg, G., Thorslund, M., Wikman, A., 1989. The prevalence of pain in the general community: The results of a postal survey in a county of Sweden. Pain 37 (1), 21–32.

Brattberg, G., Parker, M.G., Thorslund, M., 1997. A longitudinal study of pain: Reported pain from middle age to old age. Clin. J. Pain. 13 (2), 144–149.

Brescia, F.J., Portenoy, R.K., Ryan, M., et al., 1992. Pain, opioid use, and survival in hospitalized patients with advanced cancer. J. Clin. Oncol. 10 (1), 149–155.

Breivik, H., Collett, B., Ventafridda, V., et al., 2006. Survey of chronic pain in Europe: Prevalence, impact on daily life, and treatment. Eur. J. Pain 10 (4), 287–333.

Caraceni, A., Portenoy, R.K., 1999. An international survey of cancer pain characteristics and syndromes. Pain. 82 (3), 263–274.

Chakour, M.C., Gibson, S.J., Bradbeer, M., et al., 1996. The effect of age on A-delta and C-fibre thermal pain perception. Pain 64 (1), 143–152.

Cherng, C.H., Ho, S.T., Kao, S.J., et al., 1991. The study of cancer pain and its correlates. Ma Zui Xue Za Zhi 29 (3), 653–657.

Chiou, A.F., Lin, H.Y., Huang, H.Y., 2009. Disability and pain management methods of Taiwanese arthritic older patients. J. Clin. Nurs. 18 (15), 2206–2216.

Cohen-Mansfield, J., Marx, M.S., 1993. Pain and depression in the nursing home: Corroborating results. J. Gerontol. 48 (2), P96–P97.

Cole, L., Farrell, M.J., Tress, B., et al., 2006. Pain sensitivity and fMRI pain related brain activity in persons with Alzheimer's disease. Brain 129 (11), 2957–2965.

Cole, L., Farrell, M.J., Egan, G., et al., 2009. Age differences in pain sensitivity and fMRI pain related brain activity. Neurobiology of Ageing 31 (3), 494–503.

Cook, A.J., 1998. Cognitive-behavioral pain management for elderly nursing home residents. J. Gerontol. B Psychol. Sci. Soc. Sci. P51–P59.

Cook, A.J., DeGood, D.E., Chastain, D.C., 1999. Age differences in pain beliefs. In: 9th World Congress on Pain. Vienna, p. 557.

Corran, T.M., Gibson, S.J., Farrell, M.J., et al., 1994. Comparison of chronic pain experience between young and elderly patients. In: Gebhart, G.F., Hammond, D.L., Jenson, T.S. (Eds.), Proceedings of the 7th World Congress on Pain, Progress in Pain Research and Management, vol. 2. IASP Press, Seattle, pp. 895–906.

Crook, J., Rideout, E., Browne, G., 1984. The prevalence of pain complaints in a general population. Pain 18 (3), 299–305.

D'Alessandro, R., Benassi, G., Lenzi, P.L., et al., 1988. Epidemiology of headache in the republic of San Marino. J. Neurol. Neurosurg. Psychiatry 51 (1), 21–27.

Defrin, R., Lotan, M., Pick, C.G., 2006. The evaluation of acute pain in individuals with cognitive impairment: A differential effect of the level of impairment. Pain 124 (3), 312–320.

Dionne, C.E., Dunn, K.M., Croft, P.R., 2006. Does back pain prevalence really decrease with increasing age? Age Ageing 35 (3), 229–234.

Dionne, C.E., Bourbonnais, R., Frémont, P., et al., 2007. Determinants of 'return to work in good health' among workers with back pain who consult in primary care settings: a 2-year prospective study. Eur. Spine J. 16 (5), 641–655.

Edwards, R.R., Fillingim, R.B., 2001. The effects of age on temporal summation and habituation of thermal pain: Clinical relevance in healthy older and younger adults. J. Pain 6 (2), 307–317.

Edwards, R.R., Fillingim, R.B., Ness, T.J., 2003. Age-related differences in endogenous pain modulation: A comparison of diffuse noxious inhibitory controls in healthy older and younger adults. Pain 101 (1,2), 155–165.

Ersek, M., Turner, J.A., McCurry, S.M., et al., 2003. Efficacy of a self-management group intervention for elderly persons with chronic pain. Clin. J. Pain 19, 156–167.

Fahey, K.F., Rao, S.M., Douglas, M.K., et al., 2008. Nurse coaching to explore and modify patient attitudinal barriers interfering with effective cancer pain management. Oncol. Nurs. Forum 35 (2), 233–240.

Farrell, M., Gibson, S.J., 2007. Age interacts with stimulus frequency in the temporal summation of pain. Pain Med. 8 (6), 514–520.

Feldt, K.S., Warne, M.A., Ryden, M.B., 1998. Examining pain in aggressive cognitively impaired older adults. J. Gerontol. Nurs. 24 (11), 14–22.

Ferrell, B.A., 1995. Pain evaluation and management in the nursing home. Ann. Intern. Med. 123 (9), 681–695.

Gagliese, L., Farrell, M., 2005. The neurobiology of ageing, nociception and pain: An integration of animal and human experimental evidence. In: Gibson, S.J., Weiner, D. (Eds.), Progress in Pain Research and Management: Pain in the Older Person. IASP Press, Seattle, pp. 25–44.

Gagliese, L., Katz, J., 2003. Age differences in postoperative pain are scale dependent: A comparison of measures of pain intensity and quality in younger and older surgical patients. Pain 103 (1,2), 11–20.

Gagliese, L., Melzack, R., 1997. Age differences in the quality of chronic pain: A preliminary study. Pain Res. Manag. 2 (3), 157–162.

Gagliese, L., Jackson, M., Ritvo, P., et al., 2000. Age is not an impediment to effective use of patient-controlled analgesia by surgical patients. Anesthesiology 93 (3), 601–610.

Gibson, S.J., 2003. Pain and ageing. In: Dostrovsky, J.O., Carr, D.B., Koltzenburg, M. (Eds.), Proceedings of 10th World Congress on Pain. IASP Press, Seattle, pp. 767–790.

Gibson, S.J., 2007. The IASP Global Year Against Pain in Older Persons: Highlighting the current status and future perspectives in geriatric pain. Expert Rev. Neurother. 7 (6), 627–635.

Gibson, S.J., Farrell, M.J., 2004. A review of age differences in the neurophysiology of nociception and the perceptual experience of pain. Clin. J. Pain 20 (4), 227–239.

Gibson, S.J., Helme, R.D., 2000. Cognitive factors and the experience of pain and suffering in older persons. Pain 85 (3), 375–383.

Gibson, S.J., Helme, R.D., 2001. Age-related differences in pain perception and report. Clin. Geriatr. Med. 17 (3), 433–456.

Gibson, S.J., Gorman, M.M., Helme, R.D., 1990. Assessment of pain in the elderly using event-related cerebral potentials. In: Bond, M.R., Charlton, J.E., Woolf, C. (Eds.), Proceedings of the VIth World Congress on Pain. Elsevier Science Publishers, Amsterdam, pp. 523–529.

Gibson, S.J., Voukelatos, X., Flicker, L., et al., 2001. A comparison of nociceptive cerebral event related potentials and heat pain threshold in healthy older adults and those with cognitive impairment. Pain Res. Manag. 6 (3), 126–133.

Gignac, M.A., Davis, A.M., Hawker, G., et al., 2006. 'What do you expect? You're just getting older': A comparison of perceived osteoarthritis-related and aging-related health experiences in middle- and older-age adults. Arthritis Rheum. 55 (6), 905–912.

Hadjistavropoulos, T., 2005. Assessing pain in older persons with severe limitations in ability to communicate. In: Gibson, S.J., Weiner, D.K. (Eds.), Pain in Older Persons, Progress in Pain Research and Management, vol. 35. IASP Press, Seattle, pp. 135–151.

Hadjistavropoulos, T., Herr, K., Turk, D.C., et al., 2007. An Interdisciplinary Expert Consensus Statement on Assessment of Pain in Older Persons. Clin. J. Pain 23, S1–S43.

Hannan, M.T., Felson, D.T., Pincus, T., 2000. Analysis of the discordance between radiographic changes and knee pain in osteoarthritis of the knee. J. Rheumatol. 27 (6), 1513–1517.

Harkins, S.W., Price, D.D., Bush, F.M., 1994. Geriatric pain. In: Wall, P.D., Melzack, R. (Eds.), Textbook of Pain. Churchill Livingstone, New York, pp. 769–787.

Harkins, S.W., Davis, M.D., Bush, F.M., et al., 1996. Suppression of first pain and slow temporal summation of second pain in relation to age. J. Gerontol. A Biol. Sci. Med. Sci. 51A (5), M260–M265.

Helme, R.D., Gibson, S.J., 2001. The epidemiology of pain in elderly people. Clin. Geriatr. Med. 17 (3), 417–431.

Helme, R.D., McKernan, S., 1985. Neurogenic flare responses following topical application of capsaicin in humans. Ann. Neurol. 18 (4), 505–511.

Herr, K., 2005. Pain assessment in the older adult with verbal communication skills. In: Gibson, S.J., Weiner, D.K. (Eds.), Pain in Older Persons, Progress in Pain Research and Management, vol. 35, IASP Press, Seattle, pp. 111–133.

Herr, K.A., Mobily, P.R., Wallace, R.B., et al., 1991. Leg pain in the rural Iowa 65 + population: Prevalence, related factors, and association with functional status. Clin. J. Pain 7 (2), 114–121.

Hofland, S.L., 1992. Elder beliefs: blocks to pain management. J. Gerontol. Nurs. 18 (6), 19–23.

Husebo, B.S., Strand, L.I., Moe-Nilssen, R., et al., 2008. Who suffers most? Dementia and pain in nursing home patients: A cross-sectional study. J. Am. Med. Dir. Assoc. 9 (6), 427–433.

Katz, B., Scherer, S., Gibson, S.J., 2005. Multidisciplinary pain management clinics for older adults. In: Gibson, S.J., Weiner, D.K. (Eds.), Pain in Older Persons, Progress in Pain Research and Management, vol. 35, IASP Press, Seattle, pp. 45–65.

Kay, L., Jorgensen, T., Schultz-Larsen, K., 1992. Abdominal pain in a 70-year-old Danish population. J. Clin. Epidemiol. 45 (12), 1377–1382.

Kee, W.G., Middaugh, S.J., Redpath, S., et al., 1998. Age as a factor in admission to chronic pain rehabilitation. Clin. J. Pain 14, 121–128.

Keefe, F.J., Williams, D.A., 1990. A comparison of coping strategies in chronic pain patients in different age groups. J. Gerontol. 45 (4), 161–165.

Keefe, F.J., Caldwell, D.S., Martinez, S., et al., 1991. Analysing pain in rheumatoid arthritis patients: Pain coping strategies in patients who have had knee replacement surgery. Pain 46 (2), 153–160.

Kendig, H., Helme, R.D., Teshuva, K., 1996. Health status of older people project: Data from a survey of the health and lifestyles of older Australians. Report to the Victorian Health Promotion Foundation. Victorian Government, Melbourne.

Kind, P., Dolan, P., Gudex, C., et al., 1998. Variations in population health status: Results from a United Kingdom national questionnaire survey. Br. Med. J. 316 (7133), 736–741.

Konu, V., 1977. Myocardial infarction in the elderly. Acta Med. Scand. 604 (Suppl), 3–68.

Kung, F., Gibson, S.J., Helme, R.D., 2000. A community-based program that provides free choice of intervention for older people with chronic pain. J. Pain 1, 293–308.

Lautenbacher, S., Kunz, M., Strate, P., et al., 2005. Age effects on pain thresholds, temporal summation and spatial summation of heat and pressure pain. Pain 115 (3), 410–418.

Lavsky-Shulan, M., Wallace, R.B., Kohout, F.J., et al., 1985. Prevalence and functional correlates of low in the elderly: The Iowa 65+ rural health study. J. Am. Geriatr. Soc. 33 (1), 23–28.

Leong, I.Y., Nuo, T.H., 2007. Prevalence of pain in nursing home residents with different cognitive and communicative abilities. Clin. J. Pain 23 (2), 119–127.

Leveille, S.G., Gurlanik, J.M., Ferrucci, L., et al., 1998. Foot pain and disability in older women. Am. J. Epidemiol. 148 (7), 657–665.

Leung, W.S., McMillan, A.S., Wong, M.C., 2008. Chronic orofacial pain in southern Chinese people: experience, associated disability, and help-seeking response. J. Orofac. Pain 22 (4), 323–330.

Leventhal, E.A., Prohaska, T.R., 1986. Age, symptom interpretation, and health behaviour. J. Am. Geriatr. Soc. 34 (3), 185–191.

Li, Y., Duckles, S.P., 1993. Effect of age on vascular content of calcitonin gene-related peptide and mesenteric vasodilator activity in the rat. Eur. J. Pharmacol. 236 (3), 373–378.

Lichtenberg, P.A., Skehan, M.W., Swensen, C.H., 1984. The role of personality, recent life stress and arthritic severity in predicting pain. J. Psychosom. Res. 28 (3), 231–236.

Liddell, A., Locker, D., 1997. Gender and age differences in attitudes to dental pain and dental control. Community Dent. Oral. Epidemiol. 25 (4), 314–318.

MacDonald, J.B., Baillie, J., Williams, B.O., 1983. Coronary care in the elderly. Age Ageing 12 (1), 17–20.

Machin, P., de C Williams, A.C., 1998. Stiff upper lip: Coping strategies of World War II veterans with phantom limb pain. Clin. J. Pain 14 (4), 290–294.

Magni, G., Marchetti, M., Moreschi, C., et al., 1993. Chronic musculoskeletal pain and depression in the National Health and Nutrition Examination. Pain 53 (2), 163–168.

Mäntyselkä, P., Hartikainen, S., Louhivuori-Laako, K., et al., 2004. Effects of dementia on perceived daily pain in home-dwelling elderly people: A population-based study. Age Ageing 33 (5), 496–499.

McBeth, J., Jones, K., 2007. Epidemiology of chronic musculoskeletal pain. Clin. Rheumatol. 21 (3), 403–425.

McCracken, L.M., 1998. Learning to live with the pain: acceptance of pain predicts adjustment in persons with chronic pain. Pain 74 (1), 21–27.

McMillan, S.C., 1989. The relationship between age and intensity of cancer related symptoms. Oncol. Nurs. Forum 16, 237–342.

Miller, P.F., Sheps, D.S., Bragdon, E.E., 1990. Aging and pain perception in ischemic heart disease. Am. Heart J. 120 (1), 22–30.

Morrison, R.S., Ahronheim, J.C., Morrison, G.R., et al., 1998. Pain and discomfort associated with common hospital procedures and experiences. J. Pain Symptom Manage. 15 (2), 91–101.

Ochoa, J., Mair, W.G.P., 1969. The normal sural nerve in man. II. Changes in the axon and schwann cells due to ageing. Acta Neuropathol. (Berl) 13 (3), 217–253.

Oberle, K., Paul, P., Wry, J., 1990. Pain, anxiety and analgesics: A comparative study of elderly and younger surgical patients. Can. J. Aging 9 (1), 13–19.

Park, J.H., Cho, B.L., Paek, Y., et al., 2009. Development of a pain assessment tool for the older adults in Korea: The validity and reliability of a Korean version of the geriatric pain measure (GPM-K). Arch. Gerontol. Geriatr. 49, 199–203.

Parker, J., Frank, R., Beck, N., et al., 1988. Pain in rheumatoid arthritis: Relationship to demographic, medical and psychological factors. J. Rheumatol. 15, 433–447.

Parmelee, P.A., Smith, B., Katz, I.R., 1993. Pain complaints and cognitive status among elderly institution residents. J. Am. Geriatr. Soc. 41, 517–522.

Pautex, S., Herrmann, F., Le Lous, P., et al., 2005. Feasibility and reliability of four pain self-assessment scales and correlation with an observational rating scale in hospitalized elderly demented patients. J. Gerontol. A Biol. Sci. Med. Sci. 60, 524–529.

Pickering, G., 2005. Age differences in clinical pain states. In: Gibson, S.J., Weiner, D.K. (Eds.), Pain in Older Persons. IASP Press, Seattle, pp. 67–86.

Porter, F.L., Malhotra, K.M., Wolf, C.M., et al., 1996. Dementia and response to pain in the elderly. Pain 68 (2,3), 413–421.

Proctor, W.R., Hirdes, J.P., 2001. Pain and cognitive status among nursing home residents in Canada. Pain Res. Manag. 6 (3), 119–125.

Rittger, H., Rieber, J., Breithardt, O.A., et al., 2010. Influence of age on pain perception in acute myocardial ischemia: A possible cause for delayed treatment in elderly patients. Int. J. Cardiol. [epub ahead of print]

Royal College of Physicians, et al., 2007. Concise guidance to good practice series, No 8 The assessment of pain in older people: national guidelines. Royal College of Physicians, British Geriatrics Society and British Pain Society, London. Online. Available: www.britishpainsociety.org/book_pain_older_people.pdf.

Ruzicka, S.A., 1998. Pain beliefs: what do elders believe? J. Holist. Nurs. 16 (3), 369–382.

Sawyer, P., Lillis, J.P., Bodner, E.V., et al., 2007. Substantial daily pain among nursing home residents. J. Am. Med. Dir. Assoc. 8 (3), 158–165.

Scherder, E., Bouma, A., Borkent, M., et al., 1999. Alzheimer patients report less pain intensity and pain affect than non-demented elderly. Psychiatry 62 (3), 265–272.

Scherder, E., Bouma, A., Slaets, J., et al., 2001. Repeated pain assessment in Alzheimer's disease. Dement. Geriatr. Cogn. Disord. 12 (6), 400–407.

Scherder, E., Herr, K., Pickering, G., et al., 2009. Pain in dementia. Pain. 145 (3), 276–278.

Smith, B.H., Elliott, A.M., Chambers, W.A., et al., 2001. The impact of chronic pain in the community. Fam. Pract. 18 (3), 292–299.

Sorkin, B.A., Rudy, T.E., Hanlon, R.B., et al., 1990. Chronic pain in old and young patients: differences appear less important than similarities. J. Gerontol. A Biol. Sci. Med. Sci. 45 (2), 64–68.

Sternbach, R.A., 1986. Survey of pain in the United States: The Nuprin pain report. Clin. J. Pain 2 (1), 49–54.

Stoller, E.P., 1993. Interpretations of symptoms by older people: a health diary study of illness behaviour. J. Aging Health 5 (1), 58–81.

Teno, J.M., Weitzen, S., Wetle, T., et al., 2001. Persistent pain in nursing home residents. J. Am. Med. Assoc. 285 (16), 2081.

Teno, J., Bird, C., Mor, V., 2003. The prevalence and treatment of pain in US nursing homes. Centre for Gerontology and Health Care Research, Brown University.

Teno, J.M., Kabumoto, G., Wetle, T., et al., 2004. Daily pain that was excruciating at some time in the previous week: Prevalence, characteristics, and outcomes in nursing home residents. J. Am. Geriatr. Soc. 52 (5), 762–767.

Thomas, T., Robinson, C., Champion, D., 1998. Prediction and assessment of the severity of post operative pain and of satisfaction with management. Pain 75 (2,3), 177–185.

Tibblin, G., Bengtsson, C., Furness, B., et al., 1990. Symptoms by age and sex. Scand. J. Prim. Health Care 8 (1), 9–17.

Tsang, A., Von Korff, M., Lee, S., et al., 2008. Common chronic pain conditions in developed and developing countries: gender and age differences and comorbidity with depression-anxiety disorders. J. Pain 9, 883–891.

US Census Bureau DIS, 2012. National Population Projections: Summary Tables. [Internet] (cited 18 February 2013). Online. Available at: http://www.census.gov/population/projections/data/national/2012/summarytables.html.

Vigano, A., Bruera, E., Suarex-Almazor, M.E., 1998. Age, pain intensity, and opioid dose in patients with advanced cancer. Cancer 83 (6), 1244–1250.

Von Korff, M., Dworkin, S.F., Le Resche, L., et al., 1988. An epidemiologic comparison of pain complaints. Pain 32 (2), 173–183.

Von Korff, M., Dworkin, S.F., Le Resche, L., 1990. Graded chronic pain status: An epidemiologic evaluation. Pain 40 (3), 279–291.

Walid, M.S., Zaytseva, N., 2009. Pain in nursing home residents and correlation with neuropsychiatric disorders. Pain Physician 12 (5), 877–880.

Washington, L.L., Gibson, S.J., Helme, R.D., 2000. Age-related differences in the endogenous analgesic response to repeated cold water immersion in human volunteers. Pain 89 (1), 89–96.

Watkins, K.W., Shifren, K., Park, D.C., et al., 1999. Age, pain, and coping with rheumatoid arthritis. Pain 82 (3), 217–228.

Weiner, D.K., Rudy, T.E., 2002. Attitudinal barriers to effective treatment of persistent pain in nursing home residents. J. Am. Geriatr. Soc. 50 (12), 2035–2040.

Weiner, D.K., Peterson, B.L., Logue, P., et al., 1998. Predictors of pain self-report in nursing home residents. Aging Clin. Exp. Res. 10, 411–420.

Wroblewski, M., Mikulowski, P., 1991. Peritonitis in geriatric inpatients. Age Ageing 20 (2), 90–94.

Wu, N., Miller, S.C., Lapane, K., et al., 2005. Impact of cognitive function on assessments of nursing home residents' pain. Med. Care 43 (9), 934–939.

Yong, H.H., 2006. Can attitudes of stoicism and cautiousness explain observed age-related variation in levels of self-rated pain, mood disturbance and functional interference in chronic pain patients? Eur. J. Pain 10, 399–407.

Yong, H.H., Gibson, S.J., Horne, D.J., et al., 2001. Development of a pain attitudes questionnaire to assess stoicism and cautiousness for possible age differences. Journal of Gerontology: Psychological Services 56B (5), 279–284.

Yong, H.H., Bell, R., Workman, B., et al., 2003. Psychometric properties of the Pain Attitudes Questionnaire (revised) in adult patients with chronic pain. Pain 104 (3), 673–681.

Yunus, M.B., Holt, G.S., Masi, A.T., et al., 1988. Fibromyalgia syndrome among the elderly: Comparison with younger patients. J. Am. Geriatr. Soc. 36, 987–995.

Zheng, Z., Gibson, S.J., Khalil, Z., et al., 2000. Age-related differences in the time course of capsaicin-induced hyperalgesia. Pain 85 (1,2), 51–58.

Zheng, Z., Gibson, S.J., Helme, R.D., et al., 2009. The effect of local anaesthetic on age-related capsaicin-induced mechanical hyperalgesia: A randomised, controlled study. Pain 144 (1,2), 101–109.

Zwakhalen, S.M., Hamers, J.P., Berger, M.P., 2006. The psychometric quality and clinical usefulness of three pain assessment tools for elderly people with dementia. Pain 126 (1–3), 210–220.

Chapter | 20 |

Cancer pain

Sally Bennett, Geoffrey Mitchell and Jenny Strong

CHAPTER CONTENTS

LEARNING OBJECTIVES

At the end of this chapter readers will:

1. Understand the magnitude of the problem of cancer pain.
2. Understand the circumstances in the cancer journey when pain may occur.
3. Be able to describe the types of pain.
4. Understand that the experience of pain can have physical, psychological and spiritual dimensions.
5. Understand the principles of pain management.
6. Understand the barriers to good pain management.
7. Appreciate the personal issues confronted by therapists dealing with cancer pain.

OVERVIEW

Pain is one of the most common symptoms in cancer. It is also one of the most feared, and patients frequently equate cancer with intolerable pain. In the patient's mind, the onset of pain can also herald disease progression and an inexorable march towards death.

Cancer pain differs from chronic pain in some ways, and in others it is very similar. The basic mechanisms that generate pain responses are the same. Treatment will involve similar techniques, but will also include cancer-specific therapies like radiotherapy or chemotherapy.

The management of cancer-related pain differs from that of chronic pain of non-cancer origin in many ways. With cancer pain, the intensity is not static. The location and quality of the pain are more likely to change because of the dynamic nature of the illness and the treatment. The person with cancer may have multiple pain problems and interrelated symptoms that complicate management.

The meaning of changes in the pain may be more frightening and this fear can exacerbate the experience of pain. One of the biggest differences lies in the psychological, emotional and spiritual import that pain carries with it. Therapists need to be mindful of this potential and adapt their normal approach accordingly. If the pain a patient suffers is not controlled with what appears to be appropriate therapy, it is possible that there is an emotional response to the problem that needs to be addressed. Therefore, while there are many similarities in management programmes for chronic pain and cancer pain, there are elements that must be considered differently.

Further, therapists working in this area will find their own attitudes and beliefs about pain, suffering and death challenged by the experiences and responses they encounter

© 2014 Elsevier Ltd.

in their patients. It is thus important to consider personal attitudes, and consider how therapists might need to approach patients whose beliefs may differ from their own.

This chapter will consider the problem of pain experienced in cancer from a range of perspectives. The causes of cancer pain will be briefly described. Differentiating pain and suffering is important, and the therapist needs to recognize that all aspects of the person's pain experience must be addressed.

Cancer pain management will be discussed in some detail, with an overview of medication management and consideration of non-medication management of pain. However, this is not a text on how to manage pain. A useful resource is the clinical guideline entitled Adult Cancer pain (v1.2010) published by the National Comprehensive Cancer Network (NCCN) (National Comprehensive Cancer Network 2010). Box 20.1 defines some key terms.

FREQUENCY OF PAIN IN CANCER

Pain in cancer is common, with reported prevalence ranging from as low as 14% up to 100% (National Institutes of Health 2002). Most studies report a range, such as 54–92% (Teunissen et al 2007), with such differences in prevalence largely due to differences in definition, the point along the cancer journey that is being examined and the setting where the measures take place. For example, the prevalence of pain in palliative care and pain centres is higher than in oncology settings.

It is important to note that pain is not universal in people with cancer, and that some people have no pain at all. In one study concentrating on the palliative phase of cancer, 30% of people experienced no pain, 37% had minimal to mild pain, 28% described moderate to strong pain and 5% had severe to extreme pain (Wilson et al 2009).

Cancer pain is very costly, both in direct and indirect terms. Lema et al (2010) estimate that neuropathic pain costs the USA $2.4b per annum.

Types of cancer pain

Symptoms can be defined as 'subjective experience[s] reflecting changes in the biopsychosocial functioning, sensations, or cognition of an individual' (Dodd et al 2001). The *sensation* of pain arises from stimulation of pain receptors or damage to the neural tracts that carry pain. However, the *experience* of pain is modified by a range of factors.

There are three types of pain which may arise for patients with cancer: pain that is secondary to tumour growth and invasion of structures, pain that results from treatment of the cancer and pain not associated with the tumour or the treatment. Classification of pain by physiological type has been described for some time (Portenoy & Hagen 1990), but Ashby demonstrated that classifying pain by its mechanistic basis influences the type of pain treatment that is offered (Ashby et al 1992). Two major categories of pain are recognized: nociceptive pain and non-nociceptive pain. Nociceptive pain arises from the stimulation of nociceptive pain receptors (see Table 20.1 for definition), and

---

Box 20.1 Key terms defined

Adjuvant analgesia – Provided by an agent that is not primarily an analgesic, but has some analgesic properties or enhances the analgesic performance of a primary analgesic.

Palliative care – Any procedure that is performed primarily to provide symptom relief rather than to affect the primary illness. Palliative care is defined by the WHO (World Health Organization 2002) as 'an approach that improves the quality of life of patients and their families facing the problem associated with life-threatening illness, through the prevention and relief of suffering by means of early identification and impeccable assessment and treatment of pain and other problems, physical, psychosocial and spiritual'.

Ventriculostomy – A procedure in which a small morphine reservoir is inserted into the lateral cerebral ventricle. This procedure is useful for patients with cancer pain due to head or neck cancer, or those patients with bilateral, midline or diffuse cancer pain (Cramond & Stuart 1993).

Percutaneous cordotomy – A procedure performed to ablate the spinothalamic tract at C1–C2. It is done under local anaesthesia with a thermal coagulation probe. Immediate pain relief is achieved in most patients, but pain may return in

6 months in half these patients. This procedure can be useful for patients experiencing unilateral cancer pain below the head and neck (Stuart & Cramond 1993).

Radiotherapy – A procedure in which radiation is used to destroy tumour cells. Radiotherapy may reduce pain by decreasing the tumour's pressure effect on nerves, limiting a tumour's infiltration and resolving tumour inflammation (Monfardini & Scanni 1987). It is also used to help with well-localized pain due to bony metastases (Janjan 1997).

Chemotherapy – Involves the administration of cytotoxic drugs with the aim of interfering with tumour-cell division. It can relieve pain due to tumour effects such as tissue destruction, enlargement of viscera and pressure or obstruction. Because of its systemic effects, it is most helpful for relieving pain associated with diffuse metastases in chemosensitive tumours (Monfardini & Scanni 1987). Chemotherapy may provide palliation even when there is no survival benefit, in circumstances where the trade-off between symptom reduction and toxicity favours symptom relief (Archer et al 1999).

the nature of the pain varies depending on the structures where those pain receptors are located. Non-nociceptive pain is either neurogenic (arising from damage to or irritation of the neural tracts) or non-neurogenic. The physiology of pain is discussed in Chapter 6.

Cancer pain may be long-standing, of more than 3 months' duration, and so has many chronic pain features. It also changes according to tumour-growth damage to tissues and to the impact of some treatments, and so has acute pain features (Foley 1987).

Foley (1987) describes five different cancer pain types.

1. Patients with acute pain associated with the cancer or the treatment. Acute pain associated with the cancer heralds the onset or recurrence of the illness, bringing with it associated psychological ramification. In contrast, acute pain associated with treatment is self-limiting and pain tolerance is often high, with the patient is hopeful about outcome, and consequently psychological effects may be limited. In both cases, treatment needs to be targeted at the cause of pain.
2. Patients with chronic pain, either from the cancer or the therapy. Chronic pain associated with the cancer reflects tumour progression and psychological issues become much more important for these patients. Anxiety and feelings of hopelessness can further exacerbate the pain. Chronic pain may also be due to soft tissue, nerve or bony injury related to cancer treatment, and be unrelated to the tumour. Identifying this group is import in order to reassure the patient that the pain is not caused by their cancer. Treatment of patients with chronic pain is aimed at the symptom rather than the cause.
3. Patients with chronic pain from another source, generally pre-existing. These patients often already have psychological and functional limitations, and require considerable support as the presence of multiple illnesses is very taxing.
4. Patients with pain who are also actively involved with illicit drug use. These patients are very difficult to treat.
5. Patients who are dying and have cancer pain. The focus of treatment is on maximizing comfort and providing psychological care. The family must also be considered in caring for this group.

Therapists need to take into account the complexity and changing nature of cancer pain. Pain management approaches vary depending on the site of pain, chronicity of pain, characteristics of the individual patient and the stage of disease. Therapists may modify their pain-management approaches according to whether the patient is in active treatment, with the likelihood of recovery, or is dying and receiving palliative care. There are different management procedures for treatment and palliation phases. Careful assessment and flexibility in management are vital.

IMPACT OF AND RESPONSES TO CANCER PAIN

The presence of cancer pain significantly impacts on the quality of life of both the patient and their family. Pain interacts with a range of other symptoms such as fatigue, nausea and constipation, amplifying their impact and that of pain. Although the physical aspects of pain are commonly evident, people experiencing cancer pain also experience a range of psychological, social and spiritual challenges.

Anxiety, depression, anger and a sense of helplessness are common responses to unrelieved cancer pain. In turn depression and anxiety related to a cancer pain and its treatment can aggravate pain. People with advanced cancer and severe pain are twice as likely to experience clinical depression and three times more likely to have an anxiety disorder as those with less severe pain (Wilson et al 2009). Pain may also impact on a person's cognitive function, particularly placing greater demands on memory. Not surprisingly, the effect of ongoing pain is to reduce the individual's feeling of control. It is important for the therapist to acknowledge this heightened sense of loss of control and to modify their approach accordingly. The functional impact of cancer pain also limits peoples' ability to participate in meaningful activities and relationships, with pain from cancer interfering more with enjoyment of life than pain from other causes (Daut & Cleeland 1982; Ferrell et al 1995).

An individual's experience and expression of pain is partly socioculturally determined. Their previous experience of pain within their family, and their culture's perception of pain, suffering and illness influence the person's thoughts and coping styles with regard to pain. In contemporary management regimes for cancer, many patients are cared for predominantly at home and their pain management occurs at home. Therefore the patient and/or their family carers are often responsible for medication and other pain-reduction procedures. It has been found that patients are often under-medicated due to beliefs held by themselves and/or their caregivers that they should put up with pain as long as possible, and due to fear of addiction (Ferrell et al 1995; Hussein Al-Atiyyat 2008; Yeager et al 1997). Responses to cancer pain therefore clearly relate in some part to the attitudes, beliefs and knowledge of patients and carers.

Cancer pain in the later phase of the disease is a marker for patients that their disease is progressing. This opens up questions about one's mortality and related spiritual issues. Otis-Green et al (2002) note that spiritual distress may occur when there is conflict between the patient's experience of pain and suffering and their world view, leading to anxiety, depression, anger and withdrawal, as well as physical pain.

As in all pain situations, it is inappropriate to think of cancer pain as just physical. Dame Cicely Saunders used the phrase 'total pain' to describe a person's suffering from physical, psychological, social, spiritual and practical distress. All aspects need attention and should be considered in the assessment and management of cancer pain.

ASSESSMENT AND MEASUREMENT OF CANCER PAIN

Readers are advised to refer back to Chapter 7, which covered assessment and measurement issues in more depth. Inadequate cancer pain assessment results in poor control of pain. The NCCN Clinical Practice Guidelines in Oncology, Adult Cancer Pain (National Comprehensive Cancer Network 2010) recommend that pain assessment should involve assessment of factors such as:

- pain intensity
- characteristics/quality of the pain
- pain history (sites, severity, duration, mood, previous pain experience, etc.)
- factors that exacerbate or relieve pain
- psychosocial factors (patient distress, psychiatric history, social supports, etc.)
- cultural, spiritual and religious considerations
- patient's goals and expectations.

In addition, a thorough physical examination and any laboratory studies and imaging results need to be considered.

Assessment considerations

Assessment of cancer pain should be multidimensional and multidisciplinary. Pain involves a complexity of sensory, cognitive, behavioural and affective phenomena, requiring a coordinated assessment effort by different disciplines. The source of the pain can be identified by assessing the location, distribution, quality, intensity and duration (Table 20.1). Comprehensive assessment of pain should also consider other symptoms that may interact with, and exacerbate, pain, such as fatigue. Lawlor (2003) emphasizes that awareness of suffering and other psychosocial and spiritual distress in association with cancer pain is essential to palliative care. Hence a multidimensional approach to assessment that encompasses evaluation of the patient's physical, social and psychological function and spiritual needs is vital (Otis-Green et al 2002).

Anderson & Cleeland (2003) suggested that patients with cancer pain may have 'reporting biases' because cancer is an anxiety-provoking condition. They may fear that a change in pain means more than in other conditions, so there is a need to assess in a way to minimize bias, either towards under-reporting or over-reporting. Clients may under-report their pain, due to a concern about not being a nuisance to ward staff or family members, or due to denial of the increasing seriousness of their condition. A new pain in a patient with cancer should always be investigated thoroughly. It may signal a treatable new problem or the exacerbation of an existing problem that requires reassessment. A change in the patient's report of pain should be reported immediately to the treating physician and other members of the team.

One of the key recommendations for the assessment of cancer pain is that it is reassessed at frequent intervals (National Comprehensive Cancer Network 2010). Cancer pain needs to be assessed frequently to fully understand changes in the pain and underlying influences, such as proximity to or distance from time of last medication, physical activity, anxiety or time of day. In addition the time of day that pain is assessed is important because cancer pain may be worse in the early evening and better in the early morning (Klein 1983).

Frequency of assessment will depend to some extent on the setting and type of pain. If the patient's pain is stable and they are being seen as an outpatient, pain can be monitored during appointments or they can be asked to keep a diary. Patients should be given the opportunity to describe not only their pain at the moment, but also to give an overall picture of the pain at its worst and its best. In this way, the therapist is able to build up a more complete understanding of the variability in the patient's pain.

The fluctuations in pain relative to various reference points, such as the time of day, medication status, activity level or anticipation of some event, need to be charted. Patients with uncontrolled pain need frequent assessment. In this situation pain should probably be assessed at least daily, and sometimes more often is necessary, particularly to determine response to treatments (National Comprehensive Cancer Network 2010).

The implications of this type of assessment regime are that the measurement tools need to be accurate, brief and comprehensive to avoid over-taxing the client. They also need to be appropriate for multiple evaluations and still be reliable, and must be practical for use with severely ill people (Ahles et al 1984).

The guidelines produced by the NCCN (National Comprehensive Cancer Network 2010) state that since pain is subjective, the patient's self-report should be a standard source of assessment. In order for this to be an effective policy to follow, the treatment ethic of the centre must encourage accuracy in patient self-report by acting on information provided by the patient and by providing sufficient education about the aspects of illness and its treatment so that the patient is unafraid to give information about their pain. Simply asking a question such as, 'How is your pain?' does not provide enough opportunity to fully describe it. Various tools which have been shown to be sensitive and reliable should be used (see Chapter 7).

Methods for assessing pain include the Visual Analogue Scale (VAS) and the McGill Pain Questionnaire (MPQ), which were described in Chapter 7. The VAS rates pain intensity and is short and easy to use. Its reliability has been established with patients with cancer. The MPQ is longer,

Table 20.1 Mechanistic classification of cancer pain (from Ashby et al 1992)

	Nociceptive			Neurogenic
	Superficial somatic	**Deep somatic**	**Visceral**	
Origin of stimulus	1. Skin, subcutaneous tissue 2. Mucosal surfaces, e.g. mouth, urethra	1. Bone, joints, ligaments, tendons, muscles 2. Superficial lymph nodes 3. Organ capsules, pleura and peritoneum	1. Within solid or hollow organs 2. Deep tumour masses 3. Deep lymph nodes	1. Pure deafferentation 2. Mixed: nociceptive element due to tumour invasion of nerve compression
Examples	Malignant ulcers, stomatitis	Bony metastases Liver capsule distension	Gut obstruction, ureteric colic	Pure: post-herpetic neuralgia, phantom pain Mixed: brachial plexus invasion, spinal cord compression
Description	Burning Stinging	Dull, aching May be aggravated by movement (e.g. deep breath or cough in pleural involvement Capsular involvement not aggravated by movement	Dull Deep Colicky pain	1. Abnormal sensation, e.g. tingling, burning, pins and needles 2. Allodynia 3. Lancinating, shooting 4. Phantom
Localization	Very well defined	Well defined	Poor	Nerve or dermatomal distribution
Referral	No	Maybe	Maybe	Yes
Local tenderness	Yes	Yes	Maybe	No
Autonomic effects	No	No	Sweating, vomiting, nausea, BP and heart rate changes	Autonomic instability, e.g. warmth, cold, sweating, pallor

Ashby MA, Fleming BG, Brooksbank M, Rounsefell B, Runciman WB, Jackson K, et al Description of a mechanistic approach to pain management in advanced cancer. Preliminary report. PAIN, 2007. 51(2): 153–161.

but is multidimensional and also has good psychometric properties. If the patient is especially ill or fatigued, the short-form MPQ can be used.

The NCCN (National Comprehensive Cancer Network 2010) also suggest that patients be asked to describe the characteristics or quality of pain. The particular descriptive words used can give valuable clues about the cause of the pain. For example, pain described as burning or tingling is likely to involve neural structures.

Assessment of symptoms that may interact with pain may be achieved through symptom-specific measures or through measures that assess multiple prevalent cancer-related symptoms, such as the Memorial Symptom Assessment Scale (Portenoy et al 1994).

There are many approaches to the measurement of function and wider patient concerns. Disease-specific

quality-of-life instruments are one way of ascertaining the interface between cancer pain, other symptoms and functioning. Several measures of quality of life (QOL) for the patient with cancer have been developed which have acceptable psychometric properties. The Functional Assessment of Cancer Therapy Scale (FACT Scale) is a brief, 33-item, self-report measure of QOL over the past week. It covers physical well-being, social/family well-being, relationship with doctor, emotional well-being and functional well-being (Cella et al 1993).

Another measure is the European Organization for Research and Treatment of Cancer QLQ-C30 (version 2.0) (Aaronson et al 1993; Osoba et al 1997). It consists of 30 items which tap the nine subscales of function (physical, role, cognitive, emotional and social) and associated cancer-related symptoms such as fatigue, pain, nausea and vomiting, and global health, and QOL.

In general, in assessing a person's pain, a structured or semi-structured questionnaire format is preferable to interview, as it is more objective and reduces the number of details that can be inadvertently forgotten. However, incorporating an interview can be valuable to foster a good working rapport with the patient and their family.

Impact of pain on the occupations of daily life

Pain from cancer can have an impact on an individual's occupations of daily life. Associated fatigue can also impair occupational performance. Patterns of activity, ability to perform functional activities of daily living, ability to meet desired occupational goals, QOL and coping strategies should also be assessed. The impact which the pain and the cancer has had on the person's ability to perform their daily life occupations should be a particular emphasis of the occupational therapist. Again, methods for assessing these features were reviewed in Chapter 7.

Aggravating and alleviating factors of the cancer pain need to be investigated by asking the patient and by observation. A patient's attitudes towards, and beliefs about, pain and taking medication need to be taken into consideration when attempting to gather a true understanding of the patient's level of pain. Therapists should be particularly attuned to the patient's desired occupational goals and should work to enable patients to attain meaningful occupational goals that are within the capability of the patient.

Family context

The family context is another aspect to be considered. Family members may have many fears and beliefs about cancer, about the 'horror' of cancer pain, about the potential for addiction from medication and about the ways they can best care for their loved one. This requires the careful attention of the treatment team. For example, the family may be resolute in the need to care for their family member with advanced cancer within the home environment, despite seemingly major obstacles to such management. Both conscious and unconscious interactions between the patient and their family are relevant to the design and implementation of a pain-management plan. In the team, the professional responsibility for gathering information about family relationships and pain may vary. However, it is always necessary for the therapist to be at least aware of the details already gathered in designing their part of the intervention strategies. In summary, pain assessment for people with cancer needs to occur frequently and take into account the multidimensional nature of pain, factors which influence it and the impact it may have on both the person with cancer pain and their family.

PRINCIPLES OF PAIN MANAGEMENT

In all situations where pain management is required by patients, a collaborative team approach is the preferred method of practice. Beyond this, it has been determined that supporting *active* patient involvement in their therapy is important. That is, patients or clients should be involved in decisions about treatment regimes and timing of pain interventions around their lifestyle as much as possible. Such active patient involvement is important, in part, in counteracting the feelings of loss of control.

Broadly speaking, cancer pain management can be categorized into pharmacological and non-pharmacological means.

Pharmacological means of pain control

The World Health Organization devised the WHO pain ladder (Fig. 20.1) as a means of assisting in decisions around pain management (World Health Organization 2010). The ladder contains three levels: non-opioid agents, weak opioids and strong opioids. The main function of the pain ladder was to legitimize the use of opioids for chronic pain in areas of the world where access is either severely

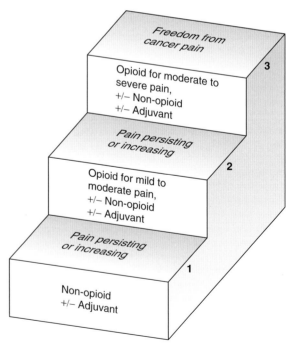

Fig. 20.1 WHO Pain Relief Ladder. Reprinted from the World Health Organization 1986, with kind permission, http://www.who.int/cancer/palliative/painladder/en/.

restricted or banned altogether. However, a more logical approach is to treat pain on the basis of the mechanism that causes the pain.

Analgesics are classified as either non-opioid or opioid. Non-opioid medications are paracetamol or aspirin. They are very effective at relieving modest pain and definitely have a place in cancer pain management. They are also very safe, although there are side effects that can occur. Paracetamol causes liver toxicity in severe overdose, but is very safe when taken as directed. Long-term aspirin can cause gastrointestinal upset and bleeding at times, and may be contraindicated in patients with a predisposition to stomach upsets or reflux, or who are at risk of bleeding. They should not be taken by people already taking anticoagulants like warfarin.

Opioids

Opioids are the mainstay of cancer treatment. They are very powerful analgesics that can be titrated from small doses to very large doses if needed. They are particularly effective when the pain is nociceptive in origin. They can be used for neurogenic pain, but the effect is less certain and other agents may need to be employed as well. The other major advantage of opioids is the range of means of delivery. They can be taken orally in short- or long-acting forms, transdermally through patches, parenterally as an injection or subcutaneously through a portable pump device. They can even be administered directly to the epidural space, the spinal cord or to the brain through a catheter and reservoir device.

They have a number of side effects. For people who have never taken them before there may be transient nausea and mental clouding. Constipation is inevitable and a constant side effect for as long as the drug is taken. It is mandatory for a laxative that stimulates bowel movement to be prescribed at the same time as an opioid. Other side effects include urinary retention, dry mouth and muscle twitches (myoclonus). In overdose, opioids can cause serious respiratory depression and loss of consciousness. Overdose is entirely avoidable if the dose is escalated slowly. Overdose can occur unintentionally in people with impaired renal function because opioids are usually excreted renally. Fentanyl is excreted through the liver and can be used in this situation.

The most common opioids used are morphine, oxycodone, fentanyl (in patches) and buprenorphine. Less commonly used opioids are methadone and hydromorphone.

Adjuvants

The term 'adjuvant' refers to medicines that modify pain without being an analgesic. In nociceptive pain they act by reducing the factors that stimulate nociceptive receptors. Hence, non-steroidal anti-inflammatory agents and steroids reduce the release of inflammatory mediators that cause nociceptive stimulation. Antispasmodic agents reduce the colicky pain that accompanies a blocked hollow organ like the gut or the bile duct.

In neurogenic pain, adjuvant therapies are the mainstay of treatment. They modify the speed of neural transmission so that the nerve damage does not lead to as many noxious stimuli reaching the brain. Groups of medicines that work in this way include anti-epileptics, anti-arrythmics and local anaesthetic agents. The other way they can work is by altering the perception of those stimuli once they reach the brain. They work much more slowly than analgesics, and have to be titrated slowly upwards to avoid unwanted side effects. Because they slow neural transmission, many of the adjuvants in this class can be sedating. However, they are used widely in this sort of pain because they can be very effective in minimizing its impact.

Comprehensive detail on the use of medicines is outside the scope of this chapter. For further detail recommended reading includes the electronic Therapeutic Guidelines series (Therapeutic Guidelines 2010) or the NCCN Clinical Practice Guidelines in Oncology – Adult Cancer Pain V.1.2010 (National Comprehensive Cancer Network 2010).

Therapists' understanding of pharmacological approaches to cancer pain management

While the management of medication regimes is the concern of physicians, pharmacists and nurses, knowledge of the commonly used drugs and methods of administration and mechanisms of action is important for therapists to understand. This knowledge can help therapists to answer questions, to support a patient's understanding of the role of medication and to structure their therapy around the most optimal times.

A therapist may realize that the patient is not taking the medication appropriately. Fear that addiction might occur or that medication should not be taken until the pain is severe, and other misunderstandings about pain medication, may result in the patient receiving poor pain relief.

Therapists should clarify and redirect the patient to their physician if this is required. Therapists may also be more aware of whether the patient has side effects, or if the medication is improving or hindering the client's occupational performance. Possible side effects of medications such as opioids may impact upon the patient's safe performance of activities of daily living (ADLs) such as stairwalking or driving. The reader is referred back to Chapter 11 for a comprehensive consideration of pharmacological methods.

Non-pharmacological medical methods

Non-pharmacological medical methods may be used for patients in whom adequate relief of pain is not achieved by pharmacological methods. Methods used include radiation therapy, ablative surgery and neurosurgical procedures such as interspinal approaches or ventriculostomy.

An understanding of the reasons for performing these procedures, in the case of each individual patient, is the professional responsibility of the therapist.

Therapists may be involved in the post-procedural rehabilitation of the patient. For example, paraesthesia or dysaesthesia may sometimes occur in patients in whom the pain recurs after a percutaneous cordotomy. Physiotherapists and occupational therapists work with such patients to maximize independence, increase safety in the activities of daily living, teach energy-conservation techniques and work with clients on attaining valued occupational goals (Tigges & Marcil 1988).

Education

Education about pain and pain-management techniques is essential for the person with cancer and the person's family and caregivers. Since much of the care is conducted on an outpatient basis, patients and families will assume considerable responsibility and should therefore be included in discussions about management of pain where possible. Yet studies attest to several misconceptions held by patients with cancer and their family members which interfere with good pain management (see Yates et al 2002; Potter et al 2003). These misconceptions include the view that pain medicines should be spared until the pain is *really* bad, the belief that they could become addicted to their medication and the fear of getting bad side effects from taking pain-relief medication (Hussien Al-Aityyat 2008). The patients were also reticent to report their pain to their doctors as they were fearful that pain was an indicator of disease progression (Yun et al 2003).

Individualized education and coaching to address misconceptions about pain and its treatment, and to encourage increased patient communication about their pain with their oncologists and healthcare team is therefore important. Recent systematic reviews and randomized controlled trials of patient education programmes for people with cancer pain have indicated modest improvements in terms of pain reduction (Bennett et al 2009; Miaskowski et al 2004; Oliver et al 2001; Yates et al 2004). A systematic review of interventions to improve patient understanding of pain compared with no intervention found improvement in knowledge and attitudes, average pain intensity and worst pain intensity by 1 point on a 10-point scale. This is evidence of a modest, but significant, improvement, and should be considered alongside other pain-relieving treatments (Bennett et al 2009).

The following aspects are usually considered de rigueur in patient education programmes:

1. Information about the principles of assessing and managing cancer pain.
2. A discussion about beliefs and misconceptions about opioid use and how these can interfere with good management.
3. Information about different pain medications, dosages and scheduling.
4. Provision of tools for monitoring pain, medication and activities, such as a pain diary.

What is not completely clear is what is the best content, delivery methods and timing of such programmes (Hoffmann 2010). Principles of effective health education and communication that use a patient-centred approach are particularly valuable in this setting. Patient-centred communication acknowledges the patients' needs, goals and expectations, and tailors communication and education to the needs, abilities and preferences of the individual (Hoffmann & Tooth 2010). Multiple methods of delivery of this education should be used, including written materials, audio-delivered information such as CDs, visual material and oral discussions (McPherson et al 2001).

More recently, patient education material has been populating the world wide web, especially via Web 2.0 technologies. For example, Hasman & Chiarella (2008) developed a pain management wiki for people with cancer pain. Web searches indicate a plethora of wikis with answers about cancer and its treatment. However, as noted by Hasman and Chiarella, such sites need monitoring to ensure the content that is uploaded is reliable and up to date.

Non-pharmacological physical methods

Other non-pharmacological physical methods that are non-invasive, and may be used by a therapist or supported by a therapist as the active choice by the patient, include acupuncture, cutaneous stimulation, cold therapy, heat, exercise, careful positioning and immobilization. The reader is referred to Chapters 12 and 14 for more detail about these techniques.

People who experience pain from cancer often protect themselves from pain by lying down or staying in certain positions for long periods of time. Gentle exercise plays an important role in reducing pain related to immobility through maximizing the use of stiff joints and developing muscle strength. Further exercise can prevent painful contractures through non-use of painful limbs. Exercise may range from a regular walking programme through to sitting out of bed in a chair or simple movements while lying in bed. Family members can encourage participation in any functional activities that also incorporate movement. Generally, some level of exercise is possible for all people with cancer throughout the varying stages of their disease but its use needs to be monitored so as not to contribute to breakthrough pain, and altered to suit individual needs.

Exercise is also effective in the management of pain due to specific nerve or tissue damage. For example, patients with head and neck cancer who have shoulder disability and pain due to spinal accessory nerve damage have been shown to benefit from progressive resistive exercise

(McNeely et al 2008). Finally, exercise has been found to improve mood and in turn this may make it easier for people to cope with chronic pain (Duijts et al 2010).

Pain may be exacerbated by pressure in the region of the tumour or from being in one position for prolonged periods of time. Attention to positioning, correct body alignment, and use of pillows and supports may relive pressure-related pain. Equipment that has adjustable features, such as reclining chairs, height-adjustable toilet seats and alternating pressure mattresses, may assist in achieving temporary pain relief.

Cutaneous stimulation includes such methods as massage, pressure, heat, cold and transcutaneous electrical nerve stimulation (TENS). TENS units operate by producing small-intensity currents. Electrodes are applied to the skin overlying the painful area or along a nerve pathway. They appear to produce stimulation that 'overrides' or 'negates' the pain stimuli. A systematic review of the efficacy of TENS in chronic pain found that it conferred some pain relief, but there was uncertainty as to what method of use was most efficacious (Nnoaham & Kumbang 2008). The stimulation may be applied to the painful area if the skin is not compromised. If the skin is not intact, application may be effectively given to the contralateral side of the body.

Massage can relieve the pain of muscle spasm around a painful joint or the back and neck. It may improve pain thresholds, relax muscles and encourage lymphatic drainage. Although it is evident massage is effective for relieving pain, its effects may be short term (Kutner et al 2008). Caution is required to avoid massage directly to tumour sites or to recently irradiated tissue that may be sensitive. General musculoskeletal pain may respond to the use of heat or cold packs and again care is required not to place these over previously irradiated areas. Cutaneous stimulation and other types of counter-stimulation may offer relief to a patient at various times through the day while providing a sense of control over the treatment for the patient. However, an increase in the use of such methods initiated by patients should be carefully monitored in case it indicates the need for further medication management. These methods are not intended to replace pharmacological methods.

Psychosocial approaches

Psychosocial approaches to the management of cancer pain encompass a range of interventions, including cognitive–behavioural therapy (CBT), relaxation, guided imagery, distraction and music, and are a powerful adjunct to physical methods of pain relief.

CBT has been found to be particularly helpful and is recommended in guidelines for cancer pain management (Miaskowski et al 2005). In short, CBT targets a person's perception of cancer pain and attempts to modify behaviours and or related cognitions. Although individualized CBT is clearly effective for managing cancer pain, there is not clear evidence of benefit from group delivery (Tatrow & Montgomery 2006). This approach has been covered in more detail in other parts of the book and will not be described again here. There is value in introducing psychosocial methods early in the course of the illness while cognitive capacity is still sufficient to understand concepts and so that the support element of intervention is developed early enough to be well established by the time the patient may need supportive psychotherapy.

A variety of relaxation methods are available, including progressive muscle relaxation (PMR), guided imagery yoga and meditation, and these are often used in conjunction or as part of cognitive–behavioural approaches (Luebbert et al 2001). Guided imagery may be used alone or in conjunction with another relaxation technique. Therapists can train patients in PMR so that they are able to use the relaxation method at any time needed. Ideally, patients need to be trained in PMR while they are pain-free or have relatively low pain intensity, but while they are still able to concentrate. Sometimes it will not be possible to teach PMR if patients are concurrently taking analgesic medication. The development of proficiency in muscle relaxation while undistracted by moderate to severe pain will increase the likelihood that the technique will be used with positive results when pain intensity increases.

In similar fashion, the therapist can introduce the patient to guided imagery techniques, which patients then have in their repertoire for use as required. Driscoll (1987) has suggested three categories of visual imagery. 'Imaginative transformation of the pain context' is a method where the pain is acknowledged and then symbolically changed to another object (e.g. a bird) to leave the patient. 'Imaginative inattention' refers to creating a pleasant and relaxing setting in one's mind, with lots of sensory aspects to attend to, but no pain. 'Imaginative transformation' is a method where the patient recodes the pain sensation as something less noxious, such as a tingling or tickling feeling. The reader is referred to Chapters 9 and 15 for earlier coverage of some of these techniques.

Mindfulness base stress reduction (MBSR) is a type of meditation that has been shown to be effective in helping to reduce anxiety and depression among people with cancer (Shennan et al 2011). Although there is no clear evidence of benefit for reducing cancer pain from MBSR, the relaxation state and acceptance states that it achieves may in turn help people to manage pain.

A caution must be sounded here. Although patients can become independent in using PMR and guided imagery, it is still valuable for the therapist to monitor use of the techniques, providing re-training and support as required. If such support is not given, the techniques may become ineffective, and the client may feel abandoned and discouraged.

Distraction is an approach that moves attention away from pain stimuli or from the negative emotions accompanying pain. People commonly use distraction in everyday life, often without thinking. It may seem that distraction would not require any particular skill. Any patient may have some methods he or she uses for distraction, which can be supplemented by suggestions from a repertoire of techniques offered by the therapist. Introducing a cognitive component to the use of distraction may be helpful. The patient can be encouraged to develop and elaborate a personal picture of their current use of distraction, and to problem solve about its effectiveness and methods of possible change.

Some activities which are useful for distraction include singing, rhythmic breathing, listening to music, playing games, talking with a specific focus, e.g. to describe a picture, and playing computer games. Distraction may be most effective when needed for relatively short periods (e.g. until medication works), and is particularly effective in coping with procedural pain.

Peer or self-help groups are a useful resource for patients with cancer. They can provide support, companionship and motivation. They are also invaluable in assisting the education process. Syntheses of numerous studies have shown that participation in a support group is associated with significant improvements in a patient's emotional state (depression and anxiety), illness adaptation and quality of life (Zabalegui et al 2005), which may subsequently assist in coping with cancer pain.

Spiritual intervention from a specialist in this area can reduce the suffering associated with the pain. This involves identifying what gives meaning and purpose for the person, and facilitating the person's capacity to tap into these things (Mitchell et al 2010). The greatest liability a life-threatening disease like cancer confers on an individual is fear – of pain, of the future, of dependence. Spiritual care provides the hope that overcomes fear, by reminding the person of those things that have greater import for them than any other circumstance. Sometimes the deepest source of spiritual support is religious beliefs and practices, but it may be something quite different – music, poetry, art or time with family and friends (Mitchell et al 2010).

Lifestyle adjustment

There are several aspects to consider when advising about adjustments to a patient's lifestyle in response to their cancer pain. Some aspects have already been covered in Chapter 23. Life goals, life roles and general everyday activities may all need adjustment. Adjustment may be achieved slowly and thoughtfully in some instances, or may be forced upon an individual quite suddenly by a radical change in health status.

Life goals are often re-determined by the patient, either privately or in discussion with the family, with a counsellor, with a spiritual advisor and with the oncologist. However, therapists have a responsibility to become aware of the patient's life goals and to provide the patient with

support in achieving them. This may occur through identifying the life roles that are important to the achievement of these goals, and helping to achieve maximum efficiency and minimum discomfort from pain in the daily activities associated with these roles.

Methods for adjusting lifestyle so that the pain is least incapacitating include the following:

- **Setting goals:** Patients can be encouraged to set goals on a daily or weekly basis, and review them frequently, until a manageable number and priority of goals is determined.
- **Adjusting timing or routine:** For example, tasks which require the most energy, or may result in the most pain, might be scheduled for earlier in the day when energy levels are higher, or may closely follow medication so that the pain will be less troublesome. Activities normally completed in one session may be paced to occur over two or more sessions, and perhaps even over more than one day.
- **Adjusting methods used in task completion:** Adapting the way in which tasks are carried out can help a patient maintain participation in important life roles essential to maintaining a sense of control. Normal principles of activity analysis and task management apply. For example, activities normally carried out while standing, such as self-care, can be adapted so they can be completed in a sitting position. Activities may be scheduled to be completed when someone is available to assist.
- **Varying the amount and type of adaptive equipment needed:** If pain is limiting the range of motion, for instance, adaptive equipment for dressing may be useful. Different seating and cushioning may be chosen to relieve pressure and so on.

In summary there is a wide range of approaches for managing cancer pain with non-pharmacological methods being used to complement pharamacological approaches. Because of this, cancer pain management is delivered by a multidisciplinary team and should be frequently reviewed.

Barriers to adequate pain management

While there are numerous pain-relief strategies, both pharmacologically based and non-pharmacologically based, pain relief remains elusive for many. According to the Australian Pain Management Association (Cousins 2010), one in five people suffer chronic pain in their lifetime, and 80% of these miss out on the treatments that would alleviate that pain. Several reasons have been proposed to explain this situation (National Institutes of Health 2002).

From the patient and family perspective in cancer pain, there is a belief that suffering pain is an integral part of having cancer, and some believe that nothing can be done to treat it. Others are aware of the existence of treatments like opioids, but have a fear of addiction or dependence. They also mistakenly believe that timely introduction of opioids will mean not having anything to fall back on as the disease progresses. Others believe that reporting symptoms may disqualify them from further treatment aimed at cure. Others do not follow treatment directions because of mis-understanding, cost or dislike of side effects.

From the therapist's perspective, there may not be an awareness of the existence of the patient's pain, stemming from time pressures impeding adequate assessment of the patient. There may be a higher priority given to curing the cancer than addressing symptom burden. This may be com-pounded by an inadequate knowledge of pain-management techniques and tools. Some clinicians are over-fearful of legal or regulatory sanctions relating to opioid use.

Finally, a lack of coordination of care and a lack of com-munication between team members and between special-ists and primary care providers can impede the identification and proper management of cancer pain. There may be regulatory barriers to access to adequate pain medication management – in some countries opioids are banned outright (University of Wisconsin Pain and Police Studies Group 2008).

DIFFERENT CONTEXTS FOR CANCER PAIN MANAGEMENT

There are many settings in which therapists may encounter patients with cancer, and with cancer pain. If cancer is the primary diagnosis, patients are likely to be either inpatients in hospital or attending an outpatient service for people with cancer. They may also be in a hospice or in hospice home-care. In each of these settings the role of the occupa-tional therapist or physiotherapist will vary according to the centre's philosophy and organization. However, the principles of pain management for patients with cancer already outlined still apply.

Therapists will also encounter patients with cancer in set-tings where cancer is not the primary diagnosis of all the patients. For instance, a community-based day centre for older people is likely to have clients with a range of diagno-ses, and some may have cancer. In such cases, it is impor-tant that the therapist does not assume the need to introduce a pain-management programme without first checking that this is not already being done by another facility. If there is a pain-management programme in exis-tence the therapist has a responsibility to follow and sup-port it while the client is in their facility.

CANCER PAIN IN CHILDREN

Children with cancer may experience pain associated with the cancer itself (e.g. bone pain), therapy-related pain (e.g. stomach pain from the side effects of chemotherapy) and/or procedure-related pain (e.g. from intramuscular injections) (Bryant 1997). A recent study at a major Austra-lian children's' hospital indicated that 46% of children who died from cancer suffered a lot or a great deal of pain in their last month of life (Heath et al 2010). The reader is referred to Chapter 18 for a comprehensive coverage of pain in childhood, its assessment, measurement and management.

PALLIATIVE-CARE PAIN MANAGEMENT

Palliative care is defined by the WHO (World Health Organization 2002) as follows:

> *'Palliative care is an approach that improves the quality of life of patients and their families facing the problem associated with life-threatening illness, through the prevention and relief of suffering by means of early identification and impeccable assessment and treatment of pain and other problems, physical, psychosocial and spiritual.'*

Palliative care involves working with the patient and their family, usually at home or in a hospice, to minimize suffer-ing, reduce the mechanization of dying, aim for agreement about treatment between the patient, family and health pro-fessionals, and reconcile interpersonal differences.

Palliative and hospice care are becoming synonymous, as physical surroundings for care are changing – patients are choosing to die at home and hospitals are establishing hos-pice units. The essential features include recognizing the terminal nature of the illness and the need for the patient to complete unfinished business, offering the patient as much choice as possible, instructing the family in the care of their dying loved one and prevention or maximum alle-viation of pain. Pain control should be organized and anticipatory, so that quality of life is enhanced for the patient and the family.

If the patient is at home, or in a situation where his or her needs and wishes and those of the close relatives and/or friends are paramount, the health professional must often adjust his or her style of practice. One may need to be pre-pared to follow a more flexible time schedule, to accept that a patient does not wish to be involved in a particular therapy procedure and to talk more openly about one's own beliefs and feelings than might be typical in some other settings.

Often palliative and hospice care involve a bereavement stage, after the patient has died, for the family and other carers. Therapists may be involved in this stage, following their previous close therapeutic involvement with the patient and the family. See Box 20.2 for a case study illus-trating many of these complex issues.

Box 20.2 **Case study: Mr NL**

Mr NL was a 61-year-old man diagnosed with prostate cancer. He was married with a 32-year-old daughter and 30-year-old son. He worked full-time as an engineer, consulting on a number of building projects.

During the early stages of his illness he underwent surgery (prostatectomy) and later received a 6-week course of radiotherapy. Mr NL experienced short-lived acute pain related to surgery which resolved within a few weeks.

After 5 years of symptom-free time, Mr NL developed an intense pain in his left hip which significantly affected his mobility. His prostate cancer had recurred with metastatic spread to his left head-of-femur. He was started on hormone treatment (androgen blockade) in an attempt to reduce the effects of the disease. In addition he was commenced on regular oral morphine until palliative radiation therapy could be arranged. He continued oral morphine for a short time until the effects of the radiation were realized, after which it was ceased.

Mr NL's pain continued to increase so that he had difficulty with weight-bearing. He restarted regular oral morphine, but in spite of escalating dosages his sleep was still being interrupted by pain in his left hip. Mr NL was then offered a percutaneous cordotomy. This provided instant relief to the pain in his left hip and he was able to mobilize more easily again.

After a few more months Mr NL started developing a central aching pain in his pelvis. On examination, it was clear the primary prostate tumour had enlarged significantly. About this time he became increasingly fatigued. The combination of pain and fatigue severely limited his ability to walk, reduced his endurance for activities of daily living such as showering, and he found it difficult to sit comfortably. He commenced oral morphine again, using a slow-release formula, and eventually needed continuous subcutaneous infusion of morphine using a subcutaneous syringe driver pump.

It was at this point that he was referred for physiotherapy and occupational therapy. Physiotherapy input focused on facilitating Mr NL's mobilization throughout this time and advice on positioning to relieve pressure to his groin when sitting, lying and toileting. As his fatigue increased, a walking frame was prescribed which took weight through his arms, decreasing pressure on weight-bearing.

Occupational therapy involvement was initially requested for home assessment, as Mr NL expressed a desire to stay at home as long as possible. The occupational therapist assessed his occupational status (that is, roles of importance to him, his functional status and performance components).

Adaptive equipment such as a shower chair and over-toilet seat were prescribed to enable him to perform self-care independently, and ways of conserving his energy were explored. In addition, the therapist worked with Mr NL and his family to find ways of adapting the environment so he could remain involved in family activities. For instance, at times when he was too uncomfortable to mobilize or sit in chairs, a bed was placed in the family room so he could participate in activities when his friends or his children visited. He also found listening to music helped to some extent to distract him from the pain. The therapist discussed other ways of maintaining a sense of control. He used the telephone and internet for some time to remain in contact with friends and work-mates, following the progress of some of the building projects he had been involved with. Support and education was also provided for his family.

As his disease progressed, he decided to go to a hospice, where his pain was closely monitored. Psychosocial and spiritual support became very important to him in the last few weeks of his life.

Mr NL presented as a patient with many common characteristics of cancer pain, that is, varying types and sites of pain as his disease progressed, changing intensities of pain that required constant re-evaluation and trialing of a number of different methods of pain relief. A multidisciplinary approach with good communication between health carers and family involvement was essential to optimal supportive care as his disease progressed.

ISSUES FACING PRACTITIONERS WHEN WORKING WITH PATIENTS WITH CANCER

When working with patients who have cancer pain, psychological aspects need to be considered. In fact, consideration of psychological aspects is important from both the patient's and the therapist's point of view. Therapists working with patients who have cancer should take some time to examine and become comfortable with their own feelings and values about, and understanding of, the issues of potentially terminal illness, dying, pain and responses to severe pain.

A number of factors can impact on a therapist and contribute to therapist stress:

1. Their own personal feelings and meanings about disease and death, including their personal philosophical or religious beliefs and values.
2. Their previous experiences and expectations about the medical system and what can be achieved.
3. The complexities, uncertainties and challenges that arise when caring for patients who are dying.

Macleod (2001) suggested similar issues for doctors entering palliative medicine.

Coping strategies therapists may use include maintaining a personal support system, examining one's own personal and professional attitudes on death and dying, having realistic expectations about what you can do, using personal stress-management techniques (such as relaxation and exercise) and re-evaluating what the criteria are for 'successful' therapy (Bennett 1991).

Patients who have cancer may exhibit the use of many defence mechanisms, which need to be understood in order to explain their behaviour and to design management and intervention. People develop a personal style of defence mechanisms over their life. For example, one person may use denial or projection more than regression or rationalization. Defence mechanisms are unconscious, and usually operate in a positive way to buffer or protect against stress. However, in some situations use of such defence mechanisms may inhibit communication and decision making, or may even affect treatment choices.

There are many defence mechanisms, but the two most commonly seen in major illness are 'projection' and 'denial'. Projection, in essence, involves attributing to others the feeling we are actually experiencing ourselves. For example, if someone is angry that he has cancer, he may see others, usually doctors or nurses or family members, as being angry with him.

Denial means being unable to accept or believe something, despite having been told about it very clearly, and acting as though it is not true. For example, a patient may insist they have not been told the diagnosis, despite having been told a number of times, or may put off treatment decisions, insisting that there is nothing wrong with their health. Denial is a common self-protection strategy for easing distress; therapists need to understand its complexity and exercise care when communicating with the patient. Treatment decisions need to be carefully facilitated, while allowing patients to face reality at a pace they can cope with.

Because of defence mechanisms and other types of psychological reaction, it is not uncommon for the patient with cancer, or the family, to react aggressively to various members of staff with whom they come into contact. It is important that the professional staff member does not take such a reaction personally, but is able to respond to what may be the underlying concern, such as a need for time to talk, a need for more information or a need to express fear and anger.

As well as the operation of defence mechanisms, there are other reasons for patients to be miserable or irritable.

There may be events occurring in their private relationships that are stressful, continual coping with pain may become wearisome or they may simply be 'having a bad day'. All patients have the right to be irritable sometimes, and the therapist has the responsibility to respond maturely and to be able to provide intervention without always requiring pleasant sociability in return.

CONCLUSION

In this chapter it has been established that there are some differences between the management of people with cancer pain and those with non-cancer pain. Cancer pain is not a static phenomenon due to only one cause. Cancer pain is of considerable import to those with cancer. It is important for occupational therapists and physical therapists working with clients with cancer to be well acquainted with the types of cancer pain, and methods for both pain assessment and measurement and management.

While there may be special management strategies to be used with people with cancer pain, such as slow-release morphine, radiotherapy and surgical procedures, therapists must remember the value of more standard therapeutic modalities, such as energy-conservation techniques. Particular issues related to working in a palliative care setting may also need to be addressed by therapists.

Q | Study questions/questions for revision

1. What are the different types of cancer pain which patients may present with?
2. Suggest two possible reasons why cancer pain may not be adequately managed in patients.
3. How often should the pain of a person with cancer be assessed?
4. What measurement tools should be routinely used with a patient with cancer pain?
5. Identify five techniques which the physiotherapist might use to help a patient with cancer pain.
6. Identify five techniques which the occupational therapist may use to help a patient with cancer pain.

REFERENCES

Aaronson, N.K., Ahmedza, S., Bergman, B., et al., 1993. The European Organization for Research and Treatment of Cancer QLQ-C30: A quality of life instrument for use in international clinical trials in oncology. J. Natl. Cancer Inst. 85, 365–376.

Ahles, T.A., Ruckdeschel, J.C., Blanchard, E.B., 1984. Cancer-related pain-II Assessment with Visual Analogue Scales. J. Psychosom. Res. 28, 121–124.

Anderson, K.O., Cleeland, C.S., 2003. The assessment of cancer pain. In:

Bruera, E.D., Portenoy, R.K. (Eds.), Cancer Pain Assessment and Management. Cambridge University Press, Cambridge, pp. 51–66.

Archer, V.R., Billingham, L.J., Cullen, M.H., 1999. Palliative chemotherapy: no longer a contradiction in terms. Oncologist. 4, 470–477.

Ashby, M.A., Fleming, B.G., Brooksbank, M., et al., 1992. Description of a mechanistic approach to pain management in advanced cancer Preliminary report. Pain. 51 (2), 153–161.

Bennett, S., 1991. Issues confronting occupational therapists working with terminally ill patients. British Journal of Occupational Therapy. 54, 8–10.

Bennett, M.I., Bagnall, A.M., Jose Closs, S., 2009. How effective are patient-based educational interventions in the management of cancer pain? Systematic review and meta-analysis. Pain. 143 (3), 192–199.

Bryant, R., 1997. Coping styles and medical play preparation of young children with leukaemia undergoing intramuscular injection. Unpublished Honours Thesis. University of Queensland Department of Occupational Therapy, Brisbane.

Cella, D.F., Tulsky, D.S., Gray, G., et al., 1993. The Functional Assessment of Cancer Therapy Scale: development and validation of the general measure. J. Clin. Oncol. 3, 570–579.

Cousins, M. (Ed.), 2010. National pain strategy: Pain management for all Australians National Pain Summit initiative. Australian and New Zealand College of Anaesthetists, St Kilda, Australia.

Cramond, T., Stuart, G., 1993. Intraventricular morphine for intractable pain of advanced cancer. J. Pain Symptom Manage. 8, 465–472.

Daut, R.L., Cleeland, C.S., 1982. The prevalence and severity of pain in cancer. Cancer. 50, 1913–1918.

Dodd, M., Janson, S., Facione, N., et al., 2001. Advancing the science of symptom management. J. Adv. Nurs. 33 (5), 668–676.

Driscoll, C.E., 1987. Pain management. Prim. Care. 14, 337–352.

Duijts, S.F., Faber, M.M., Oldenburg, H.S., et al., 2010. Effectiveness of behavioral techniques and physical exercise on psychosocial functioning and health-related quality of life in breast cancer patients and survivors – a meta-analysis. Psychooncology. Mar 24 [epub ahead of print].

Ferrell, B.R., Grant, M., Chan, J., et al., 1995. The impact of cancer pain education on family caregivers of elderly patients. Oncology Nursing. 22, 1211–1218.

Foley, K.M., 1987. Cancer pain syndromes. J. Pain Symptom Manage. 2, S13–S17.

Hasman, L., Chiarella, D., 2008. Developing a pain management resource wiki for cancer patients and their caregivers. Journal of Consumer Health on the Internet. 12, 317–326. See also http://libweb.lib.buffalo.edu/dokuwiki/hslwiki/doku.php?id=pain_management_resources_for_cancer_patients_and_their_care_givers.

Heath, J.A., Clarke, N.E., Donath, S.M., et al., 2010. Symptoms and suffering at the end of life in children with cancer: an Australian perspective. Med. J. Aust. 192, 71–75.

Hoffmann, T., 2010. Critically appraised paper. Patient-based educational interventions for cancer pain management reduce pain intensity and improve attitudes and knowledge towards cancer pain. Australian Occupational Therapy Journal 57, 146–149.

Hoffmann, T., Tooth, L., 2010. Talking with clients about evidence. In: Hoffmann, T., Bennett, S., Del Mar, C. (Eds.), Evidence based practice across the health professions. Elsevier, Sydney, pp. 276–299.

Hussein Al-Atiyyat, N.M., 2008. Patient-related barriers to effective cancer pain management. J. Hospice & Palliative Nursing 10, 198–204.

Janjan, N.A., 1997. Radiation for bone metastases: conventional techniques and the role of systematic radiopharmaceuticals. Cancer 80, 1628–1645.

Klein, M.E., 1983. Pain in the cancer patient. In: Wiernik, P.H. (Ed.), Supportive Care of the Cancer Patient. Futura Publishing, New York, pp. 173–208.

Kutner, J.S., Smith, M.C., Corbin, L., et al., 2008. Massage therapy versus simple touch to improve pain and mood in patients with advanced cancer: a randomized trial. Ann. Intern. Med. 149 (6), 369–379.

Lawlor, P., 2003. Multidimensional assessment: pain and palliative care. The assessment of cancer pain. In:

Bruera, E.D., Portenoy, R.K. (Eds.), Cancer Pain Assessment and Management. Cambridge University Press, Cambridge, pp. 67–88.

Lema, M.J., Foley, K.M., Hausheer, F.H., 2010. Types and epidemiology of cancer-related neuropathic pain: the intersection of cancer pain and neuropathic pain. Oncologist 15 (Suppl. 2), 3–8.

Luebbert, K., Dahme, B., Hasenbring, M., 2001. The effectiveness of relaxation training in reducing treatment-related symptoms and improving emotional adjustment in acute non-surgical cancer treatment: a meta-analytical review. Psychooncology 10 (6), 490–502.

Macleod, R.D., 2001. On reflection: doctors learning to care for people who are dying. Soc. Sci. Med. 52, 1719–1727.

McNeely, M.L., Parliament, M.B., Seikaly, H., et al., 2008. Effect of exercise on upper extremity pain and dysfunction in head and neck cancer survivors: a randomized controlled trial. Cancer 113 (1), 214–222.

McPherson, C., Higginson, I., Hearn, J., 2001. Effective methods of giving information in cancer: a systematic literature review of randomized controlled trials. J. Public Health Med. 23, 227–234.

Miaskowski, C., Dodd, M., West, C., et al., 2004. Randomized clinical trial of the effectiveness of a self-care intervention to improve cancer pain management. J. Clin. Oncol. 22 (9), 1713–1720.

Miaskowski, C., Cleary, J., Burney, R., et al., 2005. Guideline for the management of cancer pain in adults and children. American Pain Society, Glenview, IL, 166 pp.

Mitchell, G., Murray, J., Wilson, P., et al., 2010. 'Diagnosing' and 'managing' spiritual distress in palliative care: creating an intellectual framework for spirituality useable in clinical practice. Australasian Medical Journal 3 (6), 364–369.

Monfardini, S., Scanni, A., 1987. Chemotherapy and radiotherapy for cancer pain. In: Swerdlow, M., Ventafridda, V. (Eds.), Cancer Pain. MTP Press, Lancaster, pp. 89–96.

National Comprehensive Cancer Network, 2010. NCCN Clinical

Practice Guidelines in Oncology® – Adult Cancer Pain V.1. NCCN, Washington, DC.

National Institutes of Health, 2002. NIH State-of-the-Science Conference on Symptom Management in Cancer: Pain, Depression, and Fatigue. NIH, Bethesda, MD.

Nnoaham, K.E., Kumbang, J., 2008. Transcutaneous electrical nerve stimulation (TENS) for chronic pain. Cochrane Database Syst. Rev. 3, CD003222.

Oliver, J.W., Kravitz, R.L., Kaplan, S.H., et al., 2001. Individualized patient education and coaching to improve pain control among cancer outpatients. J. Clin. Oncol. 19 (8), 2206–2212.

Osoba, D., Aaronson, N., Zee, B., et al., 1997. Modification of the EORTC QLQ-C30 (Version 2.0) based on content validity and reliability testing in large samples of patients with cancer. Qual. Life Res. 6, 103–108.

Otis-Green, S., Sherman, R., Perez, M., et al., 2002. An integrated psychosocial-spiritual model for cancer pain management. Cancer Pract. 10 (s1), s58–s65.

Portenoy, R.K., Hagen, N.A., 1990. Breakthrough pain: definition, prevalence and characteristics. Pain. 41 (3), 273–281.

Portenoy, R.K., Thaler, H.T., Korniblith, A.B., et al., 1994. The Memorial Symptom Assessment Scale: an instrument for the evaluation of symptom prevalence, characteristics and distress. Eur. J. Cancer Care (Engl) 30A (9), 1326–1336.

Potter, V.T., Wiseman, C.E., Dunn, S.M., et al., 2003. Patient barriers to optimal cancer pain control. Psychooncology 12, 153–160.

Shennan, C., Payne, S., Fenlon, D., 2011. What is the evidence for the use of mindfulness-based interventions in cancer care: a review. Psychooncology 20 (7), 681–697.

Stuart, G., Cramond, T., 1993. Role of percutaneous cervical cordotomy for pain of malignant origin. Med. J. Aust. 158, 667–670.

Tatrow, K., Montgomery, G.H., 2006. Cognitive behavioral therapy techniques for distress and pain in breast cancer patients: a meta-analysis. J. Behav. Med. 29 (1), 17–27.

Teunissen, S.C., Wesker, W., Kruitwagen, C., et al., 2007. Symptom prevalence in patients with incurable cancer: a systematic review. J. Pain Symptom Manage. 34 (1), 94–104.

Therapeutic Guidelines, 2010. eTG. Therapeutic Guidelines, Melbourne.

Tigges, K.N., Marcil, W.M., 1988. Terminal illness and life-threatening illness: an occupational behaviour perspective. Slack, Thoroughfare, NJ.

University of Wisconsin Pain and Police Studies Group, 2008. Availability of morphine and pethidine in the world and Africa. WHO Collaborating Center of Policy and Communications in Cancer Care, Madison WI.

Wilson, K.G., Chochinov, H.M., Allard, P., et al., 2009. Prevalence and correlates of pain in the Canadian National Palliative Care Survey. Pain Res. Manage. 14 (5), 365–370.

World Health Organization, 2002. National cancer control programmes: policies and managerial guidelines, second ed WHO, Geneva. Online. Available at: www.who.int/cancer.

World Health Organization, 2010. WHO's Pain Ladder. WHO, Geneva. Online. Available at: http://www.who.int/cancer/palliative/painladder/en/20 Jun 2010.

Yates, P.M., Edwards, H.E., Nash, R.E., et al., 2002. Barriers to effective cancer pain management: a survey of hospitalised cancer patients in Australia. J. Pain Symptom Manage. 23, 385–396.

Yates, P., Edwards, H., Nash, R., et al., 2004. A randomized controlled trial of a nurse-administered educational intervention for improving cancer pain management in ambulatory settings. Patient Educ. Couns. 53, 227–237.

Yeager, K.A., Miakowski, C., Dibble, S., et al., 1997. Differences in pain knowledge in cancer patients with and without pain. Cancer Pract. 5, 39–45.

Yun, Y.H., Heo, D.S., Lee, I.G., et al., 2003. Multicenter study of pain and its management in patients with advanced cancer in Korea. J. Pain Symptom Manage. 25, 430–437.

Zabalegui, A., Sanchez, S., Sanchez, P.D., et al., 2005. Nursing and cancer support groups. J. Adv. Nurs. 51, 369–381.

Chapter | 21 |

Managing chronic spinal pain

Diarmuid Denneny

LEARNING OBJECTIVES

This chapter will enable the reader to:

1. Develop an understanding of the factors that contribute to chronicity in spinal pain.
2. Consider the importance of communication in the management of spinal pain.
3. Learn about treatment strategies for the management of persistent spinal pain.
4. Become aware of the importance of flare-up management.

OVERVIEW

Spinal pain, and in particular lower back pain, is recognized as a major usurper of healthcare resources in developed countries. Estimates suggest it costs the UK economy £10,668 million per annum, including direct costs, benefit payments and loss of productivity (Maniadakis & Gray 2000). Spinal pain is reported to have a lifetime prevalence of 80–85% (World Health Organization 2003). In the majority of cases the condition follows a natural course to resolution, requiring minimal healthcare intervention.

However, in 2–7% of cases spinal pain develops into a chronic persistent problem (Burton 2005), although more recent analysis suggests that as many as 65% of sufferers report pain after 12 months (Itz et al 2013).

It is recommended that the reader reads the chapters on the neurophysiology (Chapter 6) and psychology (Chapter 8) of pain, as well as the sections on social aspects of pain (Chapter 3) and the patient's voice (Chapter 2) prior to reading this chapter. This chapter will make little reference to specific pathophysiological mechanisms and the traditional medical model, and focuses instead on the wider issues relating to chronic spinal pain. Limiting clinical reasoning and explanations to patients of a medical model can lead to difficulties, for example when explanations do not fully address the complexity of a patient's situation or when contributing factors are largely of a psychological or behavioural nature. Maintaining a dualistic model of care may lead to reduced ownership on the part of the patient in the management of their condition (Forstmann et al 2012).

This chapter focuses on patients with chronic or persistent spinal pain, specifically low back pain. It explores factors that may contribute to persistent spinal pain and ways of assessing and managing these, and discusses how to deliver assessment findings in a helpful and constructive way. It also outlines common and emerging treatment strategies. Finally, it discusses the variable nature of persistent spinal pain and how to manage flare-ups or relapses.

THE ASSESSMENT OF CHRONIC SPINAL PAIN

The assessment of chronic spinal pain may vary depending on the setting. This section describes common considerations and some tools that may aid decision making

© 2014 Elsevier Ltd.

> **Box 21.1 Objectives of assessment'**
>
> The desired outcomes of assessment of the chronic spinal pain patient are:
> - to confirm the diagnosis of non-malignant chronic spinal pain
> - to determine the impact of the pain on the patient's life
> - to identify areas in which improvements can be made
> - to introduce the concept of chronic pain and the notion that ongoing pain does not necessarily indicate damage
> - to confirm and reassure that it is safe to move with chronic pain.

(Box 21.1). It also discusses the merits of a physical diagnosis and the relevance of special diagnostic tests. For specific physical examination techniques the reader is referred to texts for general medicine or physical therapy (e.g. Kumar & Clark 2012, Petty 2011).

Principles of examining persistent spinal pain

Initial spinal assessment, including general subjective history (history of present complaint, drug history, past medical history, etc.), objective measures of movement and red flags, are appropriate where they have not been done before (see, for example, Koes et al 2006 for further information). Standard assessment tests and questions may become unnecessary if the patient has attended before but a detailed history of the presenting condition is always important. The decision whether or not to repeat physical measures will be made on a case-by-case basis, using the following questions:

- Are the proposed tests and questions necessary and informative?
- Will they assist in determining a diagnosis which in turn could lead to an alteration to treatment?
- Could they reinforce an unhelpful model of management for the chronic pain patient?

The focus here is on the factors to consider in a chronic spinal pain condition where red flags have been ruled out. Sometimes it will be appropriate to repeat a physical examination, not just to confirm the biomedical status of musculoskeletal structures but also for the patient to feel that they are being taken seriously. In such situations a skilful examiner can communicate the purpose of specific tests and findings in a helpful way, e.g. 'This test tells me that you have some stiffness/reduced movement but it is perfectly safe for you to practise this to make it easier' rather than 'You're very stiff, which could be because of the wear and tear'. The latter may mean to the patient that moving more will cause further deterioration and even damage

and should therefore be avoided, even if this was not what the clinician intended.

Clarity and consideration of how a patient may interpret statements are key when delivering messages to a patient with chronic pain. The therapeutic relationship should be viewed in terms of a partnership where the patient's understanding, opinions and values are heard, respected and incorporated into the management plan whenever possible (Slade et al 2009). The assessment should always include explanations to the patient.

An assessment using closed questions will rarely be helpful for the chronic spinal pain patient. Although time-limited during assessment, it is important to include as many open questions as possible thus allowing the patient to fully explain their situation, interpretations and expectations. Crucial information may be missed by simply not allowing the patient to express themselves appropriately. Encouraging the patient to choose their own descriptions for their pain can reveal psychological and sensory information that might otherwise be lost.

Active listening as part of motivational interviewing techniques can be a valuable skill to develop when examining the chronic spinal patient (Rollnick et al 2010). It may help to establish whether the patient is ready to take action to change or to help them to that point (Miller & Rollnick 1991).

Being able to use language that matches the patient's can be helpful. This applies to verbal language but also to non-verbal language such as eye contact, intonation and gestures. Offering summaries of what has been said can demonstrate you have been listening as well as consolidate what you have just been told and clarify misunderstandings. There are many helpful texts for those who want to explore communication further (e.g. Main et al 2010; Miller & Rollnick 1991; Moulton 2007).

When assessing chronic spinal pain it is essential to ensure that both the clinician and the patient feel that the assessment is complete. Patients may feel that it is the clinician's job to know and that their opinion is not important, but when dealing with persistent pain the patient's view is essential. Skilful questioning can save time and ensure that the patient's needs are met. A patient who feels they have not been fully investigated will find it very difficult to assimilate key messages that the clinician may want to give them. If they remain unclear regarding their diagnosis and/or more importantly if they feel that something has been missed, this will need to be addressed. A clinician may ask a patient what they feel they need in order to be reassured about their condition. Frequently, patients will ask for an MRI, which may or may not be appropriate (see section on diagnostic tests). If an MRI scan is not appropriate, as is frequently the case, it is important to have a discussion with the patient about why this is and to check with the patient that they understand and agree. It may also be helpful to bring up difficult considerations to ensure the patient is not harbouring secret fears about their condition. For example, patients may be concerned that they may have cancer or that they will end up in a wheelchair. Other patients report thinking that they have a 'slipped disc' and the clinician should explore what the patient's interpretation of this term is. These conversations will allow the clinician to explore with the patient whether their cognitions and expectations are helpful and realistic, and provide an opportunity for explanation, reassurance and further planning.

When delivering a diagnosis it is essential to check the patient's understanding. Misunderstandings must be clarified. For example, a patient may be told that they have no serious findings on their MRI scans apart from normal age-related changes. They may take this to mean that they have 'wear and tear' and that their spine is crumbling. They may also think that they have something so sinister that it does not even show up on a scan. In other words, information that is intended to be helpful may in fact have the opposite effect. Checking how the patient interprets the diagnosis provides an opportunity to explain, reassure and start changing unhelpful behaviours. With skill, underlying fears can be unpicked and addressed in a respectful and constructive manner.

The relevance of a diagnosis

Many patients expect a diagnosis explained in terms of pathology or mechanical problems. It is important that clinicians are familiar with pain physiology so that they can also deliver a 'pain diagnosis' or description of the pain mechanisms involved (Main 2009). This is especially important when there is persistent pain despite a paucity of positive medical findings, leading some patients to wonder whether the pain is 'not real' and 'all in their head'. The urge to refer a distressed, demanding patient for more repeat tests or to another speciality rather than delivering a pain diagnosis must be resisted. Adequate time is required to deliver the information in a clear, empathic and constructive manner. The notion that nothing further that can be done must be challenged. Using examples from their values and goals can assist to demonstrate areas in which the patient can make improvements, or reverse the apparent progressive nature of their condition, despite ongoing pain.

Carers too may benefit from improved understanding of the meaning of the diagnosis, especially because over-solicitous behaviour can affect the patient's pain perception (Flor et al 1995). Conversely, a lack of understanding of family, friends or carers may maintain maladaptive pain behaviours. Involving carers in a patient's care can improve overall outcomes for the patient (Abbasi et al 2012).

The meaning of a diagnosis of chronic spinal pain can have a major impact on activities such as work or social activity. There are many myths surrounding the condition of low back pain in particular, some instigated by well-meaning healthcare professionals. For example, a patient may be told that they should never bend or lift again. They may be advised to avoid any physical exertion at work. It is not helpful to suggest that a patient is unable to carry out any activities or that certain activities must be avoided indefinitely. Instead, it is more productive to focus on what is manageable and how activities can be adapted. It is helpful to be explicit regarding the patient's ability to carry out their duties and that it is safe for them to return or continue to work. A graded return programme may be agreed with the patient and their employer, and some patients benefit from a work hardening programme tailored to their specific requirements. Patients also need advice about flare-up management.

Diagnostic tests

X-rays and MRI scans are of limited value when managing chronic spinal pain and frequently make little difference to treatment outcome (Chou et al 2009a, Kleinstück et al 2006). They are generally to be avoided unless a serious pathology such as a fracture or tumour has to be ruled out. There are numerous guidelines on the use of MRI and other diagnostic tests for patients with low back pain (Airaksinen et al 2006; NICE 2009). Evidence shows that routine spinal imaging is not associated with benefits, exposes patients to unnecessary harms and increases healthcare costs (Chou et al 2012). Disc abnormalities occur in asymptomatic people; in one study, bulges were present in 52% of people without a history of back pain, protrusions in 27%, and herniations in 1% (Jensen et al 1994). Even in symptomatic patients it is recognized that the findings on scan do not predict response to treatment (Kleinstück et al 2006). Despite this evidence these changes can be mistaken for the cause of the pain, so careful examination combined with clear clinical reasoning is required. As mentioned, the diagnosis of chronic pain and an explanation of basic pain physiology may give the patient a chance to understand pain without pathology.

When explaining diagnostic findings, clinicians should use language that the patient is familiar with, as long as relevant information is not over-simplified or omitted (Slade et al 2009).

REHABILITATION OF PERSISTENT SPINAL PAIN

Whatever approach is taken to the treatment or management of persistent spinal pain, rehabilitation is always a key component. The return to and maintenance of healthy levels of activity, along with the ability to manage flare-ups, are important goals of rehabilitation. This section describes the main considerations.

Generally, passive coping strategies can feed into the vicious cycle of pain and disability (Linton 2000). The inclusion of coping strategies is therefore recommended (Hansen et al 2010). By promoting self-management it is possible to increase patients' internal locus of control and independence, thereby reducing reliance on health services. Evidence suggests that offering too many appointments is as harmful as under-treating this population (Pike 2008). Moreover, patients with chronic low back pain benefit from fewer treatment sessions when the focus is on delivery of appropriate information, such as in cognitive–behavioural programmes, rather than on ongoing manual therapy (Critchley et al 2007; Frost et al 2004; Hansen et al 2010; Lamb et al 2010).

Patient goals

When agreeing an appropriate management plan, the patient's values and goals must be considered. A prescription of exercises, for example, no matter how evidence based or successful in research trials, is unlikely to be of benefit if the patient has no interest in setting aside the required time. Equally, if they have never previously carried out formal exercise then they are unlikely to change unless sufficient guidance and opportunity is provided. They may, however, consider activity if it is clear how it will enable them to do something that is important to them.

Goal setting may enhance adherence to rehabilitation in spinal pain (Coppack et al 2012). Generally goals can be divided into those that are enjoyable and those that make life easier. Preferably goals will fit both categories. General activities such as housework and gardening, and leisure activities such as dancing or walking the dog may also be considered exercise. The choice should take into account what the relevance of the exercise is for the patient's goals and this relevance must be made clear to them. A more extensive review of goal setting for chronic spinal pain may be found in Lee et al (2009).

Exercise

Exercise therapy is widely used as a treatment of choice for chronic spinal pain. The reader is referred to Chapter 13 for more detailed information. A recent Cochrane review of exercise for low back pain suggests that exercise is slightly effective at reducing pain and improving function in adults with chronic low back pain (Hayden et al 2011). There have been many exercise trends over the years, such as core stability, where the emphasis is on activating very specific muscle groups such as the deep abdominal and pelvic floor muscles. It is suggested that core stability is no more effective than general exercise for back pain (Cairns et al 2006; Hayden et al 2011). However, some reviews are critical of the justification of specific approaches, pointing out an overly simplistic and mechanistic view of how pain and function are linked (Lederman 2010; Schiltenwolf & Schneider 2009; Verbunt et al 2010).

The most important consideration with regard to exercise may be the patient's preferences in terms of enjoyment, practicability and relevance in terms of their goals. Enjoyment of exercise has been shown to improve adherence and motivation (Bartlett et al 2011). Patients who resist formal exercise may be provided with alternatives such as dance, vacuum cleaning or gardening, all done in ways that are safe and combined with advice regarding pain management.

Expectations

Spinal pain may be reduced or made more manageable by exercise. However, ideas that exercise should be stopped if it causes pain or continued because it is expected to reduce pain must be challenged. Exercise is generally prescribed to increase functional ability by increasing strength, endurance and flexibility. This may or may not reduce pain, but it is very likely to help the patient to achieve their goals. The patient must, however, apply the principles of activity pacing to ensure that they do not overdo their exercises, as discussed in the next section.

Pacing and other strategies to facilitate increases in activity

One of the most used physiotherapy strategies for chronic pain of any origin is pacing. The principles are useful when guiding the patient to return to activity or to break away from a detrimental cycle of periods of over-activity and under-activity (Main et al 2008). Patients often persevere with activities until high levels of pain force them to stop. This then leads to excessive periods of rest, frequently associated with frustration and deconditioning. In the long term the overall levels of activity decrease and disability increases.

Pacing is a strategy that encourages the patient to move away from using their pain as a guide to how much activity they can do by replacing pain contingent activity with activity contingent on quota (Birkholtz et al 2004). Activity pacing enables patients to maintain and increase their levels of activity without overdoing things. This can apply to:

- planning activities
- breaking activities into manageable parts
- increasing activity amounts gradually and systematically
- alternating tasks.

Activity pacing should be applied to goals that are meaningful to the patient, as described above.

Unfortunately pacing, whilst widely used, lacks a consensus definition and evidence base (Gill & Brown 2009). Care should be taken to prevent pacing from feeding into avoidance of activity and increased disability (McCracken &

Samuel 2007). Explaining the role of pacing as a method of allowing the patient to gradually increase their activity over time rather than remaining static can be helpful. Useful questions to ask the patient can include getting them to identify current activity levels and asking them to determine how much they think they could do without increasing their pain levels, even on bad days. They can be given tips to apply to their chosen activity such as practising 'little and often' even on bad days. They can be reminded to avoid pitfalls such as overdoing things on 'good days' which can lead to periods of inactivity afterwards while the patient recovers from the bursts of activity. A more in-depth explanation of pacing may be found in Lee et al (2009).

Flare-up management

The natural course of chronic pain often includes temporary increases in pain and other symptoms. Often termed 'flare-ups', these episodes tend to be managed by patients on an ad hoc basis. It is important to help patients to develop a plan for management at these times.

Encouraging patients to write down a list of possible strategies can be a valuable tool in their self-management armoury. This list will need to be specific and relevant to them, and may include information about their daily routine and priorities, what exercises to maintain or to reduce, and how to return to previous activity levels. It may also include information about medication alterations, use of modalities such as heat, ice, TENS machines, etc., and ideas regarding activities that help manage mood, such as DVDs or music that can help them to lift their mood and break out of a downward spiral. The list may also include useful telephone numbers, for example work and friends they know will encourage them, advise them or offer a sympathetic ear. The list of items on a flare-up plan is not exhaustive nor is there a right one, as long as the patient takes ownership of developing their own list. The clinician's role may be to facilitate and to help identify potential traps with any items on the list. A common example is the use of rest. There will be times when all the patient can do is rest and this is acceptable, as long as it is tempered with ways of preventing rest from developing into a downward spiral of inactivity, withdrawal, worsening mood and increasing pain. Recommendations could include using a timer to go off every hour during the waking day, reminding the patient to do some activities such as gentle stretching or sitting out for a short period of time.

The chronic pain model of central sensitization may be a useful way of explaining the importance of flare-up management. This may explain to the patient that increases in their pain are not due to more damage or a progressive and deteriorating condition. It is also useful to clarify the scope and limitations of the role of healthcare professionals such as the GP and the emergency department and what one can realistically expect them to do at times of flare-up. This may help reduce unnecessary appointments but more importantly it may prevent frustration and disappointment from feeding in to the flare-up.

PSYCHOLOGICAL APPROACHES

There is no doubt that psychological interventions are valuable in the management of chronic pain (Ecclestone 2001). There is a body of evidence to support cognitive–behavioural therapy (CBT) approaches in the management of persistent pain (Hansen et al 2010; Lamb et al 2010; NICE 2009). Terminologies such as the 'biopsychosocial model' and 'yellow flags' are now well recognized. Originally the term 'yellow flags', coined by Kendall and colleagues (1997), was used to describe prognostic factors for the development of disability following the onset of low back pain. Most of these factors turned out to be of a psychosocial rather than a physical nature (Nicholas et al 2011) and included:

- fears about pain or injury
- unhelpful beliefs about recovery
- distressed effect (e.g. despondency and anxiety)
- workers' perceptions that the workplace is unsupportive
- overly supportive healthcare providers.

Evidence suggests that targeting yellow flags, particularly when they are at high levels, is likely to lead to more consistently positive results than either ignoring them or providing interventions regardless of psychological risk factors (Nicholas et al 2011).

A more recent approach is the stratification of patients with back pain into prognostic categories (low, medium or high risk) using the StarTBack screening tool (Hill et al 2011; Main et al 2012). This simple nine-item questionnaire contains key predictive items from other assessment methods such as pain, disability, bothersomeness, catastrophizing, fear, depression and anxiety (Hill et al 2008). It reduces the risk of medicalization and overtreatment of patients at the lower end of the spectrum, while identifying the patients most likely to benefit from either one-to-one physical therapy or a psychologically informed rehabilitation approach (Hill et al 2011).

It is, however, equally important to limit the use of categorizations and management strategies based on general algorithms without truly taking account of the patient's unique pain experience and the meaning of the pain to them (Stewart et al 2011). It is known, for example, that patients with chronic low back pain more strongly endorse organic pain beliefs and catastrophizing than people without pain (Sloan et al 2008). Management must therefore address psychological issues relevant to the individual, such as catastrophic thoughts.

The psychological approaches used in pain management are often based on the CBT model. It requires skilled communication with the patient, as mentioned previously. It is known that readiness to self-manage is enhanced if the patient feels satisfied with the information they receive from their clinician (Hadjistavropoulos & Shymkiw 2007). It is equally important to be aware of our own belief systems and how they might influence our management of patients with chronic spinal pain (Daykin & Richardson 2004). Identifying our prejudices and knowledge gaps can only improve our management of this complex group.

The focus of CBT-based pain-management programmes are:

- increasing activity levels
- managing periods of over-activity
- specifically addressing catastrophizing and avoidance
- improving coping skills (Hansen et al 2010).

CBT is being developed with increasing evidence to support what is termed contextual cognitive–behavioural therapy (CCBT) in the management of chronic spinal pain (Vowels et al 2007). This umbrella term, sometimes referred to as 'third wave', includes the use of mindfulness and acceptance and commitment therapy (see Harris 2009; Kabat-Zinn 2004). Mindfulness has been shown specifically to be of benefit for chronic low back pain patients (Morone et al 2008). It has also been suggested that acceptance may be a key process involved in behaviour change in individuals with chronic low back pain (Vowels et al 2007). It can be helpful to develop links with services that can provide this specialized care if it is not something that can be provided in-house.

MEDICAL APPROACHES TO MANAGING SPINAL PAIN

The focus of this chapter is on the management rather than the treatment of persistent spinal pain. Pharmacological and interventional therapies, which can make it easier for a patient to manage their spinal pain, are discussed here.

Pharmacological management

Many guidelines include advice on the pharmacological management of spinal pain (Airaksinen et al 2006; NICE 2009; also see Chapter 11). Recommendations include advising paracetamol as a first-line treatment. If this provides insufficient relief then recommend the use of NSAIDs and weak opioids, e.g. codeine and dihydrocodeine in the short term. Be aware of the risk of certain side effects, especially with NSAIDs. Also certain tricyclic antidepressants, muscle relaxants and capsaicin plasters may be considered, although the longer-term role for many of these is unclear. If stronger opioids are required then referral to a specialist

pain-management centre should be considered. Gabapentin is generally not recommenced in the absence of radicular symptoms.

It is recommended to clarify not only what medication the patient is taking, but also what they have tried previously and what the benefits and side effects were. In order to gauge potential compliance with recommended drug regimes, it is important to determine how the patient feels about taking medication. Written information regarding effects, potential side effects and dosage can be extremely helpful. In addition, information regarding progression of dosage is important to ensure that medication is taken appropriately.

Prescriptions should be agreed with the patient and reviewed and monitored at appropriate intervals, depending on the medication prescribed (General Medical Council 2008). Non-prescribing clinicians should remind and encourage patients to arrange these reviews. It can be helpful to consider medication and prescriptions as assistance to achieving goals they have identified. Recent guidelines on the use of opioids in chronic pain recommend identifying goals other than pain reduction as a measure of the effectiveness of the medication (British Pain Society 2010; Chou et al 2009b). By using this goal-orientated approach the patient is encouraged to take an active role in the management of their condition and to set any disadvantages against more important life goals. On the other hand, it is equally important that the patient does not use medication to overdo activities.

Medication may be used to manage flare-ups in pain. Information on which medications to take or increase by what dosage and how to return to pre-flare-up levels can be useful. It also reduces reliance on the health service, particularly the inappropriate use of acute services to manage a persistent pain problem.

Interventional medicine

The options for the medical treatment of chronic spinal pain are surprisingly limited considering its incidence. Currently three possibilities exist and the efficacy of these is the subject of much debate. Medical literature is ambiguous and cost can be a reason for governments to withdraw funding, for example in the case of injection therapy.

Injections

Injections can broadly be classified into one of three types of intervention: nerve root blocks, facet joint injections or denervations, and epidural injections. The use of injection therapy for non-specific chronic low back pain is not recommended (NICE 2009).

It is important to stress the patient's active participation in the management of their condition. Injections, if beneficial, offer the potential to break into the vicious cycle of persistent pain rather than a permanent solution. The emphasis is on rehabilitation; a temporary reduction in pain can allow the patient to use strategies such as activity pacing and exercise to work towards their goals.

Surgery

Discussing surgery in detail is beyond the scope of this chapter but many reviews are available, for example Gardner and Dunsmuir (2008). Guidelines including NICE and European guidelines (Airaksinen et al 2006; NICE 2009) recommend that all other forms of treatment, especially those including psychologically based treatments such as CBT programmes, are tried before considering surgery. At present the efficacy of surgery for pain control is difficult to assess in the absence of good-quality research (Broggi et al 2012). However, structural issues such as progressive spondylolisthesis or spinal stenosis may require surgical correction.

Spinal cord stimulation

Spinal cord stimulation (SCS) consists of the surgical implantation of a battery-operated electric device. Several kinds of SCS systems are available. In general a device consists of four parts (British Pain Society 2009):

- a small computer/battery pack, which is usually situated in the abdomen
- electrodes, which are placed near the spinal cord at varying levels dependant on where the patient feels their pain
- interconnecting leads between the electrodes and the computer
- an external device for adjusting settings and/or charging the battery, depending upon which model is used.

SCS is recommended for use with chronic neuropathic and ischaemic pain, but only if other forms of treatment have been unsuccessful (NICE 2008). Currently research is investigating its usefulness with axial chronic back pain in the absence of radicular pain. SCS should only be offered as part of a multidisciplinary team (MDT) that is able to offer medical and psychological assessment and support (British Pain Society 2009; NICE 2008). Further information can be found in Kelley et al (2011).

For the purposes of this chapter similar recommendations apply to patients after receiving a stimulator implant as for medication, injection therapy and surgery: having a stimulator fitted will not instantly increase their physical ability even if the pain is more manageable. Patients need to work on gradually building up their activity in a paced manner, aided by the pain relief that the stimulator provides. The main goal is for the patient to regain optimal meaningful levels of activity and well-being.

CONCLUSION

Managing chronic spinal pain requires a sound knowledge and understanding of the patient's perception of their condition. This will only be achieved through detailed patient-centred assessment, appropriate use of diagnostics with skilled delivery of their findings and the formulation of a management plan that is not only relevant to the patient but actively developed by them. An ability to hear, explain and normalize the patient's experience without dismissing will also ensure the best possible outcomes. Checking with expectations, on the part of the patient, their carers and relatives, and yourself, is necessary to prevent a downward spiral of increasing pain, reduced mobility, frustration and despair.

Q | **Self-test questions**

1. What factors are considered important to the development of chronic spinal pain?
2. How can such risk factors be identified?
3. How can you ensure that there is no sinister explanation for a patient's chronic spinal pain?
4. What factors are important to consider when delivering a diagnosis of chronic spinal pain to a patient?
5. What are the key messages to deliver to a patient with chronic spinal pain?
6. What treatment options are available for someone with chronic spinal pain and what are the potential problems with these treatments, if any?
7. Who are the key people in the management of the chronic spinal pain patient?

REFERENCES

Abbasi, M., Dehghani, M., Keefe, F.J., et al., 2012. Spouse-assisted training in pain coping skills and the outcome of multidisciplinary pain management for chronic low back pain treatment: A 1-year randomized controlled trial. Eur. J. Pain. 16, 1033–1043.

Airaksinen, O., Brox, J.I., Cedraschi, C., et al., 2006. European guidelines for the management of chronic nonspecific low back pain. Eur. Spine J. 15 (S2), s192–s300.

Bartlett, J.D., Close, G.L., MacLaren, D.P.M., et al., 2011. High-intensity interval running is perceived to be more enjoyable than moderate-intensity continuous exercise: Implications for exercise adherence. J. Sports Sci. 29 (6), 547–553.

Birkholtz, M., Aylwin, L., Harman, R.M., 2004. Activity pacing in chronic pain management: one aim, but which method? Part two: National activity pacing survey. British Journal of Occupational Therapy 67 (11), 481–487.

British Pain Society, 2009. Spinal cord stimulation for the management of pain: recommendations for best clinical practice. BPS Professional Publications, London.

British Pain Society, 2010. Opioids for persistent pain: good practice. BPS Professional Publications, London.

Broggi, G., Acerbi, F., Broggi, M., et al., 2012. Surgical therapy for pain. In: Ellenbogen, R.G., Abdelrauf, S.I., Sekhar, L.N. (Eds.), Principles of Neurological Surgery, third ed. Elsevier Saunders, Philadelphia, pp. 737–755.

Burton, A.K., 2005. How to prevent low back pain. Best Pract. Res. Clin. Rheumatol. 19, 541–555.

Cairns, M.C., Foster, N.E., Wright, C., 2006. Randomised controlled trial of specific spinal stabilisation exercises and conventional physiotherapy for recurrent low back pain. Spine 31 (19), e670–e681.

Chou, R., Fu, R., Carrino, J.A., et al., 2009a. Imaging strategies for low-back pain: systematic review and meta-analysis. Lancet 373 (9662), 463–472.

Chou, R., Fanciullo, G.J., Fine, P.G., et al., 2009b. Clinical guidelines for the use of chronic opioid therapy in chronic non cancer pain. J. Pain 10 (2), 113–130.

Chou, R., Deyo, R.A., Jarvik, J.G., 2012. Appropriate use of lumbar imaging for evaluation of low back pain. Radiol. Clin. North Am. 50 (4), 569–585.

Coppack, R.J., Kristensen, J., Karageorghis, C.I., 2012. Use of a goal setting intervention to increase adherence to low back pain rehabilitation: a randomized controlled trial. Clin. Rehabil. 26 (11), 1032–1042.

Critchley, D.J., Ratcliffe, J., Noonan, S., et al., 2007. Effectiveness and cost effectiveness of three types of physiotherapy used to reduce chronic low back pain disability. Spine 32 (14), 1474–1481.

Daykin, A., Richardson, B., 2004. Physiotherapists' pain beliefs and their influence on the management of patients with chronic low back pain. Spine 29 (7), 783–795.

Ecclestone, C., 2001. Role of psychology in pain management. Br. J. Anaesth. 87 (1), 144–152.

Flor, H., Breitenstein, C., Birbaumer, N., et al., 1995. A psychophysiological analysis of spouse solicitousness towards pain behaviours, spouse interaction, and pain perception. Behaviour Therapy 26 (2), 255–272.

Frost, H., Lamb, S.E., Doll, H.A., et al., 2004. Randomised controlled trial of physiotherapy compared with advice for low back pain. Br. Med. J. 329 (7468), 708.

Forstmann, M., Burgmer, P., Mussweiler, T., 2012. 'The mind is willing, but the flesh is weak': The effects of mind–body dualism on health behavior. Psychol. Sci. 23 (10), 1239–1245.

Gardner, A.C., Dunsmuir, R.A., 2008. What's new in spinal surgery? Continuing Education in Anaesthesia, Critical Care and Pain 8 (5), 186–188.

General Medical Council, 2008. Good practice in prescribing medicines. Supplementary guidance.

Gill, J.R., Brown, C.A., 2009. A structured review for pacing as a chronic pain intervention. Eur. J. Pain 13, 214–216.

Hadjistavropoulos, H., Shymkiw, J., 2007. Predicting readiness to self-manage pain. Clin. J. Pain 23 (3), 259–266.

Hansen, Z., Daykin, A., Lamb, S.E., 2010. A cognitive-behavioural programme for the management of low back pain in primary care: a description and justification for the intervention used in the Back Skills Training Trial (BeST; ISRCTN 54717854). Physiotherapy 96, 87–94.

Harris, R., 2009. ACT made simple. New Harbinger Publications, Oakland.

Hayden, J., van Tulder, M.W., Malmivaara, A., et al., 2011. Exercise therapy for the treatment of non-specific low back pain (review). The Cochrane Library 2.

Hill, J.C., Dunn, K.M., Lewis, M., et al., 2008. A primary care back pain screening tool: identifying patient subgroups for initial treatment. Arthritis Rheum. 59 (5), 632–641.

Hill, J.C., Whitehurst, D.G.T., Lewis, M., et al., 2011. Comparisons of stratified primary care management for low back pain with current best practice

(STarT Back): a randomised controlled trial. Lancet 378 (9802), 1560–1571.

Itz, C.J., Geurts, J.W., van Kleef, M., et al., 2013. Clinical course of non-specific low back pain: A systematic review of prospective cohort studies set in primary care. Eur. J. Pain 17 (1), 5–15.

Jensen, M.C., Brant-Zawadzki, M.N., Obuchowski, N., et al., 1994. Magnetic resonance imaging of the lumbar spine in people without back pain. N. Engl. J. Med. 331, 69.

Kabat-Zinn, J., 2004. Full catastrophe living, 15th anniversary ed. Piatkus, London.

Kelley, G.A., Blake, C., Power, C.K., et al., 2011. The impact of spinal cord stimulation on physical function and sleep quality in individuals with failed back surgery syndromes: a systematic review. Eur. J. Pain 16, 793–802.

Kendall, N.A., Linton, S.J., Main, C.J., 1997. Guide to Assessing Psychosocial Yellow Flags in Acute Low Back Pain: Risk Factors for Long-Term Disability and Work Loss. Accident Rehabilitation and Compensation Insurance Corporation of New Zealand and the National Health Committee, Wellington.

Kleinstück, F., Dvorak, J., Mannion, A.F., 2006. Are 'structural abnormalities' on magnetic resonance imaging a contraindication to the successful conservative treatment of chronic nonspecific low back pain? Spine 31 (19), 2250–2257.

Koes, B.W., van Tulder, M.W., Thomas, S., 2006. Diagnosis and treatment of low back pain. Br. Med. J. 332, 1430–1434.

Kumar, P., Clark, M.L., 2012. Clinical Medicine. Saunders, Edinburgh.

Lamb, S.E., Hansen, Z., Lall, R., et al., 2010. Group cognitive behavioural treatment for low-back pain in primary care: a randomised controlled trial and cost-effectiveness analysis. Lancet 375, 916–923.

Lee, J., Brook, S., Daniel, C., 2009. How much activity can I do? In: Back Pain, The Facts. Oxford University Press, Oxford, pp. 77–82, 118–127.

Lederman, E., 2010. The myth of core stability. J. Bodyw. Mov. Ther. 14 (1), 84–98.

Linton, S.J., 2000. A review of psychological risk factors in back and neck pain. Spine 25 (9), 1148–1156.

Main, C.J., 2009. Talking about pain: What ever happened to "Lumbago"? Pain News Spring 30–31.

Main, C.J., Sullivan, M.J.L., Watson, P.J., 2008. Pain management. Practical applications of the biopsychosocial perspective in clinical and occupational settings. Churchill Livingstone, Edinburgh.

Main, C.J., Buchbinder, R., Porcheret, M., et al., 2010. Addressing patient beliefs and expectations in the consultation. Best Pract. Res. Clin. Rheumatol. 24 (2), 219–225.

Main, C.J., Sowden, G., Hill, P.J., et al., 2012. Integrating physical and psychological approaches to treatment in low back pain: the development and content of the STarT Back trial's 'high-risk' intervention (STarT Back; ISRCTN 37113406). Physiotherapy 98 (2), 110–116.

Maniadakis, N., Gray, A., 2000. The economic burden of back pain in the UK. Pain 84, 95–103.

McCracken, L.M., Samuel, V.M., 2007. The role of avoidance, pacing, and other activity patterns in chronic pain. Pain 130, 119–125.

Miller, W., Rollnick, S., 1991. Motivational interviewing. Preparing people to change addictive behaviour. The Guildford Press, New York.

Morone, N.E., Greco, C.M., Weiner, D.K., 2008. Mindfulness meditation for the treatment of chronic low back pain in older adults: a randomized controlled pilot study. Pain 134, 310–319.

Moulton, L., 2007. The naked consultation. Radcliff, Oxford.

NICE, 2008. Spinal cord stimulation for chronic pain of neuropathic or ischaemic origin. NICE Technology Appraisal Guidance 159. National Institute for Health & Clinical Excellence, London.

NICE, 2009. Low back pain. Early management of persistent non-specific low back pain. NICE Clinical Guideline 88. National Institute for Health & Clinical Excellence, London.

Nicholas, M.K., Linton, S.J., Watson, P.J., et al., 2011. Early identification and management of psychosocial risk factors ('yellow flags') in patients with low back pain: a reappraisal. Phys. Ther. 91 (5), 737–753.

Petty, N.J., 2011. Neuromusculoskeletal examination and assessment: a handbook for therapists, fourth ed. Churchill Livingstone, Edinburgh.

Pike, A.J., 2008. Body-mindfulness in physiotherapy for the management of long term chronic pain. Phys. Ther. Rev. 13 (1), 45–56.

Rollnick, S., Butler, C.C., Kinnersley, P., et al., 2010. motivational interviewing. Br. Med. J. 340, c1900.

Schiltenwolf, M., Schneider, S., 2009. Activity and low back pain: A dubious correlation. Pain 143 (1,2), 1–2.

Slade, S.C., Molloy, E., Keating, J.L., 2009. 'Listen to me, tell me': a qualitative study of partnership in care for people with non-specific chronic low back pain. Clin. Rehabil. 23 (3), 270–280.

Sloan, T.J., Gupta, R., Zhang, W., et al., 2008. Beliefs about the causes and consequences of pain in patients with chronic inflammatory or noninflammatory low back pain and in pain free individuals. Spine 33 (9), 966–972.

Stewart, J., Kempenaar, L., Lauchlan, D., 2011. Rethinking yellow flags. Man. Ther. 16, 196–198.

Verbunt, J.A., Smeets, R.J., Wittink, H.M., 2010. Cause or effect? Deconditioning and chronic low back pain. Pain 149 (3), 428–430.

Vowels, K.E., McNeil, D.W., Gross, R.T., et al., 2007. Effects of pain acceptance and pain control strategies on physical impairment in individuals with chronic low back pain. Behaviour Therapy 38 (4), 412–425.

WHO, 2003. The burden of musculoskeletal conditions at the start of the new millennium. World Health Organ. Tech. Rep. Ser. 919, 1–218.

Chapter | **22** |

Rehabilitation and the World Health Organization's International Classification of Functioning, Disability and Health

Karl S. Bagraith and Jenny Strong

LEARNING OBJECTIVES

At the end of this chapter readers will have an understanding of:

1. The background, development and structure of the ICF.
2. Practical tools to operationalize the ICF in clinical practice and research.
3. How to apply the ICF, and associated tools, to guide multidisciplinary rehabilitation for people with pain.
4. The utility of the ICF in practice and research outcome evaluation.

OVERVIEW

Pain is a complex and multidimensional experience. Previous chapters have highlighted the interaction that occurs between biological, psychological and social factors to produce pain. Similarly, the disability experienced by people in pain also needs to be considered from a biopsychosocial perspective. Thus the assessment and management of people living with persistent pain is often provided by collaborative multiprofessional or multidisciplinary teams. Members of these rehabilitation teams each bring their own discipline-specific terminology and frameworks to conceptualize and describe patients' health, as well as guide their management.

This chapter will focus on providing an overview of the World Health Organization's International Classification of Functioning, Disability and Health (ICF) (World Health Organization 2001) and its application to persistent (chronic) pain management. The ICF provides the first internationally agreed upon framework to define disability and health. This framework provides a universal language and classification scheme to describe health and health-related states. The ICF therefore serves as a useful tool to guide the multidisciplinary management of patients with persistent pain.

In this chapter we begin by providing an overview of previous health and disability models used in pain rehabilitation. We then summarize the ICF's development, structure and potential applications in pain practice. Next we introduce selected tools that are available to assist with

© 2014 Elsevier Ltd.

operationalizing the ICF in clinical practice and research. A clinical case study is then used to demonstrate the application and utility of the ICF, and associated tools, in multidisciplinary pain practice. This is followed by an overview of ICF-based measurement approaches. Finally, we summarize notable limitations of the ICF that should be considered when applying the framework in practice and research.

GENERIC MODELS OF HEALTH AND DISABILITY USED IN PAIN: A BRIEF HISTORICAL OVERVIEW

Pain, and particularly persistent (chronic) pain, is a condition that people have to *live with*, it is not one which people *die from*, with the symptoms and the disability experienced being the primary concerns of people with pain and their healthcare providers (Verbrugge & Jette 1994). A number of conceptual models to explain disability and health have been proposed since the 1960s that have salience for persistent pain. These models are the disablement model (Nagi 1965), the International Classification of Impairments, Disabilities and Handicaps (ICIDH) (World Health Organization 1980), the disablement process (Verbrugge & Jette 1994) and the biopsychosocial model of health and illness (Engel 1977). The key characteristics of each will be briefly described.

The disablement model (Nagi 1965) linked active pathology with impairment, functional limitation and disability; disability was seen as the person's limitation in performing socially defined roles in their particular environment. The model was linear and causal in nature. The ICIDH (World Health Organization 1980) conceptualized the key components as the disease, the impairment, the disability and the handicap. Disability in this sense was seen as a lack of ability to do activities in a normal manner, and handicap was seen as the disadvantage experienced by the person that limited normal role fulfilment. This model was a linear one, describing a causal relationship from impairments through to disability and on to handicap (Halbertsma et al 2000). The disablement process (Verbrugge & Jette 1994), while adopting the pathology, impairments, functional limitations and disability path of Nagi's model, also recognized the impact of risk factors and intra-individual factors (e.g. lifestyle and behaviour changes, psychosocial attributes and coping), and extra-individual factors (e.g. medical care and rehabilitation, external supports and environmental factors). This model also identified the difference between intrinsic disability and actual disability, with disability defined as the gap that exists between environmental demand and a person's capability.

The final model to be discussed here is the biopsychosocial model of health and illness, first described by Engel in 1977 (Engel 1977). This model provided a direct challenge to medical practice, which at the time predominantly considered only biological aspects of illness. The biomedical approach saw a linear relationship between structural abnormalities and resultant functional limitations (Engel 1977). While treatment approaches underpinned by the biomedical model have undoubtedly contributed to improvements in both morbidity and mortality outcomes in society, and in many individuals' health and well-being, the model's presumption of biological causality with regard to the relationship between bodily impairments and a person's health and functional status has been questioned (Lawrence & Jette 1996). The biopsychosocial model recognized the importance and inter-relationship between the biological, the psychological and the social in the development and maintenance of health and well-being, and the corollary, illness and lack of well-being. The biopsychosocial model is now recognized as fundamental in the understanding of pain and its impact on individuals with pain (see Gatchel et al 2007), although there is some suggestion that more attention needs to be given to the 'social' aspects of the model in pain management (Nielsen et al 2012).

INTERNATIONAL CLASSIFICATION OF FUNCTIONING, DISABILITY AND HEALTH

Development

Aspects of each of the aforementioned models of health and disability penetrated the development of the International Classification of Functioning, Disability and Health (ICF) (Bickenbach et al 1999). The ICF was developed as a successor to the ICIDH to address criticism of the classification. In particular, as community expectations changed, the ICIDH was criticized for its use of negative terminology, such as handicap, and the omission of an explicit environmental factors element (Cieza & Stucki 2008). Furthermore, it was not endorsed as an official WHO classification and adoption by end-users was limited (Cieza & Stucki 2008). Accordingly, in response to these and other criticisms, an intention to embark on the development of a new classification (now know as the ICF) was put forth with the release of the second edition of the ICIDH in 1993. The ICF, tentatively released in draft form as the ICIDH-2 in 1997, was developed through a worldwide collaborative process via the network of collaborative centres for the WHO Family of International Classifications, under the coordination of the WHO Secretariat for Classifications and Terminology (Cieza & Stucki 2008; Halbertsma et al 2000). It underwent field trials in over 50 countries during a 5-year period (World Health Organization 2001).

The ICF, as the first internationally agreed upon framework to define functioning and health, was finalized in 2000 and published the following year (World Health Organization 2001). On 22 May 2001 the 54th World Health Assembly formally endorsed the ICF and encouraged all member states of the World Health Organization to implement it in their health sectors (World Health Assembly resolution:54.21). In the relatively short time since its endorsement the ICF has made a significant impact on the disability and rehabilitation landscape (Cerniauskaite et al 2011; Jelsma 2009). For example, it has been approved by esteemed organizations (e.g. Institutes of Medicine 2007) and multidisciplinary professional associations (e.g. International Society of Physical and Rehabilitation Medicine (Jimenez & Peek 2012)). It has been employed as a basis for the conceptualization of disability in the UN Convention on the Rights of Persons with Disabilities (United Nations 2007) and the World Report on Disability (World Health Organization & World Bank 2011). Accordingly, the ICF's release, and its endorsement by the World Health Assembly, are considered to be important milestones for the care of patients (Boonen et al 2007; Cieza & Stucki 2008; Stucki et al 2007).

Overview

The ICF takes into account the biopsychosocial model in its conceptualization of functioning, disability and health (World Health Organization 2001). It is composed of two parts. The first part deals with functioning and disability, and consists of two components: the 'body' (divided into structures and functions), and 'activities and participation'. The second part addresses contextual factors, and consists of two components: 'environmental factors' (external) and 'personal factors' (internal). Figure 22.1 illustrates the proposed interactions between the ICF components

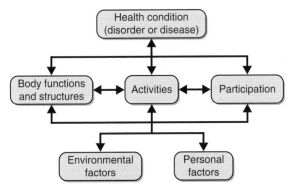

Fig. 22.1 Components of the International Classification of Functioning, Disability and Health (ICF).
Source: World Health Organization 2001, p. 18; used with permission from the World Health Organization.

and Box 22.1 provides definitions for the key features of the model.

The ICF is a broad framework intended for use by a range of disciplines assessing and managing varied health states. It has a variety of aims, two of the most salient being (World Health Organization 2001):

- to provide a basis for studying and understanding health and health-related states, outcomes and determinants
- to provide a common language for describing health and health-related states in order to improve communication between different users, such as policy-makers, health professionals, researchers and the public.

In clinical settings it has been proposed that the ICF could be used by health professionals in needs assessment, the communication of findings in multidisciplinary team meetings, matching interventions to health states, the design of clinical research studies and evaluating outcomes (Reed et al 2005). In non-clinical settings it has been proposed for use in a broad range of areas, including education, insurance, labour, health and disability policy, and medical informatics (World Health Organization 2001). Systematic literature reviews (Cerniauskaite et al

---

Box 22.1 Definitions of ICF components and key terms

Functioning

Body functions (b) are physiological functions of body systems (including psychological functions).
Body structures (s) are anatomical parts of the body such as organs, limbs and their components.
Activity (d) is the execution of a task or action by an individual.
Participation (d) is involvement in a life situation.

Environmental factors (e) make up the physical, social and attitudinal environment in which people live and conduct their lives.
Personal factors are intrinsic factors that are comprised of the background of an individual's life or living.

Disability

Impairments are problems in body function or structure such as a significant deviation or loss.

Activity limitations are difficulties an individual may have in executing activities.
Participation restrictions are problems an individual may experience in involvement in life situations.

Barriers are factors that hinder function.
Facilitators are factors that support function.

Positive factors support function.
Negative factors hinder function.

2011) and surveys (Jelsma 2009) demonstrate that the ICF has in fact been operationalized in each of these areas, and even more.

Structure

Each component of the ICF is arranged in a hierarchy (i.e. first, second, third and fourth level domains), which is reflected by codes. It is these codes (also referred to as categories) that comprise the units of the ICF and permit the classification of the impact of health conditions. Pain, for example, could be considered with the following level of detail:

Component level:	Body function	b
1st level:	Sensory functions and pain	b2
2nd level:	Sensation of pain	b280
3rd level:	Pain in a body part	b2801
4th level:	Pain in back	b28013

This hierarchical coding system is provided for each of the ICF components, with the exception of personal factors (World Health Organization 2001). In the current, and first, version of the ICF, personal factors, while important determinants of disability (Geyh et al 2011; Weigl et al 2008), are only broadly defined (e.g. age, gender, education and coping styles) rather than systematically described with a classification scheme.

Qualifier scale

A generic qualifier scale has been provided to record the presence and severity of problems at the body, person and societal level (World Health Organization 2001). This scale (see below) can be used across each of the ICF components and categories to rate function/structure impairments, activity limitations or participation restrictions. Similarly, environmental factors can be classified as barriers (mild (1) to complete (4)), facilitators (mild (+1) to complete (+4)) or neither (0). Users can incorporate information from multiple sources to quantify functioning in each category (e.g. responses to interviewer questions, self-report questionnaires, physical examinations, imaging reports and standardized functional assessments) (Grill et al 2011).

0	No problem	(0–4%)
1	Mild problem	(5–24%)
2	Moderate problem	(25–49%)
3	Severe problem	(50–95%)
4	Complete problem	(96–100%)
(8 Not specified)		
(9 Not applicable)		

For activity limitations and participation restrictions, the scale can be used to quantify functioning and disability from two related perspectives. Firstly, *performance*, which denotes what an individual actually does in their present environment. Thus performance takes into account the (positive or negative) impact of environmental factors that influence people's execution of tasks or involvement in life situations. Secondly, *capacity*, which denotes individuals' ability to execute tasks and be involved in life situations. Capacity, in contrast to performance, represents ability in a standardized environment, to permit comparison of implicit functioning without the varying influences of each individual's usual environment (i.e. environmentally adjusted functioning or disability). This distinction allows users to quantify the impact of the environment and identify modifiable factors to improve functioning, especially when capacity is greater than performance (Almansa et al 2011).

TOOLS TO OPERATIONALIZE THE ICF

ICF checklist

The ICF is exhaustive by its very nature, with 1424 categories to classify functioning, disability and health. Consequently, it is complex for daily use unless it is transformed into research- and practice-friendly tools (Ustun et al 2004). The ICF checklist (World Health Organization 2003), at 12 pages and 125 second-level categories, has been provided as a 'short' version of the ICF (Stucki et al 2008). Second-level categories were chosen because this level of the classification represents the ideal balance between breadth and depth, and is recommended as a practical level at which to apply the framework in everyday practice and research (Cieza et al 2004a, Ustun et al 2004). Experts selected categories for the checklist from each of the classified ICF components to represent the domains that are frequently used in clinical practice. It serves as a generic and thumbnail sketch of the ICF to support its application across conditions (Ustun et al 2004). Herein lies its strengths, but, particularly in speciality areas such as persistent pain, the 'one (generic) size does not fit all' (Ustun et al 2004). For example, when applying the ICF to low back pain, for the typical patient, categories from the mobility domain will tend to be more relevant than those from the communication domain. However, in language disorders, the situation would be reversed to permit comprehensive description of functioning, and especially those areas that are likely to serve as intervention targets. Thus, whilst a useful tool, the checklist does not necessarily offer the optimal balance between breadth and depth for focused applications. To this end targeted selections of categories, termed ICF core sets have been compiled for defined conditions and settings; their development and application is described below.

ICF core sets

In everyday practice clinicians and researchers are expected to use only a fraction of the entire ICF, with the general approximation being that 20% of the categories will explain roughly 80% of the variance observed for a given condition (Ustun et al 2004). Accordingly, an initiative was undertaken, the ICF Core Sets Project, to develop lists of salient (primarily) second-level categories for specific health conditions and service contexts to serve as tools to operationalize the ICF in practice, research and policy (Cieza et al 2004a; Grill et al 2005; Stucki et al 2008). This project has been led by the ICF Research Branch and is the result of partnerships between international organizations such as the International Society of Physical and Rehabilitation Medicine and collaborations with over 300 study centres across 50 countries (ICF Research Branch 2010).

The project released the first collection of core sets in 2004. This initial offering focused on 12 chronic conditions (Cieza et al 2004a), with core sets for acute and post-acute settings published in 2005 (Grill et al 2005; see Box 22.2). Several core sets have since been released, targeting conditions varying from head and neck cancer to spinal cord injury (ICF Research Branch 2010). Each core set contains only relevant codes or categories for that condition or setting. For each core set, comprehensive and brief versions have been developed. The comprehensive Low Back Pain (LBP) core set, for example, provides a list of ICF categories that includes 'as few categories as possible to be practical, but as many as required to be sufficiently comprehensive, to sufficiently describe in a comprehensive multidisciplinary assessment the typical spectrum of problems in functioning of patients with LBP' (Cieza et al 2004a,c). Whereas the brief LBP core set is a reduced selection of categories from the comprehensive core set, which are intended to serve as the minimum set of data to be collected in clinical and epidemiologic research or when management is provided by individual health professionals, as opposed to multidisciplinary teams. Accordingly, the comprehensive and brief LBP core sets contain 78 and 35 categories (at the second level), respectively, from the entire classification (Cieza et al 2004c). The LBP core set is provided in Table 22.1 (as part of a case study discussed later in this chapter) to illustrate the broad spectrum of functioning and contextual factors that are considered relevant for one complex pain condition.

Development

Each core set has been developed using a similar method established by the ICF Research Branch (Stucki et al 2008); whilst some variation exists, the following three phases have typically been undertaken. First, in the preparation phase, candidate categories for inclusion in a given core set were indentified. This phase sought to indentify ICF categories, from the whole classification, that were probably relevant for a specific condition or healthcare setting. This involved a combination of: (1) empirical data collection, generally using the ICF checklist, to identify those categories most frequently endorsed for the given condition/setting, (2) linking of items (Cieza et al 2002, 2005) from outcome measures for the condition or setting, identified from a systematic review, to ICF categories, and (3) international surveys of experts using Delphi methods to identify professionals' perspectives on important categories. In addition, individual interviews and focus groups have also been used at various stages during the process to elucidate patient perspectives on relevant categories (Coenen et al 2012).

In the second phase, candidate categories from the preparatory phase were presented to international experts, for the specific condition in which the core set was to be applied, at a consensus conference. These expert attendees represented various professional backgrounds, geographic regions and clinical, research and health policy settings. Conferences employed a structured formal decision-making and consensus process to reach agreement on the final list of ICF categories to be included in a core set. Finally, core sets, each of which is an initial offering, are required to undergo an extensive validation phase to ensure their relevance and utility. Validation is an ongoing process and as such the suite of core sets continue to be tested in different countries and regions, with varying subsets of patients, in diverse healthcare settings and from the perspectives of different health professionals as well as from the patients' perspective (Cerniauskaite et al 2011; Cieza et al 2004a; Grill et al 2005; Stucki et al 2008).

ICF core sets and pain practice

Pain, whether acute or persistent, is a feature of many health conditions. Accordingly, the majority of ICF core sets

---

Box 22.2 **Selected ICF core sets**

Chronic conditions

Low back pain	Chronic ischaemic heart disease
Chronic widespread pain	Diabetes
Osteoporosis	Obstructive pulmonary disease
Osteoarthritis	Depression
Rheumatoid arthritis	Stroke
Breast cancer	Obesity
Ankylosing spondylitis	Psoriasis or psoriatic arthritis

Acute settings

Neurological conditions
Musculoskeletal conditions
Cardiopulmonary conditions

Early post-acute settings

Neurological conditions
Musculoskeletal conditions

Cardiopulmonary conditions

Geriatric patients

343

Table 22.1 Mrs Smith's ICF Categorical Profile using the Comprehensive LBP Core Set

Initial multidisciplinary assessment of Mrs Smith: Pain Medicine Physician, Psychiatrist, Nurse, Psychologist, Occupational Therapist and Physiotherapist.

Patient Goals

Short-term 1: reduce pain intensity

Short-term 2: improve mood

Short-term 3: increase contribution to housework (e.g. vacuuming and ironing)

Short-term 4: increase participation in leisure pursuits (e.g. walking and family outings)

Long-term 1: return to paid work

ICF categories		ICF Qualifier	Problem 0	1	2	3	4	Goal Relation	Goal value
Body functions									
b126	Temperament and personality functions				▨			STG2	0
b130*	Energy and drive functions					▨		STG3,4	1
b134*	Sleep functions					▨		STG2	1
b152*	Emotional functions					▨		STG2	1
b180	Experience of self and time functions				▨				
b260	Proprioceptive function								
b280*	Sensation of pain					▨		STG 1	0
b455*	Exercise tolerance functions					▨		STG3,4	1
b620	Urination functions								
b640	Sexual functions								
b710*	Mobility of joint functions				▨				
b715*	Stability of joint functions							STG3	0
b720	Mobility of bone functions								
b730*	Muscle power functions								
b735*	Muscle tone functions								
b740*	Muscle endurance functions				▨			STG3,4	1
b750	Motor reflex functions								
b770	Gait pattern functions					▨		STG4	1
b780	Sensations related to muscles and movement functions								
Body structures									
s120*	Spinal cord and related structures								
s740	Structure of pelvic region								
s750	Structure of lower extremity								

Table 22.1 Mrs Smith's ICF Categorical Profile using the Comprehensive LBP Core Set—cont'd

ICF categories		ICF Qualifier	Problem 0	1	2	3	4	Goal Relation	Goal value
s760*	Structure of trunk		▓						
s770*	Additional musculoskeletal structures related to movement		▓						
Activities and participation									
d240*	Handling stress and other psychological demands		▓	▓				STG1,2	1
d410*	Changing basic body position		▓	▓				STG3,4	1
d415*	Maintaining a body position		▓	▓				STG3,4	1
d420	Transferring oneself		▓	▓				STG3,4	1
d430*	Lifting and carrying objects		▓	▓	▓			STG3	2
d445	Hand and arm use		▓	▓					
d450*	Walking		▓	▓	▓			STG3,4	1
d455	Moving around		▓	▓	▓			STG3,4	1
d460	Moving around in different locations		▓	▓				STG3,4	1
d465	Moving around using equipment		▓						
d470	Using transportation		▓	▓					
d475	Driving		▓	▓	▓			STG4	1
d510	Washing oneself		▓						
d530*	Toileting		▓						
d540*	Dressing		▓	▓					
d570	Looking after one's health		▓	▓					
d620	Acquisition of goods and services		▓	▓	▓				
d630	Preparing meals		▓	▓					
d640*	Doing housework		▓	▓	▓			STG3	1
d650	Caring for household objects		▓	▓	▓			STG3	1
d660	Assisting others		▓						
d710	Basic interpersonal interactions		▓	▓					
d760*	Family relationships		▓	▓					
d770	Intimate relationships		▓	▓					
d845*	Acquiring, keeping and terminating a job		▓	▓	▓			LTG1	1
d850*	Remunerative employment		▓	▓	▓			LTG1	1
d859*	Work and employment, other specified and unspecified		▓	▓	▓			LTG1	1

Continued

Table 22.1 Mrs Smith's ICF Categorical Profile using the Comprehensive LBP Core Set—cont'd

ICF categories		ICF Qualifier	Problem					Goal Relation	Goal value
			0	1	2	3	4		
d910	Community life		█						
d920	Recreation and leisure		█	█	█			STG4	1

Environmental factors		Facilitator					Barrier				Goal Relation	Goal value
		4+	3+	2+	1+	0	1	2	3	4		
e110*	Products or substances for personal consumption				█	█					STG1,2	+3
e120	Products and technology for personal indoor and outdoor mobility and transportation					█						
e135*	Products and technology for employment					█	█				LTG1	+3
e150	Design, construction and building products and technology of buildings for public use				█							
e155*	Design, construction and building products and technology of buildings for private use				█							
e225	Climate						█					
e255	Vibration							█			STG4	0
e310*	Immediate family				█							
e325	Acquaintances, peers, colleagues, neighbours and community members				█							
e330	People in positions of authority				█							
e355*	Health professionals		█									
e360	Other professionals		█									
e410*	Individual attitudes of immediate family members							█			STG3	+1
e425	Individual attitudes of acquaintances, peers, colleagues, neighbours and community members							█			STG3	+1
e450*	Individual attitudes of health professionals		█									
e455	Individual attitudes of other professionals				█							
e460	Societal attitudes					█						
e465	Social norms, practices and ideologies					█						
e540	Transportation services, systems and policies					█						
e550*	Legal services, systems and policies					█						
e570*	Social security services, systems and policies				█						LTG1	+3
e575	General social support services, systems and policies					█						

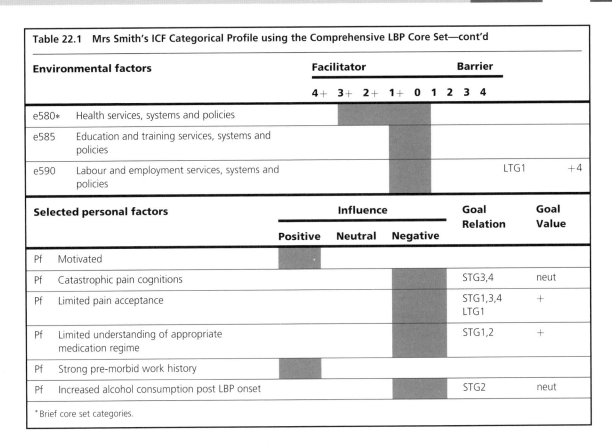

Table 22.1 Mrs Smith's ICF Categorical Profile using the Comprehensive LBP Core Set—cont'd

Environmental factors	Facilitator					Barrier				Goal Relation	Goal Value
	4+	3+	2+	1+	0	1	2	3	4		
e580* Health services, systems and policies				■							
e585 Education and training services, systems and policies				■							
e590 Labour and employment services, systems and policies				■						LTG1	+4

Selected personal factors	Influence			Goal Relation	Goal Value
	Positive	Neutral	Negative		
Pf Motivated	■				
Pf Catastrophic pain cognitions			■	STG3,4	neut
Pf Limited pain acceptance			■	STG1,3,4 LTG1	+
Pf Limited understanding of appropriate medication regime			■	STG1,2	+
Pf Strong pre-morbid work history	■				
Pf Increased alcohol consumption post LBP onset			■	STG2	neut

* Brief core set categories.

include pain (i.e. b280: Sensation of Pain) and this category has been found to account for the greatest variance in general health across conditions (Cieza et al 2006). In this regard, ICF core sets have broad utility for clinicians working with people experiencing pain related to various conditions. For many people, however, pain and its associated impact serves as a key reason for seeking health care (Gureje et al 2001) and, from an economic perspective, bears a considerable toll on society (Gaskin & Richard 2012). For those conditions in which pain is the predominant focus, a range of relevant ICF core sets exist to guide patient management. For rehabilitation clinicians who work with people living with pain and its associated factors, chronic musculoskeletal conditions constitute a great deal of the burden of disease (Woolf et al 2012). Of these conditions low back pain (LBP) is amongst the most common and costly (Hoy et al 2012; Woolf et al 2012). Thus, the utility of the ICF core sets for pain clinicians is most clearly represented by the core sets for musculoskeletal conditions.

Acute and subacute musculoskeletal conditions

In the acute and subacute phase many musculoskeletal conditions share common features and treatment goals. Their functional impact is typically characterized by pain, limitations in mobility and self-care, and restrictions in life roles (e.g. work) (Grill et al 2005; Scheuringer et al 2005; Stoll et al 2005). Similarly, management of these conditions in acute and subacute settings generally focuses on improving safety and independence to permit discharge to home (Lohmann et al 2011; Muller et al 2011). Therefore, a general comprehensive musculoskeletal conditions core set was developed for use with patients in these settings that present with multiple trauma, fractures of the upper and lower extremities, amputations, singular musculoskeletal injuries, arthropathies, spine disorders or persons who have undergone surgery due to arthropathies or spine disorders. Acute and sub-acute versions of the core set were developed to reflect setting-specific needs when treating this group of patients (Scheuringer et al 2005, Stoll et al 2005).

Chronic musculoskeletal conditions

There are currently six primary core sets that target chronic musculoskeletal conditions: LBP (Cieza et al 2004c), chronic widespread pain (Cieza et al 2004d), osteoarthritis (Dreinhofer et al 2004), rheumatoid arthritis (Stucki et al 2004), osteoporosis (Cieza et al 2004b) and anklylosing spondylitis (Boonen et al 2010). In addition, the core sets for hand conditions may be applicable (Rudolf et al 2012). For each of these, comprehensive and brief core sets exist. Many patients present with combinations of these conditions and therefore a preliminary chronic musculoskeletal conditions core set has also been considered (Schwarzkopf et al 2008).

APPLYING THE ICF IN CLINICAL PRACTICE: A CASE STUDY

Persistent pain is a complex and multidimensional experience. Similarly, the disability that people in persistent pain live with needs to be considered from a comprehensive biopsychosocial perspective. Therefore, the assessment and management of people living with persistent pain is often provided by collaborative multiprofessional or multidisciplinary teams (Scascighini et al 2008). Members of these teams each bring with them their own discipline-specific terminology and frameworks to conceptualize and describe patients' health, and guide their management (Jette 2006).

The ICF, and the core sets in particular, provide an ideal tool that can be shared by disciplines to describe and report assessment findings using a common 'yardstick' (Boonen et al 2007; Ustun et al 2004). They also provide a conceptual framework to integrate findings and guide multidisciplinary management (Stucki et al 2007). Thus, ICF core sets can be applied to manage patients in what Steiner et al (2002) have termed the 'rehab cycle'. The rehab cycle outlines a client-centred process for rehabilitation that is applicable irrespective of condition. It can be summarized in the following four steps:

1. Assessment: Assessment of patient problems.
2. Assignment: Collaborative identification of targets for intervention and assignment to team members.
3. Intervention: Planning, implementation and coordination of interventions for each targeted problem.
4. Evaluation: Evaluation of outcomes from applied interventions.

We now use a clinical case study and the rehab cycle to illustrate the utility and application of the ICF core sets, and associated tools, in pain practice.

Clinical scenario: Mrs Smith

Mrs Smith was referred by her local medical practitioner to a multidisciplinary pain centre for opinion and management of her persistent non-specific low back pain (LBP). She was 38 years old and married with two school-age children (9- and 7-year-old boys). She had been living with persistent LBP since she was 20. Her pain commenced gradually with no identifiable triggering event. Recent radiological findings were unremarkable, identifying degenerative changes in her lumbar spine that were consistent with her age and sex. Mrs Smith's use of analgesic medication had been increasing over time. Her local medical practitioner recently commenced prescribing regular low-dose oral opioid medication, in addition to continuing use of simple analgesia.

Since completing senior high school, Mrs Smith had worked in a variety of hospitality roles; most recently as a shift supervisor for a restaurant. Over the last few years her capacity to undertake work tasks had been decreasing, as her pain had increased. She had been leaving shifts early and at times calling in sick, due to pain. Nine months prior, she ceased work due to pain and was at the time of referral in receipt of a social security disability pension. For quite some time she had been avoiding the completion of household tasks that required sustained bending and twisting movements (e.g. vacuuming). Her husband completed such tasks and was generally quite supportive with running their household and looking after the children. Her participation in valued leisure pursuits (e.g. walking) had also reduced markedly in the previous year.

Upon entry to the pain centre, Mrs Smith was streamed into a 3-week intensive outpatient pain-management programme. This programme consisted of a comprehensive multidisciplinary assessment on the first day, which included input from various medical and allied health professionals. Treatment in the programme was consistent with a multifaceted cognitive–behaviourally focused rehabilitation programme (see Chapters 8 and 9 for further details on this type of treatment).

In light of her main presenting pain condition, the comprehensive ICF LBP core set (Cieza et al 2004c) was selected as an appropriate tool to operationalize the ICF in Mrs Smith's multidisciplinary assessment and treatment. Throughout each stage of the rehab cycle the LBP core set was used to support the description, documentation and evaluation of Mrs Smith during the programme.

Assessment

Mrs Smith's multidisciplinary team (MDT) assessment comprised input from six different professionals (pain medicine, psychiatry, nursing, occupational therapy, physiotherapy and psychology) on the first day of her programme. The MDT used the 78-category comprehensive ICF LBP core set categories as a basis on which to guide and document their assessments. As can be seen from Table 22.1 the team's initial assessment findings were complied into a single categorical profile across each of the core set categories and related to the goals Mrs Smith identified on entry to the service. The ICF qualifier scale was employed to quantify the extent of impairment, limitation or restriction. In the case of environmental factors the categories were rated for the extent to which the element was a facilitator or barrier. Pertinent personal factors were denoted as being positive, neutral or negative influences on functioning. Information from multiple sources was used to quantify functioning in each category (e.g. responses to interviewer questions, self-report questionnaires, physical examinations, imaging reports and standardized functional assessments) (Grill et al 2011).

Assignment

As part of her treatment Mrs Smith was to undertake a time-table of generic cognitive–behaviourally focused group sessions (see Chapters 8 and 9 for details of typical content). During the group sessions there was opportunity to tailor aspects of the content to individuals (e.g. individualized gym routines) in addition to one-on-one treatment sessions with relevant team members. During the MDT case conference meeting at the start of her programme, Mrs Smith's ICF categorical profile (Table 22.1) was used as a common basis for discussion of realistic and achievable intervention targets. With respect to her goals and assessment findings the team agreed on appropriate targets and associated interventions. Targets and interventions were assigned to appropriate team members for coordination, delivery and monitoring (see Table 22.2).

Intervention

In accordance with their assigned ICF-based targets each team member planned, implemented and coordinated interventions to work towards Mrs Smith's short- and long-term goals for functioning in each category. Table 22.2 provides an overview of selected target categories and associated interventions for each discipline. Given the intertwined nature of categories and functioning goals, some categories were assigned to multiple disciplines to affect different, but complementary, interventions.

Evaluation

At the conclusion of her programme each discipline assessed Mrs Smith again with respect to the comprehensive LBP core set categories, with particular emphasis on their assigned target ICF categories. The results were summarized and compiled into an evaluation profile (see Table 22.3) for discussion at the final MDT case conference prior to her discharge from the programme. The evaluation profile was used to assess Mrs Smith's progress and review her short- and long-term goals. A discharge plan, summarizing interventions, progress and ongoing recommendations, was formulated for dissemination to her local medical practitioner and community care providers. The evaluation profile was also used as a reference point for follow-up appointments with Mrs Smith post-programme.

Summary

Pain clinicians have traditionally relied on discipline-specific frameworks and terminology to guide and document their practice (Jette 2006). As a consequence, especially in multidisciplinary teams, such perspectives can hamper communication between team members and compromise efficient and effective care (Zwarenstein et al 2009). Given the comprehensiveness of the ICF, multidisciplinary team members are able to employ discipline-specific models or guides when approaching practice should they wish to, but are then able to 'translate' findings, for example assessment results, into the common ICF framework (e.g. Escorpizo et al 2010, Stamm et al 2006).

Mrs Smith's case study demonstrates how a number of ICF-based tools can be applied to support multidisciplinary rehabilitation, namely the LBP core set, categorical and evaluation profiles and an intervention table. Rauch et al (2008) first introduced these latter practical tools to help operationalize the ICF and range of core sets in clinical practice. Mrs Smith's case study clearly illustrates how the ICF core sets can be used as a Rosetta stone (Ustun et al 2004) by enabling different team members to document and report on their practice, in written chart notes or face-to-face case discussions for example, using the same language and framework. Accordingly, use of the ICF facilitates clear and consistent communication that fosters collaborative practice to enhance outcomes (Zwarenstein et al 2009). For interested readers, additional case studies are available which further illustrate the ICF's, and in particular the core set's, utility for clinical practice (see ICF Research Branch 2010 for papers and links to online examples).

MEASURING OUTCOMES FROM THE ICF PERSPECTIVE

Objective assessment of the efficacy and effectiveness of treatments for pain is of the utmost importance for patients, clinicians, researchers and those that fund health care. Functioning and disability are key domains for evaluating pain practice and research, and many of the key outcome measures used (some of which are described in Chapter 7) fall under these umbrella terms (Brockow et al 2004). However, just as there are many disability models, each with their own domains and definitions, there are numerous measurement frameworks that denote which concepts should be considered when measuring outcomes in pain (Turk & Melzack 2011). Accordingly, significant variability exists among outcome domains and the measures that are used to assess them in persistent pain generally (Grimmer-Somers et al 2009), and even for distinct conditions such as chronic LBP (Chapman et al 2011). Unfortunately, this has resulted in a cacophony of disparate measures, which impedes the meaningful comparison of findings across pain treatments, samples and settings; a real Tower of Babel (Fries et al 2009). As a consequence the ways in which treatment end-points are determined varies almost as much as the number of trials published (Furlan et al 2008). For example, there are

Table 22.2 ICF Intervention Table (selected goals and interventions)

Intervention Targets		Intervention	PM	Ψ	N	OT	PT	PY
Body Functions								
b152*	Emotional functions	Review medications		x	x			
		Cognitive–behavioural therapy						x
b280*	Sensation of pain	Review medication	x					
		Heat packs			x			
b455*	Exercise tolerance functions	Graded exercise programme					x	
		Core stabilization programme					x	
Activities and Participation								
d240*	Handling stress and other psychological demands	Relaxation education				x		
		Relaxation training						x
d640*	Doing housework	Graded exposure				x	x	
d430*	Lifting and carrying objects	Graded exposure				x	x	
d850*	Remunerative employment	Vocational counselling				x		
d920	Recreation and leisure	Leisure counselling				x		x
		Graded exercise programme					x	
Environmental Factors								
e110*	Products or substances for personal consumption	Pain medication review	x					
		Psychiatry medication review		x				
e410*	Individual attitudes of immediate family members	Education on pain mechanisms	x					x
e590	Labour and employment services, systems and policies	Linking patient into community vocational rehabilitation service				x		
Personal Factors								
Pf	Catastrophic pain cognitions	Education on pain mechanisms				x	x	x
		CBT						x
		Exposure to feared activities				x	x	
Pf	Limited pain acceptance	Education on pain mechanisms				x	x	x
		Acceptance and commitment therapy						x
Pf	Limited understanding of appropriate medication regime	Education on safe medication usage			x			

PM = Pain Medicine Physician; Ψ = Psychiatry; N = Nursing; OT = Occupational Therapy; PT = Physiotherapy; PY = Psychology.

approximately 165 different patient-reported measures of 'physical function' or 'disability' (Fries et al 2009) and 36 specifically for back pain alone (Grotle et al 2005). A similar myriad of measures exist for other domains such as pain intensity (Litcher-Kelly et al 2007) and psychosocial function (Pilkonis et al 2011). This creates data silos where clinicians and researchers consistently employ familiar measures, of similar constructs, that do not necessarily 'talk' to each other. This is a concern that has been repeatedly noted as a significant limitation in systematic reviews

Table 22.3 ICF Evaluation Profile

Initial-final multidisciplinary assessments of Mrs Smith: Pain Medicine Physician, Psychiatrist, Nurse, Psychologist, Occupational Therapist and Physiotherapist.

Patient Goals

Short-term 1: reduce pain intensity

Short-term 2: improve mood

Short-term 3: increase contribution to housework (e.g. vacuuming and ironing)

Short-term 4: increase participation in leisure pursuits (e.g. walking and family outings)

Long-term 1: return to paid work

ICF categories	ICF Qualifier-pre (Problem, 0–4)	Goal Relation	Goal value	ICF Qualifier-post (Problem, 0–4)	Goal Met
Body functions					
b126 Temperament and personality functions	1	STG2	0	0	√
b130* Energy and drive functions	2	STG3,4	1	1	√
b134* Sleep functions	3	STG2	1	2	×
b152* Emotional functions	2	STG2	1	1	√
b280* Sensation of pain	2	STG 1	0	2	×
b455* Exercise tolerance functions	2	STG3,4	1	1	√
b715* Stability of joint functions	1	STG3	0	0	√
b740* Muscle endurance functions	3	STG3,4	1	1	√
b770 Gait pattern functions	3	STG4	1	1	√

Continued

Table 22.3 ICF Evaluation Profile—cont'd

ICF categories	ICF Qualifier-pre (Problem 0–4)	Goal Relation	Goal value	ICF Qualifier-post (Problem 0–4)	Goal Met
Activities and Participation					
d240* Handling stress and other psychological demands		STG1,2	1		✓
d410* Changing basic body position		STG3,4	1		✓
d415* Maintaining a body position		STG3,4	1		✓
d420 Transferring oneself		STG3,4	1		✓
d430* Lifting and carrying objects		STG3	2		✓
d450* Walking		STG3,4	1		✓
d455 Moving around		STG3,4	1		✓
d460 Moving around in different locations		STG3,4	1		✓
d475 Driving		STG4	1		✓
d640* Doing housework		STG3	1		✓
d650 Caring for household objects		STG3	1		✓
d845* Acquiring, keeping and terminating a job		LTG1	1		✗
d850* Remunerative employment		LTG1	1		✗
d859* Work and employment, other specified and unspecified		LTG1	1		✗
d920 Recreation and leisure		STG$	1		✓

Environmental factors	Facilitator / Barrier (pre)	Goal Relation	Goal value	Facilitator / Barrier (post)	Goal Met
e110* Products or substances for personal consumption		STG1,2	+3		✓
e135* Products and technology for employment		LTG1	+3		✓
e255 Vibration		STG4	0		✗

Table 22.3 ICF Evaluation Profile—cont'd

Environmental factors		Facilitator 4+	3+	2+	1+	0	Barrier 1	2	3	4	Goal Relation	Goal Value	Facilitator 4+	3+	2+	1+	0	Barrier 1	2	3	4
e410*	Individual attitudes of immediate family members					▨	▨				STG3	+1									√
e425	Individual attitudes of acquaintances, peers, colleagues, neighbours and community members				▨						STG3	+1									√
e570*	Social security services, systems and policies			▨							LTG1	+3									√
e590	Labour and employment services, systems and policies	▨	▨								LTG1	+4									√

Selected personal factors		Influence-pre +	Neutral	−	Goal Relation	Goal Value	Influence-post +	Neutral	−
Pf	Catastrophic pain cognitions		▨	▨	STG3,4	neut			▨
Pf	Limited pain acceptance			▨	STG1,3,4 LTG1	+	▨		
Pf	Limited understanding of appropriate medication regime		▨	▨	STG1,2	+			
Pf	Increased alcohol consumption post LBP onset			▨	STG2	neut		▨	▨

* Brief core set categories.

353

and meta-analyses of pain treatment trials (e.g. Chou & Huffman 2007; Hayden et al 2005).

One solution to facilitate the ready comparison of research findings and clinical services is to measure the same constructs in the same way, i.e. standardization of 'what to measure' and 'how to measure' (Boonen et al 2009). International expert consensus is typically employed to develop consensus guidelines to standardize measurement in clinical practice and research, so-called 'core measures' or 'core sets' of measures. Measurement core sets are intended to provide prescriptive recommendation for what to measure and (sometimes) how to measure important constructs across treatments, samples and settings (McQuay 2005). This approach has distinct advantages: more complete investigation and reporting of outcomes, encouragement of the development of collaborative multicentre projects, simplification of the process of designing and reviewing research protocols and manuscripts, and prevention of data silos, thereby enabling data pooling (Turk et al 2003). Two of the most accepted and relevant consensus initiatives for pain are the Initiative on Methods, Measurement and Pain Assessment in Clinical Trials (IMMPACT) (Turk et al 2003) and Outcome Measures in Rheumatology (OMERACT) (Tugwell et al 2007).

IMMPACT has recommended a core set of domains (Turk et al 2003) and associated patient-reported outcome measures (Dworkin et al 2005) for trials that transcend particular pain diagnoses or affected body regions. Whereas OMERACT has provided such recommendations for specific conditions (e.g. hip, knee and hand osteoarthritis; Bellamy et al 1997). The ICF Core Sets Project, in particular the brief versions described earlier in this chapter, provides yet another collection of condition- and setting-specific recommendations for pain practice and research. Initiatives such as IMMPACT and OMERACT provide distinct advantages over the current ICF core sets because they provide practical recommendations on the 'how' as well as the 'what' to measure. In contrast, the ICF core sets chiefly provide direction on 'what' to measure, with respect to the universally agreed upon framework on which they are based, and, at present, leave the choice of 'how' to the end-user. However, almost all of the measurement tools commonly used in pain, such as those included in the IMMPACT and OMERACT core sets, were developed prior to the introduction of the ICF. Thus their conceptual underpinnings do not necessary reflect the contemporary attributes of the ICF framework or the specific nature of the components articulated in the definitions (Bagraith et al 2012). As use of the ICF grows, via application of the overarching disability conceptualization or operationalization of the classification's categories, this discord between existing (core set) measures and the ICF limits the interchangeability of findings (i.e. from the existing measures to the ICF and vice versa).

Two complementary ICF-centred approaches have been proposed to assist with this discord. Firstly, translating existing outcome measures into the ICF language and framework, and secondly, direct measurement of outcomes using the ICF qualifier scale. An overview of each approach is provided below.

Indirect applications of the ICF in outcome measurement

As clinicians and researchers embrace the ICF to conceptualize and report pain related disability, the core set measures they use need to reflect this framework. Recognizing this, steps have been taken to harmonize such recommendations with the ICF framework (e.g. the OMERACT-ICF Reference Group; Boonen et al 2009). However, at present clinicians and researchers are reluctant to move away from familiar and trusted measures (Fries & Krishnan 2009). To this end, the ICF Research Branch developed a qualitative approach to link health status measures to the ICF. These linking rules (Cieza et al 2002, 2005) have been used extensively (Fayed et al 2011) to map many common pain outcome measures to the ICF (Brockow et al 2004; Dixon et al 2007; Sigl et al 2006), therefore clinicians and researchers can continue to use existing measures, which have a wealth of psychometric support and with which they are familiar, to report results using the ICF language (e.g. Ayis et al 2010).

However, despite the advantages of such crosswalks, two limitations need to be considered when employing ICF translated measures. Firstly, linking studies have consistently demonstrated that, according to the ICF framework, existing disability instruments measure a mixture of body functions, body structures, activity and participation, and even environmental factors (Dixon et al 2007; Grotle et al 2005; Sigl et al 2006). This creates a problem when attempting to elucidate, and report on, the specific effects of treatments for people with pain when using existing measures in their original format (i.e. did the intervention reduce impairment, limitation or restriction; Ayis et al 2010; Dixon et al 2007). Secondly, the overriding conceptual underpinning of many of these measures is routed in outdated disability models (e.g. disability is typically considered to be a simple and direct consequence of pain in well-established measures, rather than the result of a complex interaction between pain and contextual factors; Bagraith et al 2012; Officer & Groce 2009).

Direct applications of the ICF in outcome measurement

At the heart of effective measurement is a clear conceptual framework to guide the development of content for tools (i.e. usually rating-scale items that tap an agreed latent construct) (Gray & Hendershot 2000; Rothman et al 2009). With its defined constructs, hierarchical scheme of categories and associated qualifier scale, the ICF itself could serve as a measurement tool. With the aid of contemporary measurement paradigms (i.e. Rasch analysis; Massof 2011) health professional ratings of 2nd level ICF categories can be summed and converted to interval-level scales (Grill & Stucki 2009). Accordingly, from a clinical perspective, ratings of categories from comprehensive ICF core sets, such as those from the categorical profile in Table 22.1, can be converted into distinct measures of body functions, body structures, activity, participation and environmental factors that cross disciplines, treatments settings and even geographic regions (Cieza et al 2009; Roe et al 2009). Similarly, for researchers, ratings of brief core sets can also serve as core measures for trials (Alguren et al 2011).

Thus, direct applications of the ICF, and associated core sets in particular, can provide both the 'how' as well as the 'what' to measure for pain practice and research. Should clinicians and researchers embrace the ICF core sets as measures, they will serve as practical tools to reduce data silos and create a uniform platform for measurement. However, whilst clinician ratings of ICF categories can produce productive measurements that meet contemporary standards (Grill & Stucki 2009), the ICF is first and foremost a hierarchical classification scheme, which, in principle, is different to a measurement system (Jette 2010). In addition, such applications are in their infancy and require much more psychometric support before they can be considered in lieu of existing outcome measures. Moreover, the majority of outcome measures in pain are necessarily self-reported (Brockow et al 2004; Chapman et al 2011, Grimmer-Somers et al 2009); to date it is unclear whether patient ratings of ICF categories (e.g. Kierkegaard et al 2009) could also constitute similar standards of measurement.

LIMITATIONS

Despite the advantages that are afforded by use of the ICF, the framework is not without limitations. These limitations need to be considered when applying the ICF in practice and research. Some of the most notable are summarized below.

First, widespread uptake of the ICF is needed to realize the benefits of its application (i.e. a critical mass of users is required for it to be able to stand as a common reference standard). Whilst there has been tremendous growth in research-based applications of the ICF (Cerniauskaite et al 2011, Jelsma 2009), it has been suggested that practice uptake is relatively lagging (Wiegand et al 2012). This creates a potential problem for clinicians who adopt the ICF, as their colleagues may not be familiar with the language and codes, which could impede interdisciplinary communication. Whilst there have been reports of large-scale education programmes (Francescutti et al 2009), further training and the implementation of policies to encourage use will be essential for widespread application. To this end detailed guidelines are available to support consistent operationalization of the framework (e.g. Australian Institute of Health and Welfare 2003).

Second, the personal factors component of the ICF remains unclassified (World Health Organization 2001). Personal factors play an integral role in functioning and disability for people with persistent pain (Weigl et al 2008). Whilst this limitation should not prevent application of the framework, as, for example, no other accepted classification is currently available for personal factors, it is a notable drawback for its operationalization. Work is progressing towards defining this component (Geyh et al 2011). The impact of this omission on the application of the ICF is unclear; for example, it is unknown to what degree clinicians focus on personal factors when assessing patients.

Third, as noted earlier in the chapter, the range of ICF core sets are currently only in their first version and require further testing. For example, when considering the LBP core sets from a critical perspective, testing could be described as being in the early stages. Research has generally confirmed that the LBP core set categories are sufficient to cover professionals' perspectives (Glocker et al 2012; Kirschneck et al 2011) and even their assessment templates (Escorpizo et al 2010). Similarly, patients' perspectives on the impact of LBP are mostly encompassed (Abbott et al 2011; Mullis et al 2007; Roe et al 2008), as are the concepts contained in frequently used LBP outcome measures (Sigl et al 2006). Furthermore, from a quantitative perspective, the majority of the core set's categories have been endorsed as relevant when classifying LBP functioning (Bautz-Holter et al 2008; Jonsdottir et al 2010) and preliminary evidence has supported its construct validity (Roe et al 2009) and inter-rater reliability (Hilfiker et al 2009). This level of validation is typical for the suite of ICF core sets that are presently available. Generally, further evidence is desirable to confirm their utility for pain practice and research (Jette 2010). In particular, from an assessment and evaluation perspective, it is unclear whether comprehensive core sets in fact fully cover the content and focus of multidisciplinary clinical assessments. Moreover, from a rehabilitation perspective, it has only recently been considered whether ICF core sets encompass patients' treatment goals (Lohmann et al 2011). Hence, additional evidence will serve to enhance clinicians' confidence in the suite of ICF core sets when using them as tools to guide, document and evaluate the rehabilitation cycle. Such evidence will also strengthen the foundations for their continued application in research.

From a specific measurement perspective there are three further limitations. First, the metric properties of the ICF qualifier scale are not yet sufficiently evaluated (Grill et al 2011). Contemporary psychometric analyses have generally supported modified three-level scales for functioning (i.e. 0 = no problem, 1 = some problem and 2 = extreme/severe problem) and environmental factors (i.e. barrier, neither barrier/facilitator and facilitator)

(Bostan et al 2012). However, qualifier scale analyses have been almost entirely post-hoc with clinician ratings on the original five- and nine-point scales respectively. Further prospective evaluations of the modified scales are needed to permit measurement, in addition to straightforward classification (Jette 2010), when using the ICF qualifiers. Second, inter-rater reliability for classifying people, using the original scales, has generally been moderate (Hilfiker et al 2009; Okochi et al 2005; Starrost et al 2008; Uhlig et al 2007) and a source of criticism for operationalization of the core sets (Jette 2010). However, recent work has suggested that with the aforementioned modified qualifier scales and additional definition for each qualifier graduation, inter-rater reliability is enhanced (Grill et al 2011; Hilfiker et al 2009). Third, the ICF manual provides end-users with the choice of which chapters and categories of the activity and participation component constitute activity, participation or both. This lack of distinction between activity and participation has led to inconsistent operationalization of this component (Whiteneck & Dijkers 2009). Whilst user guides and recommendations are available (e.g. Australian Institute of Health and Welfare 2003; Whiteneck & Dijkers 2009), the dimensionality of this component remains unclear and has generally been defined iteratively and from a statistical perspective (Ewert et al 2010; Roe et al 2009) without clear underlying theory or consensus.

In spite of these limitations the strengths and advantages of the ICF, and associated tools, support numerous calls for its operationalization, even from those raising criticisms (e.g. Jette 2010; McIntyre & Tempest 2007; Whiteneck & Dijkers 2009), albeit with the aforementioned caveats and directions for additional research.

<table>
<tr><td>**Q**</td><td>**Study questions/questions for revision**</td></tr>
</table>

1. List each of the overall ICF components.
2. List four benefits of applying the ICF in practice and research.
3. List three tools that clinicians can use to operationalize the ICF in their documentation.
4. Give one ICF core set and describe how it can support the application of the ICF in daily practice.
5. How can the ICF allow researchers to more effectively compare treatments for persistent pain?
6. What are the ICF linking rules and how can they be applied to support outcome measurement in persistent pain?
7. What are some of the limitations that should be considered when applying the ICF in practice? How could you manage these?

how they can be applied in clinical practice. The ICF provides the first universally agreed upon framework and language to describe functioning and disability. The underlying premise for this chapter was that application of the ICF can facilitate consistent description and documentation of functioning and disability across conditions, disciplines, practice settings and even geographic regions. The ICF fulfils a gap that has been present for some time in rehabilitation, and accordingly its use has grown tremendously since its release. Clinicians and researchers working in the persistent pain field should look to apply the ICF in their everyday work to enhance patient outcomes.

CONCLUSION

In this chapter we have provided an overview of the ICF and its potential applications in persistent pain rehabilitation. In doing so we have discussed the background, structure, benefits and limitations of the framework. In addition, we have introduced some of the practical tools that are available to operationalize the ICF and demonstrated

ACKNOWLEDGEMENTS

The authors thank Elizabeth Gibson for her feedback during manuscript revision. Karl Bagraith's input was supported by the RBWH Cramond Fellowship in Pain Management and Occupational Therapy, and funding from the RBWH Foundation.

REFERENCES

Abbott, A.D., Hedlund, R., Tyni-Lenne, R., 2011. Patients' experience post-lumbar fusion regarding back problems, recovery and expectations in terms of the International Classification of Functioning, Disability and Health. Disabil. Rehabil. 33, 1399–1408.

Alguren, B., Bostan, C., Christensson, L., et al., 2011. A multidisciplinary cross-cultural measurement of functioning after stroke: Rasch analysis of the brief ICF Core Set for stroke. Top. Stroke Rehabil. 18 (Suppl. 1), 573–586.

Almansa, J., Ayuso-Mateos, J.L., Garin, O., et al., 2011. The International Classification of Functioning, Disability and Health: development of capacity and performance scales. J. Clin. Epidemiol. 64, 1400–1411.

Australian Institute of Health and Welfare, 2003. ICF Australian User

Guide V1.0. Australian Institute of Health and Welfare, Canberra.

Ayis, S., Arden, N., Doherty, M., et al., 2010. Applying the impairment, activity limitation, and participation restriction constructs of the ICF model to osteoarthritis and low back pain trials: a reanalysis. J. Rheumatol. 37, 1923–1931.

Bagraith, K.S., Strong, J., Sussex, R., 2012. Disentangling disability in the fear avoidance model: more than pain interference alone. Clin. J. Pain 28, 273–274.

Bautz-Holter, E., Sveen, U., Cieza, A., et al., 2008. Does the International Classification of Functioning, Disability and Health (ICF) core set for low back pain cover the patients' problems? A cross-sectional content-validity study with a Norwegian population. European Journal of Physical and Rehabilitation Medicine 44, 387–397.

Bellamy, N., Kirwan, J., Boers, M., et al., 1997. Recommendations for a core set of outcome measures for future phase III clinical trials in knee, hip, and hand osteoarthritis. Consensus development at OMERACT III. J. Rheumatol. 24, 799–802.

Bickenbach, J.E., Chatterji, S., Badley, E.M., et al., 1999. Models of disablement, universalism and the international classification of impairments, disabilities and handicaps. Soc. Sci. Med. 48, 1173–1187.

Boonen, A., Rasker, J.J., Stucki, G., 2007. The international classification for functioning, disability and health. A challenge and a need for rheumatology. Clin. Rheumatol. 26, 1803–1808.

Boonen, A., Stucki, G., Maksymowych, W., et al., 2009. The OMERACT-ICF Reference Group: integrating the ICF into the OMERACT process: opportunities and challenges. J. Rheumatol. 36, 2057–2060.

Boonen, A., Braun, J., van der Horst-Bruinsma, I.E., et al., 2010. The ASAS/WHO ICF Core Sets for Ankylosing Spondylitis: how to classify the impact of AS on functioning and health. Annals of Rheumatic Diseases 69, 102–107.

Bostan, C., Oberhauser, C., Cieza, A., 2012. Investigating the dimension functioning from a condition-specific perspective and the qualifier scale of the International Classification of Functioning, Disability, and Health based on Rasch analyses. Am. J. Phys. Med. Rehabil. 91, S129–S140.

Brockow, T., Cieza, A., Kuhlow, H., et al., 2004. Identifying the concepts contained in outcome measures of clinical trials on musculoskeletal disorders and chronic widespread pain using the International Classification of Functioning, Disability and Health as a reference. J. Rehabil. Med. (Suppl. 44), 30–36.

Cerniauskaite, M., Quintas, R., Boldt, C., et al., 2011. Systematic literature review on ICF from 2001 to 2009: its use, implementation and operationalisation. Disabil. Rehabil. 33, 281–309.

Chapman, J.R., Norvell, D.C., Hermsmeyer, J.T., et al., 2011. Evaluating common outcomes for measuring treatment success for chronic low back pain. Spine (Phila Pa 1976) 36, S54–S68.

Chou, R., Huffman, L.H., 2007. Nonpharmacologic therapies for acute and chronic low back pain: a review of the evidence for an American Pain Society/American College of Physicians clinical practice guideline. Ann. Intern. Med. 147, 492–504.

Cieza, A., Stucki, G., 2008. The international classification of functioning disability and health: Its development process and content validity. European Journal of Physical and Rehabilitation Medicine. 44, 303–313.

Cieza, A., Brockow, T., Ewert, T., et al., 2002. Linking health-status measurements to the International Classification of Functioning, Disability and Health. J. Rehabil. Med. 34, 205–210.

Cieza, A., Ewert, T., Ustun, T.B., et al., 2004a. Development of ICF Core Sets for patients with chronic conditions. J. Rehabil. Med. (Suppl. 44)44, 9–11.

Cieza, A., Schwarzkopf, S.R., Sigl, T., et al., 2004b. ICF Core Sets for osteoporosis. J. Rehabil. Med. (Suppl. 44), 81–86.

Cieza, A., Stucki, G., Weigl, M., et al., 2004c. ICF Core Sets for low back pain. J. Rehabil. Med. (Suppl. 44), 69–74.

Cieza, A., Stucki, G., Weigl, M., et al., 2004d. ICF Core Sets for chronic widespread pain. J. Rehabil. Med. (Suppl. 44), 63–68.

Cieza, A., Geyh, S., Chatterji, S., et al., 2005. ICF linking rules: An update based on lessons learned. J. Rehabil. Med. 37, 212–218.

Cieza, A., Geyh, S., Chatterji, S., et al., 2006. Identification of candidate categories of the International Classification of Functioning Disability and Health (ICF) for a Generic ICF Core Set based on regression modelling. BMC Med. Res. Methodol. 6, 36.

Cieza, A., Hilfiker, R., Chatterji, S., et al., 2009. The International Classification of Functioning, Disability, and Health could be used to measure functioning. J. Clin. Epidemiol. 62, 899–911.

Coenen, M., Stamm, T.A., Stucki, G., et al., 2012. Individual interviews and focus groups in patients with rheumatoid arthritis: a comparison of two qualitative methods. Qual. Life Res. 21, 359–370.

Dixon, D., Pollard, B., Johnston, M., 2007. What does the chronic pain grade questionnaire measure? Pain 130, 249–253.

Dreinhofer, K., Stucki, G., Ewert, T., et al., 2004. ICF Core Sets for osteoarthritis. J. Rehabil. Med. (Suppl. 44), 75–80.

Dworkin, R.H., Turk, D.C., Farrar, J.T., et al., 2005. Core outcome measures for chronic pain clinical trials: IMMPACT recommendations. Pain 113, 9–19.

Engel, G.L., 1977. The need for a new medical model: a challenge for biomedicine. Science 196, 129–136.

Escorpizo, R., Davis, K., Stumbo, T., 2010. Mapping of a standard documentation template to the ICF core sets for arthritis and low back pain. Physiother. Res. Int. 15, 222–231.

Ewert, T., Allen, D.D., Wilson, M., et al., 2010. Validation of the International Classification of Functioning Disability and Health framework using multidimensional item response modeling. Disabil. Rehabil. 32, 1397–1405.

Fayed, N., Cieza, A., Bickenbach, J.E., 2011. Linking health and health-related information to the ICF: a systematic review of the literature from 2001 to 2008. Disabil. Rehabil. 33, 1941–1951.

Francescutti, C., Fusaro, G., Leonardi, M., et al., 2009. Italian ICF training programs: describing and promoting human functioning and research. Disabil. Rehabil. 31 (Suppl. 1), S46–S49.

Fries, J.F., Krishnan, E., 2009. What constitutes progress in assessing patient outcomes? J. Clin. Epidemiol. 62, 779–780.

Fries, J.F., Krishnan, E., Bruce, B., 2009. Items, Instruments, Crosswalks, and PROMIS. J. Rheumatol. 36, 1093–1095.

Furlan, A.D., Tomlinson, G., Jadad, A.R., et al., 2008. Examining heterogeneity in meta-analysis: Comparing results of randomized trials and nonrandomized studies of interventions for low back pain. Spine 33, 339–348.

Gaskin, D.J., Richard, P., 2012. The economic costs of pain in the United States. J. Pain 13 (8), 715–724.

Gatchel, R.J., Peng, Y.B., Peters, M.L., et al., 2007. The biopsychosocial approach to chronic pain: scientific advances and future directions. Psychol. Bull. 133, 581–624.

Geyh, S., Peter, C., Muller, R., et al., 2011. The Personal Factors of the International Classification of Functioning, Disability and Health in the literature – a systematic review and content analysis. Disabil. Rehabil. 33, 1089–1102.

Glocker, C., Kirchberger, I., Glabel, A., et al., 2012. Content validity of the comprehensive international classification of functioning, disability and health (ICF) core set for low back pain from the perspective of physicians: a Delphi survey. Chronic. Illn. Jun 11 [epub ahead of print].

Gray, D.B., Hendershot, G.E., 2000. The ICIDH-2: developments for a new era of outcomes research. Arch. Phys. Med. Rehabil. 81, S10–S14.

Grill, E., Stucki, G., 2009. Scales could be developed based on simple clinical ratings of International Classification of Functioning, Disability and Health Core Set categories. J. Clin. Epidemiol. 62, 891–898.

Grill, E., Ewert, T., Chatterji, S., et al., 2005. ICF core sets development for the acute hospital and early post-acute rehabilitation facilities. Disabil. Rehabil. 27, 361–366.

Grill, E., Gloor-Juzi, T., Huber, E.O., et al., 2011. Assessment of functioning in the acute hospital: operationalisation and reliability testing of ICF categories relevant for physical therapists interventions. J. Rehabil. Med. 43, 162–173.

Grimmer-Somers, K., Vipond, N., Kumar, S., et al., 2009. A review and critique of assessment instruments for patients with persistent pain. J. Pain Res. 2, 21–47.

Grotle, M., Brox, J.I., Vollestad, N.K., 2005. Functional status and disability questionnaires: What do they assess? A systematic review of back-specific outcome questionnaires. Spine 30, 130–140.

Gureje, O., Simon, G.E., von Korff, M., 2001. A cross-national study of the course of persistent pain in primary care. Pain 92, 195–200.

Halbertsma, J., Heerkens, Y.F., Hirs, W.M., et al., 2000. Towards a new ICIDH. International Classification of Impairments, Disabilities and Handicaps. Disabil. Rehabil. 22, 144–156.

Hayden, J.A., van Tulder, M.W., Malmivaara, A.V., et al., 2005. Meta-analysis: Exercise therapy for nonspecific low back pain. Ann. Intern. Med. 142, 765–775.

Hilfiker, R., Obrist, S., Christen, G., et al., 2009. The use of the comprehensive International Classification of Functioning, Disability and Health Core Set for low back pain in clinical practice: a reliability study. Physiother. Res. Int. 14, 147–166.

Hoy, D., Bain, C., Williams, G., et al., 2012. A systematic review of the global prevalence of low back pain. Arthritis Rheum. 64, 2028–2037.

ICF Research Branch, 2010. ICF Research Branch. Home page. Online. Available:http://www.icf-research-branch.org/(5.03.12).

Institutes of Medicine, 2007. The Future of Disability in America. The National Academies Press, Washington, DC.

Jelsma, J., 2009. Use of the International Classification of Functioning, Disability and Health: a literature survey. J. Rehabil. Med. 41, 1–12.

Jette, A.M., 2006. Toward a common language for function, disability, and health. Phys. Ther. 86, 726–734.

Jette, A.M., 2010. Invited commentary on the ICF and physical therapist practice. Phys. Ther. 90, 1064–1065; author reply 1066–1067.

Jimenez, J., Peek, W., 2012. International Society of Physical and Rehabilitation Medicine (ISPRM): Archives and History. Online. Available: http://www.isprm.org/?CategoryID=232&ArticleID=93&SearchParam=icf (15.06.12).

Jonsdottir, J., Rainero, G., Racca, V., et al., 2010. Functioning and disability in persons with low back pain. Disabil. Rehabil. 32 (Suppl. 1), S78–S84.

Kierkegaard, M., Harms-Ringdahl, K., Widen Holmqvist, L., et al., 2009. Perceived functioning and disability in adults with myotonic dystrophy type 1: a survey according to the International Classification Of Functioning, Disability and Health. J. Rehabil. Med. 41, 512–520.

Kirschneck, M., Kirchberger, I., Amann, E., et al., 2011. Validation of the comprehensive ICF core set for low back pain: the perspective of physical therapists. Man. Ther. 16, 364–372.

Lawrence, R.H., Jette, A.M., 1996. Disentangling the disablement process. J. Gerontol. B Psychol. Sci. Soc. Sci. 51, S173–S182.

Litcher-Kelly, L., Martino, S.A., Broderick, J.E., et al., 2007. A systematic review of measures used to assess chronic musculoskeletal pain in clinical and randomized controlled clinical trials. J. Pain 8, 906–913.

Lohmann, S., Decker, J., Muller, M., et al., 2011. The ICF forms a useful framework for classifying individual patient goals in post-acute rehabilitation. J. Rehabil. Med. 43, 151–155.

Massof, R.W., 2011. Understanding Rasch and item response theory models: applications to the estimation and validation of interval latent trait measures from responses to rating scale questionnaires. Ophthalmic Epidemiol. 18, 1–19.

McIntyre, A., Tempest, S., 2007. Two steps forward, one step back? A commentary on the disease-specific core sets of the International Classification of Functioning,

Disability and Health (ICF). Disabil. Rehabil. 29, 1475–1479.

McQuay, H., 2005. Consensus on outcome measures for chronic pain trials. Pain 113, 1–2.

Muller, M., Strobl, R., Grill, E., 2011. Goals of patients with rehabilitation needs in acute hospitals: goal achievement is an indicator for improved functioning. J. Rehabil. Med. 43, 145–150.

Mullis, R., Barber, J., Lewis, M., et al., 2007. ICF core sets for low back pain: do they include what matters to patients? J. Rehabil. Med. 39, 353–357.

Nagi, S.Z., 1965. Some conceptual issues in disability and rehabilitation. In: Sussman, M.B. (Ed.), Sociology and Rehabilitation. American Sociological Association, Washington, DC.

Nielsen, M., Forster, M., Henman, P., et al., 2012. Talk to us like we're people, not an X-ray': the experience of receiving care for chronic pain. Australian Journal of Primary Health 18, A–F.

Officer, A., Groce, N.E., 2009. Key concepts in disability. Lancet 374, 1795–1796.

Okochi, J., Utsunomiya, S., Takahashi, T., 2005. Health measurement using the ICF: test-retest reliability study of ICF codes and qualifiers in geriatric care. Health Qual. Life Outcomes 3, 46.

Pilkonis, P.A., Choi, S.W., Reise, S.P., et al., 2011. Item Banks for Measuring Emotional Distress From the Patient-Reported Outcomes Measurement Information System (PROMIS(R)): Depression, Anxiety, and Anger. Assessment 18, 263–283.

Rauch, A., Cieza, A., Stucki, G., 2008. How to apply the international classification of functioning, disability and health (ICF) for rehabilitation management in clinical practice. European Journal of Physical and Rehabilitation Medicine 44, 329–342.

Reed, G.M., Lux, J.B., Bufka, L.F., et al., 2005. Operationalizing the International Classification of Functioning, Disability and Health in clinical settings. Rehabil. Psychol. 50, 122–131.

Roe, C., Sveen, U., Bautz-Holter, E., 2008. Retaining the patient perspective in the International Classification of Functioning, Disability and Health

Core Set for low back pain. Patient Prefer Adherence 2, 337–347.

Roe, C., Sveen, U., Geyh, S., et al., 2009. Construct dimensionality and properties of the categories in the ICF Core Set for low back pain. J. Rehabil. Med. 41, 429–437.

Rothman, M., Burke, L., Erickson, P., et al., 2009. Use of existing patient-reported outcome (PRO) instruments and their modification: the ISPOR Good Research Practices for Evaluating and Documenting Content Validity for the Use of Existing Instruments and Their Modification PRO Task Force Report. Value Health 12, 1075–1083.

Rudolf, K.D., Kus, S., Chung, K.C., et al., 2012. Development of the International Classification of Functioning, Disability and Health core sets for hand conditions – results of the World Health Organization International Consensus process. Disabil. Rehabil. 34, 681–693.

Scascighini, L., Toma, V., Dober-Spielmann, S., et al., 2008. Multidisciplinary treatment for chronic pain: a systematic review of interventions and outcomes. Rheumatology (Oxford) 47, 670–678.

Scheuringer, M., Stucki, G., Huber, E.O., et al., 2005. ICF Core Set for patients with musculoskeletal conditions in early post-acute rehabilitation facilities. Disabil. Rehabil. 27, 405–410.

Schwarzkopf, S.R., Ewert, T., Dreinhofer, K.E., et al., 2008. Towards an ICF Core Set for chronic musculoskeletal conditions: commonalities across ICF Core Sets for osteoarthritis, rheumatoid arthritis, osteoporosis, low back pain and chronic widespread pain. Clin. Rheumatol. 27, 1355–1361.

Sigl, T., Cieza, A., Brockow, T., et al., 2006. Content comparison of low back pain-specific measures based on the International Classification of Functioning, Disability and Health (ICF). Clin. J. Pain 22, 147–153.

Stamm, T.A., Cieza, A., Machold, K., et al., 2006. Exploration of the link between conceptual occupational therapy models and the International Classification of Functioning, Disability and Health. Aust. Occup. Ther. J. 53, 9–17.

Starrost, K., Geyh, S., Trautwein, A., et al., 2008. Interrater reliability of the extended ICF core set for stroke applied by physical therapists. Phys. Ther. 88, 841–851.

Steiner, W.A., Ryser, L., Huber, E., et al., 2002. Use of the ICF model as a clinical problem-solving tool in physical therapy and rehabilitation medicine. Phys. Ther. 82, 1098–1107.

Stoll, T., Brach, M., Huber, E.O., et al., 2005. ICF Core Set for patients with musculoskeletal conditions in the acute hospital. Disabil. Rehabil. 27, 381–387.

Stucki, G., Cieza, A., Geyh, S., et al., 2004. ICF Core Sets for rheumatoid arthritis. J. Rehabil. Med. (Suppl. 44), 87–93.

Stucki, G., Cieza, A., Melvin, J., 2007. The International Classification of Functioning, Disability and Health (ICF): a unifying model for the conceptual description of the rehabilitation strategy. J. Rehabil. Med. 39, 279–285.

Stucki, G., Kostanjsek, N., Ustun, B., et al., 2008. ICF-based classification and measurement of functioning. European Journal of Physical and Rehabilitation Medicine 44, 315–328.

Tugwell, P., Boers, M., Brooks, P., et al., 2007. OMERACT: An international initiative to improve outcome measurement in rheumatology. Trials 8, 38.

Turk, D.C., Melzack, R., 2011. Handbook of pain assessment. Guilford Press, New York.

Turk, D.C., Dworkin, R.H., Allen, R.R., et al., 2003. Core outcome domains for chronic pain clinical trials: IMMPACT recommendations. Pain 106, 337–345.

Uhlig, T., Lillemo, S., Moe, R.H., et al., 2007. Reliability of the ICF Core Set for rheumatoid arthritis. Ann. Rheum. Dis. 66, 1078–1084.

United Nations, 2007. Convention on the Rights of Persons with Disabilities. Online. Available: http://www.un.org/disabilities/convention/conventionfull.shtml(12.06.12).

Ustun, B., Chatterji, S., Kostanjsek, N., 2004. Comments from WHO for the Journal of Rehabilitation Medicine special supplement on ICF core sets. J. Rehabil. Med. (Suppl. 44), 7–8.

Verbrugge, L.M., Jette, A.M., 1994. The disablement process. Soc. Sci. Med. 38, 1–14.

Weigl, M., Cieza, A., Cantista, P., et al., 2008. Determinants of disability in chronic musculoskeletal health conditions: A literature review. European Journal of Physical and Rehabilitation Medicine 44, 67–79.

Whiteneck, G., Dijkers, M.P., 2009. Difficult to measure constructs: conceptual and methodological issues concerning participation and environmental factors. Arch. Phys. Med. Rehabil. 90, S22–S35.

Wiegand, N.M., Belting, J., Fekete, C., et al., 2012. All Talk, No Action?: The Global Diffusion and Clinical Implementation of the International Classification of Functioning, Disability, and Health. Am. J. Phys. Med. Rehabil. 91 (7), 550–560.

Woolf, A.D., Erwin, J., March, L., 2012. The need to address the burden of musculoskeletal conditions. Best Pract. Res. Clin. Rheumatol. 26, 183–224.

World Health Organization, 1980. International Classification of Impairments, Disabilities, and Handicaps: A Manual of Classification Relating to the Consequences of Disease. World Health Organization, Geneva.

World Health Organization, 2001. International classification of functioning, disability and health: ICF. World Health Organization, Geneva.

World Health Organization, 2003. ICF Checklist v2.1a – Clinician Form. Online. Available: http://www.who.int/classifications/icf/training/icfchecklist.pdf(14.05.12).

World Health Organization & World Bank, 2011. World report on disability. World Health Organization & World Bank, Geneva.

Zwarenstein, M., Goldman, J., Reeves, S., 2009. Interprofessional collaboration: effects of practice-based interventions on professional practice and healthcare outcomes. Cochrane Database Syst. Rev. (3).

Chapter | 23 |

Participating in life roles

Jenny Strong

LEARNING OBJECTIVES

At the end of this chapter readers will have an understanding of:

1. Why people with pain may discontinue participation in life roles.
2. The way in which a client-centred approach assists clients re-engage in life roles.
3. Methods that can be used to facilitate re-engagement in life roles.

This chapter should be read in conjunction with Chapters 8, 9 and 17, which explained a number of strategies therapists can use with clients, including client education, goal-setting, self-efficacy enhancement, self-esteem development, exercise prescription and coping-skills enhancement.

OVERVIEW

As detailed in Chapter 22, human beings are at their peak of health when they are actively participating in life roles of value to them. This is definitely the case for the person with pain, especially persistent pain. Many people with chronic pain have disruptions to several of these pre-pain occupational roles, and hence to aspects of their lifestyle that are important to them. This chapter will help the reader to understand why such role disruption occurs, and ways in which people with chronic pain can be assisted to re-engage and participate in life roles beyond the paid worker role, which was covered in Chapter 16.

MANAGING LIFE WITH PERSISTENT PAIN

One of the first patients living with chronic pain that I had the privilege to work with was a 50-year-old woman who had suffered facial pain for 12 years due to post-hepatic neuralgia in the distribution of her trigeminal nerve. This case was published in Patient Management (Strong 1989), and republished with permission in 1996 (Strong 1996). Mrs P taught me how, for some people, chronic pain could overtake all valued life roles, leaving one with only the role of 'patient'. I learnt the importance of not working with the patient in isolation. Each patient or client has an environmental context, which may facilitate or limit participation. While I focused on Mrs P and her valued occupations, I ignored environmental factors, to my peril. The person–environment–occupation model (PEO) provides an important heuristic to guide our work with clients to ensure maximum and sustainable outcomes for our clients (Law et al 1996).

The two scenarios from Reflective exercise 23.1 are almost identical, apart from the first person having a demonstrable and accepted badge of injury, and the second person having no overt sign of injury or disability. People in pain find that others in the community may treat them

© 2014 Elsevier Ltd.

Reflective exercise 23.1

1. Imagine that you have broken your leg playing weekend sport. After your visit to accident and emergency, you are discharged home with your leg in a full-length plaster and a set of crutches. You are not to weight-bear on that leg for a number of weeks. Initially you rest at home, but after a week has passed you need to get food into the house, and it would be nice to have a cup of coffee at a coffee shop. At this point, you cannot drive and so you phone a friend, who drives you to the shopping centre. It is so hard to walk with the crutches, so you tell your friend to park in the disabled parking spot. He is reluctant, as he does not have a disabled parking sticker. You say to him, 'Of course people will see that I have a temporary disability, so it will be fine.' And so it is. People see you getting out of the car and hobbling in to the shop using your crutches, and continue on with their activities. You get to the coffee shop and it is crowded, but your friend finds a table in the far corner. So you crutch walk over and people politely move out of your way, so you have room to pass.

2. Let's replay the story, only this time, we will consider the scenario in which you have chronic back pain. You don't use crutches to walk and you do have a disabled parking sticker on your car. One day, you drive to the shopping centre, planning to meet a friend for coffee in the same coffee shop. You park your car in the disabled parking bay and as you get out of the car a passer-by comes up to you and yells at you, 'What are you doing? You are so selfish! Get out of the disabled parking space.' You try to point out that you do have a disabled parking sticker and that you have a disability, but the person mutters at you some more and walks away. You go into the shopping centre, somewhat shaken by this experience. You see your friend in the far corner of the coffee shop, and you gingerly make your way through the crowd to reach him. A number of people bump into you, as they push past you, each bump making your pain increase. When you get to your friend, you say, 'This is too hard to do,' and you feel like weeping and/or punching someone.

in a disrespectful way because the others can see no demonstrable badge of injury. People with pain must learn to manage feelings of delegitimacy, which arise when their pain and suffering is not regarded as credible by others (Rhodes et al 1999). One management strategy in this situation would be to withdraw from social settings where one is likely to experience such insensitivity. A number of life roles could be relinquished for this reason, such as instrumental activities of daily living like shopping, social outings and attending sporting events with children.

Chronic pain, like chronic fatigue syndrome, is a condition where people frequently experience stigma (Cohen et al 2012). While stigma refers to a visible mark of disgrace or a stain, such as in leprosy, the invisibility of pain and the incredulity of others creates the stigma for people with chronic pain. Stigmatization is the process whereby the way the community reacts to a person's pain results in the person being devalued and ostracized (Berger et al 2005, Cohen et al 2012, Goffman 1963).

Additionally, as was illustrated in Chapter 9, the fear of pain escalation or further injury can play a big part in the person in pain giving up doing activities where they might be bumped or jostled. The fear of pain has been seen as more disabling than the pain itself (Vlaeyen & Linton 2000). We well know that inactivity, and more specifically the disuse of muscles, contributes to muscle weakness. Too soon, people with chronic pain may find themselves in a downward spiral, also known as the chronic pain cycle (Strong 1989). They avoid activities or situations where their pain may increase or where they may be subjected to uninformed comment, they do less, they feel less satisfied, they may gain weight, they become socially isolated, their mood is depressed, they begin to feel worthless and lose hope. Once in this cycle, it can be difficult to escape, with the result that people with chronic pain may relinquish all meaningful life roles and be left with only the role of patient. Reflective exercise 23.2 gives the reader an inside perspective to coming to terms with chronic pain.

Unfortunately, at a time when scientific knowledge is expanding at an exponential rate, there is still no one panacea or cure for chronic pain. At the current stage of our knowledge and skill in assessing and treating people with chronic pain, there remain many people for whom a 'cure' is not available. The reality for such individuals is that they must *learn to manage with pain*. Such management typically involves a combination of pharmacological agents, exercises, lifestyle modifications and cognitive adjustments. People with chronic pain must learn to adjust their patterns of living, their dreams and aspirations, and their expectations, to accommodate a chronic pain problem, in much the same way as someone newly diagnosed with multiple sclerosis or a spinal injury must learn to accommodate and adjust. When the person learns to live with the pain, without reaction, disapproval or trying to reduce it, then they have accepted the pain. It has been posited by McCracken (1998) that acceptance is an important step in successful adjustment. The acceptance of pain has been shown to be associated with less pain, less disability, less depression and anxiety, and better activity engagement (McCracken & Eccleston 2003, 2006). Acceptance has been posited as more therapeutic than active coping with the pain condition.

Those seeking help are not representative of those experiencing pain in the general population. Many will be capable of working out individual and highly effective ways to manage their pain and maintain the most satisfying lifestyle possible, while others will require considerable help and still manage only a minimally rewarding lifestyle. For each of these two ends of the spectrum the therapist will

Reflective exercise 23.2

One way of understanding the experience of a patient with chronic pain is to imagine yourself arriving for work, expecting not only a normal day, but also a normal future, only to be told by a stranger that you are never again allowed to work, ever, in any capacity for which you are trained.

Most people in this situation would initially dismiss this as untrue, unbelievable, and try to ignore it. However, when it became evident that not only were you not allowed to work, but also you were unable to dress easily, sit, stand or work in comfort, you could manage only basic household tasks with difficulty and discomfort, you could not concentrate to read, you could not maintain sufficient activity and interest to sustain friendships, and you had to move out of your house to different accommodation more suitable because of physical and financial reasons, then this would start to hurt.

Most people would vigorously and energetically try to identify the cause of such a catastrophe to reverse it, to return to their normal lifestyle, to fulfil the hopes, dreams and expectations they held for themselves, their family and friends.

When no cause or explanation can be identified, even after considerable effort, it is not unreasonable to consider such a situation as unreasonable, unfair and undeserved. Most people would be *very* distressed, angry, confused and apprehensive, and not confident about what to do next. This is a grief reaction to the multitude of losses involved.

If, during one's life, there had been similar losses and/or hardships, the current events may trigger one to remember, and to re-experience, various aspects of those previous difficulties. The connection may be obscure because the association is usually highly variable; while the concepts involved are the same (loss, deprivation, injustice, powerlessness, etc.), one's experience of it may be highly individual. For example, a divorce may mean devastation to one person and release to another. The recall of these past associations may be only partial. Perhaps it may be experienced only by similar emotions rather than a clear, readily identifiable picture of thoughts, ideas and images, such that the reasons for one being so upset may not be immediately apparent, either to the therapist or to oneself.

After many struggles, trials, disappointments and frustrations, the search for an answer may give way to acceptance that there is none. The ability of a person to negotiate this difficult course is very reliant on him or her having developed sufficient skills, knowledge, confidence and supports to cope with such problems earlier in life.

take a different approach. Those who are active in working out solutions will need less support but may profit most from technical advice and information. Clients who are less able to see solutions will require considerable support and encouragement, and possibly cognitive restructuring, as well as information, technical advice and ongoing support.

GOAL SETTING

One of the first responsibilities of the therapist is to assist the client with chronic pain to identify personally meaningful goals. Goal setting involves a collaborative process between the client and the therapist (Law et al 1995, Neistadt 1995). Clients are more likely to be satisfied with the service if they have been able to participate in decision making. For people who have lived with chronic pain for many years, and who have relinquished almost all of their goals, goal setting may take some time. The goal-setting process may include both formal and informal methods to set goals. A useful strategy can be to ask the client to tell you about their life before they had pain. An alternative, more formal method of setting goals involves the use of a questionnaire or scale, such as the Occupational Performance History Questionnaire (Kielhofner & Henry 1988) or the Neuropsychiatric Institute (NPI) Interest Checklist (Matsutsuyu 1969). These assessments assist therapists in identifying activities that are important to the client; moreover they can assist the client in remembering the things that were previously important to them. The Canadian Occupational Performance Measure (COPM) (Law et al 1991) is another useful tool for goal setting. The COPM utilizes a client-centred philosophy in assisting clients to identify their priorities for therapy (Law et al 1994, Lidstone 1996, Toomey et al 1995) and addresses the client's functioning in the areas of self-care, productivity and leisure (Pollock 1993).

Key questions to consider when setting goals include:

- the client's daily living routines
- the client's life roles
- the client's interests, values and goals
- the client's perception of ability and assumption of responsibility
- human and non-human components of the client's environment (Kielhofner & Henry 1988).

ACTIVE INVOLVEMENT OF THE CLIENT IN DECISION MAKING

Increasingly, health services are moving away from the traditional medical model in which health professionals define problems and make decisions for their clients, to an enablement model that aims to shift autonomy, control and responsibility back to the client. Pollock (1993) argues that if the client is not the problem definer then it will be unlikely that she or he will be the problem solver either. The concept of client involvement in decision making reflects a core philosophy of occupational therapy and physiotherapy, and is a recurring theme throughout this book.

An approach in which clients become active participants in their health care acknowledges aspects of the patient's lifestyle which are unique to the individual. One person's occupational needs and abilities will not be the same as any other person's. When clients are actively involved in decision making, treatment is likely to be more meaningful for the patient, as it reflects the importance of their roles, environments and culture. This is important when working with clients with chronic pain, as chronic pain is a multidimensional phenomenon involving physical, psychological and social domains.

The role of the occupational therapist and physiotherapist, in the client-centred approach, is to provide information and guided experience to enable the client to make appropriate decisions regarding therapy. While clients are considered to be experts about their occupational function, the occupational therapist possesses the expertise to facilitate solutions to a broad range of occupational performance issues associated with chronic pain. Information should be provided in a format that is understandable and that will enable clients to make decisions about their needs.

It is important that clients recognize that all activities, and avoidance of activities, have both a possibility of benefit and a risk of failure of varying degree (Law et al 1995). Practice can be used as a valuable learning experience, provided that the client is able to understand the risks associated with the decision (Law et al 1995). However, therapists need to be able to openly discuss such issues with clients. Obviously therapists cannot support actions which are unethical, could involve excessive risk of harm or are considered malpractice. In such instances therapists must firmly state that they cannot support the client's plan. On the other hand, some clients may be reluctant to assume responsibility for their care.

It is important to explore reasons why clients are reluctant to accept responsibility in their treatment. Lack of confidence, anger, excessive reliance on others, fear of pain, depression, lack of knowledge regarding pain or belief in a medical 'cure' are just some of the reasons which may affect a client's willingness to accept responsibility in their treatment. Occupational therapists and physiotherapists must discuss these issues with the client and work together towards potential solutions. An important role of the occupational therapist and physiotherapist is to help the client develop a judgement that is useful and appropriate to their changed situation. The judgements and practices of the past, or of others, are no longer necessarily applicable.

Client involvement in decision making during therapy has been shown to facilitate the development of rapport, promote treatment participation and satisfaction, and empower the patient by encouraging independence, personal control, self-determination and self-esteem (Mew & Fossey 1996). Studies have demonstrated that active involvement of clients in decision making can result in shorter hospital stays (Shendell-Falik 1990), and better goal attainment and outcomes for the patient (Czar 1987) than a traditional medical model approach. Considering the escalating costs associated with treatment of clients with chronic pain, approaches that enhance the effectiveness of therapy are important (Access Economics 2007). Involving the patient in decision making is a relatively simple, yet effective, means of achieving more effective outcomes.

ACTIVITY ENGAGEMENT

'The level and pattern of daily activities performed by persons with chronic pain are regarded as central determinants of their overall physical, social and emotional functioning.' (McCracken & Samuel 2007, p. 119). Two important aspects of assisting the person with chronic pain to re-engage in activities are, firstly, the choice of sequential, achievable goals, and the approach to the activities adopted by the client. Both short-term and long-term goals need to be considered. It is essential that the goals are realistic and meaningful to the client, and that the client gradually introduces them to their lifestyle. Rather than an umbrella (and possibly unachievable) goal of 'getting rid of the pain', the person can be assisted to identify and focus on other life goals involving useful functioning, such as travelling to visit family or friends, or starting a vocational course to learn new skills.

The practical implications of an approach to lifestyle management based on a 'living despite' pain philosophy are the need to gradually introduce more activities into the client's lifestyle and the need to ensure that managing these activities is both rewarding and enjoyable for the client. Clients with chronic pain often experience a change in their usual activity pattern, in addition to changes in expectations about what they can achieve while they have pain. Many clients with chronic pain underestimate their functional abilities. Often this results in a reduction in activity level, although some clients may increase their level of activity in an attempt to 'cope' with their pain. Too much inactivity can lead to physical deconditioning, which may contribute to muscle pain and stiffness.

Alternatively, overdoing oneself can exacerbate symptoms and cause setbacks for several days. This is why it is important for therapists to assist clients to develop healthy approaches to activity. The three types of activity engagement observed in people with chronic pain are avoidance of activity, pacing and overuse (Andrews et al 2012, McCracken & Samuel 2007). While it has been demonstrated that avoidance of activity is associated with poorer outcomes, there have been few studies that have shown the benefits of activity pacing (McCracken & Samuel 2007). A recent systematic review and meta-analysis has found that while pacing was linked to better psychological functioning, it was also associated with more pain and disability (Andrews et al 2012). However, it could be that people who had more positive psychological health but greater levels of pain and disability used pacing to help them cope. In the absence of conclusive evidence about the benefits of pacing, the principles will be outlined here, due to popularity of the technique in pain management programmes and the intuitive sense such an approach makes. As Nicholas et al (2006) say, 'Pacing: an essential technique for mastering chronic pain (p. 79).

Therapists encourage clients with chronic pain to re-establish more normal levels of activity (Moran & Strong 1995). Clients are encouraged to change daily activity patterns so that they may function successfully in spite of pain. This may involve challenging beliefs that activity is 'bad' for pain and providing clients with advice about spreading out their activities so they avoid a boom–bust cycle, where they overdo the activity and then either spend the next week in bed or need to go to the accident and emergency department for strong pain relief. Therapists may also encourage family members to shift their responses from concerns about the patient's pain to interest in activity performance.

Once the client has decided on their goals, they may need to adjust the activity level in order to achieve them. This involves an approach referred to as 'pacing'. Pacing involves breaking tasks down into a smaller set of activities and then introducing the task in a graded manner, in order for the client to build skills, confidence and tolerance for the activity, so that activity level may be increased. Gradual increases in activity are expected (Harding & Williams 1995). This is particularly important in clients with chronic pain who may be physically deconditioned as a result of reduced activity. The pacing techniques which women with fibromyalgia found helpful in managing everyday activities were the following:

- Organizing – The majority of women learned to organize their daily schedule to allow more time to complete tasks and to include necessary rest breaks. Many required several hours to get ready in the morning due to morning stiffness. Activities were often spaced out to ensure adequate 'downtime'.
- Prioritizing – Many women would complete the most important tasks first, while pain levels were relatively low. Tasks which were deemed most important varied between the women, reflecting differences in the women's roles and values.
- Flexibility – Many women found that they developed more flexibility in the way they approached tasks. For example, they were able to alternate between light and heavy tasks, change work positions frequently and adjust their level of activity according to fluctuating pain levels (Henriksson 1995).

Therapists need both to monitor clients' progress in achieving their goals and to help clients develop the skills to do this themselves, for future use. Barriers to achieving goals will need to be identified and clients should be encouraged to develop problem-solving skills to overcome these barriers. It is also important that the client and therapist re-evaluate their goals to determine whether they are still relevant to the patient's lifestyle.

An important aspect of pacing is taking an overall approach to an activity, to a single day, a week and, indeed, to life activities in the long term. People without their full fitness, agility and freedom of movement may have to accept a reduction in the ability to be as spontaneous and to act when the desire tempts them, and learn to organize their whole lives in a much more predictable and regular manner. This recommended reduced spontaneity and freedom is a significant loss and intrusion on quality of life for many people. Clients may need guidance to gain confidence in adjusting to a way of thinking that considers the long term, delayed, benefits of more successful functioning. This requires a shift from a short-term perspective and measure to a long-term view, something that is challenging for people whose confidence and trust may be rather battered by their current and past life experiences.

Box 23.1 provides an example of the integration of goal setting and pacing strategies in the rehabilitation of a 53-year-old man with low back pain and headache.

SELF-MANAGEMENT

Professor Kate Lorig was a champion of the self-management approach, firstly, for people living with rheumatoid arthritis, and, secondly, for people with chronic back pain. Randomized controlled trials have demonstrated the effectiveness of Lorig's Stanford programme in improving health outcomes and decreasing service usage for people with arthritis and back pain (Lorig et al 2006). The Stanford programme involves lay leaders, with group activities run over six consecutive weeks. Topics addressed include managing emotions, exercise, medication use, nutrition, communicating with others, approach to activities and evaluating new treatments. The self-management approach was later adopted for use with many other client groups who live with chronic conditions. Self-management refers to the individual being able to take charge of all the aspects of living with a chronic health condition, such as dealing with healthcare providers and managing their condition emotionally and physically.

A recent systematic review of self-management programmes for people with chronic musculoskeletal pain concluded that courses that were led by health professionals, lasted for less than 8 weeks and included a psychological component had more beneficial results (Carnes et al 2012). Self-management programmes using the Internet have also been developed, for example the painACTION-Back Pain self-management programme, and have shown encouraging results (Chiauzzi et al 2010).

Box 23.1 Case example

Name: Mr S
Age: 53 years
Marital status: Married
Employment: Senior public servant, administrative
History – presenting illness: Low back pain and headache

These complaints related to degenerative vertebral changes for which no curative surgical or medical option was available.

He was supported by his wife who tolerated, but did not support, his obsessive attitudes to almost all activities.

He previously prided himself on putting 110% into all endeavours, including his job, football coaching and gardening. This approach had been instrumental to his considerable early career advancement, with early promotions, great responsibility, commendations and great expectations. He had similarly been given great recognition and responsibility with football coaching.

He routinely worked very long hours, after hours at home and on weekends. Holidays, when they were taken, were usually focused on catching up even further on these tasks, leaving little time for rest and recovery, which was increasingly required because of both his condition and the loss of the reserves of youth.

He was a friendly, gregarious but busy gentleman, very generous and well liked, but with little insight regarding the contribution of his approach to his difficulties, especially about how he could aggravate his physical condition by his excessive expectations and habits.

In his usual tendency to extremes, he completely ceased working, coaching and mowing the lawn, berating himself for his inadequacies.

He did, however, have a very good set of standards when advising others, particularly those close to him, and for whom he believed he had a duty of care. He accepted the wisdom of other employees not routinely arriving early, not leaving late, not taking work home and not having holidays, and saw that this provided them with an opportunity for recovery and to enjoy their lives.

Using his very overgrown lawn as an easily available and controllable project, he gradually accepted the proposition that doing the overall task in steps was a better option than doing nothing, and without the necessity to achieve the level of perfection he had previously demanded. In the past, he did not stop until he had mown all of the considerable lawn, cut and trimmed the edges, and weeded all the garden beds, all in one effort. Following his injury, he needed several days of bed-rest to recover from this task.

Accepting that it would be useful for him to use his considerable skills in good management and coaching, with a graduated programme, with built-in review and encouragement on a 'current personal best' basis, he was eventually able to start the mower and complete a square yard only, as a planned first step.

He learned how to stop the task when it was useful for him, without a period of extended recovery required, rather than being 'externally' dictated to in his activity by the amount of work available.

Again, using his skills of perseverance and self-discipline, he mapped out a plan of graduated increase, based on his demonstrated recovery time, to do the lawn, edges and garden in sections, as well as to deal with the considerable emotional turmoil this programme precipitated within him as he battled against his own obsessive impulses. To accomplish this, he had to confront and control emotional pressures based on a personal value system that was no longer useful.

Having achieved control of his 'lawn project' he was then able to generalize and to apply the new conceptual approach to coaching, accepting new limitations, developing new techniques and being mindful to develop a balance of his activities such that he no longer worked to exhaustion before he allowed himself to stop.

Replenishment of his reserves had particularly been a more recent issue because of his age and because of the development of employment and business practices that placed less value on the encouragement from senior management, but which relied on individually competitive outputs. Being somewhat dependent, he was not adept at encouraging himself but excessively reliant on the praise of others.

Returning to work was more difficult. Initially, he experienced considerable nausea approaching his workplace. The nausea itself was disabling and required a behavioural desensitization programme to eliminate this problem. This programme used initially very small goals with a very high probability of achievement, in his own estimation, then increasingly more complicated steps as he became more comfortable.

He initially drove past his building, then walked, then entered it after hours and later visited during hours, before he recommenced work. He returned to work in a different capacity, with the support of his superior, who was also informed about the usefulness of a step-wise approach for returning to work. It is worthwhile remembering that Mr S had been a very successful worker prior to being overcome by his chronic pain condition. He had been consumed by his work and derived great benefits from it, both economic and personal. And yet the anxiety he felt about returning to his work was a big issue for him, one that needed a sensitive and supportive approach from his therapist (who in this case was a consultant psychiatrist).

Graduated duties recommenced, with an emphasis on having precisely formulated the details of the project before he left home, based on the degree of confidence (not desire) he had developed from his recent level of functions, with many small increments planned. The finishing point had to be defined *before he started each step*, not continuing on the basis of how he felt at the time but on the basis of the track record he had recently established. He had to guard against continuing while he felt good to the point of failure again.

Relapses occurred, giving an opportunity for review, further learning and a re-commitment to a disciplined approach to resist the temptation to yield to previously well-established old desires, which were once cued by the old environment and which arose again to challenge the new order. Implementing life-long changes is often a challenge, especially for a person with chronic pain.

SOCIAL SUPPORT

The type and degree of social support available to an individual with chronic pain will have influence on their lifestyle. In most chronic conditions the presence of social support is a positive factor. Linton (2000) suggested that the family might provide a source of social support that provides a buffer to the problems associated with chronic pain. For example, family members are able to offer encouragement, distraction, praise and compassionate listening. In addition to support, family members can also provide tangible assistance to an individual with chronic pain. On the other hand, support from family members may sometimes serve as positive reinforcement of pain behaviours. An individual with chronic pain may learn that displays of pain behaviour lead to positive social consequences such as attention, sympathy and avoidance of unwanted marital or family responsibilities (Gil et al 1987). Consequently, family support may actually sustain pain behaviours and encourage disability in individuals with chronic pain.

An example of an appropriate response may be for family members to allow clients with chronic pain more time to complete an activity, rather than completing the activity on the patient's behalf. Families need to appreciate the importance of focusing on an individual's achievements and adaptive behaviours. This strategy fits in well with the operant–behavioural model, and has an overall goal of reducing pain behaviours and increasing activity levels in clients with chronic pain (further discussion of the operant–behavioural approach can be found in Chapter 8).

Individuals with chronic pain may find some support from those in a similar situation. Support or self-help groups for people with chronic pain may provide fertile ground for the exchange of ideas and information regarding techniques for lifestyle management (Baptiste & Herman 1982; Herman & Baptiste 1981). Shared problem solving and positive role modelling are other potential benefits.

There is considerable evidence in the literature regarding the buffering effect of social support gained from outside family networks. Social support has been found to buffer against the adverse effects of life stress on physical and mental health (Iso-Ahola & Park 1996). This is particularly important for clients with chronic pain as for many ongoing pain is a source of considerable stress and can lead to isolation (Nielsen et al 2012; Turner et al 1987). Individuals with chronic pain, however, often experience a limited social network as a result of withdrawing from activities due to pain or depression. The use of social media has been suggested as an important tool for people with chronic pain to connect with others and gain social support (Strong et al 2012).

The maintenance of social contacts and involvement in leisure activities is an important component of a pain management programme, assisting towards the balanced lifestyle that most people aspire to.

CONCLUSION

In this chapter, consideration was given to the reasons why many people living with chronic pain may relinquish life roles, and ways in which therapists may assist clients to identify and re-engage in valued activities. Given the chronicity of many pain problems, it is important that therapists broaden their focus beyond the mere elimination of the person's pain. This is, of course, not to deny the value of a focus on pain relief. However, for many of the clients with whom therapists work, a more fruitful focus is to participate in meaningful occupations.

Q Study questions/questions for revision

1. Why do some people with chronic pain become incapacitated by the pain?
2. What are the effects of the invisibility of pain?
3. How can you assist a person with chronic pain to re-engage in activities?
4. Why is social support important for people with chronic pain?

REFERENCES

Access Economics, 2007. The high price of pain: the economic impact of persistent pain in Australia. Access economics, with MBF Foundation, in collaboration with University of Sydney Pain Management Research Institute, Sydney.

Andrews, N.E., Strong, J., Meredith, P.J., 2012. Activity pacing, avoidance, endurance, and associations with patient functioning in chronic pain: a systematic review and meta-analysis. Arch. Phys. Med. Rehabil. 93, 2109–2121.

Baptiste, S., Herman, E., 1982. Group therapy: A specific model. In: Roy, D., Tunks, E. (Eds.), Chronic Pain – Psychosocial Factors in Rehabilitation. Williams & Wilkins, Baltimore, pp. 166–177.

Berger, M., Wagner, T.H., Baker, L.C., 2005. Internet use and stigmatized illness. Soc. Sci. Med. 61, 1821–1827.

Carnes, D., Homer, K.E., Miles, C.L., et al., 2012. Effective delivery styles and content for self-management interventions for chronic musculoskeletal pain. A systematic literature review. Clin. J. Pain. 28 (4), 244–254.

Chiauzzi, E., Pujol, L.A., Wood, M., et al., 2010. PainAction-Back Pain: a self-management website for people with chronic back pain. Pain Med. 11, 1044–1058.

Cohen, M., Quinter, J., Buchanan, D., et al., 2012. Stigmatization of patients with chronic pain: the extinction of empathy. Pain Med. 12, 1637–1643.

Czar, M., 1987. Two methods of goal setting in middle-aged adults facing critical life changes. Clin. Nurse Spec. 1, 171–177.

Gil, K.M., Keefe, F.J., Crisson, J.E., et al., 1987. Social support and pain behaviour. Pain. 29, 209–217.

Goffman, E., 1963. Stigma: notes on the management of spoiled identity. Prentice Hall, New York.

Harding, V., Williams, A.C., de, C., 1995. Extending physiotherapy skills using a psychological approach: cognitive-behavioral management of chronic pain. Physiotherapy. 81, 681–687.

Henriksson, C.M., 1995. Living with continuous muscular pain – patient perspectives. Part II: Strategies for daily life. Scand. J. Caring Sci. 9, 77–86.

Herman, E., Baptiste, S., 1981. Pain control: mastery through group experience. Pain. 10, 79–86.

Iso-Ahola, S.E., Park, C.J., 1996. Leisure-related social support and self-determination as buffers of stress-illness relationship. Journal of Leisure Research. 28, 169–187.

Kielhofner, G., Henry, A., 1988. Development and investigation of the occupational performance history interview. Am. J. Occup. Ther. 42, 489–498.

Law, M., Baptiste, S., Carswell-Opzoomer, A., et al., 1991. Canadian Occupational Performance Measure. Canadian Association of Occupational Therapists, Toronto.

Law, M., Polatajko, H., Pollock, N., et al., 1994. Pilot testing of the Canadian Occupational Therapy Performance measure: clinical and measurement issues. Can. J. Occup. Ther. 61, 191–197.

Law, M., Baptiste, S., Mills, J., 1995. Client-centered practice: What does it mean and does it make a difference? Can. J. Occup. Ther. 62, 225–250.

Law, M., Cooper, B., Strong, S., et al., 1996. The person–environment–occupational model: a transactive approach to occupational performance. Can. J. Occup. Ther. 63, 9–23.

Lidstone, P.J., 1996. Family-centred assessment and goal-setting for occupational therapy in early education. Honours Thesis, Department of Occupational Therapy, University of Queensland, Brisbane.

Linton, S.J., 2000. A review of psychological risk factors in back and neck pain. Spine. 25, 1148–1156.

Lorig, K., Ritter, P., Laurent, D., et al., 2006. Internet-based chronic disease self-management: a randomized trial. Med. Care. 4, 964–971.

Matsutsuyu, J., 1969. The Interest Checklist. Am. J. Occup. Ther. 23, 368–373.

McCracken, L.M., 1998. Learning to live with the pain: acceptance of pain predicts adjustment in persons with chronic pain. Behav. Ther. 13, 363–375.

McCracken, L.M., Eccleston, C., 2003. Coping or acceptance: what to do about chronic pain? Pain. 105, 197–204.

McCracken, L.M., Eccleston, C., 2006. A comparison of the relative utility of coping and acceptance-based measures in a sample of chronic pain sufferers. Eur. J. Pain. 10, 23–29.

McCracken, L.M., Samuel, V.M., 2007. The role of avoidance, pacing, and other activity patterns in chronic pain. Pain. 130, 119–125.

Mew, M.M., Fossey, E., 1996. Client-centered aspects of clinical reasoning during an initial assessment using the Canadian Occupational Performance Measure. Aust. J. Occup. Ther. 43, 155–166.

Moran, M., Strong, J., 1995. Outcomes of a rehabilitation program for patients with chronic back pain. Br. J. Occup. Ther. 58, 55–60.

Neistadt, M.E., 1995. Methods of assessing clients' priorities: A survey of adult physical dysfunction settings. Am. J. Occup. Ther. 49, 428–436.

Nicholas, M., Molloy, A., Tonkin, L., et al., 2006. Practical and positive ways of adapting to chronic pain. Manage your pain, second ed. Australian Broadcasting Corporation, Sydney.

Nielsen, M., Forster, M., Henman, P., et al., 2012. 'Talk to us like we're people, not an X-ray': the experience of receiving care for chronic pain. Australian Journal of Primary Health. Online. http://ax.doi.org/10.1071/PY11154.

Pollock, N., 1993. Client-centered assessment. Am. J. Occup. Ther. 47, 298–301.

Rhodes, L.A., McPhillips-Tangum, C.A., Markham, C., et al., 1999. The power of the visible: the meaning of diagnostic tests in chronic back pain. Soc. Sci. Med. 48, 1189–1203.

Shendell-Falik, N., 1990. Creating self-care units in the acute care setting: a case study. Patient Educ. Couns. 15, 39–45.

Strong, J., 1989. The occupational therapist's contribution to the management of chronic pain. Patient Manag. 13, 43–50.

Strong, J., 1996. Chronic Pain: The occupational therapist's perspective. Churchill Livingstone, Edinburgh.

Strong, J., Nielsen, M, Wales, C., et al., 2012. The power of social media for empowering people with chronic pain. The Inaugural Social Media in Healthcare Conference (www.informa.com.au/SMhealthcare), Sydney, Australia.

Toomey, M., Nicholson, D., Carswell, A., 1995. The clinical utility of the Canadian Occupational Performance Measure. Can. J. Occup. Ther. 62, 242–249.

Turner, J.A., Clancy, S., Vitaliano, P.P., 1987. Relationships of stress, appraisal and coping to chronic low back pain. Behav. Res. Ther. 25, 281–288.

Vlaeyen, J.W.S., Linton, S.J., 2000. Fear avoidance and its consequences in chronic musculoskeletal pain: a state of the art. Pain. 85, 317–332.

Chapter 24

Persistent pain and the law: clinical and legal aspects of chronic pain

George Mendelson and Danuta Mendelson

CHAPTER CONTENTS

OVERVIEW

'Pain and suffering' have been among the traditional 'heads of damages' in personal injury claims for a long time, and the relationship between pain and personal injury litigation is the most frequently recognized association of pain and the law. There are, however, other important areas in which clinical aspects of pain management interact with the law, including in relation to valid consent to treatment and allegations of malpractice or professional negligence in the management of patients with pain.

Considerations concerning disclosure of potential material risks apply to all treatment procedures undertaken for pain management, for example nerve blocks, and it has been considered that such disclosure is essential for the patient's consent to treatment to be valid. Swerdlow (1982) reviewed a variety of problems following such procedures that have led to legal action and found that lack of valid consent was one of the five grounds on which such litigation had arisen. Others were medical complications due to the procedure, incompetence in carrying out the specific procedure, the wrong procedure being performed and inadequate treatment of the complication. While Swerdlow only discussed litigation against medical practitioners in relation to a specific treatment modality, these concerns also relate to physiotherapists (Osborne 1983),

occupational therapists (Jarvis 1983; Ranke & Moriarty 1997; Wright 1985) and other healthcare practitioners.

In this chapter we shall discuss professional negligence with respect to consent and alleged malpractice in relation to the potential risks of certain types of treatment and procedures undertaken for pain relief, and some aspects of personal injury claims in which pain is a significant complaint.

LEGAL LIABILITY AND PAIN MANAGEMENT

Shapiro (1994) discussed liability that might arise in the management of pain under the following five headings:

1. Liability to patients and/or exposure to professional discipline for inappropriate pain management.
2. Liability to third parties for injury caused by patients treated for pain.
3. The legal distinction between pain management and euthanasia or physician-assisted suicide.
4. Healthcare payers' liability to patients for cost-containment decisions that impact on pain management.
5. Manufacturers' and healthcare providers' liability for the risks and side effects of prescription drugs and pain-management devices.

Other legal aspects of pain management relate to the use of placebo medications (Rushton 1995), generally in a misguided attempt to demonstrate that the pain 'is not real', and obtaining valid consent before initiating treatment.

The impact of cost-containment decisions, responsibility to third parties and product liability matters will not be discussed in this review. Euthanasia and physician-assisted suicide have been the topic of numerous articles and

© 2014 Elsevier Ltd.

symposia over the past few years, and the interested reader is referred to the medical (Ashby 1995), psychiatric (Buchanan 1995), coronial (Ranson 1995) and moral (Kuhse & Singer 1995; Mullen 1995) concerns raised. Other reviews have considered the position in the USA (Thomasma 1996), including constitutional (Linville 1996), legal (Schwartz 1996), regulatory (Coleman & Fleischman 1996; Miller et al 1996) and nursing (Kjervik 1996) aspects.

This section will discuss issues involving direct liability to patients, such as obtaining valid consent to treatment, and claims alleging malpractice and negligence related to pain management. We shall not discuss issues relevant to the misdiagnosis of acute pain in emergency settings (such as myocardial infarction or acute appendicitis) (Rusnak et al 1994), as these generally are pertinent to acute care and emergency physicians (Karcz et al 1996) rather than those working in specialized pain clinics.

Valid consent to treatment and medical duty of adequate disclosure

As a general rule, except in cases of necessity (emergency treatment) [1] or under statutory exceptions (for example in relation to persons who refuse treatment for a notifiable infectious disease), valid consent of the legally competent patient is essential for lawful administration of treatment.

Legal competence to give such consent involves the person's capacity to understand 'the general nature and effect of the proposed procedure or treatment' and capacity to 'indicate whether or not he or she consents or does not consent to the carrying out of the proposed procedure or treatment' (*Guardianship and Administration Act 1986 (Vic), s 36(2)*).

If the patient is legally competent, administering treatment in the face of his or her refusal will, prima facie, amount to an actionable wrong even if the treatment is efficacious and the motive benevolent [2], although prosecution for criminal battery or a civil action for trespass to the person in relation to non-consensual treatment for the purpose of pain relief would probably only occur in exceptional circumstances.

Negligent advice

Under the law of negligence, where there exists a legal duty of care towards another person, one must guard against creating risks that might result in an injury to that person. If a particular foreseeable risk cannot be eliminated or minimized, then the risk ought to be disclosed to those who might be harmed by it. The duty of clinicians towards their patients involves the exercise of reasonable care and skill in the provision of diagnosis, advice and treatment to the patient. Consequently, except in the case of emergency, and subject to 'therapeutic privilege' [3], healthcare practitioners must advise their patients not only about the nature of the proposed procedure but also about the material risks inherent in the proposed treatment.

When controversial procedures or treatments are involved, or treatments with recognized potential adverse long-term consequences, it would be prudent for clinicians to initiate a discussion with the patient about any inherent risks that might be involved. Discussions about alternative treatments, and the risks and benefits of the proposed management must be documented in the patient's contemporaneous clinical records.

Given the recent publications concerning the lack of clinical effectiveness of acupuncture for relief of chronic pain, and the risks of this procedure (Ernst 2010; Ernst et al 2011; Heo et al 2011), it will be interesting to see whether those subjected to such 'treatment' without benefit or where a clinically significant complication had occurred will initiate legal action against the healthcare practitioners who used acupuncture in pain management. For example, there was adverse publicity in the media concerning the epidural injection of steroids, although the accepted view in the medical literature was that such injections were safe and effective in the management of specific conditions (Benzon 1986; Pawl et al 1985). Claims to the contrary were made by Nelson (1988), whose article has been criticized and attention drawn to his misquotation of the relevant literature (Abram 1989; Wilkinson 1989). The Health Department of Western Australia (1990) issued guidelines for the use of epidural steroids that set out the indications for this treatment and the appropriate procedure for obtaining valid consent, including the relevant information that should be provided to the patient.

Tennant & Uelmen (1983) have suggested that written consent be obtained from patients prior to the prescription of opiate analgesics for the treatment of chronic non-cancer pain. They recommended that the patient be advised of the potential for becoming dependant on the medication, and of the medical and legal consequences should this occur in the context of discussion about the potential benefits and risks of possible long-term therapy with opiate analgesics (Savage 1996). Tennant and Uelmen suggested that female patients of childbearing age also require explanation that in the event of pregnancy the child will experience withdrawal symptoms after birth. Warning about the nature of withdrawal symptoms is also recommended by these authors, as well as warning about the interaction between opiate analgesics and other medications, and between such analgesics and alcohol.

The authors recommended that such explanations and warnings should feature on a consent form. It should be noted that even a detailed pro-forma consent form is merely an adjunct to, and not a substitute for, the treating practitioner's clinical records documenting that these issues were discussed with the patient. The guidelines suggested by Tennant and Uelmen have been set out in Table 24.1, with some modifications.

Table 24.1 Guidelines for use and monitoring of opioid analgesics

1. Identify cause of chronic pain.
2. Document that non-narcotic therapy has been inadequate.
3. Obtain and document in clinical notes valid consent of patient.
4. Initially select a weak oral narcotic combined with a non-narcotic analgesic.
5. Use a more potent oral narcotic if weaker agent ineffective.
6. Raise daily dosage gradually to achieve a stable maintenance dose that effectively controls pain.
7. Monitor patient regularly (at least monthly) for sedation, motor function and side effects.
8. Concurrently use adjuvant medications and other pain therapies.
9. Avoid benzodiazepines and sedative-hypnotics.

*Based on Tennant & Uelmen (1983).

Portenoy & Foley (1986) reviewed the risk of opioid abuse among patients initially prescribed these agents for therapeutic purposes. Group studies of drug addicts showed that between 4 and 27% began opioid abuse after being treated as medical patients. However, follow-up studies of patients who had been prescribed narcotic analgesics for therapeutic reasons have provided different findings. Thus, Porter & Jick (1980) have shown that only four of 11,882 patients without a prior history of drug dependence treated with opioids went on to become drug abusers. Another review of 2369 patients with chronic headache treated with narcotic analgesics found that only three were abusing the drugs (Medina & Diamond 1977).

A systematic review of the literature dealing with iatrogenic addiction concluded that, apart from case reports, there are no 'definitive data regarding the evidence for or against iatrogenic addiction in patients treated for acute or subacute pain' (Wasan et al 2006). A subsequent 'structured evidence-based review' led to the conclusion that 'chronic opioid analgesic therapy ... will lead to abuse/addiction in a small percentage of chronic pain patients, but a larger percentage will demonstrate aberrant drug-related behaviours and illicit drug use' (Fishbain et al 2008). The authors of this review also stated that 'these percentages appear to be much less if chronic pain patients are preselected for the absence of a current or past history of alcohol/illicit drug use or abuse/addiction.'

Although the risk of iatrogenic opioid addiction is thus very small, the potential problem of dependency needs to be discussed with patients before these drugs are prescribed, and this should be either acknowledged on a consent form or entered in the clinical notes.

The prescription of opioids for pain management in patients 'with addictive disease' was specifically discussed by Wesson et al (1993) with a recommendation that such patients be managed jointly by a 'pain specialist' and an 'addiction specialist'. A 'written treatment plan should be negotiated with the patient', specifying details of medications, frequency of visits, prohibitions on obtaining prescriptions from other physicians, addiction treatment and the consequences of the patient not complying with the treatment plan.

Malpractice claims and pain management

The American Society of Anesthesiologists Closed Claims has monitored malpractice claims against anaesthetists since 1977. A review of 284 malpractice claims related to management of chronic pain during the period 1977–1999 found that 2% were associated with medication use, while a subsequent interim review of data for the period 1995–2004 found that medication management claims increased to 8%. The most recent report of this ongoing study (Fitzgibbon et al 2010), for the period 2005–2008, found that there were 295 claims involving chronic pain management, indicating a very significant rise in such claims since 1977.

During the 2005–2008 period there were 51 claims related to medication management, representing 17% of all chronic pain claims. Of the 51 claims, 94% involved opioids (predominantly controlled-release oxycodone, methadone or hydrocodone). Of the 51 claims involving medication management, death occurred in 57% of cases. The authors commented that 'The increasing use of long-acting opioids is associated with an increase in drug-related deaths in the general population, and it is reflected in the high proportion of deaths in our malpractice claims.'

Iatrogenic narcotic addiction

Another group of malpractice claim cases ia those in which the plaintiff alleged that the prescription of an opiate analgesic caused iatrogenic addiction (Musto 1985). The rate of addiction following the therapeutic use of opioids is very low. As noted above, Porter and Jick found four such cases among 11,882 patients, and Medina and Diamond found only three instances of opioid abuse among 2369 patients treated with opiate analgesics for headache.

Steven (1995) drew attention to what seems to be an increased risk of dependence among patients treated with an opiate analgesic for pain following a work injury, particularly where this caused persistent low back pain. This report highlighted the need for careful evaluation of patients, early rehabilitation and return to work performing modified duties, and the importance of non-pharmacological approaches to chronic pain management.

Although there have been relatively few reported successful claims for iatrogenic addiction, this is probably because most of these cases were settled rather than proceeding to a verdict. In general, reported cases have held that iatrogenic opioid addiction is a legitimate cause of action (*Los Alamos Medical Center, Inc. v. Coe* 1954; Rigelhaupt 1982). It is imperative for doctors to inform patients about the benefits and risks inherent in management involving opiate analgesic preparations, including the risk of addiction. They must document these warnings in their clinical notes.

Allegations of clinician malpractice can also follow death while the patient was taking long-term opioid analgesic medication.

Rich & Webster (2011) reported on a series of 35 cases 'of patients with chronic pain who overdosed, 20 of them fatally, while consuming therapeutic opioids, leading to lawsuits against physicians for malpractice'. Ten deaths were related to methadone, whereas the use of hydrocodone was associated with four deaths. The authors commented that a number of 'knowledge deficits' were considered to have contributed to the overdoses, including initiating too high a starting dose, titrating doses too rapidly, converting to a different opioid using inadequate guides, and failing to screen and monitor for medical or psychiatric co-morbidities that can compromise opioid therapy.

Failure to provide adequate pain relief

At least since the case of *R. v Adams* (1957), the courts have declined to impose legal liability for death that may occur following the provision of reasonably necessary pain relief treatment. In this case, an English general practitioner, Dr John Bodkin Adams, was charged with murder when it was discovered that a number of elderly patients who had died were treated by him with high doses of opiate analgesics. Lord Justice Devlin focused on the intention of the physician, which distinguished palliative treatment aimed at enhancing the patient's well-being by relieving the pain and symptoms of an advanced disease from actions specifically aimed at ending the patient's life. According to Devlin (1986), a physician 'is entitled to do all that is proper and necessary to relieve pain and suffering, even if the measures he takes may incidentally shorten life' (at 71).

Conversely, leaving patients in pain may amount to negligence as well as unethical and unprofessional conduct. It is regrettable that, as Cherny & Catane (1995) commented, too many patients with pain due to cancer receive inadequate pain relief because oncologists 'commonly underestimate the prevalence and severity of pain' experienced by their patients. They noted that there were oncologists in clinical practice who had inadequate knowledge about pain management and, moreover, 'in many cases these knowledge deficits are not appreciated by the clinicians involved'.

Angarola & Donato (1991) drew attention to a North Carolina jury verdict in November 1990 that awarded

$15 million in damages to the family of a man whose opioid analgesic medication, ordered by his physician for treatment of pain due to terminal cancer of the prostate with bony metastases, was withheld in a nursing home by a nurse and her employer who considered the patient to be 'addicted to morphine'. As a consequence of withholding of morphine, prior to his death the patient suffered 'increased pain and suffering, as well as emotional and mental anguish'. During the trial reference was made to the existence of a 'Patients' Bill of Rights' in nursing homes which, the jury agreed, gave the patient 'a right to appropriate pain treatment'. The jury verdict was appealed, and prior to the matter being reconsidered by the court it was 'resolved by an undisclosed settlement between the parties'.

In June 2001, a California jury awarded the family of a patient who died of cancer US$1.5 million in damages for pain and suffering of the patient. The treating physician was found liable for recklessness and abuse because he had failed to prescribe adequate pain-relieving medication for the patient (CNN 2001). In this particular case the physician was sued for failure to prescribe sufficient medication to ease the patient's pain, and for 'elder abuse' in not providing adequate treatment.

Drug-specific liability issues

The use of opioid analgesics can give rise to legal claims arising from complications other than addiction.

Several years ago one of us (GM) was asked to undertake a psychiatric assessment of a woman who had been given an excessive dose of morphine for post-operative pain relief following surgery for a fractured hip, then developed respiratory depression. She experienced bizarre 'out of body' sensations during the episode of hypoxia (which had been documented) and when evaluated some years later described continuing symptoms of post-traumatic stress disorder arising from that episode. The case was settled out of court.

The use of pethidine (known as meperidine in the USA) in the management of chronic pain can give rise to neurotoxicity due to an accumulation of the toxic metabolite norpethidine (Hermes & Hare 1993). Manifestations of norpethidine neurotoxicity range from agitation to grand mal convulsions. It has also been suggested that pethidine is more likely than other opiate analgesics to give rise to addictive behaviour following therapeutic use. For these reasons, it has been recommended that pethidine only be used on a short-term basis in specific situations, such as during labour. Until relatively recently it was considered that pethidine was the opiate of choice in the management of severe pain in cases of biliary tract and pancreatic disease. Research has shown that parenteral ketorolac produces analgesia equal to that of pethidine and butorphanol in the management of biliary colic (Dula et al 2001; Olsen et al 2008) and renal colic (Sandhu et al 1994), as well as the control of severe acute pain in general (Koenig et al 1994), with fewer side effects. In the treatment of pain due to pancreatitis, it has been argued that morphine is preferable to pethidine because it offers longer pain relief with less risk of seizures (Thompson 2001).

Patients are usually warned about the risk of excessive use of ergotamine, and advised about the upper limit of dosage that may be taken. The risk of gangrene due to excessive use of ergotamine and similar compounds has been known for a considerable time. However, where there is no such warning and the patient develops such a complication legal liability will lie with the prescribing physician and the dispensing pharmacist (*Dwyer v. Roderick & Others* 1983).

In this case the patient, Mrs Dwyer, was prescribed an ergotamine preparation for treatment of migraine headaches. The prescribing doctor advised the patient to take two tablets every 4 hours, without any further instructions, and failed to warn the patient that no more than four tablets should be taken for any one attack of migraine, and no more than 12 tablets should be taken in a week. The patient was provided with 60 tablets. Over a 6-day period after the tablets were dispensed Mrs Dwyer took 36 tablets, suffered gangrene of the toes and lower limbs, and amputation was required.

In the lower court judgment was given against the defendants for £100,000, that is, against the prescribing doctor, a second doctor who had visited the patient at home and had failed to notice that incorrect instructions had been given to Mrs Dwyer concerning the dosage of the medication, and the two pharmacists who dispensed the medication with incorrect instructions. On appeal, it was held that no liability attached to the second doctor, and ultimately 45% of the damages were apportioned against the prescribing doctor and the remainder against the pharmacists.

PERSONAL INJURY CLAIMS AND PERSISTENT PAIN

As has been noted above, healthcare practitioners who treat patients with chronic non-cancer pain will frequently encounter individuals who are involved in personal injury litigation or workers' compensation claims.

Hadler has noted that 'to experience regional musculoskeletal pain at work is as unavoidable as it is outside the workplace'. Based on many surveys in many countries, it is clear that the experience of backache is ubiquitous and, along with episodes of neck and/or arm pain, irrespective of the physical demands of the workplace (Hadler 2004).

Workers' compensation is an insurance scheme that is charged with the task of making an award only to those who have suffered a loss that is indemnified. Chronic pain is a frequent complaint among claimants for personal injury (Mendelson 1988). Workers' compensation provides that any worker who has suffered an injury that arose out of and in the course of employment be afforded all medical and rehabilitative care that might put the injury right and provide financial recompense for any loss in income.

The injured worker, or the personal injury litigant, with chronic pain is placed in the position of having to 'prove' his or her illness and thus, again in Hadler's (1996) conceptualization, show that that person 'can't get well'.

The illness manifested by the workers' compensation claimant or litigant with chronic pain is qualitatively different from that suffered by individuals whose chronically painful illness is not confounded by such factors. Where the pain complained of by the patient is deemed disproportionate to the extent of objectively demonstrable organic abnormality, the clinician is expected to consider whether the individual is manifesting 'learned pain behaviour' (Tyrer 1986) or whether the diagnosis of 'persistent somatoform pain disorder' (in accordance with ICD-10 1992, published by the World Health Organization) or one of the sub-types of 'pain disorder' (using the categories of DSM-IV-TR 2000, published by the American Psychiatric Association (2000)) is appropriate.

Clearly, there is no 'magic formula' to determine whether the degree of pain described by a patient, and the extent of alleged disability, is 'in proportion' or 'disproportionate' to demonstrable organic abnormalities or continuing evidence of physical injury. The opinion of the clinician can only be based on experience with a wide range of patients with similar organic pathology, taking into consideration individual variations in the experience of, and response to, disease or injury.

In a discussion of the possible relationships between chronic pain and litigation, Weintraub (1995) drew attention to what he termed 'the surge in fraudulent claims' in the USA. There are, however, no objective tests to determine whether or not an individual does or does not subjectively experience pain, and each patient with a complaint of pain, whether or not involved in litigation or in receipt of compensation benefits, requires a comprehensive evaluation. It is ultimately for the court to determine whether or not a claim is fraudulent. There is no such diagnosis as 'malingering' (Mendelson & Mendelson 2000), and any such putative 'diagnosis' offered by a clinician usurps the function of the trier of fact.

Of relevance is the trend identified by Merskey & Teasell (2000) and described as 'the disparagement of pain'. According to these authors, there are three factors that encourage physicians to underestimate patients' pain. These are the requirement for doctors to control the issue of opiate analgesics, circumstances in which patients might benefit from compensation by exaggeration of pain severity and the development of attitudes that understate the importance of the relief of pain and overstate the importance of activity, exercise and not complaining.

Despite anecdotal and single-case reports, whether or not fibromyalgia can be caused by traumatic injury remains unresolved, and similarly it is unclear whether it can be considered to be a cause of work disability (Hadler 1997; Wolfe et al 1995). The apparent increasing prevalence of fibromyalgia might be attributable to the new-found respectability and validation, both medical and social, of the diagnostic term.

The effect of compensation on pain treatment outcome

In general, compensation payments have an adverse effect on response to treatment. For example, Fowler & Mayfield (1969), in a study comparing 327 patients receiving disability compensation with 613 patients not in receipt of compensation, found that compensation beneficiaries, although manifesting fewer symptoms, had a significantly poorer occupational adjustment than the no-compensation group.

In a similar study, Leavitt (1990) found that among a group of 1373 patients with pain following a work injury 23.7% were disabled for longer than 12 months, whereas among 417 patients with similar pain not receiving compensation benefits 13.2% were off work for longer than 12 months.

The surgical literature is replete with the observation that elective orthopaedic procedures are met with less success when the patient is a workers' compensation claimant. This outcome has been shown repeatedly following lumbar spine (Atlas et al 2010), carpal tunnel (Higgs et al 1995) and rotator cuff surgery (Holtby & Razmjou 2010), and confirmed in a meta-analysis (Harris et al 2005). Reporting on long-term outcomes of lumbar fusion, Nguyen et al (2011) concluded that 'lumbar fusion for the diagnoses of disc degeneration, disc herniation, and/or radiculopathy in a WC setting is associated with significant increase in disability, opiate use, prolonged work loss, and poor RTW status.'

A recent study of spinal cord stimulation (SCS) following 'failed back surgery syndrome' similarly concluded that in 'workers' compensation recipients, the high procedure cost of SCS was not counterbalanced by lower costs of subsequent care, and SCS was not cost-effective. The benefits and potential cost savings reported in RCTs may not be replicated in workers' compensation patients treated in community settings' (Hollingworth et al 2011).

Although receipt of compensation has a negative effect on treatment outcome and tends to prolong work disability, specific treatment programmes can reduce the likelihood of progression to pain chronicity following work injuries (Fordyce et al 1986; Ryan et al 1995; Wiesel et al 1984). Programmes which stress early mobilisation and return to the workplace, appropriate activity and exercises, and avoidance of other factors that might promote 'learned pain behaviour' have had good outcomes.

Malingering

Malingering is discussed in Chapter 24.

This section considers only those aspects of malingering that pertain to securing possible financial advantages following a compensable injury, and particularly in relation to persistent pain.

In a wide-ranging study of the limits of psychiatric expertise, Bursten (1984) listed several domains of data which need to be considered when evaluating the consistency of the clinical presentation, namely:

1. symptoms (as described by the individual)
2. signs (as observed by the doctor or by others)
3. laboratory data
4. reported limitations of activity
5. corroboration and 'the verification of the activities report given by the patient'.

Bursten noted that, in relation to this last area of assessment, 'psychiatric expertise may be of less importance than good detective work' and 'if the psychiatrist diagnoses a conversion disorder on the basis of a patient's inability to move his or her legs, and other witnesses have moving pictures of the patient riding a bicycle, society's representatives may be justified in wresting the power of making the diagnosis from the psychiatrist'.

Two points require emphasis. First, clinicians are not trained to assess the veracity of the patient. Diagnosis is made on the presumption that the patient is truthful in describing his or her subjective symptoms and that the signs elicited on clinical examination are not feigned. Second, the clinician as an expert witness formulates a professional opinion based, in part, on information provided by the person being examined or assessed. Unless contrasting information is made available to the examining clinician, she/he is entitled to assume that the history and symptoms described during the consultation are true. If the 'assumed facts' on which the clinician has relied are not accepted as true by the court, the expert opinion becomes invalid.

If the symptoms described by the patient are improbable or even absurd, or the combination of symptoms is unlikely or contradictory, the clinician may consider the possibility of malingering in the absence of an alternative explanation. In such a situation, a diagnosis might not be possible, and the report should specify this and draw attention to aspects of the individual's presentation during the interview and the symptoms that appear implausible.

While non-organic signs elicited in patients with low back pain have been clearly delineated by Waddell et al (1980), the distinction between the 'disproportionate' experience and the description of pain due to emotional factors and malingering remains, as ever, unclear (Main & Waddell 1998). Chronic pain, in particular, frequently arouses suspicion of deceit among medical and other healthcare practitioners, who are accustomed to assessing and treating patients with acute pain (Greve et al 2008, 2009a; Hackett 1971).

Some efforts have been made to assess malingering (e.g. Scale et al 1984).

Given that malingering is fraud in a healthcare setting, it is striking that not one of the numerous putative 'methods' for the determination of alleged malingering has been independently validated against a judicial finding of fraud that was arrived at independently of the opinion of the clinician promoting the specific psychometric test or symptom checklist.

It is also appropriate to caution against the use of some of these methodologies by clinicians who use them selectively, and who in their expert witness reports and testimony fail to make clear the limitations of the methods and their interpretation. An Australian case that achieved a degree of notoriety in this regard was *Mustac v. Medical Board of Western Australia* (2004), in which a consultant psychiatrist lost an appeal against that State's Medical Board. The Board had suspended Dr Mustac for 6 months for using the Test of Malingered Memory (TOMM) (Tombaugh 1996) in a manner for which it was not designed, and for having drawn conclusions about the veracity of two personal injury litigants in relation to their complaints of symptoms other than memory problems.

There is a group of authors who claim to be able to detect 'malingered pain-related disability' on the basis of the Word Memory Test (Greve et al 2008), the Portland Digit Recognition Test (Greve et al 2009b) and the TOMM (Greve et al 2009c). These claims have not been validated by any empirical studies, a criticism that also applies to the methods described by Rogers (2008). While some tests, such as the Rey Complex Figure Test, have been used to detect suboptimal effort (Blaskewitz et al 2009), there is a qualitative difference between an opinion concerning suboptimal effort and an expert witness asserting that a litigant is malingering (Freckelton 2004).

While the clinician acting as an expert witness may draw attention, if appropriate, to certain inconsistencies in the history and examination, lack of motivation and poor treatment compliance, the ultimate question of veracity of the claimant is a legal one and dependent on the judicial finding based on the facts of the case.

This view was also reflected in a judgment given by Lawton L J which, although written in a criminal appeal, in our view applies with equal validity to civil proceedings (*R v. Turner* 1975):

> 'We do not consider that . . . in all cases psychologists and psychiatrists can be called to prove the probability of the accused's veracity. If any such rule was applied in our courts, trial by psychiatrists would be likely to take the place of trial by jury and magistrates. We do not find that prospect attractive and the law does not at present provide for it.'

Thus, similarly, the question of the veracity of the plaintiff in a personal injury case is not an issue to be decided by the expert witness.

Table 24.2 Legitimate role of the healthcare professional in the assessment of personal injury/disability claimants

1. Is there a diagnosable disorder/disease?
2. If so, what is the aetiology of the condition?
3. What is the extent of impairment? Is it temporary or permanent?
4. Is the history consistent? Is it plausible?
5. Are findings on physical examination/mental status examination consistent/credible?
6. Has there been compliance with treatment and treatment recommendations?
7. Has there been cooperation and motivation during rehabilitation?

In our view healthcare professionals do have a legitimate role in the assessment of personal injury and disability claimants, but this role has to be confined to relevant clinical matters and must not usurp the function of the trier of fact, be it a jury, tribunal or judge. The relevant clinical questions that may be answered by the healthcare professional have been listed in Table 24.2.

While lawyers might attempt to seduce the clinician expert witness to express an opinion that is beyond the legitimate limits of his or her professional expertise, it is part of the healthcare professional's task to avoid that trap (Mendelson & Mendelson 1993).

The rating of pain-related impairment

In the context of the medicolegal evaluation of a compensation recipient or litigant with chronic pain, it is important to distinguish between the concepts of impairment and disability, as defined by the World Health Organization (1980). Impairment is defined as the 'loss or abnormality of psychological, physiological, or anatomical structure or function', whereas disability is defined as the 'restriction or lack (resulting from an impairment) of ability to perform an activity in the manner or within the range considered normal for a human being'.

It is generally accepted that the evaluation and rating of impairment is the task of the clinician, whereas the determination of disability is an administrative and legal matter that depends on the specific circumstances of the claimant and the relevant statutory provisions. Curran (1990) argued that evaluation of impairment is a medical responsibility but determination of disability requires examination of legal, social, psychological and vocational issues.

Turk & Rudy (1991) suggested that the focus of impairment and disability evaluation be on the injured worker rather than on biomedical diagnosis, and that psychological, behavioural and job-related factors also need to be considered.

The benefits of such an approach in the vocational rehabilitation of injured workers have been demonstrated by the success of functional restoration (Mayer et al 1987; Moreno et al 1991) and work-hardening programmes (Matheson et al 1985). In relation to such programmes, it is relevant to note that 'disability exaggeration' is a poor predictor of the success of a functional restoration programme for patients with chronic low back pain (Hazard et al 1991). These authors have commented that when disability exaggeration did correlate significantly with a positive treatment outcome, the correlation was negative.

It is clear that any proposed system of rating of impairment due to chronic pain needs to take into consideration relevant occupational factors in translating impairment into disability. McBride (1963), in an important yet relatively neglected work on the evaluation of disability, provided an extensive listing of various occupations, indicating those parts of the body which may be functionally impaired but the individual can 'still work at the designated job'. Nachemson (1983) emphasized that, with respect to chronic low back pain, return to work is possible and indeed 'well justified from a medical, psychologic, and economic point of view' for the approximately 80% of patients who do not have an objectively demonstrable organic cause for the pain complaint or significant physical impairment.

If it is considered that the pain complained of by the patient cannot be attributed to a specific demonstrable physical cause, the problem of determining the extent of any pain-related impairment thus becomes a difficult one, and the method initially suggested by Turk, Loeser and Robinson (all from the University of Washington's multidisciplinary pain clinic) in the American Medical Association *Guides to the Evaluation of Permanent Impairment* (5th edition) appears the most appropriate (American Medical Association 2000). As set out in Chapter 18 of the AMA *Guides*, the evaluation of pain-related impairment involves six steps. Three of these use questionnaires and thus rely on the individual's self-report. These questionnaires rate pain severity, activity limitation and effect of pain on mood. The examiner rates the individual on the presence of pain behaviours and is also required to make 'a global assessment of the person's credibility', although there is no guidance as to how this should be determined. The final step involves the calculation of the 'total pain-related impairment score' and determining the 'impairment class' on the basis of that score.

It will be apparent that the method of assessment of pain-related impairment in the AMA *Guides* is quite different from those in relation to other conditions. One of the principles of impairment assessment is that it should have an objective basis. While Chapter 18 is an improvement on earlier editions of the AMA *Guides*, it is crucially dependent not only on the subjective responses of the person being evaluated but also on the subjective responses of the examiner, both in relation to observations of pain behaviour and in deciding that person's credibility.

There are indications that in many jurisdictions the courts and tribunals are becoming increasingly familiar with advances in the understanding of pain mechanisms, and are beginning to use this knowledge in the decision-making process (Ontario Workers' Compensation Appeals Tribunal 1987). In other cases, such as the requirement in Victoria, Australia, that clinicians 'disentangle' pain and suffering due to 'psychological and psychiatric consequences' from that due to 'an organic or physical basis' (see *Mutual Cleaning and Maintenance Pty Ltd v. Stamboulakis* 2007), it could be argued that the Courts have adopted a dualism that is inconsistent with recent advances in the clarification of pain physiology. It is therefore equally important that clinicians who treat patients with chronic pain and who are likely to become involved as expert witnesses in the legal process keep abreast of new developments in the understanding and management of chronic pain problems.

ENDNOTES

1. For example, the *Guardianship and Administration Act 1986 (Vic)*, s 42A provides immunity from prosecution and civil liability for registered practitioners in relation to battery and assault .'.. if the practitioner believes on reasonable grounds that the procedure or treatment is necessary, as a matter of urgency – (a) to save the patient's life; or (b) to prevent serious damage to the patient's health; or (c) in the case of a medical research procedure or medical or dental treatment, to prevent the patient from suffering or continuing to suffer significant pain or distress.'

2. 'The incision made by the surgeon's scalpel need not be and probably is most unlikely to be hostile, but unless a defence of justification is established it must in my judgment fall within a definition of a trespass to person.' *T v. T* [1988] 2 WLR 189 at 203 per Wood J.

3. Under therapeutic privilege, treating clinicians retain discretion to decide whether or not, and if so, when, to disclose disturbing information directly to the patient who is unusually nervous, disturbed or volatile. When a decision is made against the disclosure, a relative or a close associate who regularly attends the patient is provided with the relevant information. See *Battersby v. Tottman* [1985] 37 SASR 524; *Di Carlo v. Dubois* [2004] QCA 150 at [80]–[81]; *Sheppard v. Swan* [2004] WASCA 215 at [41]–[42]; *Rooke v. Minister for Health* [2009] WASCA 27 at [41]–[42]. See also Mulheron T 2003 The defence of therapeutic privilege in Australia. Journal of Law and Medicine 11:201–213.

4. *Civil Liability Act 2002* (Tas), s 21(1); *Civil Liability Act 2003* (Qld), s 21(1): 'In this section patient, when used in a context of giving or being given information, includes a person who has the responsibility for making a decision about the medical treatment to be

undergone by a patient if the patient is under a legal disability.'

5. *Civil Liability Act 2002* (Tas), s 21(2) and *Civil Liability Act 2003* (Qld), s 21(2) further provide that: 'This section does not apply where a registered medical practitioner has to act promptly to avoid serious risk to the life or health of the patient and (a) the patient is not able to hear or respond to a warning about the risk to the patient; and (b) there is not sufficient time for the registered medical practitioner to contact a person responsible for making a decision for the patient.'

6. *Civil Liability Act 2002* (NSW), s 5P. Duty to Warn of Risk: 'This Division [s 5O: standard of care for professionals] does not apply to liability arising in connection with the giving of (or the failure to give) a warning, advice or other information in respect of the risk of death of or injury to a person associated with the provision by a professional of a professional service.'

7. *Wrongs Act 1958* (Vic), s 60. Duty to warn of risk: 'Section 59 [standard of care for professionals] does not apply to a liability arising in connection with the giving of (or the failure to give) a warning or other information in respect of a risk or other matter to a person if the giving of the warning or information is associated with the provision by a professional of a professional service.'

8. *Civil Liability Act 2003* (Qld), s 22(5): Failure to give a warning: 'This section [standard of care for professionals] does not apply to liability arising in connection with the giving of (or the failure to give) a warning, advice or other information, in relation to the risk of harm to a person, that is associated with the provision by a professional of a professional service.'

9. *Civil Liability Act 1936* (SA), s 41(5): 'This section [standard of care for professionals] does not apply to liability arising in connection with the giving of (or the failure to give) a warning, advice or other information in respect of a risk of death of or injury associated with the provision of a health care service.'

10. *Civil Liability Act 2002* (Tas), s 22(5): 'This section [standard of care for professionals] does not apply to liability arising in connection with the giving of (or the failure to give) a warning, advice or other information in relation to the risk of harm associated with the provision by a professional of a professional service to a person.'

11. See *Hammond v Heath* [2010] WASCA 6.

12. *Civil Liability Act 2002* (NSW), s 5P. Duty to warn of risk: 'This Division [s 5O: standard of care for professionals] does not apply to liability arising in connection with the giving of (or the failure to give) a warning, advice or other information in respect of the risk of death of or injury to a person associated with the provision by a professional of a professional service.'

13. *Wrongs Act 1958* (Vic), s 60. Duty to warn of risk: 'Section 59 [standard of care for professionals] does not apply to a liability arising in connection with the giving of (or the failure to give) a warning or other information in respect of a risk or other matter to a person if the giving of the warning or information is associated with the provision by a professional of a professional service.'

14. *Civil Liability Act 2003* (Qld), s 22(5). Failure to give a warning: 'This section [standard of care for professionals] does not apply to liability arising in connection with the giving of (or the failure to give) a warning, advice or other information, in relation to the risk of harm to a person, that is associated with the provision by a professional of a professional service.'

15. *Civil Liability Act 1936* (SA), s 41(5): 'This section [standard of care for professionals] does not apply to liability arising in connection with the giving of (or the failure to give) a warning, advice or other information in respect of a risk of death of or injury associated with the provision of a health care service.'

16. *Civil Liability Act 2002* (Tas), s 22(5): 'This section [standard of care for professionals] does not apply to liability arising in connection with the giving of (or the failure to give) a warning, advice or other information in relation to the risk of harm associated with the provision by a professional of a professional service to a person.'

17. See *Di Carlo v. Dubois* [2004] QCA 150 at [80]–[81]; *Sheppard v. Swan* [2004] WASCA 215 at [41]–[42]; *Rooke v. Minister for Health* [2009] WASCA 27 at [41]–[42].

18. *Civil Liability Act 2002* (Tas), s 13(3); *Civil Liability Act 2002* (NSW), s 5D(3).

19. The text of the *Civil Liability Act 2003* (WA), s 5C(3) follows more closely the Ipp Report Recommendation 29(g)(i): 'For the purposes of sub-paragraph (ii) of this paragraph, the plaintiff's own testimony, about what he or she would have done if the defendant had not been negligent, is inadmissible.'

REFERENCES

Abram, S.E., 1989. Perceived dangers from intraspinal steroid injections [letter]. Arch. Neurol. 46, 719–720.

American Medical Association, 1993. Guides to the evaluation of permanent impairment, fourth ed. American Medical Association, Chicago.

American Medical Association, 2000. Guides to the evaluation of permanent impairment, fifth ed. American Medical Association, Chicago.

American Psychiatric Association, 2000. Diagnostic and statistical manual of mental disorders, fourth ed, text revision American Psychiatric Association, Washington, DC.

Angarola, R.T., Donato, B.J., 1991. Inappropriate pain management results in high jury award [letter]. J. Pain Symptom Manage. 6, 407.

Ashby, M., 1995. Hard cases, causation and care of the dying. J. Law Med. 3, 152–160.

Atlas, S.J., Tosteson, T.D., Blood, E.A., et al., 2010. The impact of workers' compensation on outcomes of surgical and nonoperative therapy for patients with a lumbar disc herniation: SPORT. Spine. 35, 89–97.

Ballenger v. Crowell. 1978 247 S.E.2d 287.

Banja, J.D., Wolf, S.L., 1987. Malpractice litigation for uninformed consent Implications for physical therapists. Phys. Ther. 67, 1226–1229.

Benzon, H.T., 1986. Epidural steroid injections for low back pain and lumbosacral radiculopathy. Pain 24, 277–295.

Blaskewitz, N., Merten, T., Brockhaus, R., 2009. Detection of suboptimal effort with the Rey Complex Figure Test and Recognition Trial. Appl. Neuropsychol. 16, 54–61.

Buchanan, J., 1995. Euthanasia: the medical and psychological issues. J. Law Med. 3, 161–168.

Bursten, B., 1984. Beyond psychiatric expertise. Charles C Thomas, Springfield, IL.

Chappel v. Hart, [1998] HCA 55.

Chatterton v. Gerson, [1981] 1 All ER 257.

Cherny, N.I., Catane, R., 1995. Professional negligence in the management of cancer pain. Cancer. 76, 2181–2185.

Clayer, J.R., Bookless, C., Ross, M.W., 1984. Neurosis and conscious symptom exaggeration: Its differentiation by the Illness Behaviour Questionnaire. J. Psychosom. Res. 28, 237–241.

Clayer, J.R., Bookless-Pratz, C.L., Ross, M.W., 1986. The evaluation of illness behaviour and exaggeration of disability. British Journal of Psychiatry. 148, 296–299.

CNN, 2001. Doctor liable for not giving enough pain medicine. Online. Available: http://edition.cnn.com/ 2001/LAW/06/13/elderabuse. lawsuit/index.html (18.08.11).

Coleman, C.H., Fleischman, A.R., 1996. Guidelines for physician-assisted suicide: can the challenge be met? J. Law Med. Ethics. 24, 217–224.

Curran, W.J., Hall, M.A., Kaye, D.H., 1990. Health care law, forensic science, and public policy, fourth ed. Little Brown, Boston.

Devlin, P., 1986. Easing the Passing: The Trial of Dr John Bodkin Adams. Faber and Faber, London.

Dula, D.J., Anderson, R., Wood, G.C., 2001. A prospective study comparing I.M. ketorolac with I.M. meperidine in the treatment of acute biliary colic. J. Emerg. Med. 20, 121–124.

Dwyer v. Roderick & Others, [1983] 127 Solicitors' Journal 805; [1983] 80 Law Society Gazette 3003.

Ellis v. Wallsend District Hospital, [1989] Australian Tort Reports 80–289.

Ernst, E., 2010. Acupuncture – a treatment to die for? J. R. Soc. Med. 103, 384–385.

Ernst, E., Lee, M.S., Choi, T.Y., 2011. Acupuncture: does it alleviate pain and are there serious risks? A review of reviews. Pain 152, 755–764.

Fishbain, D.A., Cole, B., Lewis, J., et al., 2008. What percentage of chronic nonmalignant pain patients exposed to chronic opioid analgesic therapy develop abuse/addiction and/or aberrant drug-related behaviors? A structured evidence-based review. Pain Med. 9, 444–459.

Fishbain, D.A., Lewis, J.E., Gao, J., 2010. Allegations of medical malpractice in chronic opioid analgesic therapy possibly related to collaborative/split treatment and the P-450 enzyme system: forensic case report. Pain Med. 11, 1419–1425.

Fitzgibbon, D.R., Rathmell, J.P., Michna, E., et al., 2010. Malpractice claims associated with medication management for chronic pain. Anesthesiology 112, 948–956.

Fordyce, W.E., Brockway, J.A., Bergman, J.A., et al., 1986. Acute back pain: a control group comparison of behavioral vs. traditional management methods. J. Behav. Med. 9, 127–140.

Fowler, D.R., Mayfield, D.G., 1969. Effect of disability compensation: disability symptoms and motivation for treatment. Arch. Environ. Health 19, 719–725.

Freckelton, I., 2004. Regulating forensic deviance: the ethical responsibilities of expert witness report writers and witnesses. J. Law Med. 12, 141–149.

Gregory, P., 1996a. Hospital sued over patient's addiction. The Age, Melbourne p. 8.

Gregory, P., 1996b. Pethidine damages claim settled. The Age, Melbourne p. 3.

Greve, K.W., Ord, J., Curtis, K.L., et al., 2008. Detecting malingering in traumatic brain injury and chronic pain: a comparison of three forced-choice symptom validity tests. Clin. Neuropsychol. 22, 896–918.

Greve, K.W., Ord, J.S., Bianchini, K.J., et al., 2009a. Prevalence of malingering in patients with chronic pain referred for psychologic evaluation in a medico-legal context. Arch. Phys. Med. Rehabil. 90, 1117–1126.

Greve, K.W., Bianchini, K.J., Etherton, J.L., et al., 2009b. Detecting malingered pain-related disability: classification accuracy of the Portland Digit Recognition Test. Clin. Neuropsychol. 23, 850–869.

Greve, K.W., Etherton, J.L., Ord, J., et al., 2009c. Detecting malingered pain-related disability: classification accuracy of the test of memory malingering. Clin. Neuropsychol. 23, 1250–1271.

Hackett, T.P., 1971. Pain and prejudice: why do we doubt that the patient is in pain? Med. Times. 99, 130.

Hadler, N.M., 1996. If you have to prove you are ill, you can't get well. The object lesson of fibromyalgia. Spine. 21, 2397–2400.

Hadler, N.M., 1997. Fibromyalgia: La maladie est morte. Vive le Malade!. J. Rheumatol. 24, 1250–1251.

Hadler, N.M., 2004. The semiotics of backache. Spine. 29, 1289.

Hamilton, J.C., Feldman, M.D., Cunnien, A.J., 2008. Factitious disorder in medical and psychiatric practices. In: Rogers, R. (Ed.), Clinical assessment of malingering and deception. third ed Guilford Press, New York, pp. 128–144.

Harris, I., Mulford, J., Solomon, M., et al., 2005. Association between compensation status and outcome after surgery: a meta-analysis. JAMA 293, 1644–1652.

Hazard, R.G., Bendix, A., Fenwick, J.W., 1991. Disability exaggeration as a predictor of functional restoration outcomes for patients with chronic low-back pain. Spine. 16, 1062–1067.

Health Department of Western Australia, 1990. Guidelines for medical practitioners for the epidural administration of Depo-Medrol. Perth.

Heo, J.H., Bae, M.H., Lee, S.J., 2011. Intracranial hemorrhage and cerebral infarction caused by acupuncture. [Letter]Neurol. India. 59, 303–304.

Hermes, E.R., Hare, B.D., 1993. Meperidine neurotoxicity: three case reports and a review of the literature. Journal of Pharmaceutical Care in Pain & Symptom Control 1 (3), 5–20.

Higgs, P.E., Edwards, D., Martin, D.S., et al., 1995. Carpal tunnel surgery outcomes in workers: effect of workers' compensation status. J. Hand Surg. [Am]. 20, 354–360.

Hollingworth, W., Turner, J.A., Welton, N.J., et al., 2011. Costs and cost-effectiveness of spinal cord stimulation (SCS) for failed back surgery syndrome: an observational study in a workers' compensation population. Spine. (epub ahead of print).

Holtby, R., Razmjou, H., 2010. Impact of work-related compensation claims on surgical outcome of patients with rotator cuff related pathologies: a matched case-control study. J. Shoulder Elbow Surg. 19, 452–460.

In re W (a Minor), [1992] 3 W.L.R. 758 at 765.

Jarvis, J., 1983. Professional negligence and the occupational therapist. Can. J. Occup. Ther. 50, 45–48.

Karcz, A., Korn, R., Burke, M.C., et al., 1996. Malpractice claims against emergency physicians in Massachusetts: 1975–1993. Am. J. Emerg. Med. 14, 341–345.

Kjervik, D.K., 1996. Assisted suicide: the challenge to the nursing profession. J. Law Med. Ethics. 24, 237–242.

Koenig, K.L., Hodgson, L., Kozak, R., et al., 1994. Ketorolac vs meperidine for the management of pain in the emergency department. Acad. Emerg. Med. 1, 544–549.

Kuhse, H., Singer, P., 1995. Active voluntary euthanasia, morality and the law. J. Law Med. 3, 129–135.

Leavitt, F., 1985. Pain and deception: use of verbal pain measurement as a diagnostic aid in differentiating between clinical and simulated low-back pain. J. Psychosom. Res. 29, 495–505.

Leavitt, F., 1990. The role of psychological disturbance in extending disability time among compensable back injured industrial workers. J. Psychosom. Res. 34, 447–453.

Leavitt, F., Sweet, J.J., 1986. Characteristics and frequency of malingering among patients with low back pain. Pain. 25, 357–364.

Linville, J.E., 1996. Physician-assisted suicide as a constitutional right. J. Law Med. Ethics. 24, 198–206.

Los Alamos Medical Center, Inc. v. Coe, [1954] 275 P.2d 175.

Main, C.J., Waddell, G., 1998. Behavioral responses to examination. A reappraisal of the interpretation of 'nonorganic signs'. Spine. 23, 2367–2371.

Marion's Case (Department of Health & Community Services v JWB & SMB), [1992] 175 C.L.R. 218.

Matheson, L.N., Ogden, L.D., Violette, K., et al., 1985. Work hardening: occupational therapy in vocational rehabilitation. Am. J. Occup. Ther. 39, 314–321.

Mayer, T., Gatchel, R., Mayer, H., et al., 1987. A prospective two year study offunctional restoration in industrial low back injury: an objective assessment procedure. JAMA. 258, 1763–1767.

McBride, E.D., 1963. Disability evaluation and principles of treatment of compensable injuries, sixth ed. J.B. Lippincott, Philadelphia.

McCarroll v. Reed, [1983] 679 P.2d 851 (Okl. App.).

Medical Treatment Act. 1988(Vic). (See also: *Medical Treatment (Enduring Power of Attorney) Act* 1990 (Vic), ss 5 (1); 7(3); Schedule 1 Note; *Consent to Medical Treatment and Palliative Care Act* 1995 (SA) s 8(7)).

Medina, J.L., Diamond, S., 1977. Drug dependency in patients with chronic headache. Headache. 17, 12–14.

Mendelson, G., 1987. Measurement of conscious symptom exaggeration by questionnaire: a clinical study. J. Psychosom. Res. 31, 703–711.

Mendelson, G., 1988. Chronic pain. In: Psychiatric aspects of personal injury claims. Charles C. Thomas, Springfield, IL, pp. 91–111 (See also: Mendelson G 1986 Chronic pain and compensation: a review. J Pain Symptom Manage 1:135–144; Mendelson G 1991 Chronic pain, compensation and clinical knowledge. Theor Med 12:227–246; Mendelson G 1992 Compensation and chronic pain. Pain 48:121–123).

Mendelson, D., 1995. The Northern Territory's euthanasia legislation in historical perspective. J. Law Med. 3, 136–144.

Mendelson, D., 1998. Euthanasia. In: Smith, R. (Ed.), Health Care Crime and Regulatory Control. The Australian Institute of Criminology, Hawkins Press, Sydney, pp. 149–166.

Mendelson, G., Mendelson, D., 1993. Legal and psychiatric aspects of malingering. J. Law Med. 1, 28–34.

Merskey, H., Teasell, R.W., 2000. The disparagement of pain: social influences on medical thinking. Pain Res. Manag. 5, 259–270.

Miller, F.G., Brody, H., Quill, T.E., 1996. Can physician-assisted suicide be regulated effectively? J. Law Med. Ethics. 24, 225–232.

Moreno, R., Cunningham, A.C., Gatchel, R.J., et al., 1991. Functional restoration for chronic low back pain: changes in depression, cognitive distortion, and disability. J. Occup. Rehabil. 1, 207–216.

Mullen, P.E., 1995. Euthanasia: an impoverished construction of life and death. J. Law Med. 3, 121–128.

Mustac v. Medical Board of Western Australia, [2004] WASCA 156.

Musto, D.F., 1985. Iatrogenic addiction: the problem, its definition and history. Bull. N. Y. Acad. Med. 61, 694–705.

Mutual Cleaning and Maintenance Pty Ltd v. Stamboulakis, [2007] 15 VR 649; [2007] VSCA 46.

Nachemson, A., 1983. Work for all – for those with low back pain as well. Clin. Orthop. 179, 77–85.

National Health and Medical Research Council, 1993. General guidelines for medical practitioners on providing information to patients. Australian Government Publishing Service, Canberra.

Nelson, D.A., 1988. Dangers from methylprednisolone acetate therapy by intraspinal injection. Arch. Neurol. 45, 804–806.

Nguyen, T.H., Randolph, D.C., Talmage, J., et al., 2011. Long-term outcomes of lumbar fusion among workers' compensation subjects: a historical cohort study. Spine. 36, 320–331.

Olsen, J.C., McGrath, N.A., Schwarz, D.G., et al., 2008. A double-blind randomized clinical trial evaluating the analgesic efficacy of ketorolac versus butorphanol for patients with suspected biliary colic in the emergency department. Acad. Emerg. Med. 15, 718–722.

Ontario Workers' Compensation Appeals Tribunal, 1987. Decision no. 915. Research Publications Department, Workers' Compensation Appeals Tribunal, Toronto

Osborne, P.H., 1983. Malpractice: a perspective for physiotherapists. Physiother. Can. 35, 258–260.

Osterweis, M., Kleinman, A., Mechanic, D. (Eds.), 1987. Pain and disability: clinical, behavioral, and public policy perspectives. National Academy Press, Washington, DC.

Parker, N., 1979. Malingering: a dangerous diagnosis. Med. J. Aust. 1, 568–569.

Pawl, R.P., Anderson, W., Shulman, M., 1985. Effect of epidural steroids in the cervical and lumbar region on surgical intervention for discogenic spondylosis. Adv. Pain Res. Ther. 9, 791–798.

Pilowsky, I., 1985. Malingerophobia. Med. J. Aust. 143, 571–572.

Pilowsky, I., 1994. Abnormal illness behaviour: a 25th anniversary review. Aust. N. Z. J. Psychiatry 28, 566–573.

Portenoy, R.K., Foley, K.M., 1986. Chronic use of opioid analgesics in non-malignant pain: report of 38 cases. Pain 25, 171–186.

Porter, J., Jick, H., 1980. Addiction rare in patients treated with narcotics [Letter]. N. Engl. J. Med. 302, 123.

R. v. Adams, [1957] Crim LR 365.

R. v. Turner, [1975] 1 QB 834.

Ranke, B.A., Moriarty, M.P., 1997. An overview of professional liability in occupational therapy. Am. J. Occup. Ther. 51, 671–680.

Ranson, D., 1995. The coroner and the Rights of the Terminally Ill Act 1995 (NT). J. Law Med. 3, 169–176.

Reilly, P.A., Littlejohn, G.O., 1991. A glossary of pain terms for medicolegal work. Med. J. Aust. 155, 264–266.

Rich, B.A., 1997. Pain management: legal risks and ethical responsibilities. Journal of Pharmaceutical Care in Pain & Symptom Control. 5 (1), 5–20.

Rich, B.A., Webster, L.R., 2011. A review of forensic implications of opioid prescribing with examples from malpractice cases involving opioid-related overdose. Pain Med. 12, S59–S65.

Rigelhaupt, J.L., 1982. Physician's liability for causing patient to become addicted to drugs. 16 ALR 4th 999.

Robinson, D.D., 1990. Occupations potentially appropriate for persons with low back pain [Abstract]. Pain Suppl. 5, S394.

Rogers, R. (Ed.), 2008. Clinical assessment of malingering and deception, third ed. Guildford Press, New York.

Rogers v. Whitaker. 175 C.L.R. 479 at 490. (See also: Chatterton v. Gerson [1981] 1 All ER 257; Sidaway v. The Board of Governors of the Bethlem Royal Hospital and the Maudsley Hospital [1985] 1 A.C. 871 (Lord Scarman dissenting); Secretary, Department of Health & Community Services (NT) v. JWB and SMB [1992] 175 CLR 218; Malette v. Shulman [1990] 67 DLR (4th) 321).

Rosenberg v. Percival, [2001] 205 CLR 434.

Rushton, C.H., 1995. Placebo pain medication: ethical and legal issues. Pediatr. Nurs. 21, 166–168.

Rusnak, R.A., Borer, J.M., Fastow, J.S., 1994. Misdiagnosis of acute appendicitis: common features discovered in cases after litigation. Am. J. Emerg. Med. 12, 397–402.

Ryan, W.E., Krishna, M.K., Swanson, C.E., 1995. A prospective study evaluating early rehabilitation in

preventing back pain chronicity in mine workers. Spine. 20, 489–491.

Sandhu, D.P., Iacovou, J.W., Fletcher, M.S., et al., 1994. A comparison of intramuscular ketorolac and pethidine in the alleviation of renal colic. Br. J. Urol. 74, 690–693.

Savage, S.R., 1996. Long-term opioid therapy: assessment of consequences and risks. J. Pain Symptom Manage. 11, 274–286.

Schwartz, J., 1996. Writing the rules of death: state regulation of physician-assisted suicide. J. Law Med. Ethics. 24, 207–216.

Shapiro, R.S., 1994. Liability issues in the management of pain. J. Pain Symptom Manage. 9, 146–152.

Sidaway v. The Board of Governors of the Bethlem Royal Hospital and the Maudsley Hospital, [1985] 1 A.C. 871.

Steven, I.D., 1995. Opioid dependence in 15 patients after a work injury. Med. J. Aust. 163, 193–196.

Swerdlow, M., 1982. Medico-legal aspects of complications following pain relieving blocks. Pain 13, 321–331.

Szasz, T.S., 1956. Malingering: diagnosis or social condemnation? Analysis of the meaning of 'diagnosis' in the light of some interrelations of social structure, value judgment, and the physician's role. Arch. Neurol. Psychiatry. 76, 432–443.

Tennant, F.S., Uelmen, G.F., 1983. Narcotic maintenance for chronic pain: medical and legal guidelines. Postgrad. Med. 73, 81–94.

Thomasma, D.C., 1996. When physicians choose to participate in the death of their patients: ethics and physician-assisted suicide. J. Law Med. Ethics 24, 183–197.

Thompson, D.R., 2001. Narcotic analgesic affects on the sphincter of Oddi: a review of the data and therapeutic implications in treating pancreatitis. Am. J. Gastroenterol. 96, 1266–1272.

Tombaugh, T.N., 1996. The test of memory malingering (TOMM). Multi Health Systems, North Tonawanda, NY.

Turk, D.C., Rudy, T.E., 1991. Pain and the injured worker: integrating biomedical, psychosocial and behavioral factors in assessment. J. Occup. Rehabil. 1, 159–179.

Turk, D.C., Rudy, T.E., Stieg, R.L., 1988. The disability determination dilemma: toward a multiaxial solution. Pain 34, 217–229.

Tyrer, S.P., 1986. Learned pain behaviour. BMJ. 292, 1–2.

Waddell, G., McCulloch, J.A., Kummel, E., et al., 1980. Nonorganic physical signs in low back pain. Spine. 5, 117–125.

Wasan, A.D., Correll, D.J., Kissin, I., et al., 2006. Iatrogenic addiction in patients treated for acute or subacute pain: a systematic review. J. Opioid Manag. 2, 16–22.

Weintraub, M.I., 1995. Chronic pain in litigation. What is the relationship? Neurol. Clin. 13, 341–349.

Wesson, D.R., Ling, W., Smith, D.E., 1993. Prescription of opioids for treatment of pain in patients with addictive disease. J. Pain Symptom Manage. 8, 289–296.

Wiesel, S.W., Feffer, H.L., Rothman, R.H., 1984. Industrial low back pain: a prospective evaluation of a standardized diagnostic and treatment protocol. Spine. 9, 199–203.

Wilkinson, H., 1989. Dangers from methylprednisolone acetate therapy by intraspinal injection [Letter]. Arch. Neurol. 46, 721.

Witztum, E., Grinshpoon, A., Margolin, J., et al., 1996. The erroneous diagnosis of malingering in a military setting. Mil. Med. 161, 225–229.

Wolfe, F., Aarflot, T., Bruusgaard, D., et al., 1995. Fibromyalgia and disability. Report of the Moss International Working Group on medico-legal aspects of chronic widespread musculoskeletal pain complaints and fibromyalgia. Scand. J. Rheumatol. 24, 112–118.

World Health Organization, 1980. International classification of impairments, disabilities, and handicaps. WHO, Geneva.

World Health Organization, 1992. The ICD-10 classification of mental and behavioural disorders: clinical descriptions and diagnostic guidelines. WHO, Geneva.

Wright, M., 1985. Legal liability for occupational therapists. Can. J. Occup. Ther. 52, 16–19.

Chapter | 25 |

Chronic pain and psychiatric problems

Harold Merskey

LEARNING OBJECTIVES

At the end of this chapter readers will have an understanding of:

1. The relationship between chronic pain and psychiatric disorders.
2. Psychiatric disorders coincidental with pain.
3. Chronic pain causing psychiatric disorders.
4. Specific psychiatric syndromes and pain.

OVERVIEW

Patients with chronic pain often face many life difficulties. Such patients can benefit not only from conventional medical therapies, but also psychological therapies. An awareness of the particular physical, psychological and social problems that accumulate for people with long-term pain and disability, and an ability to identify and appropriately manage these problems, allows healthcare professionals to obtain more successful outcomes and satisfaction for patients.

In this chapter, the manner in which psychosocial disturbances can develop and present in people with chronic pain will be described. An overview will be given of the association between chronic pain and psychiatric disorders, before a number of specific psychiatric syndromes will be described. Key terms are defined in Box 25.1.

THE ASSOCIATION BETWEEN PAIN AND PSYCHIATRIC DISORDERS

Chronic pain occurs in about 10–15% of the general population, with many also having a psychiatric disorder, either pre-existing or consequential (Dworkin & Caligor 1988). Merskey & Spear (1967) reported that pain is as frequent a complaint in the psychiatric clinic as it is in medical clinics. Spear (1967) found that 45–50% of patients with psychiatric problems attending a psychiatric clinic reported pain problems, with the highest incidence occurring in patients with anxiety states. These problems were not such as to lead to consultations, and were not compared to any appropriate group without pain. Large (1986) found that, in a consecutive series of 50 patients presenting for psychosocial evaluation at a pain clinic, 94% had a psychiatric disorder and 96% had a physical disorder. In other words, most had both psychiatric and physical disorders. Associations between chronic pain and psychiatric disorders can be psychiatric disorders coincidental with pain, pre-existing factors which predispose to both chronic pain and psychiatric disorders, and/or chronic pain causing psychiatric disorders.

© 2014 Elsevier Ltd.

PSYCHIATRIC DISORDERS COINCIDENTAL WITH PAIN

An illness such as schizophrenia is associated with difficulty defining, understanding and resolving problems. The illness leads patients to have major perceptual, affective and cognitive impairment, which can lead to misinterpretations, at times to a psychotic degree. This distortion might lead to over-reporting or under-reporting of problems. Pain can be a confounding experience for a person with a major psychiatric illness. Occasionally someone with a delusional illness, such as schizophrenia, may develop a delusional misinterpretation of a physical symptom. For example, a patient who had excruciating back pain from degenerative spinal disease 'knew' that this was caused by aliens having implanted electronic stimulators in his spine that they turned on and off at will.

Box 25.1 **Key terms defined**

Somatization – The presentation of emotional problems as if they are symptoms of physical disorders.

Post-traumatic stress disorder – A condition that develops after a person is exposed to a major life-threatening event whereby the event is frequently re-experienced, with symptoms of persisting arousal.

Dissociation – Where a person reacts to some part of their conscious experience as if detached.

Kinesiophobia – The fear and avoidance of activity.

In rare cases the pain may be a true 'psychogenic' phenomenon, a hallucination, which is associated with a delusional interpretation. Chronic patients hospitalized with schizophrenia tend to complain less about pain than patients with depression. However, it has been demonstrated (Whitlock 1967) that when a major psychiatric disorder such as schizophrenia, major depression or conversion disorder is diagnosed, then it is in fact more likely that the person will also have an underlying physical illness, rather than the reverse. Increased vigilance in assessing possible physical contributions is indicated, rather than prematurely attributing the patient's complaints to their psychiatric disorder. The case study in Box 25.2 is illustrative of the difficulties people with a major mental illness can face when a coincidental pain problem arises.

When depressed, a person's judgement is clouded by a very bleak, pessimistic outlook, a withdrawn, narrow focus, such that the person has difficulty concentrating and conceptualizing, and difficulty shifting focus sufficiently to accurately interpret new information. This point is illustrated by the case study in Box 25.3.

PRE-EXISTING FACTORS PREDISPOSING TO BOTH CHRONIC PAIN AND PSYCHIATRIC DISORDERS

A person's chronic pain and behaviour may be affected by psychosocial factors, many of which are present well before the onset of the pain. This psychosocial contribution to a person's pain is consistent with the IASP definition of pain and with the knowledge of the interaction between

---

Box 25.2 **Case study: Mrs DB**

Mrs DB had been at an international conference in Europe. Post-conference, she sustained a fractured humerus after a bicycle accident. Her arm was set and she returned home. She went to her GP for further management. Her regular doctor was unavailable, so she was seen by another doctor.

He couldn't understand why she was in pain. The surgery had a computer system which allowed the doctor to see what medications she was prescribed. He saw that she was taking some psychotropic medication and asked who her psychiatrist was.

Mrs DB couldn't understand that he needed to speak with the psychiatrist as it was her arm that was broken and not her head. He inferred that the pain she was experiencing was due to her mental illness.

He sent her for an X-ray, commenting that if she insisted on being referred to an orthopaedic surgeon he would do this, but that he was too busy that day to make the referral.

She became angry and decided that she wouldn't push the matter with this doctor.

The pain did not abate and eventually she rang the surgery for a referral to an orthopaedic surgeon after her family and friends insisted that she do this.

Fortunately, she was seen quickly by the orthopaedic surgeon, who expressed surprise at how the bone had been set, and told her that if she had left it much longer she would have had irreversible damage in her left arm. He operated the next day, placing two pins in the break.

Mrs DB was impressed at how the orthopaedic surgeon explained the pros and cons of operating prior to the operation and included her in the decision-making process. This involvement allowed her to own the outcome and the rehabilitation process involved.

The surgeon carefully explained to Mrs DB the possible risks involved in surgery and took considerable time in fully explaining these risks. Mrs DB felt like any other person with a broken arm and not a person with a mental illness with a broken arm.

This was in stark contrast to the way Mrs DB felt after her encounter with the GP.

Box 25.3 **Case study**

A gentleman sat with a handkerchief carefully laid out between the hem of his shorts and his legs, because he found the discomfort of the touch of his shorts against his legs quite intolerable.

He had a recurring unipolar depressive illness, and complained of headache, chest pain and many other physical symptoms with each episode, with relief coinciding with effective treatment of his depression.

It was as if he became exquisitely aware of his body whenever he was depressed.

physical and psychosocial factors as explained in the gate control theory of pain (Melzack & Wall 1965), albeit rare in our experience.

Problems such as family dysfunction, abuse (substance, emotional, physical, sexual), unemployment, personal and family illness, poverty, isolation and deprivation are all over-represented in the histories of chronic pain patients (Feuerstein et al 1985; Goldberg et al 1999; Katon et al 1985). Such predisposing problems may result in the patient taking excessive risks, insufficient attention to personal welfare and isolation. However, such problems may not have any strong intrinsic link with pain. In fact, they may often arise because of independent concomitant difficulties and the same problems occur as complications of other physical or psychological disorders – if not as some of their causes. A sense of entrapment, and perceived loss of control over one's destiny and well-being, may lead to 'fight or flight' defences, including depression and anxiety, dependency or over-activity, instability and aggression. Patients may be distrustful and reluctant to accept reasonable advice regarding well-being, their pain becoming a symbol of ongoing dissatisfaction and conflict with the world.

People who have been disadvantaged in life are more likely to have occupations and lifestyles with higher rates of injury and illness, and often have fewer personal, financial and social resources to cope with these experiences. In fact, nearly all physical and psychological illnesses occur more frequently in lower socioeconomic groups. For example, illiteracy is often associated with considerable early life disruption and is over-represented among patients with chronic pain. The disadvantage of illiteracy is magnified considerably when needing to participate in learning processes that are required for rehabilitation. It is worthwhile considering the mechanisms by which these factors can impact on a person. A person who is stressed, insecure and distracted does not learn well. Unhelpful attitudes and habits may be acquired. This limits the person's ability to develop the academic, vocational, personal and social skills and resources that would best equip her for life.

The predisposing factors may not have actually caused any problems, distress or dysfunction before the illness or accident, especially as people very often develop coping strategies. However, these factors do make people vulnerable while still able to continue functioning, in the same manner as rust affects a car. At the moment of illness or accident, with the preoccupation of the immediate trauma, the importance of pre-existing factors is often not considered, even though the impact of the trauma is worse because of them.

Accepting a particular behaviour as predisposing to problems can be difficult for a patient, especially if a person previously had a very high level of functioning, such as working 16 hours per day, 6 days per week, sick or not. This socially encouraged behaviour might conceal significant problems with pacing, time-management, self-care, anxiety, excessive worry about others' approval or poor management skills.

Many people disregard the effects of earlier life experiences, focusing only on the physical aspects of pain. Others become very sensitive to further disruptions to life, and may find it difficult to muster and maintain the personal strength necessary to confront and deal with further problems.

In the health system, the dependency of the socially accepted sick role can be a welcome refuge from life's cruelty, especially as the price of continuing illness may remain hidden. Unfortunately, at times the supports offered, such as compensation payments, can have the unintended effect of prolonging illness, a contradiction that continues to trouble society at large.

Therapies aimed at improving function, when accepted, can have a powerful effect in overcoming any sense of threat, in turn decreasing levels of depression, anxiety and anger in the patient. The benefits of occupational therapy and physiotherapy in relieving the emotional distress experienced by patients should not be underrated.

The case study in Box 25.4 illustrates the unexpected ways in which the crisis of a pain syndrome can uncover pre-morbid psychopathology, which then requires treatment in its own right.

CHRONIC PAIN CAUSING PSYCHIATRIC DISORDERS

In its own right, pain is a potent cause of depression, particularly when combined with a disability that presents a series of losses – job, lifestyle, friends, interests, income, status, etc. Hopelessness, helplessness and fear of the future become major challenges, along with frustration and irritability, which in turn tend to worsen the situation by discouraging those offering help. Insomnia, fatigue, poor appetite and limited activity, as well as many prescribed medications, can have a biological 'depressogenic' effect.

Box 25.4 **Case study: AM**

AM was a 35-year-old rock musician. Her career was terminated by a debilitating forearm pain and weakness. Occupational overuse syndrome was diagnosed. She faced the grief of losing not only her career, but also the joy of playing the keyboards. She changed to a career of sound engineering, and made some adjustment to her loss, with gradual alleviation of her arm pain.

In the course of treatment, AM revealed intermittent self-mutilation, stormy arguments with her partner and intense mood swings. Psychiatric assessment revealed an atypical dissociative disorder, with significant early childhood sexual abuse.

She engaged in long-term psychotherapy, which helped her gradually integrate her fragmented memories, and she settled into a more stable pattern and relationship with her partner.

Very often people remain focused on treatments that may have been unsuccessful, inappropriate or even substandard. People become desperate and vulnerable. Judgement may be impaired due to distress and fear, and people may accept approaches offering very dubious promises of return of their health, hopes and wealth.

SPECIFIC PSYCHIATRIC SYNDROMES AND PAIN

Adjustment disorder

Learning to live with pain is a major task. It is remarkable how well most people with chronic pain succeed with this, and most often without any specific professional help. This reflects a general acceptance of some changes, such as ageing and 'wear and tear', with change being less threatening when not premature, sudden, unexplained or surrounded by conflict, and when occurring in the context of a good life.

The risk factors for an adjustment disorder are essentially the same as for morbid grief. Unrelated personal issues, such as family role changes, might inadvertently reinforce an unhelpful pattern of behaviour. Although people may have entitlements to financial support and compensation in some circumstances, there is ongoing concern regarding the effects of compensation and litigation processes on the welfare of the individual involved. Experience suggests that, at best, such involvement does not improve the physical and psychological well-being of patients and, at worst, such involvement may result in increased pain and disability, and delayed recovery (Greenough & Fraser 1988; Fraser 1996).

A feature of adjustment disorders is emotional distress, which is more severe and/or prolonged than would usually

be expected, especially if the distress becomes worse or interferes with a person's recovery process.

Other manifestations of the disorder can be detected from an understanding of a reasonable and recommended process of adjustment to permanent impairment and suffering. People with chronic pain are more likely to be physically, mentally and socially underactive. They may occasionally be overactive, as if attempting to deny and defy their predicament.

The lack of a widely accepted model for appropriate adjustment to chronic pain has led to some justified criticism of diagnosing an adjustment disorder. It is understandably difficult to cope with chronic pain, but pain is not considered a psychiatric disorder.

Medical practitioners are commonly not aware of, or do not take into account, the important differences between acute and chronic pain. However, it may be reasonable to use the diagnosis of adjustment disorder because it refers to a pattern of behaviour that interferes with the patient's task of reorganizing life to maximize his or her potential for functioning, and carries considerable risk of future harm. Treatment involves identifying the points where a person's progress has departed from that which would be most likely to give the best long-term result, identifying the reasons for the departure and addressing these.

Lack of appropriate information about pain management is the most common reason for adjustment difficulties. Hence, pain education programmes can be very useful. Associated personal and social problems can be dealt with in the usual way, with the occasional use of psychotropic medication to ease distress, to allow attention to the process of learning how to develop a new life.

Adjustment disorders can become complicated by the development of other disorders such as depression. Depressive disorders are differentiated from adjustment disorders by being more intense and pervasive, and not necessarily related to the issues of pain and disability, although most often they are related to pain when it is present.

Depression

Patients with chronic pain are often depressed (Brown 1990; Kerns & Haythornthwaite 1988; Rudy et al 1988). The actual incidence of depression among pain patients varies, with reports ranging from 10 to 100% (Brown 1990; Magni 1987; Rudy et al 1988; Turk et al 1987). Merskey (1999) has suggested that the prevalence of depression in people with pain is approximately 10–30%, while the incidence of depression in the general population ranges from 9 to 14% (Turk et al 1987). It is likely that the variance observed in surveys reflects different inclusion and exclusion criteria, different definitions of 'depression' and the use of different survey tools.

Some would argue that depression is commonly underdiagnosed in patients with chronic pain, and that treating patients with antidepressants significantly relieves chronic pain. Others point out that some antidepressants are also analgesic agents (e.g. amitriptyline), and that the mild, grumbling depression seen in chronic pain is not the same as the primary depression seen in psychiatric clinics. Very frequently, the presenting picture is a manifestation of grief, demoralization, disillusionment and frustration, rather than a typical melancholic depression. However, these psychological responses can lead on to the development of the more typical pattern of 'biological' depression, especially if a person is also genetically predisposed.

Many different measures have been used to detect depression in the patient with chronic pain. The Beck Depression Inventory (BDI) (Beck 1967; Beck et al 1961) and the Zung Self Rating Depression Scale (Zung 1965) are sensitive and specific, and correctly classify according to a DSM III (American Psychiatric Association 1980) diagnosis (Turner & Romano 1984). However, the problem with these measures is that they contain somatic items that are also commonly associated with chronic pain and disability, even in the absence of depression, raising the issue of their appropriateness for a chronic pain population (Love & Peck 1987; Merskey 1999; Turk et al 1987).

Although there has been much discussion about which comes first, the depression or the chronic pain, recent research supports the view that depression mostly develops after or concurrently with pain, rather than preceding it (Cohen & Marx 1993; Fishbain et al 1997; Merskey 1999). Fishbain et al (1997) have thoroughly reviewed this issue and concluded that the evidence for pain causing depression is quite strong, while the evidence that depression causes pain is relatively weak, although there is some support for the 'scar' hypothesis, that previous depression may predispose patients to recurrence of depression if they develop pain.

The primary focus of intervention may depend upon which problem is more severe and troublesome for the patient: the pain or the depression. However, because the pain itself can have such a profound effect on a person's mood, it is useful to not prescribe antidepressant therapy before there has been an attempt to treat the underlying physical disorder and the pain. The case study in Box 25.5 illustrates this point.

However, the clinical situation is frequently such that removal of the pain and return to normal ability and lifestyle is not possible. In such situations, treatment of the depression cannot, and should not, be further delayed once initial physical interventions have been adequately tried.

It is also important to recognize that the management of depression encompasses far more than pharmacotherapy. Depression for people with chronic pain is significantly improved by involvement in a comprehensive pain-management programme (Maruta et al 1989). Cognitive–behavioural therapy (CBT) is a cornerstone to many comprehensive pain-management programmes and is efficacious in the treatment of depression (Flor et al 1992).

Box 25.5 Case study

A 67-year-old lady was experiencing low back pain from osteoporotic crush fractures. She was a widow, lived alone and was relatively isolated in her high-set house.

Not surprisingly, she was depressed, although this was severe with imminent suicidal threat, refusal of food and fluids, rejection of visitors, and intense pessimism and self-criticism, such that her life was in danger from self-harm and neglect.

Urgent ECT was discussed with the patient and her relatives, with trepidation because of the osteoporosis. During the few days of these discussions, a narcotic infusion was introduced.

Not only did she obtain relief from the pain after being given adequate analgesia, but her usual mood also returned to the extent that even antidepressant medication was no longer required.

The challenge is to find the right balance of pharmacological and non-pharmacological therapies.

Therapists must be aware of the suicide risk that may be present for patients who have depression in association with chronic pain. Talk about 'the future seeming hopeless' or 'ending all this pain', should never be minimized or disregarded. Messages of distress should be recognized, potential suicide risks evaluated and concerns reported to the patient's doctor.

Therapists need to be aware that *enquiring* about these issues with patients is unlikely to *cause* them to attempt suicide, whereas *not enquiring* may lead to a serious risk going undetected. The case study in Box 25.6 illustrates the importance of secondary depression arising in a patient with chronic pain, and the danger of suicide.

Anxiety disorders

Anxiety disorders can also be associated with chronic pain, and each can reinforce the other (Gross & Collins 1981). Anxiety makes pain less tolerable, and for many anxious patients it is the anxiety about the pain itself that becomes the major source of distress and the main stumbling block to rehabilitation.

This anxiety may present as a heightened state of tension, with persistent worrying without an obvious focus (generalized anxiety disorder), with discrete episodes of overwhelming fear and with profound sympathetic arousal (palpitations, sweating, nausea, vomiting, diarrhoea, hyperventilation – panic disorder) and/or 'kinesiophobia'.

Kinesiophobia refers to the fear of activity because of the pain it may cause, particularly if the pain is misinterpreted as a signal of more damage. A major thrust of pain-management programmes is to help patients overcome their fear of movement and/or re-injury, and to correctly

---

Box 25.6 Case study: Mr Brown

Mr Brown was a 45-year-old farmer, married, with three children ranging from 5 to 10 years old. He sustained a lifting injury while baling hay 5 years ago. A disc herniation was shown on imaging and he had back surgery that failed to relieve his pain. He became progressively more disabled, with continuing pain and restriction in activities. He sold his farm because he felt incapable of the tough physical work involved.

He continued to search for a surgical solution to his pain and shied away from offers of non-interventional pain management. When first seen in the pain clinic he was depressed, with continuous ruminations about his pain, loss of appetite, sleep disturbance and suicidal ideation (but he said he would not act on these ideas because of his commitment to his children).

He was also highly kinesiophobic and had become physically deconditioned.

He declined treatment for depression because he did not feel he should have to 'accept' his pain. Management consisted of further orthopaedic consultation, where the surgeon fully discussed the surgical facts and confronted him with the reality that further surgery would not cure his pain.

When reviewed in the pain clinic his depression was worse, he was anhedonic and he showed the slowing of talk and movement seen in severe depression (psychomotor retardation). He had, however, reached the point of accepting that his pain was chronic and expressed a willingness to attend an intensive 4-week programme of pain management involving education, relaxation and activation.

In the initial week of the programme, staff felt that his depression was limiting his ability to participate and benefit from the programme. He was prescribed an antidepressant, but he did not take it. Consistent with his work ethic, and now with improved judgement as the result of the counselling with the surgeon, he elected instead to throw himself more fully into the programme. He also began sharing more of his personal anguish in individual and group sessions.

Within another week his mood started lifting and he made rapid progress in the gym, with significant gains in activity levels by the end of 4 weeks. At 1-month follow-up, he was smiling, animated and actively planning his return to work, now managing his back pain much better.

---

interpret the pains they continue to experience as not necessarily indicating disaster.

Sometimes the withdrawal and loss of confidence associated with pain can lead to the onset of a more generalized social phobia and agoraphobia, and in children to school phobia. Occasionally, when the underlying disorder is adequately treated and when the 'nociception' is reduced or better controlled, the learned phobic behaviours persist regardless. Unless these problems are recognized, therapists may be puzzled as to why patients remain reluctant to leave their house or to try suggested therapy activities.

Post-traumatic stress disorders

The events of an accident, illness or treatment can lead to a post-traumatic stress disorder (PTSD), particularly if people regard themselves as having been in a life-threatening situation, with no sense of control.

The experience of ongoing pain, particularly when it is poorly controlled and interferes with a person's normal functioning, is a major obstacle to a person regaining the confidence to recover from PTSD. Pain management is difficult, as each new advance in a person's therapy involves confronting a reminder of their trauma, potentially arousing considerable distress, particularly with 'flashbacks' that intrude and overwhelm the person's consciousness. In cases of PTSD, patients may have the experience of 'reliving' the events which caused the pain. They may have panic

attacks and nightmares about the event, and they may have a pervasive fear of being hurt.

Up to 10% of patients with chronic pain may have features of PTSD (Muse 1985). Pilowsky (1985) has written about 'crypto trauma', referring to those cases where a significant psychological trauma has gone unrecognized because of the emphasis on the physical presentation. The case study in Box 25.7 illustrates this situation.

The circumstances of injury and its immediate consequences can have long-standing effects on the course of recovery. DeGood and Kiernan (1996) have found that people who attribute blame to others have a worse prognosis

---

Box 25.7 Case study

A plumber fell off a roof and injured his back. It was not until the detailed history of the accident was taken that it was revealed he had clung to the guttering for approximately half an hour before he lost his grip and fell. He had struggled in this time to climb back onto the roof, all the while only too aware of the height of the drop.

His reluctance to return to roofing was understandable in light of his history, although before more detailed consideration he had attributed his difficulty returning to work to his pain, despite reasonable functional recovery.

There are many aspects of this man's frightening experience that would have 'hurt' him apart from the impact with the ground.

---

than those who do not. Even though at times a person does suffer because of the actions of others, a person needs to accept at least some degree of responsibility for their own future welfare, no matter what the original cause of their problems. This acceptance is vital for successful rehabilitation. It involves the patient adopting an approach where she perceives her 'locus of control' as being within her own resources, has the confidence that she can actually *do* things and can make things happen rather than relying on others.

In the therapeutic relationship, the essential element in deciding an appropriate approach is what is in the best long-term interests of the patient, especially in terms of functioning. It may be necessary to use some temporary compromises along the way. For example, a patient may need to accept some dependency temporarily, such as depending initially on adaptive equipment or the advice of professionals. She can then become increasingly independent. If the treatment does not assist progress towards this effect, it needs review.

CHRONIC PAIN, SUBSTANCE ABUSE AND DEPENDENCE

The issue of substance abuse in patients with chronic pain creates many difficulties in management, with prevalence rates for substance abuse in people with chronic pain ranging from 15 to 40% (Cohen 1995).

There is a range of presentations of patients in this category.

Long-standing prior history of illicit drug abuse

Patients with a long-standing prior history of illicit drug abuse, including opioids, are already familiar with the effects of opioids and may have a high tolerance to these medications. Patients who have been alcohol dependent also have a high tolerance for opioids because of the induction of liver enzymes for the metabolism of the alcohol. The consequence of this is that such patients will need higher than usual doses of analgesic medications for acute pain. They are also likely to have a focus on symptom control, with a low tolerance of distress, particularly relying on opioids and benzodiazepines, with all the attendant problems of overuse, abuse and, sometimes, diversion of supplies for trafficking.

The physical focus of such patients may be in the context of very limited social skills, problem-solving skills and personal skills, frequently with a distorted sense of responsibility and entitlement, and low levels of self-esteem and confidence, although of course no one pattern exists for all cases. People with these problems are usually rather

'damaged' and present extra difficulties in management, with less likelihood of resolving problems by themselves.

Patients who have a history of drug abuse or alcohol addiction prior to the onset of chronic pain have an increased risk of developing addiction when taking opioids for pain. In these cases, analgesic medications need to be offered with extra supervision to ensure appropriate pain management and reduce the risk of inappropriate drug use.

When working with patients with chronic pain who have a history of illicit drug abuse, therapists should be aware of the potential additional issues of transmissible infectious diseases associated with physical contact, especially if this involves body fluids such as blood or chest secretions.

Prior history of inappropriate use of prescription drugs

Prescription drugs include analgesic and hypnotic-sedative medications, most notably the benzodiazepines group. People misusing these drugs may have similar limitations in the personal skills required to solve their own difficulties and tend to depend inappropriately on 'external agencies', including medication, rather than developing their own non-pharmaceutical approaches. But others among them can justifiably claim to have been given the drugs on appropriate prediction and to have developed tolerance that leads them to need increased dosages. It may be futile and inappropriate to attempt withdrawal, and to encourage use of such approaches requires considerable explanation and encouragement, often because these patients lack confidence, experience excessive self-criticism, and have a substantial and partly warranted fear of failure.

Clinicians working in the area of pain need to be as knowledgeable as possible about the effects, short-term and long-term, of analgesic medications. They also need to understand the distinctions between proper use and abuse, drug dependence, addiction and 'pseudo addiction'.

Some early evaluations of pain-management programmes showed that drug withdrawal alone, without any other therapy, resulted in significant improvements in well-being and a reduction in the pain experienced. These findings convinced many workers that chronic management called for analgesic withdrawal in most cases. This view has been challenged by clinicians experienced in cancer pain management, who have campaigned against the under-usage of opioids (Portenoy & Foley 1986). Their view is that some patients with chronic pain of non-malignant origin may be denied adequate pain control if opioids are withheld.

The few systematic and controlled studies done in this area offer only limited support to the hope that ongoing opioid therapy would be effective for chronic pain of non-malignant origin. The situation is currently unproven. Nevertheless, limited use of moderate doses of long-acting forms, especially fentanyl patches, may be of use for some and, where legally permitted, the same may apply to other opioids, particularly those with a long half-life, like methadone.

Patients may wait until their pain is severe before taking medication, thinking this to be the right approach, but then use excessively large doses because of the increased pain severity at a time when their ability to tolerate it has been exhausted. This approach is more likely to involve patients in an unstable 'boom and bust' approach, with a tendency to be excessively preoccupied by their experience, rather than being able to focus their intentions and energies on functioning and the future (Butler & Moseley 2003; McCracken & Samuel 2007).

Patients may have been advised by multiple specialists, who may have adopted different approaches and prescribed different medications. Caution is needed at times, as patients with chronic pain who are not using their medication properly may be unfairly regarded as having a problem with addiction, although taking this medication might be at the direction of the prescriber (Fuchs & Gamsa 1997).

Addiction to medication occurs when a person who is taking medication seeks opioid medication to achieve a psychological high rather than pain relief. This process may involve physical dependence, as indicated by the development of tolerance, with a decreasing effect from the same dose and a physical withdrawal syndrome if the medication is ceased abruptly.

A well-balanced comprehensive management plan is important. Any single focus approach, whether medication or a particular form of therapy, poses the risk of inappropriate dependency by suggesting that there are no other solutions.

Unfortunately, such situations usually reflect good intentions, but indicate a lack of knowledge and appropriate judgement of both the patient and the practitioner with respect to the management of chronic pain disorders. Often remedies that are appropriate for short-term disorders can have unrecognized and unwarranted complications when applied to long-term conditions. In short-term situations such complications are inconsequential, easily tolerated, with quick recovery. Over the long term, such complications have a much greater cumulative effect.

SOMATOFORM DISORDERS

The somatoform disorders are a group of disorders in which the physical complaints are the major presenting focus of the patient, but where the major difficulty is thought to be psychological. The Diagnostic and Statistical Manual (DSM IV) of the American Psychiatric Association (1994) includes pain disorder in this group, but with diagnostic criteria which make it possible to fit most people with chronic pain into this category (Merskey 1988). Historically, this was 'hysteria'. The concept of hysterical

bodily pain should probably be dropped as a misdiagnosis of regional musculoskeletal pain (Merskey 2004).

Pain disorder

The DSM IV criteria signify a pain disorder as:

- pain presenting in one or more sites
- pain causing clinically significant distress and impairment
- pain in which psychological factors play a role
- experiencing symptoms that are not intentional
- pain for which there is no other psychiatric disorder that better accounts for the pain.

Unfortunately this definition is so broad that it is arguably of little use. Also, the attribution of psychological factors is now largely unwarranted.

Conversion disorder

Some people present with conversion disorders, which involve a loss of function related to somatic nervous control, such as paralysis, anaesthesia, blindness, deafness, aphonia, etc. Great care is needed when diagnosing these situations. For example, features such as paralysis may be associated with pain secondary to poor posture. The hallmark of conversion disorder is its sudden onset in relation to conflict or emotional trauma, and its symptoms typically resolve a problem for the patient. Box 25.8 outlines an example of this.

It was previously considered that some pain syndromes were manifestations of a conversion disorder. We recognize that we really do not have the expertise to precisely separate psychological and physical contributions to a person's pain, but it is now considered inappropriate to regard pain as a conversion disorder.

Somatization disorder

A more extreme presentation of the somatoform disorders is somatization disorder. This term is used to describe a presentation previously labelled 'Briquet's syndrome', and has been included in older descriptions of 'hysteria'.

Box 25.8 Case study

One patient developed a sudden onset of paraplegia immediately after her first attempt at Christian witnessing. She knocked on a door; no one opened it, after which she experienced relief, but then immediate guilt. She felt giddy and her paraplegia commenced. Her symptoms effectively ended her continuing witnessing, even though, despite exhaustive investigation, no physical explanation was revealed.

Essentially, this is a pattern of presenting with physical complaints involving multiple organ systems, including pain. Repeated examinations and investigations fail to show sufficient organic cause to explain the extent of the symptoms.

Psychosocial evaluation usually reveals a history of interpersonal problems, emotional deprivation in childhood and past abuse, including sexual abuse. This pattern is recognized more often in women. The presentation of physical symptoms is thought to be a manifestation of abnormal illness behaviour, in which the need for care is expressed through illness.

Regular evaluation, at the same time limiting the number of investigations performed to those that have a clear medical indication rather than as a continuing attempt to appease the patient, appears to contain these patients, perhaps preventing iatrogenic harm, but it does little to change the underlying dynamics. These patients usually do not respond to any radical treatment but benefit from a supportive approach which, without denying their symptoms, encourages them to manage within their limits.

Factitious disorders

Uncommonly, there are dramatic presentations of illness in patients who deliberately induce symptoms and who falsify investigations to gain care (Kelly & Loader 1997). Those with factitious disorders have a complex motivation to enter the sick role and may go to extremes by swallowing sharp objects, taking medications, adding blood to urine, etc. to mimic a clinical syndrome. This is otherwise known as 'Munchausen's syndrome', as described by Asher (1951).

In 'Munchausen's by proxy', a caregiver induces signs and symptoms in a child. This is considered a form of child abuse. Fabricated signs and symptoms may be physical, such as rashes, seizures, facial pain or headaches, but in some cases the fabricated signs and symptoms will be characteristic of psychiatric disease, such as reporting of multiple personalities, delusions and hallucinations (Schreier 1997; Solomon & Lipton 1999).

Malingering has similar manifestations and presentations, the difference being a demonstration that the deliberate presentation of illness is motivated by material gain, such as obtaining money or being excused from duty, rather than by more obscure personal motivation.

Diagnosis of factitious disorder and malingering can be difficult. Suspicion can be aroused by inconsistencies, although it is important not to prematurely come to such a conclusion as there are many other potential explanations for inconsistencies between expectations and observations.

With chronic pain management, a focus on functioning is important, rather than only on symptom relief. For example, contrary to popular belief, prolonged rest can be very harmful, disabling and potentially fatal. Physical interventions, particularly if there is a likelihood of irreversible consequences, such as with surgery, need to be based on an identified physical disorder, rather than responding only on the basis of the person's level of distress. The more speculative the understanding of the physical basis, the greater the risk of failure. The more classical the syndrome, the better the result is likely to be.

'DIFFICULT PATIENTS' OR PATIENTS WITH DIFFICULT PROBLEMS?

Difficult patient behaviour may be a relationship problem between the professional and the patient, which is exacerbated by the subjectivity of pain, the apparent inconsistencies between the pain complaint and the pain behaviour, poor communications, frustration and resentment at times because of difficulties dealing with the sense of failure following a patient's lack of progress (DeGood & Dane 1996).

DeGood & Dane (1996) suggested four principles to guide interaction with patients:

1. Therapists need to recognize that patients may complain about their pain until they feel they have been heard and taken seriously.
2. Therapists should avoid treating all patients with pain in a stereotypical and automated fashion. Taking the time to understand the patient and his or her context is important to avoid misunderstanding.
3. Therapists need to avoid personalizing or blaming other health professionals or patients for failures. It is important to decide on first-hand information where possible, rather than other people's recall, perspectives and interpretations of what transpired. Therapists also need to learn to accept their own limitations and the need for review, revision and/or referral when progress stops prematurely.
4. Therapists need to remember that changes in behaviour and functioning are likely to be gradual and incremental. Realistic expectations are important for both therapists and patients. Therapists need to be mindful that their own experiences and preferences may influence their reactions to the problems with which the patients present.

CONCLUSION

The vast majority of people with chronic pain are honest, well intentioned and well motivated, but have difficulty managing their pain, particularly because they have not yet made the appropriate life adjustments to their new state. The fact that they have attended probably indicates that they are receptive to advice, but it is important not to expect rapid change. It is often only with the proof that comes from actual performance, especially when carefully guided by an occupational therapist and/or physiotherapist, that such people regain confidence, optimism and a willingness to take the ordinary risks necessary to emerge from one's 'comfort zone' to again enjoy life.

Understanding the contribution of psychiatry to pain management means understanding the essence of psychiatric methods. This means listening carefully, setting aside preconceptions, 'bracketing' one's biases and attempting to stand in the other person's shoes. Only when this has been done are we free to relate the individual's story to the pattern of presentations built by descriptions documented over the past century.

Health professionals need to use reflection to ensure that their assessment and management strategies are influenced by patient need, rather than by the bias that all people, including therapists, inevitably have.

The relationship between psychiatric illness and pain is complex. The challenge for clinicians is to deal with the main complaint in the context of the person's understanding and reaction to his or her predicament, while still taking physical factors into account.

Management of chronic pain is unfortunately often bedevilled by attempts to distinguish between the components of the disorder. Studies demonstrate a very high degree of overlap between the psychiatric and physical diagnosis, which suggests that it is far more practical to consider both psychiatric and physical morbidity concurrently when assessing patients with pain. Pain is pain, and attempting to tease out the causation in a dualistic framework does little to predict appropriate management for the patient. It is more feasible to assess each dimension on its merits and to develop a management approach addressing each of the issues concurrently.

Q   Study questions/questions for revision

1. In what way can the onset of pain as a result of physical illness contribute to a psychiatric problem?
2. Describe the relationship between chronic pain and psychiatric illness.
3. What should you do if a patient with chronic pain whom you are treating refers to a desire to 'end it all'?
4. You are referred a patient with chronic pain and you are unable to find a demonstrable pathology to explain the pain complaint, despite repeated assessment and treatment sessions. What should you do next?

REFERENCES

American Psychiatric Association, 1980. Diagnostic and Statistical Manual of Mental Disorders, third ed. American Psychiatric Association, Washington, DC.

American Psychiatric Association, 1994. Diagnostic and Statistical Manual of Mental Disorders, fourth ed. American Psychiatric Association, Washington, DC.

Asher, R., 1951. Munchausen's syndrome. Lancet 1, 339–341.

Beck, A.T., 1967. Depression: Causes and Treatment. University of Pennsylvania Press, Philadelphia.

Beck, A.T., Ward, C.H., Medelson, M., et al., 1961. An inventory for measuring depression. Arch. Gen. Psychiatry. 4, 561–571.

Brown, G.K., 1990. A causal analysis of chronic pain and depression. J. Abnorm. Psychol. 99, 127–137.

Butler, D.S., Moseley, G.L., 2003. Explain Pain. Noigroup Publications, Adelaide.

Cohen, M.J., 1995. Psychosocial aspects of evaluation and management of chronic low back pain. Physical Medicine and Rehabilitation 9, 725–746.

Cohen, J.M., Marx, M.C., 1993. Pain and depression in the nursing home: corroborating results. J. Gerontol. 48, 96–97.

DeGood, D.E., Dane, J.R., 1996. The psychologist as a pain consultant in outpatient, inpatient, and workplace settings. In: Gatchel, R.J., Turk, D.C. (Eds.), Psychological Approaches to Pain Management – A practitioner's handbook. Guilford Press, London, pp. 403–437.

DeGood, D.E., Kiernan, B., 1996. Perception of fault in patients with chronic pain. Pain. 64, 153–159.

Dworkin, R.H., Caligor, E., 1988. Psychiatric diagnosis and chronic pain: DSM-III-R and beyond. J. Pain Symptom Manage. 3, 87–98.

Feuerstein, M., Sult, S., Houle, M., 1985. Environmental stressors and chronic low back pain: life events, families and work environment. Pain. 22, 295–307.

Fishbain, D.A., Cutler, R., Rosomoff, H.L., et al., 1997. Chronic pain-associated depression: antecedant or consequence of chronic pain? A review. Clin. J. Pain. 13, 116–137.

Flor, H., Fydrich, T., Turk, D.C., 1992. Efficacy of multidisciplinary pain treatment centres: a meta-analytic review. Pain 49, 221–230.

Fraser, R.D., 1996. Compensation and recovery from injury. Med. J. Aust. 165, 71–72.

Fuchs, P.N., Gamsa, A., 1997. Chronic use of opioids for nonmalignant pain: a prospective study. Pain Res. Manag. 2, 101–107.

Goldberg, R.T., Pachas, W.N., Keith, D., 1999. Relationship between traumatic events in childhood and chronic pain. Disabil. Rehabil. 21, 23–30.

Greenough, C.G., Fraser, R.D., 1988. The effects of compensation on recovery of low back injury. Spine. 14, 947–955.

Gross, R.T., Collins, F.L., 1981. On the relationship between anxiety and pain: a methodological confounding. Clin. Psychol. Rev. 1, 375–386.

Katon, W., Egan, K., Miller, D., 1985. Chronic pain: lifetime psychiatric diagnoses and family history. Am. J. Psychiatry 142, 1156–1160.

Kelly, C., Loader, P., 1997. Factitious disorder by proxy: the role of the child mental health professionals. Child Psychology and Psychiatry Review 2, 116–124.

Kerns, R.D., Haythornthwaite, J.A., 1988. Depression among chronic pain patients: cognitive–behavioural analysis and effect on rehabilitation outcome. J. Consult. Clin. Psychol. 56, 870–876.

Large, R.G., 1986. DSM-III Diagnoses in chronic pain: confusion or clarity. J. Nerv. Ment. Dis. 174, 295–303.

Love, A.W., Peck, D.L., 1987. The MMPI and psychological factors in chronic low back pain: a review. Pain 28, 1–12.

Magni, G., 1987. On the relationship between chronic pain and depression when there is no organic lesion. Pain 31, 1–21.

Maruta, T., Vatterott, M.K., McHardy, M.J., 1989. Pain management as an antidepressant: long-term resolution of pain-associated depression. Pain 36, 335–337.

McCracken, L., Samuel, V.M., 2007. The role of avoidance, pacing, and other activity patterns in chronic pain. Pain 130, 119–125.

Melzack, R., Wall, P.D., 1965. Pain mechanisms; a new theory. Science 150, 971–976.

Merskey, H., 1988. Regional pain is rarely hysterical. Arch. Neurol. 45, 915–918.

Merskey, H., 1999. Pain and psychological medicine. In: Wall, P.D., Melzack, R. (Eds.), Textbook of Pain. fourth ed. Churchill Livingstone, New York, pp. 929–949.

Merskey, H., 2004. Pain disorder: hysteria or somatization. Pain Res. Manag. 9, 67–71.

Merskey, H., Spear, F.G., 1967. Pain: Psychological and Psychiatric Aspects. Baillière Tindall & Cassell, London.

Muse, M., 1985. Stress-related, posttraumatic chronic pain syndrome: criteria for diagnosis and preliminary report on prevalence. Pain 23, 295–300.

Pilowsky, I., 1985. Cryptotrauma and 'accident neurosis'. Br. J. Psychiatry. 147, 310–311.

Portenoy, R.K., Foley, K.M., 1986. Opioid therapy for chronic nonmalignant pain. Pain Res. Manag. 1, 17–28.

Rudy, T.E., Kerns, R.D., Turk, D.C., 1988. Chronic pain and depression: toward a cognitive–behavioural model. Pain. 35, 129–140.

Schreier, H.A., 1997. Factitious presentation of psychiatric disorder: when is it Munchausen by proxy? Child Psychology and Psychiatry Review 2, 108–115.

Solomon, S., Lipton, R.B., 1999. Headaches and face pains as a manifestation of Munchausen syndrome. Headache 39, 45–50.

Spear, F.G., 1967. Pain in psychiatric patients. J. Psychosom. Res. 11, 187–193.

Turk, D.C., Rudy, T.E., Steig, R.L., 1987. Chronic pain and depression: I 'Facts'. Pain Management 1, 17–26.

Turner, J.A., Romano, J.M., 1984. Self-report screening measures for depression in chronic pain patients. J. Clin. Psychol. 40, 909–913.

Whitlock, F.A., 1967. The aetiology of hysteria. Acta Psychiatr. Scand. 43, 144–162.

Zung, W.W.K., 1965. A self-rating depression scale. Arch. Gen. Psychiatry 12, 63–70.

Chapter 26

Acute pain

Stephan A. Schug, Deborah Watson and Esther M. Pogatzki-Zahn

LEARNING OBJECTIVES

At the end of this chapter readers will have an understanding of:

1. The principles underlying acute pain management for post-operative patients.
2. Various pharmacological options for pain management, including the use of systemic opioid and non-opioid analgesics.
3. Principles, benefits and potential problems relating to patient-controlled analgesia.
4. Regional techniques for analgesia.
5. Some non-pharmacological options for pain management, including physical and cognitive treatment techniques.
6. The role of an acute pain service in dealing with post-operative pain.

OVERVIEW

Acute pain is seen in a multitude of clinical situations: in the post-operative and post-trauma setting, following burns, in acute medical diseases (e.g. pancreatitis, myocardial infarction) and as obstetric pain. Post-operative pain is the most common form of acute pain (and of major relevance for therapists), therefore this chapter will direct its focus towards management of post-operative patients.

There is widespread agreement in the literature on the inadequacy of acute pain management. On the other hand, there is also a wide body of evidence which suggests that relief of acute pain is not only an integral part of humane health care, but can also have profound effects on patient outcomes. Only over the last decade has a considerable amount of scientific and clinical effort been invested in providing the patient in acute pain with the best quality analgesia, at the same time ensuring safety from potentially life-threatening adverse events for each modality of analgesia (Macintyre et al 2010).

This chapter focuses on the importance of effective management of acute pain. It incorporates the most important pharmacological and non-pharmacological modalities of analgesia in the treatment of acute pain (for definitions see Box 26.1); reference will be made to comparison of the efficacy, benefits and adverse effects of these modalities. Some of the newer techniques used have accumulated substantial evidence demonstrating an improvement not only in quality of analgesia and patient satisfaction, but also in short- and long-term morbidity, and, potentially, even mortality. In addition, there is now increasing evidence

© 2014 Elsevier Ltd.

Box 26.1 **Key terms defined**

Systemic analgesia: The provision of pain relief by administration of medications systemically, usually by the parenteral, oral, transdermal or rectal route.

Regional analgesia: Techniques which administer local anaesthetics or other adjuvants in such a way that they act locally or regionally, e.g. by administration close to a peripheral nerve or the spinal cord.

Patient-controlled analgesia (PCA): A technique using a programmable infusion device that can be activated by the patient to deliver small bolus doses of analgesics on demand.

Epidural analgesia: A technique whereby drugs are administered into the epidural space, close to the spinal cord but outside the spinal meninges.

Intrathecal analgesia: A technique whereby drugs are administered into the intrathecal space, close to the spinal cord and inside the meninges.

Pre-emptive analgesia: Techniques administered where it has been shown that preoperative treatment is more effective than the identical treatment being administered after incision or surgery.

Preventive analgesia: An analgesic intervention wherein the effect lasts longer than the expected duration of action of the intervention.

of a relative association between the experience of acute pain and the development of chronic pain. Prevention of such progression is another important goal of adequate acute pain management.

However, despite the theoretical availability of a wide range of appropriate agents and techniques, the cause of poor acute pain management is often their insufficient, inappropriate or unsupervised application. Therefore, the chapter would be incomplete without a discussion of appropriate organizational structures to provide acute pain relief, that is, the concept and the role of the acute pain service.

PRINCIPLES OF ACUTE PAIN MANAGEMENT

Post-operatively, up to 80% of patients experience pain, and it is moderate, severe or extreme in 86% of these cases (Apfelbaum et al 2003). The Apfelbaum et al study also found pain to be the most common concern of patients after surgery (59%). Psychological factors such as pre-operative anxiety, depression, catastrophizing, expectation of pain, fear of death and associated sleep deprivation influence post-operative pain control, and attention must therefore be given to individual patient differences, which may lead to an improved outcome.

Traditionally, post-operative pain has been managed using fixed doses of intramuscularly (IM) administered opioids on an as-needed basis; this treatment approach has led to unrelieved pain in more than 50% of post-operative

patients (Oden 1989). The major problem with this approach is explained by the huge interindividual variation in dose requirements, which can vary more than ten-fold for patients of similar age and weight having the same operation. Furthermore, opioid concentrations following IM bolus doses exhibit a pronounced peak and trough pattern, with periods of inadequate analgesia, but also the associated risk of delayed overdose (Cashman & Dolin 2004).

A more appropriate approach to acute pain management should therefore consider a much wider array of techniques and their combination. These include the following pharmacological options:

- administration of systemic opioids (intravenously [IV], subcutaneously [SC], orally [PO], transmucosally or transdermally) on a regular and/or as-required basis or via patient-controlled analgesia (PCA)
- administration of non-opioid analgesics, such as paracetamol, non-steroidal anti-inflammatory drugs (NSAIDs) and cyclo-oxygenase-2 (COX-2) inhibitors
- administration of other systemic agents that have uses in particular settings, such as nitrous oxide (Entonox), ketamine, adrenergic drugs, antidepressants and anticonvulsants
- neuraxial analgesia (epidural or intrathecal administration of opioid and/or local anaesthetic drugs)
- intermittent or continuous peripheral neural blockade with local anaesthetic drugs.

Besides these, there are many non-pharmacological options, which are often under-utilized, despite their simplicity:

- explanation, reassurance and discussion of analgesic options
- cognitive–behavioural interventions such as relaxation, distraction and imagery, which can be taught preoperatively
- various physical interventions such as splints, massage, application of heat or cold, acupuncture and transcutaneous electrical nerve stimulation (TENS).

The majority of this chapter focuses on the pharmacological options, discussing their efficacy, benefits, side-effect profiles and combination therapy possibilities with other analgesic agents.

Systemic Pharmocological Modalities

SYSTEMIC OPIOIDS

Systemic opioids are the treatment of choice in the management of moderate to severe acute pain. They include the 'gold-standard' morphine as well as other opioids such as fentanyl, oxycodone, hydromorphone and methadone.

They all bind to opioid receptors within and outside the central nervous system, with the μ-receptor being the most important because of morphine's affinity for it. While this receptor activation explains the analgesic effect of opioids, it also explains most of the adverse effects of these agents, intrinsically linked to their analgesic effect (Schug et al 1992). The most common side effects are nausea and vomiting, sedation, pruritus, slowing of gastrointestinal function (constipation), urinary retention and sometimes – surprisingly – dysphoria (see Chapter 11 for more details). The most serious, but rare, complication of opioid usage is respiratory depression and subsequent hypoxia, which can be potentially life-threatening or even fatal.

Systemic opioids can be given by a wide variety of routes. The decision on which route to use is dependent upon the individual situation of the patient, the acuteness of the pain and the infrastructure of the hospital. The traditional routes of opioid administration are PO, SC and IM, but there is an increasing trend towards IV administration, in particular following opioid protocols or via PCA devices. Other routes of administration, for example transmucosal, intra-nasal and transdermal, are increasingly utilized.

Oral opioids

Oral opioids are an option only after return of gastric motility, that is, when the patient is able to tolerate fluids freely. Evidence suggests that oral opioids are as effective as parenteral opioids in appropriate doses, and should be used as soon as oral medication is tolerated. In such a scenario, this is the route of choice for acute pain management.

Codeine is used widely, but it might not be the drug of choice as its efficacy is limited and some patients (ca. 10%) lack the enzyme needed to generate its active metabolite morphine. On the other hand, subjects carrying a gene duplication are predisposed to life-threatening opioid intoxication (Stamer & Stuber 2007).

One useful alternative to codeine is the compound trama-dol, a centrally acting analgesic with a mixed mechanism of action (opioid, noradrenergic, serotonergic). This mecha-nism of action explains its adverse effect profile, which is dif-ferent from conventional opioids; in particular, there is a reduced risk of respiratory depression, constipation and sedation (Scott & Perry 2000). Furthermore, the abuse potential is lower than that of classical opioids. However, similar to codeine, polymorphisms of the cytochrome P450 enzymes influence the analgesic efficacy of tramadol (Stamer & Stuber 2007).

Morphine itself can be used here, initially often in immediate- (ca. 20 minutes to onset) and short-acting preparations such as morphine elixir or immediate-release tablets. There is an increasing trend to avoid morphine due to some of its untoward effects, in particular its metabolism leading to active metabolites, which can complicate treat-ment, particularly in patients with renal impairment. Strong opioid alternatives in this case are oxycodone and hydromorphone, which lack such metabolites and are available in a wide range of preparations.

Tramadol and all the other opioids mentioned above are available in sustained-release formulations, which, given at defined time intervals, can provide long-term analgesia, in particular once the ongoing need for opioid analgesia in the post-operative and, more commonly, the post-trauma rehabilitation period is established.

The use of pethidine (meperidine) should be discour-aged in acute and chronic pain settings, as it has a high abuse potential and a neurotoxic metabolite that can potentially induce seizures (Latta et al 2002).

Intramuscular opioids

As mentioned above, IM opioids have, until recently, been the mainstay of post-operative pain management using opi-oids. Traditionally, standard doses (commonly '10 mg for everyone') were administered by intermittent IM injections, usually no more frequently than every 4 hours, hence the infamous prescription: '10 mg morphine IM, PRN (as required) 4 hourly'. Such a 'one-dose-fits-all' approach leads to some patients being left in extreme pain and others at risk of suffering from major side effects such as respiratory depression. The incidence of respiratory depression using this route has been found to range from 0.8 to 37% depend-ing on its definition (Cashman & Dolin 2004). In addition, IM injections are painful, disliked by patients, and carry the risk of tissue damage (e.g. to nerves) and infection (e.g. abscesses). Finally, absorption from an IM injection site is slow, unpredictable and delayed by physical factors such as hypothermia, hypovolaemia and immobility, commonly encountered in the early post-operative period.

The current recommendation and standard practice is to avoid this route if at all possible (Macintyre et al 2010). If, for organizational, political or training (better: lack of training) reasons, IM injections are the only parenteral route of administration permitted or – inappropriately – deemed safe in a certain environment, then the dose used should be based on age and medical condition, and the administration interval should be shortened to 2 hourly PRN, to increase flexibility (Macintyre & Schug 2007).

Subcutaneous opioids

Opioids can be given intermittently or as a low-volume continuous infusion via the SC route. The absorption profile is similar to that of IM administration (Semple et al 1997), and both routes have similar analgesic and side-effect profiles. However, patients prefer the SC route, particularly if used via an indwelling SC cannula, for obvious reasons (Cooper 1996). The approach has been shown to be beneficial as a continuous infusion (volu-mes < 1–2 ml/h) in severe cancer pain and in post-operative patients in whom IV access is not, or not easily, available. Morphine and hydromorphone are used preferentially as they are low-irritants to the SC tissue; treatment algorithms in this area have been published (Macintyre & Schug 2007). For patients with an indwelling IV line (i.e. most early post-operative patients), there are no advantages, but some disadvantages (delayed onset of analgesia, second access) of the SC route in comparison to the IV route.

Intravenous opioids

Opioids can be given as boluses (e.g. 0.5–4 mg morphine every 3–5 minutes as directed by a formal IV protocol; Aubrun et al 2001), as a continuous infusion or via PCA devices through the IV route. The IV route is the route of choice following major surgery, but there is a risk of respiratory depression with inappropriate dosing, and close monitoring and safety precautions are therefore required.

Intermittent IV boluses

Intermittent IV boluses provide a rapid, predictable and observable response compared to other parenteral routes. This is the rationale behind use of IV PCA. The IV route is particularly useful for:

- obtaining initial and rapid pain relief such as in the immediate post-operative period and in acute trauma (Aubrun et al 2001)
- patients who are hypovolaemic and/or hypotensive, and will absorb IM/SC opioids in a delayed and unpredictable fashion
- treating so-called 'incident pain' caused by events such as dressing changes, mobilization and physiotherapy.

Intermittent boluses are also an ideal path to titrated pain relief in the recovery room, and bridge times of severe pain until medical review and/or more appropriate analgesic methods become accessible. Most commonly, nurse-administered bolus doses, prescribed according to a protocol or algorithm, are used. Such protocols specify (or permit some flexibility with regard to) bolus size, assessments and 'lock-out' time (Macintyre & Schug 2007).

Continuous IV infusion

This form of infusion avoids the peaks and troughs in blood concentrations associated with intermittent administration, but it has proven difficult to predict the required individual blood concentration for optimal analgesia. A continuous infusion requires reliable infusion devices and frequent assessment and monitoring by staff who are trained to monitor patients with an emphasis on level of sedation, and who are authorized to adjust the infusion rate and give bolus doses. To provide adequate analgesic blood concentrations can take up to 20 hours (five half-lives); consequently, if analgesia is inadequate, a bolus is given as well as the rate of infusion being increased.

The risk of respiratory depression using a continuous morphine infusion (up to 1.65%) is the highest of all parenteral routes (Schug & Torrie 1993). This needs to be considered carefully, as fatal outcomes are reported, in particular in sleeping or sedated patients (Macintyre & Schug 2007).

Patient-controlled analgesia

PCA was introduced to overcome the variability in individual morphine dose requirements and the problems associated with insufficient analgesia and potentially serious adverse outcomes. This is primarily a concept granting a patient control of his/her pain relief, and can be utilized by various routes of systemic and regional drug administration, but is commonly associated with IV drug administration.

A PCA device is a sophisticated, programmable infusion instrument that can be activated by the patient to self-administer small bolus doses of IV opioid on demand, separated by a lock-out period, during which the device does not respond to further activation. As such, the PCA concept overcomes the interindividual variation in opioid requirements, and allows the patient to adjust the level of analgesia to their own desired level of comfort, balanced to an individually acceptable severity of side effects. Intravenous opioids administered by PCA improve analgesia and patient satisfaction (Hudcova et al 2006). It has been demonstrated that, for morphine, a bolus dose of 1 mg with a 5-minute lock-out period is ideal for most patients; other programmes are associated with either inadequate analgesia or sedation and increased respiratory compromise (Owen et al 1989). However, some patients might need different programmes, depending on age, co-morbidity, pain intensity and previous opioid exposure, therefore regular review of all patients using PCA devices by experienced personnel is mandatory for a good outcome. Other opioids such as fentanyl, hydromorphone or tramadol can also be used.

Following surgery, the average patient will require PCA for 2–4 days. Drug consumption is maximal within the first 24 hours and thereafter rapidly declines. Use after abdominal surgery tends to be increased and relatively prolonged (Sidebotham et al 1997), which reflects the major physiological insult and the additional pain associated with mobilization and physiotherapy. Women use 20–30% more morphine early after surgery than men (Aubrun et al 2005), but less morphine thereafter (Sidebotham et al 1997). Age is the best predictor of post-operative opioid requirements (Macintyre & Jarvis 1996), but there is little correlation between patient weight and levels of consumption (Burns et al 1989).

The technique provides effective, steady analgesia and is popular with patients. However, analgesia at rest and on movement is not perfect. About 40% of patients using PCA have a pain score >3/10 at rest on day one post-operatively. The occurrence of unpleasant side effects from increased opioid usage may be responsible for some of this inadequate analgesia, which prevents 20% of patients from complying with physiotherapy on day one post-operatively

(Schug & Fry 1994; Sidebotham et al 1997). It requires special infusion pumps and staff education. In addition, patients require instructions preoperatively to be able to understand the principles underlying the PCA technique and how/when to activate it (Chumbley et al 2002).

Although PCA is the safest method of administering systemic opioids, there still remains a small risk of respiratory depression (incidence in the range 0.1–0.8%) (Macintyre 2001). This risk is much smaller than that associated with continuous IV infusion or intermittent IM injection. This advantage with regard to safety is due to the fact that acute pain causes stimulation of respiratory centres in the brain and, consequently, respiratory depression does not occur simultaneously with acute pain. As patients use the PCA device by titrating opioids to effect, there is less likelihood of respiratory depression. This is even more the case as the sedated patient will stop using the device. In the rare cases of respiratory depression, the causes are commonly:

- operator error (e.g. inappropriate prescription, incorrect programming of PCA device, incorrect dilution of medication)
- patient-related error (e.g. relatives using PCA button instead of the patient)
- equipment failure (e.g. cracked syringes with gravity siphoning of opioid solution [rare]) (Macintyre 2001).

Other side effects associated with PCA administration of opioids are nausea and vomiting in 35% of cases (Sidebotham et al 1997), occurring mainly on the first post-operative day, as well as sedation in 18% and confusion in 12% of cases (Schug & Fry 1994). These problems occur with similar incidence to other methods of opioid administration and are not reduced by the PCA approach (Hudcova et al 2006).

Continuous low-dose IV infusion, when given together with PCA, has been shown to increase the risk of side effects (Schug & Torrie 1993; Sidebotham et al 1997) without significantly improving analgesia (Dal et al 2003, Parker et al 1992); the incidence of respiratory depression is five to eight times higher than in the case of PCA alone, as the inherent safety concept of PCA is violated. Hence, the only patients who should be prescribed a background opioid infusion are those already receiving opioids. These patients already have some degree of opioid tolerance as well as increased requirements (e.g. chronic pain, recreational abuse, methadone substitution) (Mitra & Sinatra 2004).

All routes of opioid administration, especially parenteral routes, need to be carefully monitored for side effects, notably respiratory depression. Specific protocols are written for each route of administration so that patients receive optimal analgesia whilst always being safeguarded against respiratory depression and monitored for other side effects of opioids. Safe and appropriate use of the PCA method requires frequent and informed monitoring by nurses who have undergone relevant education and accreditation in the management of these devices. Standard orders and drug dilutions are suggested to maximize the effectiveness of the PCA and minimize complications.

The risk of opioid addiction is often cited as a reason for provision of inadequate analgesia. However, it has been demonstrated that addiction to opioids is rare when used in the treatment of acute pain. Patients choose not to fully relieve their pain, despite free access to drugs, and demands tend to be conservative, with patients opting to remain alert and in a small amount of discomfort (Macintyre 2001). There is at present no evidence that opioid use in the management of acute pain leads to opioid dependence or addiction (Chapman & Hill 1989; Schug & Torrie 1993).

Summary

Opioids delivered via a PCA device provide better analgesia and higher levels of patient satisfaction, with less risk of respiratory depression than conventional routes of opioid administration. Patients' preference for PCA is possibly caused by the degree of control it affords them over their own pain management. However, PCA offers no reduction of opioid-related adverse effects and no difference in duration of hospital stay.

To improve the analgesia provided by IV PCA, the technique should be integrated into a concept of multimodal analgesia using other appropriate techniques and medications.

SYSTEMIC NON-OPIOID ANALGESICS

Paracetamol/acetaminophen

Paracetamol, also called acetaminophen, has analgesic and -anti-pyretic effects, but is not anti-inflammatory (see Chapter 11). It is an effective analgesic in its own right, but not as effective as the other non-opioids. As a component of multimodal analgesia, it reduces opioid requirements by 20–30%, but it does not result in an increase in pain relief or a decrease in opioid-related adverse effects (Remy et al 2005). However, with short-term use in appropriate doses, there is a side effect profile comparable to placebo. Therefore, many of the contraindications to NSAIDs, in particular renal impairment, do not relate to the use of paracetamol. Combining paracetamol with NSAIDs improves analgesia and increases patient satisfaction in comparison to the sole use of paracetamol (Remy et al 2006).

Non-steroidal anti-inflammatory drugs

Non-selective non-steroidal anti-inflammatory drugs (NSAIDs) and COX-2 selective inhibitors, so-called coxibs, are effective analgesics in the management of mild and moderate acute pain, and also most useful components of multimodal analgesia. These drugs reduce the level of inflammatory mediators generated at the site of tissue injury. They have this effect by inhibiting the enzyme cyclo-oxygenase. Non-selective NSAIDs inhibit both iso-enzymes COX-1 and COX-2, while coxibs selectively inhibit COX-2.

With regard to efficacy, both groups of drugs are similar. As components of multimodal analgesia, they are opioid-sparing, improve analgesia and reduce the incidence of opioid-related adverse effects such as nausea, vomiting and sedation (Marret et al 2005). Because of their selectivity for the iso-enzyme COX-2, coxibs have a better adverse effect profile than non-selective NSAIDs (Schug 2006). In short-term use they result in gastric ulceration rates similar to those of a placebo, even in higher-risk populations. They do not impair platelet function and this leads to reduced perioperative blood loss in comparison with non-selective NSAIDs. They also do not appear to induce bronchospasm in patients with aspirin-exacerbated asthma. They might have similar adverse effects on renal function, although recent data contradict this statement (Lafrance & Miller 2009). Nevertheless, they should be used with care and consideration in situations of pre-existing renal impairment, hypovolemia or hypotension, and when used together with other nephro toxic agents and angiotensin-converting enzyme (ACE) inhibitors. While there has been an ongoing debate about the risk of cardiovascular adverse events with the long-term use of coxibs, this could not be proven for short-term use of paracoxib and/or valdecoxib used after non-cardiac surgery (Schug et al, 2009). However, coxibs, like other non-selective NSAIDs, should not be used after coronary artery bypass surgery or possibly after all cardiac surgery due to an increased incidence of cardiovascular events. There is a theoretical concern that these compounds impair wound and bone healing, but this could not be shown conclusively in the data available to date (Boursinos et al 2009).

Overall, these compounds play an important role in the management of post-operative pain, particularly as a component of multimodal analgesia, as they do not cause typical opioid adverse effects such as sedation, respiratory depression or impaired bowel recovery. At the same time, they are particularly effective in the treatment of pain with a major inflammatory component and pain on movement (Schug & Manopas 2007).

OTHER SYSTEMIC AGENTS

Entonox

Entonox is a mixture of 50% oxygen and 50% nitrous oxide. It provides a safe way to administer the analgesic inhalational anaesthetic nitrous oxide in a subanaesthetic concentration. The agent is usually given by self-administration via a face mask or mouth piece. Self-administration enhances safety, as the patient will stop usage in the unlikely case of loss of consciousness. Entonox is particularly useful as a safe short-term analgesic with a rapid onset of action, therefore it is commonly used for painful procedures such as dressing changes or passive mobilization, and during labour (Macintyre et al 2010).

Clonidine

Clonidine is an α2-receptor agonist and thus potentiates the descending inhibitory pathways within the spinal cord that act on pain transmission at the dorsal horn. It reduces opioid requirement and is therefore potentially useful as an adjunct to PCA. It also reduces the incidence of opioid-induced nausea and vomiting, and does not cause respiratory depression per se. Potential problems resulting from the use of clonidine are sedation and hypotension (Macintyre & Schug 2007). Its administration in neuraxial analgesia techniques (Elia et al 2008) and peripheral nerve blocks (Murphy et al 2000) is also useful.

Ketamine

Ketamine is an antagonist at the N-methyl-D-aspartate (NMDA) receptor within the central nervous system. This receptor is involved in the production of 'wind-up' during excitation of the dorsal horn with repetitive pain impulses (Visser & Schug 2006). Ketamine, in combination with PCA, has been shown to reduce opioid consumption, improve pain control and reduce nausea and vomiting (Bell et al 2006). It has a specific role in the management of procedural and neuropathic pain, the management of pain that is poorly responsive to opioids and opioid-tolerant patients (Urban et al 2008).

Tricyclic antidepressants and anticonvulsants

These drugs are commonly used in chronic pain management, in particular in the treatment of neuropathic pain (their role is discussed more extensively in Chapters 10 and 11). However, they also play a role in the management of acute and subacute neuropathic pain, that is, sciatica pain caused by nerve or spinal cord injury and stroke. For the acute emergency treatment of such situations, IV ketamine in low subanaesthetic doses, or IV lidocaine in anti-arrhythmic doses or by continuous infusion can be used (Challapalli et al 2006). The anticonvulsants gabapentin and pregabalin, which inhibit the release of excitatory amino acids, have recently gained an increasing role in the management of acute pain. Given as pre-medication, they improve analgesia and reduce opioid requirements and opioid-related adverse effects. However, ideal doses and duration of treatment to achieve maximum benefit without untoward side effects like sedation are unknown (Tiippana et al 2007). Given for longer periods perioperatively, they may prevent the development of persistent post-surgical pain states (Buvanendran et al 2010).

REGIONAL TECHNIQUES

Neuraxial analgesia

The two types of neuraxial analgesia used in acute care are:

- **intrathecal** analgesia: drugs are administered into the intrathecal space
- **epidural** (extradural) analgesia: drugs are administered into the epidural space.

The intrathecal space lies inside the spinal meninges, which hold the cerebrospinal fluid (CSF), and the epidural space lies outside the meninges (dura mater). The spinal nerve roots traverse both spaces; as they pass through the epidural space, they are surrounded by a cuff of dura. The neuraxial route provides access to nerve roots supplying the thorax, abdomen, pelvic organs, perineum and lower limbs. Drugs administered by this route can affect pain transmission in the dorsal horn of the spinal cord, the somatic afferent (sensory) and efferent (motor) nerve roots, and the sympathetic efferent nerves.

Intrathecal analgesia

Intrathecal (i.e. spinal) anaesthesia is usually given pre-operatively as a 'single-shot' technique, which involves insertion of a spinal needle through a lumbar intervertebral space, gentle advancement of the needle until CSF back-flow occurs through the needle, and subsequent injection of local anaesthetic ± opioid. This method provides good surgical anaesthesia for up to 4 hours, but a long-acting opioid can provide ongoing post-operative analgesia for 12–24 hours and more (Boezaart et al 1999). The technique is often used for urological and orthopaedic operations, as it primarily covers the pelvis and lower limbs. The use of continuous intrathecal techniques is an option, primarily in cancer pain management, and only in an experimental state for provision of post-operative analgesia (Rathmell et al 2005).

Epidural analgesia

If analgesia is required for a prolonged period post-operatively, notably following upper abdominal surgery or thoracic surgery, it is better to have a continuous infusion as opposed to a single shot. Under these circumstances, epidural techniques are commonly employed; a needle is inserted into the epidural space, which is usually identified by a 'loss-of-resistance' technique, and a catheter is fed into the space, allowing longer-term infusion or repeated bolus doses of analgesic agents.

Drugs that are commonly given by the spinal route are:

- local anaesthetics (e.g. bupivicaine, lidocaine, ropivacaine)

- opioids (e.g. morphine, fentanyl, sufentanil, pethidine, diamorphine).

Local anaesthetics

Local anaesthetics block axonal conduction and hence prevent transmission of nociceptive (pain) impulses into the dorsal horn of the spinal cord (see Chapter 11). Dependent on which level is selected for the insertion of the epidural catheter (dermatomal level), they preferentially block those dermatomes closer to the site of catheter insertion. Hence, lumbosacral epidural catheters are inserted for lower limb surgery, low-thoracic epidurals for lower abdominal surgery and mid-thoracic epidurals for upper abdominal surgery.

As local anaesthetic agents block axonal conduction in all nerves to some extent, when used spinally, most of their side effects (see Chapter 11) are basically an extension of this property:

- inadvertent overdose or injection into an epidural vessel, which can lead to local anaesthetic toxicity, the most serious consequences being central nervous system toxicity (convulsions and coma) and cardiovascular toxicity (fatal arrhythmias)
- urinary retention
- 'total spinal anaesthesia' as a result of an excess of local anaesthetic being inadvertently administered directly into the CSF (i.e. intrathecally), rather than into the epidural space – this blocks the sympathetic outflow from the spinal cord and constitutes an emergency situation; the patient rapidly develops total body paralysis and is unable to breathe, followed by cardiovascular collapse, loss of consciousness and, if untreated, death
- variable haemodynamic effects of sympathetic blockade, commonly resulting in hypotension as a result of vasodilatation –this often requires treatment with vasoconstrictors and/or increased volumes of IV fluid
- motor blockade, which can impair mobilization, and, in combination with sensory blockade, may contribute to the development of pressure areas, if nursing care is inadequate.

Opioids

Opioids administered neuraxially block opioid receptors in the dorsal horn of the spinal cord. Lower doses than those needed for systemic analgesia are required for provision of neuraxial analgesia and, as a result, opioid side effects may be reduced. Epidural opioids can cause analgesia by:

- diffusion through the dural membrane of the spinal root cuffs into the CSF, and then to the opioid receptors in the dorsal horn and to the brain (cephalad spread)
- direct transfer from the epidural space to the spinal cord via spinal arteries
- vascular uptake into the bloodstream, thus providing systemic analgesia (Bernards 2002).

If morphine or other hydrophilic (water-soluble) opioids are used, they stay in the CSF for a longer period of time and are more commonly associated with cephalad migration. The advantages of a single dose providing analgesia for 12–24 hours are traded off by the potential for delayed respiratory depression 12–24 hours after the dose is administered, as a result of cephalad migration to the respiratory centres in the brain. Conversely, fentanyl and other lipophilic (fat-soluble) opioids do not stay in the CSF as long, and consequently provide a shorter duration of analgesia and less risk of respiratory depression. As such, epidural fentanyl or sufentanil can and should be given as an infusion.

Other side effects of neuraxial opioids, particularly morphine, are pruritus, nausea and urinary retention.

Epidural opioids are rarely given as the sole analgesic agent, as it has been demonstrated that there is no clear advantage of using spinal opioids over IV opioids. Both provide the same quality of analgesia and the same risk of side effects. However, it has been demonstrated that, if local anaesthetic drugs are used in combination with opioids in the epidural space, they reduce the requirement for opioids and therefore the risk of opioid side effects (i.e. they are opioid-sparing). They may in fact improve the quality of analgesia and reduce the incidence of patchy/unilateral blocks. Such a combination of low-dose epidural opioid and local anaesthetic allows low concentrations of local anaesthetic to be used, providing good-quality analgesia with minimal motor blockade (seen as limb weakness and inability to mobilize), and less sympathetic blockade. Continuous infusions of these combinations, often amalgamated with a patient-controlled bolus dose as patient-controlled epidural analgesia (PCEA), are currently the most common way to provide epidural analgesia (Standl et al 2003).

Benefits of neuraxial techniques

Epidural analgesia is used after a wide variety of surgical operations, ranging from thoracic surgery to vascular surgery on the lower limbs. It can also be used for acute pain secondary to medical disease, such as angina or pancreatitis.

Local anaesthetics supplied via epidural catheters provide better analgesia than systemic opioids (Wu et al 2005), in particular for mobilization and coughing.

In contrast to systemic opioid administration, there is increasing evidence that epidural analgesia offers the potential for improved outcomes, that is, reduced morbidity and possibly mortality (Guay 2006; Rodgers et al 2000; Wu et al 2006). Data for such results show the following benefits:

- *Preservation of gastrointestinal function*: Epidurals significantly reduce the incidence of ileus (reduced gut motility) (Liu et al 1995), allowing early oral feeding, and decrease the incidence of breakdown of surgical bowel anastomoses. Also, they reduce the breakdown

of body protein and energy sources (catabolism), thus preventing protein loss.
- *Preservation of pulmonary function*: Epidurals significantly reduce the incidence of pulmonary infections, atelectasis and hypoxaemia (Popping et al 2008).
- *Reduced incidence of thromboembolic complications*: Epidurals reduce the incidence of deep venous thrombosis (DVT), pulmonary embolism (PE) and graft thrombosis after vascular reconstruction (Christopherson et al 1993).
- *Reduced neuroendocrine response (stress response) to surgery*: This is a physiological response to surgery and is caused by hormones (catecholamines) and cytokines being released during surgical trauma. This forces the body into a catabolic state (having an increased metabolic rate), whereby the body's nutritional state is depleted and blood clots more readily, increasing the risk of DVT and PE. This may contribute to immunosuppression and increased risk of infection. An epidural is extremely effective in reducing the stress response (Guay 2006).
- *Increased protection of the heart*: Epidurals reduce the oxygen requirement of the heart and increase its blood supply. It has recently been demonstrated that epidurals reduce the incidence of fatal arrhythmias and myocardial ischaemic events, and prevent myocardial infarction following upper abdominal surgery (Beattie et al 2001).

Modification of surgical and nursing protocols, to ensure early oral feeding, improved nutrition and active mobilization, is required to maximize the effects of neural blockade on pain, the stress response and organ dysfunction. A multidisciplinary approach (fast-track surgery), which incorporates all aspects of perioperative rehabilitation, is likely to offer the best chances of improving outcomes, reducing the length of hospital stays and ensuring cost–benefit advantages (Kehlet 2008; Wind et al 2006).

Complications of neuraxial techniques

In addition to adverse effects of drugs, neuraxial techniques have other potential complications related to the insertion of an epidural needle and subsequent presence of an epidural catheter (Macintyre et al 2010):

- Dural puncture is the inadvertent puncturing of the dural membrane during insertion of an epidural catheter, allowing leakage of CSF into the epidural space. This occurs during ~1% of epidural catheter insertions. There is a high chance of developing a postdural puncture headache following this, particularly if the patient is young and mobilizing soon after epidural insertion.

- Neurological deficit with regional numbness as a consequence of nerve injury by needle or catheter occurs in 0.013–0.023% of cases (Macintyre et al 2010). This is usually a temporary deficit, and complete recovery occurs at least within 3 months.
- Epidural haematoma that results in neurological deficit due to compression of the spinal cord can occur. Unless surgical intervention (decompression) takes place within hours of first symptom presentations, permanent neurological injury in the form of paraplegia can result. Fortunately, this complication is an extremely rare event, with an estimated incidence in the range of 1/10,000–15,000 (Macintyre et al 2010).
- Epidural abscess or meningitis can be the result of contamination on insertion or haematogenic colonization of the indwelling catheter. This is another extremely rare complication requiring antibiotic treatment and possibly surgical intervention. The incidence can be reduced by maintenance of appropriate asepsis during catheter placement and handling, as well as careful consideration of risks and benefits in septic patients (Horlocker & Wedel 2008);
- Many different drugs have been mistakenly administered into epidural catheters, commonly as a result of nursing error or system failure. Consequences depend on the type of drug injected, but can be severe.

Peripheral neural blockade

Neuraxial analgesia is just one method by which local anaesthetics can be used to provide analgesia. Other types of peripheral neural blockade that are commonly used improve analgesia with minimal adverse effects. They also reduce the requirements for opioid analgesia and thus the incidence of opioid side effects.

Wound infiltration

This is an extremely simple technique, usually performed by the surgeon at the end of the operation. Use of long-acting local anaesthetics such as bupivacaine and ropivacaine can provide good analgesia, lasting for many hours after surgery. It is a particularly useful technique following minor operations such as hernia repair, paediatric surgery or trauma surgery, but high-volume infiltration after knee replacement has also proved to be very successful (Andersen et al 2008). Leaving a catheter in the wound area to perform continuous infusion with local anaesthetics results in improved analgesia, reduced opioid consumption and other beneficial outcomes (Liu et al 2006).

Femoral nerve blocks

These can be performed as a single-shot technique with a long-acting local anaesthetic. Alternatively, a catheter can be placed in the fascial sheath of the femoral nerve and analgesia can be provided by bolus injections or continuous infusion of local anaesthetics. This technique is useful for relief of pain and muscle spasm following knee surgery, arthroplasty and fractures of the femur neck (Fowler et al 2008).

Brachial plexus blocks

For these a single-shot injection can be delivered, or a catheter placed, near the brachial plexus. Access is possible through the axilla, around the clavicle or via an interscalene approach by a variety of techniques. Depending on access and catheter position, analgesia covers nearly the entire upper limb, also providing sympathetic blockade with resulting vasodilatation. This is a desired effect in plastic surgery (skin flaps, retransplantations, etc.) and in vascular surgery (e.g. shunt formation). The block is also useful for orthopaedic surgery to the arm and the shoulder, particularly when early mobilization is required (Evans et al 2005).

Intercostal nerve blocks, interpleural blocks and paravertebral blocks

These blocks can be used to treat pain due to rib fractures, thoracotomies and upper abdominal surgery. Continous paravertebral analgesia via a catheter is as effective as thoracic epidural analgesia for thoracotomies, with a better adverse effect profile (Davies et al 2006).

NON-PHARMACOLOGICAL MODALITIES

These techniques are used to *supplement* pharmacological modalities, but can sometimes be sufficient on their own:

- physical
  - superficial heat/cold
  - massage
  - exercise
  - immobilization
  - electroanalgesia (e.g. TENS)
- cognitive
  - behavioural approaches
  - preparatory information
  - simple relaxation
  - imagery
  - hypnosis
  - biofeedback.

Although evidence for the efficacy of non-pharmacological modalities in acute pain management is largely at the expert opinion level, certain patients may derive benefit from them as a result of reducing drug therapy, and also if they are likely to experience a prolonged interval of pain. (See Chapters 8, 9, 12, 13 and 14 for a more complete description of these therapies.)

Physical modalities

These techniques may provide comfort, correct physical dysfunction, alter physiological responses and reduce fears associated with pain-related immobility or activity restriction. However, there is only very limited evidence for their effectiveness in acute pain. There is contradictory evidence for the use of massage in the treatment of acute pain. While some studies have described benefits, others could not find an effect.

The situation is comparable with regard to the benefits of post-operative local cooling. Two meta-analyses of the use of cooling for pain relief from perineal trauma after childbirth and in low back pain came to similar inconsistent conclusions. Again, there is only weak evidence for the effectiveness of heat application in acute or subacute musculoskeletal pain. Static magnet therapy, millimetre wave therapy and healing touch have been found to be ineffective. On the other hand, there are data showing that acupuncture reduces post-operative pain and opioid consumption in the post-operative setting, but also treats pain during childbirth and dental pain. However, this has been contradicted by a meta-analysis of all types of pain, which did not show a benefit. Similarly, the evidence for TENS is contradictory, with no indicated benefit in labour pain but some evidence of improvement in some acute pain situations. With regard to psychological interventions, there is inconsistent evidence relating to hypnosis and relaxation techniques. Benefits have been shown from listening to music, receiving training in coping methods or behavioural instructions, and distraction from procedure-related pain for children.

Exercise, activation and early mobilization are important components of management in the post-operative period, aimed at achieving a rapid return to normal function and life after surgery, with as little deconditioning of physical function as possible (Allen et al 1999). The aim is the establishment of a normal routine for post-operative patients as quickly as possible, allowing pain relief prior to intervention and scheduled rest, but with a consistent approach encouraging restoration of function and clear guidelines as to how to mobilize out of bed, how far to mobilize and how frequently to mobilize.

Progression from acute to chronic pain

The risk of chronic pain as a consequence of surgery is underestimated, as it can occur quite often and represents a significant source of ongoing disability. Estimates of chronic pain after certain surgeries, such as amputation, thoracotomy and mastectomy, range between 5 and 80%, with an estimated incidence of chronic severe pain in the range of 5–10% (Kehlet et al 2006). Even inguinal hernia repair carries a 2–4% risk of developing chronic severe pain. This pain is often of neuropathic nature, and a number of risk factors have been identified. These include preoperative moderate to severe pain, particularly with longer duration, as well as female gender, psychological vulnerability and preoperative anxiety, and possibly also genetic predisposition. A surgical approach with danger of nerve damage increases the risk, as do moderate to severe post-operative pain, the psychological factors mentioned above and, possibly, radiation therapy. Current research is focusing on attempts to reduce the incidence of chronic pain after surgery; some specific anaesthetic and/or analgesic interventions may reduce the incidence (Macintyre et al 2010). Here, in particular, the use of regional anaesthesia techniques and the use of antihyperalgesic medications (such as gabapentin or pregabalin) look promising. These approaches seem to be most effective if administered during surgery and for a certain time thereafter (preventive analgesia). There is, however, no evidence-based recommendation possible for how long the treatment should last. Hopefully, future studies will lead to drugs and treatment protocols able to successfully prevent chronic pain after surgery (Rappaport et al 2010).

THE ACUTE PAIN SERVICE

Acute pain is an area of growing interest in all specialities involved with inpatient care. As shown above, the benefits the patient receives from effective analgesia extend beyond patient comfort into areas that often result in reduced morbidity.

An increasing body of knowledge covering the mechanism of acute pain and its effects on the dorsal horn of the spinal cord has emerged. This has resulted in an increased availability of better and more sophisticated techniques to treat acute pain, that is, regional blockade and PCA. However, until recently, provision of optimal analgesia for acute pain has been moving at a much slower pace. Before the late 1980s, most surveys demonstrated that 60–80% of post-operative patients suffered considerable pain in the early post-operative period (Marks & Sachar 1973). Even in 1991 (Semple & Jackson 1991) and 2003 (Apfelbaum et al 2003), many patients were still dissatisfied with their post-operative analgesia. This was in part due to a large number of traditionally held (and incorrect) beliefs concerning the provision of effective analgesia, such as the common idea that pain is merely a symptom and not harmful in itself, the mistaken impression that analgesia makes accurate diagnosis difficult or impossible

(Manterola et al 2007), fear of potential for addiction to opioids, and concerns about respiratory depression and other opioid-related side effects, such as nausea and vomiting.

Another reason for inadequate provision of analgesia was that, although more sophisticated methods of providing analgesia were being introduced, such as regional blockade and PCA, there was a lack of appropriate organizational structures for safe and effective use of this equipment. Reports of shortened hospital stays, reduced morbidity and mortality, and increased patient satisfaction in association with effective pain relief from those using these new analgesic techniques led to increased medical and public awareness of the importance of effectively managing acute pain. There developed a need for a service to manage acute pain patients, hence the introduction of the acute pain service (APS).

In 1986, Ready set up the first 'anesthesiology-based post-operative pain management service' in Seattle, USA (Ready et al 1988), with the rapid subsequent development of other similar services worldwide (for further descriptions see Macintyre et al 1990; Schug and Haridas 1993; Wheatley et al 1991).

The Royal Australasian College of Surgeons summarized the following topics as prerequisites for effective pain control:

- patient education
- assessment of pain
- appropriate prescribing
- use of special techniques
- individualization of treatment.

In order to provide the above service, a coordinated, organized team approach is necessary. This team should include anaesthetists, surgeons, nurses and pharmacists, not to mention a multitude of other specialists such as physiotherapists, occupational therapists, infection control specialists and psychologists – an APS. Recommendations were made that acute pain teams be established in all major hospitals and that there should be a formal, team approach to the management of acute pain with 'clear lines of responsibility'. In summary, the role of an APS is to:

- provide education about pain management, as well as more specialized analgesic techniques
- introduce the newer and more specialized methods of pain relief (epidural and PCA), and provide guidance to improve the more traditional methods
- provide and standardize orders, procedures and methods of pain assessment for all pain-relief strategies, and carry out ongoing improvement to these based on the results of audit activity
- provide daily supervision and 24-hour cover for patients under the care of the APS, as well as for patients with any other acute pain management problems
- undertake audit and clinical research activity.

Thus, the management of acute pain has really only been fully addressed over the last 20 years. As further scientific evidence emerges outlining the benefits and safety of the more recently introduced analgesic techniques, together with the establishment of the APS, the occurrence of inadequate relief of acute pain should eventually become less frequent.

APSs have now been introduced into many hospitals worldwide. However, they have quite a diverse structure, with no clear agreement on what constitutes the best model or the definition of such a service. The organizational structures range from 'low-cost' nurse-based services, via anaesthesia-led but primarily nurse-run services, to comprehensive and multidisciplinary services with 24-hour cover by an anaesthetist and supervising nurses, and involving other staff such as pharmacists. Similarly, their range of involvement extends from input to all forms of acute pain management in a hospital, to services that only look after advanced techniques. In addition, many APSs have moved on to become comprehensive pain services dealing with all pain-management issues in a hospital from the acute to the subacute to the chronic. Overall, there are some data to suggest that APSs have benefits in achieving reduced pain scores and side effects of analgesia in a hospital. This aligns with other data that suggest that the development of an APS in a hospital is accompanied by significant improvement in post-operative pain management. Other potential beneficial outcomes are the reduction of post-operative morbidity or even mortality, and the use of techniques that reduce the incidence of persistent pain after surgery. In this context, it is important that comprehensive pain services are, in particular, able to diagnose early-onset neuropathic pain and deal with it appropriately, but that they can also manage patients with complex issues, such as opioid-tolerant or opioid-abusing patients, in the framework of a multidisciplinary setting.

Q	**Study/revision questions**

1. How can systemic opioids be administered and what are the arguments for and against each method?
2. What are the potential benefits and dangers of patient-controlled analgesia?
3. What alternatives to systemic opioid use exist and what are the features of each treatment type?
4. By what methods can neuraxial analgesia be achieved and how do these methods compare and contrast?
5. By what methods can peripheral neural blockade be achieved and how do these methods compare and contrast?
6. What evidence exists for and against the use of non-pharmacological treatment modalities?
7. What is the function of an acute pain service?

REFERENCES

Allen, C., Glasziou, P., Del Mar, C., 1999. Bed rest: A potentially harmful treatment needing more careful evaluation [see comments]. Lancet 354 (9186), 1229–1233.

Andersen, L.O., Husted, H., Otte, K.S., et al., 2008. High-volume infiltration analgesia in total knee arthroplasty: A randomized, double-blind, placebo-controlled trial. Acta Anaesthesiol. Scand. 52 (10), 1331–1335.

Apfelbaum, J.L., Chen, C., Mehta, S.S., et al., 2003. Postoperative pain experience: Results from a national survey suggest postoperative pain continues to be undermanaged. Anesth. Analg. 97 (2), 534–540, table of contents.

Aubrun, F., Monsel, S., Langeron, O., et al., 2001. Postoperative titration of intravenous morphine. Eur. J. Anaesthesiol. 18 (3), 159–165.

Aubrun, F., Salvi, N., Coriat, P., et al., 2005. Sex- and age-related differences in morphine requirements for postoperative pain relief. Anesthesiology 103 (1), 156–160.

Beattie, W.S., Badner, N.H., Choi, P., 2001. Epidural analgesia reduces postoperative myocardial infarction: A meta-analysis. Anesth. Analg. 93 (4), 853–858.

Bell, R.F., Dahl, J.B., Moore, R.A., et al., 2006. Perioperative ketamine for acute postoperative pain. Cochrane Database Syst. Rev. (1),CD004603.

Bernards, C.M., 2002. Understanding the physiology and pharmacology of epidural and intrathecal opioids. Best Pract. Res. Clin. Anaesthesiol. 16 (4), 489–505.

Boezaart, A.P., Eksteen, J.A., Spuy, G.V., et al., 1999. Intrathecal morphine: Double-blind evaluation of optimal dosage for analgesia after major lumbar spinal surgery. Spine 24 (11), 1131–1137.

Boursinos, L.A., Karachalios, T., Poultsides, L., et al., 2009. Do steroids, conventional non-steroidal anti-inflammatory drugs and selective Cox-2 inhibitors adversely affect fracture healing? J. Musculoskelet. Neuronal. Interact. 9 (1), 44–52.

Burns, J.W., Hodsman, N.B., McLintock, T.T., et al., 1989. The influence of patient characteristics on the requirements for postoperative analgesia: A reassessment using patient-controlled analgesia. Anaesthesia 44 (1), 2–6.

Buvanendran, A., Kroin, J.S., Della Valle, C.J., et al., 2010. Perioperative oral pregabalin reduces chronic pain after total knee arthroplasty: A prospective, randomized, controlled trial. Anesth. Analg. 110 (1), 199–207.

Cashman, J.N., Dolin, S.J., 2004. Respiratory and haemodynamic effects of acute postoperative pain management: Evidence from published data. Br. J. Anaesth. 93 (2), 212–223.

Challapalli, V., Tremont-Lukats, I., McNicol, E., et al., 2006. Systemic administration of local anesthetic agents to relieve neuropathic pain. Online. Available:http://www.cochrane.org/reviews/en/ab003345.html.

Chapman, C.R., Hill, H.F., 1989. Prolonged morphine self-administration and addiction liability: Evaluation of two theories in a bone marrow transplant unit. Cancer. 63 (8), 1636–1644.

Christopherson, R., Beattie, C., Frank, S.M., et al., study group, 1993. Perioperative morbidity in patients randomized to epidural or general anesthesia for lower extremity vascular surgery: Perioperative Ischemia Randomized Anesthesia Trial Study Group [see comments]. Anesthesiology 79 (3), 422–434.

Chumbley, G.M., Hall, G.M., Salmon, P., 2002. Patient-controlled analgesia: What information does the patient want? J. Adv. Nurs. 39 (5), 459–471.

Cooper, I.M., 1996. Morphine for postoperative analgesia: A comparison of intramuscular and subcutaneous routes of administration. Anaesth. Intensive Care 24 (5), 574–578.

Dal, D., Kanbak, M., Caglar, M., et al., 2003. A background infusion of morphine does not enhance postoperative analgesia after cardiac surgery. Canadian Journal of Anesthesia. 50 (5), 476–479.

Davies, R.G., Myles, P.S., Graham, J.M., 2006. A comparison of the analgesic efficacy and side-effects of paravertebral vs epidural blockade for thoracotomy: A systematic review and meta-analysis of randomized trials. Br. J. Anaesth. 96 (4), 418–426.

Elia, N., Culebras, X., Mazza, C., et al., 2008. Clonidine as an adjuvant to intrathecal local anesthetics for surgery: Systematic review of randomized trials. Reg. Anesth. Pain Med. 33 (2), 159–167.

Evans, H., Steele, S.M., Nielsen, K.C., et al., 2005. Peripheral nerve blocks and continuous catheter techniques. Anesthesiol. Clin. North America. 23 (1), 141–162.

Fowler, S.J., Symons, J., Sabato, S., et al., 2008. Epidural analgesia compared with peripheral nerve blockade after major knee surgery: A systematic review and meta-analysis of randomized trials. Br. J. Anaesth. 100 (2), 154–164.

Guay, J., 2006. The benefits of adding epidural analgesia to general anesthesia: A metaanalysis. J. Anesth. 20 (4), 335–340.

Horlocker, T.T., Wedel, D.J., 2008. Infectious complications of regional anesthesia. Best Pract. Res. Clin. Anaesthesiol. 22 (3), 451–475.

Hudcova, J., McNicol, E., Quah, C., et al., 2006. Patient controlled opioid analgesia versus conventional opioid analgesia for postoperative pain. Cochrane Database Syst. Rev. (4), CD003348.

Kehlet, H., 2008. Fast-track colorectal surgery. Lancet. 371 (9615), 791–793.

Kehlet, H., Jensen, T.S., Woolf, C.J., 2006. Persistent postsurgical pain: Risk factors and prevention. Lancet 367 (9522), 1618–1625.

Lafrance, J.P., Miller, D.R., 2009. Selective and non-selective non-steroidal anti-inflammatory drugs and the risk of acute kidney injury. Pharmacoepidemiol. Drug Saf. 18 (10), 923–931.

Latta, K.S., Ginsberg, B., Barkin, R.L., 2002. Meperidine: A critical review. Am. J. Ther. 9 (1), 53–68.

Liu, S.S., Carpenter, R.L., Mackey, D.C., et al., 1995. Effects of perioperative analgesic technique on rate of recovery after colon surgery. Anesthesiology. 83 (4), 757–765.

Liu, S.S., Richman, J.M., Thirlby, R.C., et al., 2006. Efficacy of continuous wound catheters delivering local anesthetic for postoperative analgesia: A quantitative and qualitative systematic review of randomized controlled trials. J. Am. Coll. Surg. 203 (6), 914–932.

Macintyre, P.E., 2001. Safety and efficacy of patient-controlled analgesia. Br. J. Anaesth. 87 (1), 36–46.

Macintyre, P.E., Jarvis, D.A., 1996. Age is the best predictor of postoperative morphine requirements. Pain 64 (2), 357–364.

Macintyre, P.E., Schug, S.A., 2007. Acute Pain Management: A practical guide. Saunders, London.

Macintyre, P.E., Runciman, W.B., Webb, R.K., 1990. An acute pain service in an Australian teaching hospital: The first year. Med. J. Aust. 153, 417–421.

Macintyre, P.E., Schug, S.A., Scott, D.A., et al., 2010. Acute Pain Management: Scientific Evidence. ANZCA & FPM, Melbourne.

Manterola, C., Astudillo, P., Losada, H., et al., 2007. Analgesia in patients with acute abdominal pain. Cochrane Database Syst. Rev. (3), CD005660.

Marks, R.M., Sachar, E.J., 1973. Undertreatment of medical inpatients with narcotic analgesics. Ann. Intern. Med. 78, 173–181.

Marret, E., Kurdi, O., Zufferey, P., et al., 2005. Effects of nonsteroidal antiinflammatory drugs on patient-controlled analgesia morphine side effects: Meta-analysis of randomized controlled trials. Anesthesiology 102 (6), 1249–1260.

Mitra, S., Sinatra, R.S., 2004. Perioperative management of acute pain in the opioid-dependent patient. Anesthesiology 101 (1), 212–227.

Murphy, D.B., McCartney, C.J., Chan, V.W., 2000. Novel analgesic adjuncts for brachial plexus block: A systematic review. Anesth. Analg. 90 (5), 1122–1128.

Oden, R., 1989. Acute postoperative pain: Incidence, severity and etiology of inadequate treatment. Anesthesiol. Clin. North America 7, 1–5.

Owen, H., Plummer, J.L., Armstrong, I., et al., 1989. Variables of patient-controlled analgesia: 1. bolus size. Anaesthesia 44, 7–10.

Parker, R.K., Holtmann, B., White, P.F., 1992. Effects of a nighttime opioid infusion with PCA therapy on patient comfort and analgesic requirements after abdominal hysterectomy. Anesthesiology 76 (3), 362–367.

Popping, D.M., Elia, N., Marret, E., et al., 2008. Protective effects of epidural analgesia on pulmonary complications after abdominal and thoracic surgery: a meta-analysis. Arch. Surg. 143 (10), 990–999, discussion 1000.

Rappaport, B.A., Cerny, I., Sanhai, W.R., 2010. ACTION on the prevention of chronic pain after surgery: Public–private partnerships, the future of analgesic drug development. Anesthesiology. 112 (3), 509–510.

Rathmell, J.P., Lair, T.R., Nauman, B., 2005. The role of intrathecal drugs in the treatment of acute pain. Anesth. Analg. 101 (Suppl. 5), S30–S43.

Ready, L.B., Oden, R., Chadwick, H.S., et al., 1988. Development of an anesthesiology-based postoperative pain management service. Anesthesiology 68 (1), 100–106.

Remy, C., Marret, E., Bonnet, F., 2005. Effects of acetaminophen on morphine side-effects and consumption after major surgery: Meta-analysis of randomized controlled trials. Br. J. Anaesth. 94 (4), 505–513.

Remy, C., Marret, E., Bonnet, F., 2006. State of the art of paracetamol in acute pain therapy. Curr. Opin Anaesthesiol. 19 (5), 562–565.

Rodgers, A., Walker, N., Schug, S., et al., 2000. Reduction of postoperative mortality and morbidity with epidural or spinal anaesthesia: results from overview of randomised trials. Br. Med. J. 321 (7275), 1493–1504.

Schug, S.A., 2006. The Role of COX-2 Inhibitors in the Treatment of Postoperative Pain. J. Cardiovasc. Pharmacol. 47 (Suppl. 1), S82–S86.

Schug, S.A., Fry, R.A., 1994. Continuous regional analgesia in comparison with intravenous opioid administration for routine postoperative pain control. Anaesthesia 49 (6), 528–532.

Schug, S., Haridas, R., 1993. Development and organizational structure of an acute pain service in a major teaching hospital. Aust. N. Z. J. Surg. 63 (1), 8–13.

Schug, S.A., Manopas, A., 2007. Update on the role of non-opioids for postoperative pain treatment. Best Pract. Res. Clin. Anaesthesiol. 21 (1), 15–30.

Schug, S., Torrie, J., 1993. Safety assessment of postoperative pain management by an acute pain service. Pain 55 (3), 387–391.

Schug, S.A., Zech, D., Grond, S., 1992. Adverse effects of systemic opioid analgesics. Drug Saf. 7 (3), 200–213.

Schug, S.A., Joshi, G.P., Camu, F., et al., 2009. Cardiovascular safety of the cyclooxygenase-2 selective inhibitors parecoxib and valdecoxib in the postoperative setting: An analysis of integrated data. Anesth. Analg. 108 (1), 299–307.

Scott, L.J., Perry, C.M., 2000. Tramadol: A review of its use in perioperative pain. Drugs 60 (1), 139–176.

Semple, P., Jackson, I.J., 1991. Postoperative pain control: A survey of current practice. Anaesthesia 46 (12), 1074–1076.

Semple, T.J., Upton, R.N., Macintyre, P.E., et al., 1997. Morphine blood concentrations in elderly postoperative patients following administration via an indwelling subcutaneous cannula. Anaesthesia. 52 (4), 318–323.

Sidebotham, D., Dijkhuizen, M.R., Schug, S.A., 1997. The safety and utilization of patient-controlled analgesia. J. Pain Symptom Manage. 14 (4), 202–209.

Stamer, U.M., Stuber, F., 2007. Genetic factors in pain and its treatment. Curr. Opin Anaesthesiol. 20 (5), 478–484.

Standl, T., Burmeister, M.A., Ohnesorge, H., et al., 2003. Patient-controlled epidural analgesia reduces analgesic requirements compared to continuous epidural infusion after major abdominal surgery. Canadian Journal of Anesthesia 50 (3), 258–264.

Tiippana, E.M., Hamunen, K., Kontinen, V.K., et al., 2007. Do surgical patients benefit from perioperative gabapentin/pregabalin? A systematic review of efficacy and safety. Anesth. Analg. 104 (6), 1545–1556, table of contents.

Urban, M.K., Ya Deau, J.T., Wukovits, B., et al., 2008. Ketamine as an adjunct to postoperative pain management in opioid tolerant patients after spinal fusions: A prospective randomized trial. HSS Journal 4 (1), 62–65.

Visser, E., Schug, S.A., 2006. The role of ketamine in pain management. Biomed. Pharmacother. 60 (7), 341–348.

Wheatley, R.G., Madej, T.H., Jackson, I.J., et al., 1991. The first year's experience of an acute pain service. Br. J. Anaesth. 67 (3), 353–359.

Wind, J., Polle, S.W., Fung Kon Jin, P.H., et al., 2006. Systematic review of enhanced recovery programmes in colonic surgery. Br. J. Surg. 93 (7), 800–809.

Wu, C.L., Cohen, S.R., Richman, J.M., et al., 2005. Efficacy of postoperative patient-controlled and continuous infusion epidural analgesia versus intravenous patient-controlled analgesia with opioids: A meta-analysis. Anesthesiology 103 (5), 1079–1088, quiz 109–110.

Wu, C.L., Rowlingson, A.J., Herbert, R., et al., 2006. Correlation of postoperative epidural analgesia on morbidity and mortality after colectomy in Medicare patients. J. Clin. Anesth. 18 (8), 594–599.

Chapter | 27 |

Conclusions: the future

Anita M. Unruh, Jenny Strong and Hubert van Griensven

In the 12 years since *Pain: A Textbook for Therapists* was published, much new knowledge has been gained about pain. Gatchel et al (2007) have described an 'explosion' of research into chronic pain, in particular, with a resultant increase in knowledge about its cause, assessment and management.

Much more is understood about the complex physiological mechanisms which happen at the periphery when we are injured, and what is happening in the central nervous system of the individual in pain. The poor correspondence between disease and resulting symptoms has led to a call for treatment, based on the underlying pathophysiological mechanisms (Woolf & Max 2001). This has led to revolutionary changes in the investigation of neuropathic pain and complex regional pain syndrome (CRPS) (Maier et al 2010). Meanwhile, advances in real-time brain imaging have enabled us to link subjective pain experiences with physiological changes (Bushnell et al 2004). These and other developments are giving us a better array of pharmacological agents than ever before. Our understandings about how to minimize or prevent acute pain from transitioning into persistent pain have grown. As identified in Chapter 9, our understandings of the psychology of pain has expanded greatly, as has the psychological armamentarium now at our fingertips. We are better at educating our clients and patients about their pain and now, we value the people who suffer pain more, and even at times, work in partnership *with* them, rather than doing *to* them. This is clearly amplified in Mandy Nielsen's chapter (Chapter 2).

We have a plethora of Clinical Guidelines to assist us in our work. There are numerous Clinical Guidelines and Consensus Statements, of which clinicians worldwide can avail themselves. For example, the American Pain Society published its *Guideline for Management of Cancer Pain in Adults and Children* in 2005 and the *Clinical Guidelines for the Use of Chronic Opioid Therapy in Chronic Noncancer Pain* in 2009 (Chou 2009). In Australia, the National Health & Medical Research Council published the 3rd edition of its *Acute Pain Management: Scientific Evidence* guidelines in 2010 (Macintyre et al 2010) and the Australian Pain Society published its *Evidence-based Recommendations for the Pharmacological Management of Neuropathic Pain* in 2008. Similarly, the British Pain Society has published a range of guidelines covering spinal cord stimulation, cancer pain management, acute pain in children and paediatric anaesthetics. The UK's National Institute for Health and Clinical Excellence (NICE) continues to produce guidance for treatment based on current evidence. Consensus statements abound, for example, *An Interdisciplinary Expert Consensus Statement on Assessment of Pain in Older Persons* (Hadjistavropoulos et al 2007). There is indeed a wealth of knowledge out there.

Yet, as has been frequently mentioned in previous chapters of this new book, and in other literature such as Cousins (2007), our pain management practices remain patently inadequate in many quarters. As Brennan and Cousins stated in 2004, 'The gap between an increasingly sophisticated knowledge of pain and its treatment and the effective application of that knowledge is large and widening'. Such gaps exist across the spectrum of acute and chronic pain; across pain in the elderly and pain in the young; pain in developed countries and pain in developing countries. Wittink and colleagues opined, in 2008, that the best treatments for people with chronic pain remain 'elusive'. There is also inadequate acute pain management. Surveys of patients who undergo surgery repeatedly reveal unrelieved post-operative pain (see, e.g. Apfelbaum et al 2003). Apfelbaum and his colleagues (2003), in a national telephone survey in the USA, of a random sample of 250 adults who had undergone surgery, found that almost

© 2014 Elsevier Ltd.

80% had pain after their surgery, with 39% of these people experiencing severe to extreme pain. Some 88% of patients who had received pain medication were satisfied with the medication. Three-quarters of this sample believed that pain after surgery was a necessary evil, with 72% saying they would prefer a non-narcotic drug due to fears of addiction or bad side-effects of narcotics.

Pain management for children, including those children who are dying from cancer, is insufficient. For example, in an interview study of parents of children who had died from cancer over a 9-year period and who had attended one of the biggest children's hospitals in Australia, 37 families (46% of respondents) reported that their child had suffered a lot or a great deal from pain in the last month of their life (Heath et al 2010). The comprehensive Access Economics report *The High Price of Pain* (2007) identified a lack of data on the prevalence of chronic pain among children in Australia.

For the increasingly ageing population around the world, our record of pain management is far from excellent: Finne-Soveri and Pitkälä (2007) and Gagliese (2009) have highlighted several important issues about the under-treatment of pain among elderly people. Additionally, the social suffering of people who live with persistent pain is not well understood or serviced.

After posing the question, 'How important is knowledge translation to the area of pain, chronic or persistent pain in particular?' (2008 p 465), Henry pointed to unacceptable levels of unrelieved or under-treated pain, suffering and lost productivity in Canada, and declared an urgent need for knowledge translation in this field. In Australia, the *The High Price of Pain* report (2007), commissioned by the MBF Foundation in collaboration with the University of Sydney Pain Management Research Unit, projected that, in 2007, 3.2 million Australians would experience chronic pain, with the costs of this pain totalling AU$34.3 billion. In the USA, Von Korff et al (2005) estimated that the prevalence of chronic pain was 19%.

Furthermore, differential access to pain management services may be experienced by patients of different racial or ethnic backgrounds, gender or age (Nguyen et al 2005, Green 2004). A telephone survey of a nationally representative sample of white, African-American and Hispanic people in the USA, with persistent pain, indicated that being Hispanic was a significant factor in low access to care for chronic pain (Nguyen et al 2005).

In some developing countries, there is a lack of access opioids for relief of pain in patients with cancer (Anderson 2010). This problem occurs despite the existence of the World Health Organization's (WHO 2000) guidelines on the treatment of cancer pain, which prominently articulate the need for morphine for the relief of moderate to severe cancer pain.

Henry (2008) urged that all stakeholders come together 'within a focused community of practice' to combat the impact of chronic pain. The Australian National Pain Strategy, launched at the 2010 National Pain Summit, has now grown to become the International Pain Summit, held in Montreal in 2010 in conjunction with the International Association for the Study of Pain (IASP) World Congress on Pain. The aim of the International Pain Summit is to help improve the quality of life for people who live with pain, and to reduce the burden of pain around the world (IASP 2010). This focused endeavour, which is designed to deliver partnership between health professional organizations such as the IASP, health professionals, governments, human rights advocates, consumers and the WHO, is a potentially powerful mechanism to mobilize all to action.

The call to regard persistent (chronic) pain as a disease entity in its own right, also augers well for the better management of persistent pain (Cousins 2007). Considering it a disease symbolically legitimizes persistent pain as being a real phenomenon, one which may perpetuate long after the disease or injury which triggered the pain to develop (Cousins 2007). Such a re-conceptualization can direct clinicians to treat not only the initiating problem, but also the secondary pathology that develops.

Education of clinicians remains a significant challenge, as many persist in believing that painful activity must be avoided, possibly reflecting a pervasive acute biomedical model (Linton et al 2002). In Canada, an extensive survey study highlighted that only a third of health science programmes could identify time dedicated to pain (Watt-Watson et al 2009). Courses in veterinary medicine spent far more time on pain than medical programmes (Watt-Watson et al 2009). The British Pain Society reported similar findings, with veterinary courses allocating twice and physiotherapy courses three times as much time to pain-related subjects (British Pain Society 2009). Now that the inadequacies in the curricula are being identified, there is a real opportunity for universities to take action. The IASP has published guidelines for pain education programmes and introduced a special interest group, which will help course leaders to integrate pain into the curricula.

In our small way, we urge therapists and health professionals to utilize the knowledge contained within the chapters of this book, to aid in the prevention of chronic pain, to participate in the rehabilitation of those who have persistent pain, and also, importantly, to advocate for people who have pain, especially those who are unable or unwilling to speak for themselves – particularly our children, older people, those who have cognitive deficits and people who have linguistic and cultural differences from the dominant culture. We as health professionals have an ethical, moral and professional imperative to assist in the relief of suffering for all. Let us do our bit to ensure people are not swallowed up in the enormity of pain.

REFERENCES

Access Economics Pty Limited, 2007. The high price of pain: the economic impact of persistent pain in Australia. MBF Foundation in collaboration with University of Sydney Pain Management Research Institute.

American Pain Society, 2005. Guideline for the Management of Cancer Pain in Adults and Children. American Pain Society.

Anderson, T., 2010. Pain control: the politics of pain. Br. Med. J. 341, c3800.

Apfelbaum, J.L., Chen, C., Mehta, S.S., et al., 2003. Postoperative pain experience: results from a national survey suggest postoperative pain continues to be undermanaged. Anesth. Analg. 97, 534–540.

Australian Pain Society, 2008. Evidence-Based Recommendations for the Pharmacological Management of Neuropathic Pain. APS.

Brennan, F., Cousins, M.J., 2004. Pain relief as a human right. Pain: Clinical Updates. 12, 1–4.

British Pain Society, 2009. Survey of undergraduate pain curricula for healthcare professionals in the United Kingdom. Pain News, Winter, pp. 38–42.

Bushnell, M., Villemure, C., Duncan, G., 2004. Psychophysical and neurophysiological studies of pain modulation by attention. In: Price, D., Bushnell, M. (Eds.), Psychological Methods of Pain Control: Basic Science and Clinical Perspectives. IASP Press, Seattle, pp. 99–116.

Chou, R., Fanciullo, G.J., Fine, P.G., et al., the American Pain Society – American Academy of Pain Medicine Opioids Guidelines Panel, 2009. Clinical guidelines for the use of chronic opioid therapy in chronic noncancer pain. J. Pain. 10, 113–130.

Cousins, M.J., 2007. Persistent pain: a disease entity. J. Pain Symptom Manage. 33 (Suppl. 2), S4–S10.

Finne-Soveri, H., Pitkälä, K., 2007. Is older age a blessing for persons with painful conditions? Pain. 129, 3–4.

Gagliese, L., 2009. Pain and aging: the emergence of a new subfield of pain research. J. Pain. 10, 343–353.

Gatchel, R.J., Bo Peng, Y., Peters, M.L., et al., 2007. The biopsychosocial approach to chronic pain: scientific advances and future directions. Psychol. Bull. 133, 581–624.

Green, C.R., 2004. Racial disparities in access to pain treatment. Pain: Clinical Updates. 12, 1–4.

Hadjistavropoulos, T., Herr, K., Turk, D.C., et al., 2007. An interdisciplinary expert consensus statement on assessment of pain in older persons. Clin. J. Pain. 23 (Suppl. 1), S1–S43.

Heath, J.A., Clarke, N.E., Donath, S.M., et al., 2010. Symptoms and suffering at the end of life in children with cancer: an Australian perspective. Med. J. Aust. 192, 71–75.

Henry, J.L., 2008. The need for knowledge translation in chronic pain. Pain Res. Manag. 13, 465–476.

International Association for the Study of Pain, 2010. IASP International Pain Summit. Online. Available: http://www.iasp-pain.org/AM/Template.cfm?Section=Home&TEMPLATE=/CM/HTMLDisplay.cfm&CONTENTID=10974(accessed 13.08.10.).

Linton, S., Vlaeyen, J., Ostelo, R., 2002. The back pain beliefs of health care providers: are we fear avoidant? J. Occup. Rehabil. 12, 223–232.

Macintyre, P.E., Schug, S.A., Scott, D.A., et al., the Working Group of the Australian and New Zealand College of Anaesthetists and Faculty of Pain Medicine, 2010. Acute Pain Management: Scientific Evidence, 3rd ed. ANZCA & FPM, Melbourne.

Maier, C., Baron, R., Tölle, T., et al., 2010. Quantitative sensory testing in the German Research Network on Neuropathic Pain (DNFS): somatosensory abnormalities in 1236 patients with different neuropathic pain syndromes. Pain. 150, 439–450.

Nguyen, M., Ugarte, C., Fuller, I., et al., 2005. Access to care for chronic pain: racial and ethnic differences. J. Pain. 6, 301–314.

Von Korff, M., Crane, P., Lane, M., et al., 2005. Chronic spinal pain and physical-mental comorbidity in the United States: results from the national comorbidity survey replication. Pain. 113, 331–339.

Watt-Watson, J., McGillion, M., Hunter, J., et al., 2009. A survey of pre-licensure pain curricula in health science faculties in Canadian universities. Pain Res. Manag. 14, 439–444.

Wittink, H., Nicholas, M., Kralik, D., et al., 2008. Are we measuring what we need to measure? Clin. J. Pain. 24, 316–324.

Woolf, C., Max, M., 2001. Mechanism-based pain diagnosis: issues for analgesic drug development. Anesthesiology. 95, 241–249.

World Health Organization, 2000. Narcotic and Psychotropic Drugs: Achieving Balance in National Opioids Control Policy: Guidelines for Assessment. Online. Available: http://www.painpolicy.wisc.edu/publicat/00whoabi/00whoabi.pdf (accessed 25.08.10.).

Appendix

Glossary of pain physiology terms

For a full list of definitions with extended commentary, please refer to the IASP Taxonomy (International Association for the Study of Pain 2011).

Aδ fibre A small-diameter myelinated afferent axon.

Allodynia Pain as a result of a stimulus that normally does not provoke pain, such as a light touch or a gentle stretch.

C fibre An unmyelinated afferent axon.

C-tactile A subclass of unmyelinated afferents mediating pleasant touch.

Catecholamines The neurotransmitters dopamine, adrenaline (epinephrine) and noradrenaline (norepinephrine).

Chemokines Small proteins, secreted by cells, that induce movement of cells according to a chemical gradient.

Dysaesthesia An unpleasant abnormal sensation. Could be called painful paraesthesia (paraesthesia in itself is not).

Hyperaesthesia Increased sensitivity to sensory stimulation.

Hyperalgesia An increased pain response to a stimulus that can be expected to be painful.

Hyperpathia An abnormally painful response to sensory stimulation in an area that has an increased stimulation threshold.

Hypoaesthesia Decreased sensitivity to sensory stimulation.

Hypoalgesia A decreased response to a stimulus that can be expected to be painful.

Modulation A term used to indicate the actions of neurotransmitters that do not directly evoke postsynaptic potentials in a neuron, but which modify its responses to other synaptic inputs.

Neuropathic pain Pain caused by a lesion or disease of the somatosensory nervous system. The IASP no longer lists the term 'neurogenic pain'. See Chapter 10 for discussion.

Neurotransmitter A chemical that is released by a presynaptic element following stimulation and activates postsynaptic receptors.

Nociceptive pain Pain as a result of the activation of type C and Aδ nociceptive neurones. The receptors of these neurones have high stimulation thresholds, making them sensitive to stimuli that are damaging to normal tissues or may become damaging if prolonged.

Nociceptor A receptor preferentially sensitive to noxious stimuli or to stimuli that would become noxious if prolonged.

Pain An unpleasant sensory and emotional experience associated with actual or potential tissue damage, or described in terms of such damage. Alternative definition: pain is whatever the patient says it is (McCaffrey & Beebe 1989).

Paraesthesia An abnormal sensation, typically described as pins and needles or crawling insects.

Polymodal nociceptor A nociceptor that is responsive to a range of stimuli (mechanical, thermal, chemical).

Receptive field The region of a sensory surface (e.g. skin) that, when stimulated, changes the membrane potential of a neuron.

Sensitization An increased responsiveness to stimuli.

REFERENCES

International Association for the Study of Pain, 2011. IASP Taxonomy. Onine. Available: http://www.iasp-pain.org/ Content/NavigationMenu/GeneralResourceLinks/PainDefinitions/default.htm.

McCaffrey, M., Beebe, A., 1989. Pain: Clinical manual for nursing practice. Mosby, St Louis.

Index

Index